Public Health, Nutritional Behavior and Nutritional Status

Public Health, Nutritional Behavior and Nutritional Status

Guest Editors

Sabina Lachowicz-Wiśniewska
Wioletta Zukiewicz-Sobczak
Agata Kotowska

Basel • Beijing • Wuhan • Barcelona • Belgrade • Novi Sad • Cluj • Manchester

Guest Editors
Sabina Lachowicz-Wiśniewska
Department of Medical and Health Science
University of Kalisz
Kalisz
Poland

Wioletta Zukiewicz-Sobczak
Department of Food and Nutrition
Calisia University
Kalisz
Poland

Agata Kotowska
Department of Social Policy
University of Rzeszow
Rzeszow
Poland

Editorial Office
MDPI AG
Grosspeteranlage 5
4052 Basel, Switzerland

This is a reprint of the Special Issue, published open access by the journal *Nutrients* (ISSN 2072-6643), freely accessible at: https://www.mdpi.com/journal/nutrients/special_issues/039W177H74.

For citation purposes, cite each article independently as indicated on the article page online and as indicated below:

Lastname, A.A.; Lastname, B.B. Article Title. *Journal Name* **Year**, *Volume Number*, Page Range.

ISBN 978-3-7258-6408-9 (Hbk)
ISBN 978-3-7258-6409-6 (PDF)
https://doi.org/10.3390/books978-3-7258-6409-6

Contents

About the Editors

Sabina Lachowicz-Wisniewska

Sabina Lachowicz-Wisniewska, Associate Professor, received her Doctor Habilitation (DSc) in Health Science at the Institute of Rural Health, specializing in natural products and dietetics. She completed her PhD at Wroclaw University of Environmental and Life Sciences in natural product technology and chemistry. Currently, she carries out research at the University of Kalisz as part of the Kalisz Microbiota Research Team, focusing on prebiotic and probiotic functional foods and the bioavailability of their bioactive compounds for the prevention of oxidative stress and inflammation. Since 2024, she has carried out research at the IMDEA Materials Institute in Madrid, Spain, as part of the Accelerated Materials Discovery Team, on the encapsulation and interaction of edible biopolymers and the bioavailability of bioactive compounds for the prevention of metabolic disease. Meanwhile, she also carries out research at Wroclaw University of Economics and Business on innovative and functional food from colored corn. Her past research has focused on the general area of functional foods and pharmaceutical and medicinal plant chemistry, with over 100 peer-reviewed scientific papers covering research fields such as (i) the production of innovative functional foods designed to have health-promoting properties; (ii) the bioavailability and digestibility of bioactive compounds in simulated digestive systems created using in vitro methods; (iii) the determination of antioxidant, anti-diabetic, anti-obesity, and anti-inflammatory potential; and (iv) the identification and assessment of the health-promoting properties of bioactive compounds from plant materials based on chromatographic techniques. She has collaborated as part of the Dekaban Foundation with Prof. Anubhav Pratap Singh (Faculty of Land and Food Systems (LFS), University of British Columbia), Prof. Antonio J. Melendez-Martin, the Food Colour and Quality Laboratory, Universidad de Sevilla, and with many European research centers.

Wioletta Zukiewicz-Sobczak

Wioletta Zukiewicz-Sobczak is a Professor at the University of Kalisz and the University of Life Sciences in Lublin. In 2009, she obtained a PhD in the field of food and nutrition technology from the University of Life Sciences in Lublin. In 2014, she received a postdoctoral degree in health sciences at the Medical University of Poznan. Currently, she is a professor and an academic teacher at the Department of Food and Nutrition. As a researcher, she conducts research in the field of health sciences, dietetics, food, nutrition, and sustainable development. She has been the author and co-author of over 200 peer-reviewed publications and 2 patents. She has also acted as a reviewer in foreign and Polish journals. She has also been a Guest Editor for five Special Issues in collaboration with MDPI, two of which are finished. Within the framework of scientific cooperation, Prof. Wioletta Zukiewicz-Sobczak has participated in internships at institutions such as the University of Bari (Italy) and the University of Lund (Sweden), as well as at the Institute of Sustainability in Rio de Janeiro (Brazil). She is currently the manager of two research projects.

Agata Kotowska

Agata Kotowska is an Assistant Professor at the Faculty of Social Sciences, University of Rzeszów. In 2012, she obtained a PhD in the field of Sociology from the University of Rzeszów. Currently, she works at the Department of Sociology of Education, Institute of Sociology. As a researcher, she conducts research in the field of health sociology and social policy, social communication, and socio-psychological determinants of public health. She has received awards for her teaching work and publications. She has also been a Guest Editor for three Special Issues in collaboration with MDPI, two of which are finished. Within the framework of scientific cooperation, Dr. Agata Kotowska has visited the University of Auckland, New Zealand, and the University of the Peloponnese, Greece.

Preface

This volume, drawn from the *Nutrients* Special Issue "Public Health, Nutritional Behavior and Nutritional Status," presents cutting-edge research at the nexus of public health, dietary behavior, and nutritional status. Building on WHO-recommended dietary patterns and increasing consumer awareness of bioactive-rich, high-quality foods, this collection asks a pressing question: why does population health continue to deteriorate despite this awareness? This Special Issue demonstrates the centrality of dietary behavior and nutritional status in public health and highlights the scientific challenge of monitoring their changes over time to provide clinicians and dietitians with clear, up-to-date evidence and practical guidance.

Gathering rigorously peer-reviewed articles, this volume tracks shifts in eating behaviors, assesses nutritional status, and probes the mechanisms behind adverse trends. The contributions synthesize new indicators, methodologies, and interventions, offering tools for monitoring and improving diet-related health at both the individual and population levels and providing actionable strategies for healthcare professionals, dietitians, and policy makers. By mapping current trends and outlining responses to counter unfavorable changes, this Special Issue advances the field and has attracted strong interest from readers across disciplines and research areas.

Sabina Lachowicz-Wiśniewska, Wioletta Zukiewicz-Sobczak, and Agata Kotowska
Guest Editors

nutrients

Editorial

Precision Nutrition for Public Health

Sabina Lachowicz-Wiśniewska [1,2,*] and Agata Kotowska [3,*]

1 Department of Medical and Health Science, University of Kalisz, W. Bogusławskiego 2 Square, 62-800 Kalisz, Poland
2 Department of Biotechnology and Food Analysis, Wroclaw University of Economics and Business, Komandorska 118/120 Street, 53-345 Wroclaw, Poland
3 Institute of Sociology, University of Rzeszów, Rejtana 16C, 35-959 Rzeszów, Poland
* Correspondence: s.lachowicz-wisniewska@uniwersytetkaliski.edu.pl (S.L.-W.); akotowska@ur.edu.pl (A.K.)

1. Introduction

Public health—understood as both a science and a practice aimed at preventing disease, prolonging life, and promoting health—has become one of the most critical domains of institutional action, shaped by both nation-states and international organizations. These activities include, in particular, population health assessment, epidemiological surveillance, health promotion, disease prevention (environmental and infectious), and emergency preparedness. Conducting interdisciplinary research across these domains underpins key public health decisions—both ad hoc and those concerning the formulation of long-term policies designed to protect and support population health. In view of rapid societal change and the emergence and consolidation of phenomena that adversely affect human health, undertaking in-depth scientific studies and implementing the resulting recommendations are especially warranted.

In this special issue of *Nutrients* entitled "Public Health, Dietary Behaviors, and Nutritional Status," we present findings generated by scholars from multiple disciplines using diverse research methodologies. Some contributions are reviews, while others report original studies (pilot, representative, and non-representative). The papers identify selected determinants of population health and correlations among variables, addressing health-related social behaviors including established habits, knowledge, self-perception, and the societal perception of individuals with obesity.

2. Results

Considerable attention is devoted to obesity, a highly prevalent disease in contemporary societies associated with numerous serious health consequences. The contributors argue that conventional indices (body mass index and waist circumference) are insufficient for characterizing early metabolic risk in patients with obesity, and that the development of new, more precise indicators is warranted. Accordingly, the studies focus on the impact of abdominal adipose tissue (subcutaneous and visceral) on disturbances of carbohydrate and lipid metabolism in individuals with obesity. This impact proved to be significant; however, ambiguous findings regarding dyslipidemia warrant further research in larger populations [contribution 1]. At the same time, mHealth practices—by intervening in users' lifestyles—may facilitate health promotion and reduce the risk of cardiometabolic syndrome. Study participants demonstrated improvements in health behaviors, with improved healthy-eating scores and increased physical activity indices. Health risk factors declined substantially, and the proportion of individuals with three or more components of the metabolic syndrome was halved (from 42.3% at baseline to 19.2% at endline) [contribution 2].

 https://doi.org/10.3390/nu17183004

Obesity, in addition to its adverse effects on physical health, also affects mental health and self-esteem. Cultural beauty standards often subject individuals living with obesity to social stigmatization, and bias and stigma may even be observed at times among physicians, dietitians, and other healthcare professionals [contribution 3]. Overweight and obesity markedly reduce the likelihood of satisfaction with one's body and health, and among women, a history of depression and emotional eating increased the odds of overweight/obesity [contribution 4]. Body satisfaction is higher among physically active individuals, although its distribution is shaped differently in women and men. Studies in strength-training populations have revealed significant sex differences across multiple domains, including body satisfaction, dietary patterns, and psychological traits [contribution 5].

Lifestyle is among the most important determinants of health, with diet constituting a principal component and dietary modification therefore being a common strategy for improving quality of life, well-being, self-image, and social acceptance. The crucial roles of the gut microbiota, dietary habits, and physical activity have been demonstrated in the management of co-occurring depression and obesity [contribution 6]. In the media (particularly online), one frequently encounters vigorous promotion by proponents of various elimination diets; however, their use carries the risk of deficiencies in essential nutrients. Studies among healthy adults adhering to omnivorous, vegetarian, vegan, and low-carbohydrate–high-fat diets indicate that micronutrient deficiencies are common—regardless of dietary pattern—even though participants believe their diets are balanced and health-promoting. In such cases, appropriately selected dietary supplements may increase the likelihood of meeting micronutrient intake recommendations [contribution 7]. Research on diet and nutrient deficiencies in Brazilian adults shows that, despite high rates of adequacy for macronutrients (over 99% for protein, 84.7% for carbohydrates, and 80.7% for total fat), there remains a substantial prevalence of micronutrient inadequacy, to which women and older adults are particularly vulnerable. The population exhibited a high probability of inadequacy for vitamins D and E (above 90%) and for calcium and magnesium (above 85%), irrespective of age group. Except for iron, the probability of inadequacy for other minerals increased with age [contribution 8]. Similarly, in the United States population, inadequate calcium intake is widespread; moreover, dietary calcium intake declined between 2009 and 2018 [contribution 9].

One dietary approach gaining worldwide popularity is intermittent fasting, which has favorable effects on metabolic health and weight reduction. In a Spanish cohort, individuals practicing intermittent fasting reported better body image and exhibited greater discipline with respect to lifestyle and diet. Most participants were middle-aged men, and no significant differences were observed by educational attainment or place of residence [contribution 10]. In Spain, plant-based eating is also becoming increasingly common, gradually supplanting the Mediterranean dietary pattern, and studies indicate that sociodemographic variables do not influence its prevalence. Compared with adherents of the Mediterranean diet, individuals following vegetarian or vegan diets have lower BMI, consume less processed food, and lead healthier lifestyles (sleep longer, exercise more, smoke less, and consume alcohol less frequently); however, they display a higher prevalence of diagnosed eating disorders [contribution 11].

Given adverse public health trends in Lebanon—rising rates of obesity, undernutrition, and other noncommunicable diseases among adults—an assessment of dietary habits was undertaken. The findings indicate that the Lebanese diet is characterized by high energy intake, elevated consumption of sugars, sodium, and saturated fats, and insufficient intake of healthy fats and vitamins A, D, and E. Most respondents were overweight or obese, and adult women failed to meet daily intake requirements for calcium, vitamin D, iron, and vitamin B12, increasing the risk of anemia, osteoporosis, and other health problems [contribution 12].

Excessive alcohol consumption—linked to elevated risks of cancer, mental disorders, and aggression—represents a particularly detrimental population health phenomenon. In Brazil, alcohol use is hazardous and exceeds the global average by nearly 30%. A study comparing the costs of consuming the most popular alcoholic beverages with expenditures on basic food staples showed unequivocally that all modeled scenarios of high alcohol consumption cost less—or far less—than a basic 2000 kcal/day diet. This analysis underscores the urgent need for fiscal policy establishing a minimum unit price for alcohol to reduce its affordability [contribution 13].

Access to safe drinking water is an increasingly important global health issue. A study of Italians' consumption of tap water—premised on the notion that the production and consumption of bottled water contribute to water scarcity and pollution—evaluated attitudes toward drinking tap water in relation to sociodemographic factors, obesity, and self-perceived health status [contribution 14].

Because a large share of daily life occurs at work or school, there is a clear need to shape and improve dietary habits within occupational and educational settings [contribution 15]. For example, a study of Portuguese university students found comparable levels of two behaviors: regular use of vending machines and bringing lunches from home (70% and 60%, respectively) [contribution 16].

Despite educational programs, public campaigns, and relatively easy access to information, knowledge about how nutrition affects human functioning and health should be continuously disseminated, as in many cases understanding may depend substantially on sociodemographic variables. Nutritional knowledge is also highly useful for improving quality of life and alleviating certain conditions—for example, dietary patterns can mitigate or exacerbate menstrual symptoms [contribution 17]. In the context of women's health, research has also examined the association between cervical cancer and dietary habits [contribution 18].

Possessing nutrition knowledge is particularly important for individuals with specific dietary needs, such as adolescents engaged in sports. A study assessing sports nutrition knowledge among parents and guardians of male academy footballers in the United Kingdom demonstrated both the feasibility and the necessity of intervention in this area, with nutrition knowledge classified as "poor" overall [contribution 19]. Because athletes' nutrition involves specialized and often costly requirements, meeting these needs becomes a critical issue for both health and athletic performance. Studies among student athletes in the United States indicate that food insecurity (FI) is a real and pressing problem: depending on the region, FI prevalence ranged from 9.9% to 65%, influenced by limited financial resources, time management, meal-plan structures, and housing location/amenities [contribution 20]. Public health challenges do not stem solely from excess or poor-quality food; they are equally tied to scarcity. An analysis of children under five in various agro-ecosystems of northwestern Ethiopia found an overall undernutrition prevalence of 49% in the study population, with marked variation by agro-ecosystem (from 36.1% in highland areas to 59% in lowland areas) [contribution 21].

In this context, pediatric data are particularly important in showing that excess body weight is not the only determinant of early cardiometabolic risk. A study of Polish children aged 5–11 years born small for gestational age (SGA; $n = 93$), compared with appropriate-for-gestational-age (AGA) peers ($n = 47$), found that, despite no differences in body weight or BMI, SGA children exhibited an adverse metabolic profile: higher total cholesterol, LDL cholesterol, and triglycerides, as well as higher fasting glucose. No differences in the lipid profile were observed between SGA subtypes (symmetric vs. asymmetric IUGR), and the only significant difference was higher fasting glucose in symmetric SGA. These findings strengthen the argument that, in public health practice, cardiometabolic markers should be routinely assessed in children with an SGA history—irrespective of their current anthropometric indices—aligning with the logic of early cardiovascular disease (CVD) prevention [contribution 22].

The broad spectrum of issues addressed in the contributions presented here not only illustrates how wide-ranging the field of public health is, but it may also provide a foundation for formulating long-term policies and for taking concrete practical actions at local and global levels.

3. Conclusions

This Special Issue synthesizes current public health themes at the intersection of nutrition, lifestyle, and the prevention of chronic diseases. The authors emphasize that conventional indices (BMI, waist circumference) are insufficient for early cardiometabolic risk assessment and call for more precise markers, including the evaluation of fat distribution (subcutaneous and visceral). They highlight the effectiveness of mHealth interventions in modifying health behaviors and reducing metabolic syndrome components, as well as the psychosocial consequences of obesity (stigma, effects on self-esteem), with sex differences in body satisfaction and habits. The studies presented demonstrate the widespread nature of micronutrient deficiencies across diverse dietary patterns (from omnivorous to vegan and low-carbohydrate–high-fat), the growing interest in intermittent fasting and plant-based diets, and the national and environmental determinants of diet (Lebanon, Brazil, Ethiopia, Italy). In the area of nutrition education, the contributions underscore knowledge gaps (e.g., among parents of youth athletes), food insecurity among student athletes, and the importance of diet in menstrual symptoms and cancer prevention. A particularly important pediatric point is that children born SGA exhibit an unfavorable metabolic profile despite normal BMI, which justifies early cardiometabolic screening in this group. Taken together, the evidence supports multilevel, systemic actions—from fiscal and environmental policies to personalized nutrition and education strategies.

The key theses and practical implications are as follows:

- Beyond BMI: There is a need for markers that more precisely reflect risk (visceral adiposity, metabolic indicators).
- mHealth works: Digital interventions effectively improve diet and physical activity, reducing components of MetS.
- Psychosocial dimension: Obesity stigma (including within healthcare) undermines well-being, and anti-bias measures are needed.
- Diets and deficiencies: Micronutrient shortfalls persist across many dietary patterns—supporting targeted supplementation and education.
- National context: Food and fiscal policies (e.g., minimum unit pricing of alcohol), improving population dietary habits, and access to healthy food/safe water should be public health priorities.
- Pediatrics (SGA): Routine lipid–glucose screening is indicated in children with an SGA history, regardless of BMI.

Overarching conclusion: This Special Issue outlines a "public health 2.0" agenda—integrating population-level policies with precision prevention, and treating biology (markers), behaviors (diet/physical activity), psychology (stigma), and environment (availability of healthy choices) as co-equal pillars.

Author Contributions: Conceptualization, S.L.-W. and A.K.; writing—original draft preparation, S.L.-W. and A.K.; writing—review and editing, S.L.-W. and A.K.; visualization, S.L.-W. All authors have read and agreed to the published version of the manuscript.

Funding: This research received no external funding.

Institutional Review Board Statement: Not applicable.

Informed Consent Statement: Not applicable.

Conflicts of Interest: The authors declare no conflicts of interest.

List of Contributions:

1. Witczak-Sawczuk, K.; Ostrowska, L.; Cwalina, U.; Leszczyńska, J.; Jastrzębska-Mierzyńska, M.; Hładuński, M.K. Estimation of the impact of abdominal adipose tissue (subcutaneous and visceral) on the occurrence of carbohydrate and lipid metabolism disorders in patients with obesity—A pilot study. *Nutrients* **2024**, *16*, 1301. https://doi.org/10.3390/nu16091301.
2. Park, N.-Y.; Jang, S. Effects of mHealth practice patterns on improving metabolic syndrome using the information–motivation–behavioral skills model. *Nutrients* **2024**, *16*, 2099. https://doi.org/10.3390/nu16132099.
3. Baska, A.; Świder, K.; Zgliczyński, W.S.; Kłoda, K.; Mastalerz-Migas, A.; Babicki, M. Is obesity a cause for shame? Weight bias and stigma among physicians, dietitians, and other healthcare professionals in Poland—A cross-sectional study. *Nutrients* **2024**, *16*, 999. https://doi.org/10.3390/nu16070999.
4. Suwalska, J.; Łukasik, S.; Cymerys, M.; Suwalska, A.; Bogdański, P. Determinants of weight status and body, health and life satisfaction in young adults. *Nutrients* **2024**, *16*, 1484. https://doi.org/10.3390/nu16101484.
5. Jimenez-Morcillo, J.; Clemente-Suárez, V.J. Gender differences in body satisfaction perception: The role of nutritional habits, psychological traits, and physical activity in a strength-training population. *Nutrients* **2024**, *16*, 104. https://doi.org/10.3390/nu16010104.
6. Sochacka, K.; Kotowska, A.; Lachowicz-Wiśniewska, S. The role of gut microbiota, nutrition, and physical activity in depression and obesity—Interdependent mechanisms/co-occurrence. *Nutrients* **2024**, *16*, 1039. https://doi.org/10.3390/nu16071039.
7. Bogataj Jontez, N.; Šik Novak, K.; Jenko Pražnikar, Z.; Petelin, A.; Kenig, S.; Mohorko, N. Does dietary supplement use increase micronutrient intake adequacy in healthy adults with habitual omnivorous, vegetarian, vegan, and low-carbohydrate high-fat diets? *Nutrients* **2024**, *16*, 1832. https://doi.org/10.3390/nu16121832.
8. Fisberg, M.; Batista, L.D.; Previdelli, A.N.; Ferrari, G.; Fisberg, R.M. Exploring diet and nutrient insufficiencies across age groups: Insights from a population-based study of Brazilian adults. *Nutrients* **2024**, *16*, 750. https://doi.org/10.3390/nu16050750.
9. Yu, Z.; Li, Y.; Ba, D.M.; Veldheer, S.J.; Sun, L.; Geng, T.; Gao, X. Trends in calcium intake among the US population: Results from the NHANES (1999–2018). *Nutrients* **2024**, *16*, 726. https://doi.org/10.3390/nu16050726.
10. Sandri, E.; Borghesi, D.; Cantín Larumbe, E.; Cerdá Olmedo, G.; Vega-Bello, M.J.; Bernalte Martí, V. Intermittent fasting: Socio-economic profile of Spanish citizens who practice it and the influence of this dietary pattern on the health and lifestyle habits of the population. *Nutrients* **2024**, *16*, 2028. https://doi.org/10.3390/nu16132028.
11. Sandri, E.; Sguanci, M.; Cantín Larumbe, E.; Cerdá Olmedo, G.; Werner, L.U.; Piredda, M.; Mancin, S. Plant-based diets versus the Mediterranean dietary pattern and their socio-demographic determinants in the Spanish population: Influence on health and lifestyle habits. *Nutrients* **2024**, *16*, 1278. https://doi.org/10.3390/nu16091278.
12. Hoteit, M.; Khattar, M.; Malli, D.; Antar, E.; Al Hassani, Z.; Abdallah, M.; Hachem, D.; Al Manasfi, E.; Chahine, A.; Tzenios, N.; et al. Dietary intake among Lebanese adults: Findings from the updated LEBANese natiONal food consumption survey (LEBANON-FCS). *Nutrients* **2024**, *16*, 1784. https://doi.org/10.3390/nu16111784.

13. Nóbrega, I.C.C.; Marques, R.V.L.; Ferreira, M.A.; Lachenmeier, D.W. The paradox of alcohol and food affordability: Minimal impact of leading beer and cachaça brands on Brazilian household income amid hazardous drinking patterns. *Nutrients* **2024**, *16*, 1469. https://doi.org/10.3390/nu16101469.
14. Dolcini, J.; Chiavarini, M.; Ponzio, E.; Firmani, G.; D'Errico, M.M.; Barbadoro, P. Consumption of tap water and sociodemographic-associated characteristics: A nationwide cross-sectional study. *Nutrients* **2024**, *16*, 944. https://doi.org/10.3390/nu16070944.
15. Hyży, A.; Jaworski, M.; Cieślak, I.; Gotlib-Małkowska, J.; Panczyk, M. Improving eating habits at the office: An umbrella review of nutritional interventions. *Nutrients* **2023**, *15*, 5072. https://doi.org/10.3390/nu15245072.
16. Oliveira, L.; BinMowyna, M.N.; Alasqah, I.; Zandonadi, R.P.; Teixeira-Lemos, E.; Chaves, C.; Alturki, H.A.; Albaridi, N.A.; Alribdi, F.F.; Raposo, A. A pilot study on dietary choices at universities: Vending machines, canteens, and lunch from home. *Nutrients* **2024**, *16*, 1722. https://doi.org/10.3390/nu16111722.
17. Ciołek, A.; Kostecka, M.; Kostecka, J.; Kawecka, P.; Popik-Samborska, M. An assessment of women's knowledge of the menstrual cycle and the influence of diet and adherence to dietary patterns on the alleviation or exacerbation of menstrual distress. *Nutrients* **2024**, *16*, 69. https://doi.org/10.3390/nu16010069.
18. Meneses-Urrea, L.A.; Vaquero-Abellán, M.; Villegas Arenas, D.; Benachi Sandoval, N.; Hernández-Carrillo, M.; Molina-Recio, G. Association between cervical cancer and dietary patterns in Colombia. *Nutrients* **2023**, *15*, 4889. https://doi.org/10.3390/nu15234889.
19. Callis, L.; Russell, M.; Hurst, H.; Hardwicke, J.; Roberts, C.J. Room for improvement in sports nutrition knowledge amongst parents and caregivers of male academy soccer players in the UK: A cross-sectional study. *Nutrients* **2023**, *15*, 4331. https://doi.org/10.3390/nu15204331.
20. Pacenta, J.; Starkoff, B.E.; Lenz, E.K.; Shearer, A. Prevalence of and contributors to food insecurity among college athletes: A scoping review. *Nutrients* **2024**, *16*, 1346. https://doi.org/10.3390/nu16091346.
21. Wubetie, B.Y.; Tsunekawa, A.; Haregeweyn, N.; Tsubo, M.; Nigussie, Z.; Meshesha, T.M.; Abe, T. Analysis of malnutrition among children under five years across contrasting agroecosystems of northwest Ethiopia: Application of structural equation modeling. *Nutrients* **2024**, *16*, 1208. https://doi.org/10.3390/nu16081208.
22. Zamojska, J.; Niewiadomska-Jarosik, K.; Kierzkowska, B.; Gruca, M.; Wosiak, A.; Smolewska, E. Lipid profile in children born small for gestational age. *Nutrients* **2023**, *15*, 4781. https://doi.org/10.3390/nu15224781.

nutrients

MDPI

Review

Prevalence of and Contributors to Food Insecurity among College Athletes: A Scoping Review

Jamie Pacenta [1,*], Brooke E. Starkoff [1], Elizabeth K. Lenz [2] and Amanda Shearer [2]

1 The Ohio State University, School of Health and Rehabilitation Sciences, Columbus, OH 43210, USA
2 SUNY Brockport, Department of Kinesiology, Sport Studies, and Physical Education, Brockport, NY 14420, USA; egrimm@brockport.edu (E.K.L.)
* Correspondence: pacenta.11@osu.edu

Abstract: Given the financial demands of attending college, the transition to new living situations, abrupt changes in social support, and overall lifestyle adjustments, college students are at an increased risk of food insecurity (FI) compared to the general population. Collegiate athletes experience an even greater risk of FI as a result of greater time commitments and energy demands associated with their sports. This heightened vulnerability poses a tremendous threat to student-athletes' academic and athletic achievements. This study aims to address the prevalence and primary determinants of FI among collegiate athletes while providing potential solutions to navigate and alleviate the effects of diminished food security among this demographic. To address these aims, a total of 18 articles were selected from both peer-reviewed and gray literature. The U.S. Household Food Security Survey Module (US-HFSSM) survey tools were predominantly utilized across universities throughout the United States to gather data on FI. Student-athletes reported experiencing FI across various regions of the United States, including universities in the northeastern states (n = 5), the southwest region (n = 3), the southeast region (n = 3), the northwest (n = 1), and the Midwest (n = 1). Overall, FI prevalence rates ranged from 9.9% to 65%, and the most significant contributors included limited financial resources, time management, meal plans, and housing location/amenities. These findings highlight a need for screening, education, and interventions to address FI among collegiate athletes.

Keywords: food insecurity; food security; collegiate athlete; student-athlete

1. Introduction

Despite national concerns regarding food insecurity (FI), which affects 12.8% of the U.S. population, it remains a significantly underestimated issue among college students [1]. Food insecurity often goes undetected among college students, particularly amidst the demands of academia and the transition to independent living. Studies reveal that, on average, approximately 30% of college students experience FI during their academic careers, a rate more than double the national average [1–7]. Further research across diverse institutions identifies additional groups at greater risk of FI, including those living in urban communities, students of color, Pell Grant recipients, athletes without meal plans, first-generation students, and those with pre-existing FI [8,9].

Among the vulnerable population of college students are student-athletes, encompassing individuals engaged in intercollegiate athletic programs supported by their respective institutions. The Hope Center's Real College Survey found that 24% of Division I athletes experience FI, with higher rates in Division II (26%), and two-year colleges (39%) [10]. Student-athletes face unique barriers to food access due to demanding academic and athletic schedules, specialized dietary needs, and regular travel away from home. Balancing demanding academic and athletic schedules poses a unique challenge for college athletes, often impacting their ability to access adequate nutrition to fuel their sports performance [8,11,12]. Although various factors influence food access for all college students, recognizing the distinct challenges faced by student-athletes is crucial for developing effective interventions tailored to this specific demographic.

Collegiate athletes are at even greater risk of FI particularly due to the increased energy demands associated with physical performance. The reduced caloric intake, specifically of nutrient-dense foods, associated with FI can impair athletic performance and potentially increase injury risk [13]. Moreover, FI-related decreases in energy and nutrient intake raise the risk of Relative Energy Deficiency in Sport (REDs), contributing to physical and psychological harm in athletes [14]. This vulnerability emphasizes the urgent need for research on FI in college athletes. Despite the growing awareness of FI among college students, this unique population with specific nutritional challenges has been largely overlooked.

Understanding the distinct barriers to adequate nutrition faced by college athletes compared to the general student population is essential for tailoring effective interventions. Although comprehensive studies exist for non-athlete students, a critical knowledge gap remains regarding FI among college athletes. This scoping review aims to shed light on the prevalence of FI in college athletes, explore the specific factors contributing to this issue within their unique context, and offer prospective solutions to mitigate FI in this population. Through this investigation, we sought to: (1) elucidate the prevalence of FI among college athletes from a variety of institutions; (2) identify the specific contextual factors that contribute to FI in this cohort; and (3) propose target solutions to mitigate FI and its negative consequences. Addressing these issues will not only directly benefit college athletes but also inform our broader understanding of FI within higher education.

2. Materials and Methods

2.1. Search Strategy

All procedures for the scoping review were conducted based on guidelines within the JBI Manual for Evidence Synthesis [15]. The protocol for the review was registered on 22 August 2023, and is publicly available on the Open Science Framework register (https://osf.io/3bhgx/?view_only=ab875b81858e4ed4b9d552b6a55b21a7 accessed on 26 April 2024). A total of four databases were used for the initial identification of primary research articles: (1) PubMed/Medline; (2) EBSCOHost; (3) SportDiscus; and (4) GoogleScholar. In each database, every combination of the following keywords was used: "food insecurity" OR "food security" OR "access to health* foods" OR "food supply" OR "healthy food availability" AND athlete* OR "athlete* college" OR "college athlete*". To identify gray literature (unpublished reports of studies), theses/dissertations, abstracts, and newspaper articles were included in the database searches. To extend the comprehensiveness of searches, citations selected for full-text review were also used for a reference list search (backward reference search) and a cited reference search (forward reference search). All database searches, reference searches, and author communications were conducted between 10 August 2023 and 19 March 2024.

2.2. Study Eligibility Criteria

Eligibility criteria were constructed with the following inclusion criteria: (1) college students in the United States; (2) collegiate athletes (including NCAA and others); and (3) the examination of food insecurity. The title and abstract results from the systematic searches were imported into Covidence systematic review software (Veritas Health Innovation, Melbourne, Australia) (www.covidence.org) and were independently screened by two researchers. Those meeting the eligibility criteria underwent a full-text review, in which the full texts of all citations considered for further review were screened independently by two researchers based on the inclusion criteria. Any discrepancies during this process were considered by a third researcher acting as a tiebreaker. The records were reviewed and organized to represent individual study samples. Although eighteen records reported on studies that met the eligibility criteria, only eight primary, peer-reviewed, original research articles were included. An additional ten resources were included as gray literature, including theses, dissertations, and abstracts (Figure 1).

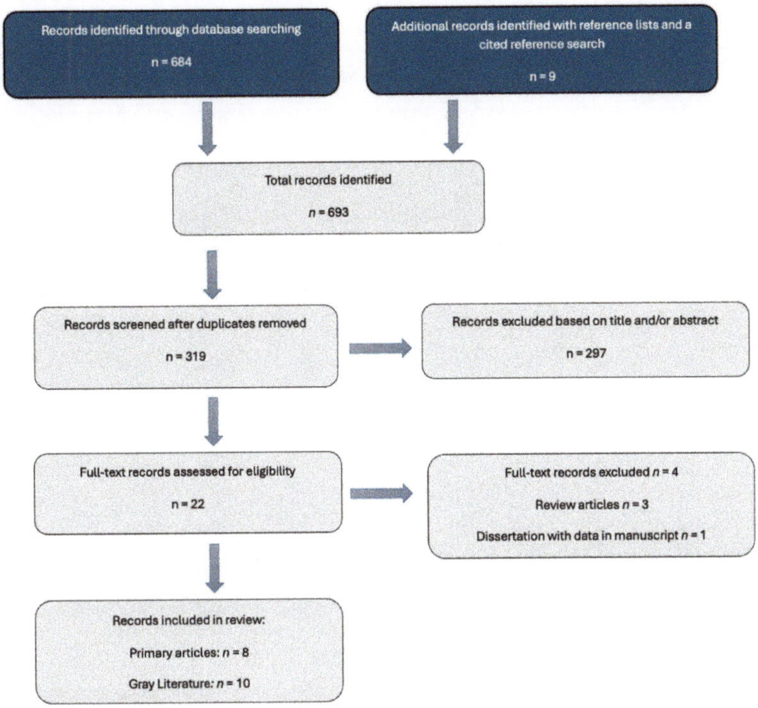

Figure 1. Study selection flow diagram.

2.3. Data Extraction

Data were extracted from each study and independently checked for accuracy by one other researcher. Using a standardized form, the extracted characteristics included the authors, publication year, whether the source was gray literature or peer-reviewed, year/month of data collection, study design, study population, sampling and recruitment strategies, sample size, sample demographics, size and location of the university, FI measurement tool used, FI reference period, medium (online, in-person, etc.) of FI assessment, prevalence of FI, and contributors to FI.

3. Results

3.1. Study Characteristics

The basic characteristics of the eighteen studies, which met all eligibility criteria, are outlined in Table 1. Less than half of the studies were considered primary articles, whereas the majority (56%) of the included studies were gray literature, including academic theses and dissertations. All publications included in this review were cross-sectional, and the sample sizes ranged from 10 to 3506 participants, with a median of 88 participants per study. To understand the prevalence of and the main contributors to FI, the results included institution types, participation demographics, and the tools used to collect and assess FI.

Table 1. Description of the included studies (n = 18).

Citation	Type of Institution	Participant Demographics	Tool to Assess FI	Prevalence of FI	Contributors to FI
		Peer-Reviewed Articles			
Anziano & Zigmont, 2023 [11]	Public university in New England	-NCAA athletes (division not noted) -N = 10 -Food insecure -White: 90% -Females: 50% -On campus: 80.0%	6-item US-HFSSM	100%: only surveyed those with FI	-Lack of time -Special dietary needs -Limited campus dining options -Lack of healthy options in dining hall -Limited kitchen access -Limited access to transportation
Brown et al., 2023 [8]	-Multiple institutions -Unspecified location and type	-NCAA DIII -N = 787 -Female: 63.3% -White: 81.5% -First generation: 19% -Pell recipient: 18.2% -Live on campus: 81% -Have a meal plan: 83.3% Family Income: -<$25,000: 5.4% -$25,000–49,999: 6.5% -$50,000–74,999: 16.5% -$75,000–99,999: 12.9% -$100,000+: 39.8%	5 questions from 6-item US-HFSSM and 17 researcher-created questions	Overall: 14.7% By ethnicity: -White: 13.3% -Hispanic: 18.3% -Black: 31% -Asian: 8.5% -NHPI: 100% By meal plan: -With: 11.5% -Without: 29.9% By Pell Grant: -Yes: 26.5% -No: 11.1% First Generation: -Yes: 27.2% -No: 11.3% FI before college: -Yes: 52.5% -No: 11.5%	-Games during dining hours -Living off campus and/or limited money -Practice during dining hours -Regulation and restriction of feeding in DIII
Daniels & Hanson, 2021 [16]	Public land-grant research university in Kansas	-Army ROTC cadets -N = 37 -Female: 30% -White: 86.5%	6-item US-HFSSM	27%	-Social -Access -Personal
Douglas et al., 2022 [4]	Public university in rural East Texas	-NCAA DI -N = 78 -Female -White: 75.6%	6-item US-HFSSM	32%	-Timing of practice -Limited dining hall hours -Lack of financial resources -Lack of cooking skills and equipment
Goldrick-Rab et al., 2020 [10]	171 2-year and 56 4-year institutions across the U.S.	-13 NCAA DI -11 NCAA DII -24 NCAA DIII -124 2-Year Colleges -N = 3506	18-item US-HFSSM	-DI: 24% -DII: 26% -DIII: 21% -2-Year institutions: 39%	Limited financial resources
Hickey et al., 2019 [13]	Public liberal arts university in New Hampshire	-NCAA DIII -N = 371 (not all athletes) -Female: 65.8% -Athletes: 78.17% -White: 89.8% -Have a meal plan: 80.8% -First generation: 24.9%	Survey developed specifically for the study	34.6%	None reported
Poll et al., 2020 [17]	Public research university in Mississippi	-NCAA DI -N = 111 -Male	Childhood History of Food Insecurity Questionnaire	9.9%	FI before college

Table 1. *Cont.*

Citation	Type of Institution	Participant Demographics	Tool to Assess FI	Prevalence of FI	Contributors to FI
Reader et al., 2022 [7]	State University in Northwest U.S.	-NCAA DI -*N* = 45 -Female: 73.33% -White: 68.89% -On campus: 44.4%	10-item US-HFSSM	60%	-Balancing academics and athletics -Elevated energy needs -COVID-19 -Living location -Lack of financial resources
			Abstracts		
Chimera et al., 2022 [9]	Public university in rural North Carolina and public research university in urban Alabama	-NCAA DI -None reported	10-item US-HFSSM	50%	Greater in urban vs. rural
Dellana et al., 2023 [18]	Public university in rural North Carolina and public research university in urban Alabama	-NCAA DI -*N* = 404 -LGBTQ+: *N* = 24	10-item US-HFSSM	45.6%	None reported
Gagnon et al., 2023 [19]	Not reported	-*N* = 124 -Female: 55% -White: 66%	Researcher developed survey	65%	-Financial insecurity -Dining hall hours -COVID isolation
Mayeux et al., 2020 [20]	Public university in rural East Texas	-NCAA (no division noted) -*N* = 91 -Female: 85.7% -White: 67%	6-item US-HFSSM	39.6%	-Lack of financial resources -Lack of time
Poll et al., 2017 [21]	University in southeast	-NCAA DI -*N* = 93 -Male -White: 48.4%	6-item US-HFSSM	16%	None reported
			Theses/Dissertations		
Anziano, 2020 [22]	Public university in Connecticut	-NCAA DII -*N* = 18 -White: 88.9% -Live on campus: 83.3% -Female: 50% Hours worked per week: -0: 66.7% -1–12: 22.2% -12+: 11.1% Financing college: -Self-pay: 27.8% -Scholarships/grants: 55.6% -Loans: 38.9% -Assistance from others: 50% Meal plan: -None: 5.6% -Unlimited: 61.1% -Declining balance: 33.3%	6-item US-HFSSM	44.4%	-Lack of time -Family history -Spending priorities -Transportation -Limitations of dining halls -Meal plan -Limited kitchen access -Lack of assistance from coaches/universities
Bowman, 2020 [23]	Private Catholic university in Pennsylvania	-NCAA DII -*N* = 31 -First generation -Male: 71% -White: 55%	10-item US-HFSSM	40%	-Older students -Male -Female

Table 1. *Cont.*

Citation	Type of Institution	Participant Demographics	Tool to Assess FI	Prevalence of FI	Contributors to FI
Misener, 2020 [24]	Private liberal arts college in northeast	-NCAA DIII -N = 424 -Female: 46.5% -White: 79%	6-item US-HFSSM	31.8% in season	-Greater in male vs. female -Greater in white vs. non-white -Based on sport -Ran out of money for swipes -Ran out of money for campus food court -Unable to afford balanced meals -Correlated with receiving grant money -Correlated with being first-generation
Nilsson, 2023 [25]	University in southwest	-NCAA (division not noted -N = 70 -Female: 56.25% -Living location:-Campus housing: 28.13% -Off-campus, walking distance: 26.56% -Off-campus, driving distance: 45.31%	10-item US-HFSSM	Not reported	-Dining hall hours conflict with practice/game times -Living location -Limited resources (money)
Stowers et al., 2022 [26]	University in southeast	-NCAA DI -Football players -N = 85 -Male	10-item US-HFSSM	63%	Greater in black vs. white

Note: FI = food insecurity; NCAA = National Collegiate Athletics Association; 6-/10-/18-item US-HFSSM = U.S. Household Food Security Survey Module: 6-/10-/18-Item Short Form [16]; NHPI = Native Hawaiian/Pacific Islander.

3.2. Institution Types

Overall, the majority of the included studies were conducted at National Collegiate Athletics Association (NCAA) institutions (n = 16), with one reporting on Army Reserve Officers' Training Corps (ROTC) cadets and another with no description of the type of university. Of the sixteen studies including NCAA institutions, seven focused on DI, two focused on DII, three were completed at DIII institutions, and four included multiple divisions or did not note a specific division. Furthermore, nine studies occurred at public universities, two at private institutions, and three reported on students from multiple institutions. Four of the reported studies did not include information about the type of institutions where the research was conducted. The locations of the institutions were throughout the United States, including the northeastern states (n = 5), the southwest region (n = 3), the southeastern region (n = 3), the northwest (n = 1), and the Midwest (n = 1), with one study not reporting the location and four reporting on multiple institutions.

3.3. Participant Demographics

The demographic information included race/ethnicity, sex, sexual orientation, housing situation, income, meal plan access, and first-generation student status. Although three studies reported on all males, one reported on all females, and three did not include information regarding sex, 47% of the participants self-reported as female. Among the twelve studies that reported race and ethnicity, the median was 77.3% white students. One study reported the sexual orientation of their students, which included LGBTQ+ individuals. Of the five studies examining housing, the majority of participants lived on campus, with a median of 80% living on campus. Three studies assessed the relationship between FI and first-generation students, with Bowman et al. (2020) [23] reporting solely on first-generation college student-athletes. Additionally, three studies examined meal plan status and found, on average, that 86.2% had a meal plan.

3.4. Assessment Tools for FI

The USDA screens individuals for FI by analyzing results from food security survey modules [27]. The 18-item U.S. Household Food Security Survey Module (US-HFSSM) is a three-stage survey that allows for minimal respondent burden with the benefit of reliable data. In addition to this screening tool, a 10-item U.S. Adult Food Security Survey Module and a 6-item Short Form of the Food Security Survey Module provide a more condensed version of the survey. Goldrick-Rab et al. (2020) [10] utilized the 18-item survey, four studies employed the 10-item survey, and eight studies used the 6-item survey. In addition to the US-HFSSM, Brown et al. (2023) [8] utilized a series of researcher-created questions for students to answer regarding FI, whereas Hickey et al. (2019) [13] utilized a hunger survey developed specifically for assessing food security. Poll et al. (2020) [17] used a questionnaire on the childhood history of FI to gather further information on food security status.

3.5. Prevalence

Apart from one study highlighting only students identifying as food insecure, one describing the prevalence based on the type of institution, and another not reporting FI prevalence, fifteen reported a range of FI from 9.9% to 63%, with a median of 39.6% of participants identifying as food insecure. The lowest prevalence rate, reported at 9.9%, was observed among male-only participants attending the University of Mississippi, an NCAA DI institution, and the highest rate, 63%, was also observed among male-only participants attending an NCAA DI institution located in the southeastern United States. Furthermore, Brown et al. (2023) [8] identified trends in FI, with the greatest rates among participants identifying as Native Hawaiian or Pacific Islander (100%), without a meal plan (29.9%), receiving a Pell Grant (26.5%), first-generation (27.2%), and having a history of FI before college (52.5%). Lastly, Goldrick-Rab et al. (2020) [10] found the prevalence of FI to be greater among those attending two-year institutions (39%) compared to DI (24%), DII (26%), and DIII (21%) institutions.

3.6. Contributors

The most significant contributors to FI included limited financial resources, time management, and housing location/amenities. Overall, 50% of the studies reported limited financial resources as their primary cause for FI. Time management was another major contributor, with 44.4% of studies reporting that athletic commitments disrupted mealtimes and the ability to access campus dining resources. Lastly, 38.8% of the included studies reported the location of dining facilities and/or access to kitchen amenities and 22.2% reported the lack of options for specific dietary needs as the most substantial hurdle to food security.

Other less commonly reported contributing factors to FI included race/ethnicity (11.1%), sex (11.1%), age (5.6%), sport (5.6%), a history of FI (11.1%), social/access/personal factors (5.6%), location (5.6%), meal plans (11.1%), assistance from coaches and the institution (5.6%), being first-generation (5.6%), identifying as a Pell Grant recipient (5.6%), NCAA policy changes in the regulation of feeding among DIII institutions (5.6%), and the change in campus routines during and following COVID-19 (11.1%).

4. Discussion

This review aims to shed light on the prevalence of FI among college athletes, to explore the specific factors contributing to this issue within their unique context, and to offer prospective solutions to alleviate and prevent further FI among this population. The overall prevalence rates of FI ranged from 9.9% to 65%. Food insecurity rates were primarily captured using the US-HFSSM 18-, 10-, and 6-item surveys. The results indicate that the most reported contributors to FI among athletes included limited financial resources (50%), limited time (44.4%), the location of eateries (38.8%), and a lack of options for their dietary needs (22.2%). The evidence of FI among these universities highlights the need for immediate intervention.

4.1. Financial Challenges

The demands of playing a college sport and managing finances are challenging tasks for student-athletes across all collegiate levels and types of universities. One study examining 91 female student-athletes found that 25% of participants reported limited finances as the primary barrier to adequate food intake [20]. Similar studies have reported limited financial resources as the major contributor to FI for student-athletes [4,7,10,11,19,20,24]. Student-athletes often face additional expenses, such as equipment and travel fees, that the general college population is not expected to pay, which may partly explain these financial challenges [10]. To further compound the financial strain, the considerable time commitment to sports and academics often prevents collegiate athletes from working to earn more money.

The challenges of juggling an athletic schedule, coursework, and employment often force student-athletes to prioritize spending. As a result of financial prioritization, student-athletes may resort to eating less, skipping meals, or eating more affordable but less nutritious meals [7,10,11,19,24]. Based on the results from a food security questionnaire, 72% of participants stated that they often or sometimes worried about food running out before obtaining enough money to buy more, 73% stated that they often or sometimes felt that the food they bought did not last because there was not enough money to get more, and 38% stated that they were hungry but avoided eating because there was not enough money to buy more food [25].

These results demonstrate how the overall intake of nutritious and balanced meals among student-athletes is often sacrificed to save money. A survey conducted in the California University system found that food-insecure students were more likely to purchase food based on cost and not nutritional quality when compared to food-secure students [28]. An additional study found that 55% of polled student-athletes were not able to afford balanced meals due to their limited financial resources [25]. Even with the help of scholarships and supplemental food assistance program participation, these factors, which have been linked to assisting lower-income individuals, are not protective enough to prevent FI among students [20]. Although the prevalence of student-athletes receiving aid has not been investigated, Goldrick-Rab et al. (2020) [10] found that 18% of college students received food assistance benefits despite the significant list of eligibility criteria, which include working at least 20 h per week, being a single parent, or participating in on-the-job training [10,29].

4.2. Meal Plans

Meal plans are often not effective enough on their own to prevent FI among college athletes [30]. A study that looked at FI among four-year colleges reported a staggering prevalence of 43%, even though students had access to a meal plan and campus dining locations [30]. Out of the students enrolled in the meal plan option, those reporting higher rates of FI reported consuming fewer meals in the dining hall compared to their peers, with 69% of participants eating nine or fewer meals in a dining hall each week [30]. The same report also found that individuals consuming five to nine meals per week at a dining hall reported 7% higher rates of FI compared to individuals who consumed fewer than five meals per week, which shows that the number of meals per week and meal plans alone are not predictive of FI [30]. Lower rates of meals consumed per week while on a meal plan may decrease because off-campus students use swipes on top of purchasing groceries and cooking at home. One of the main concerns is that although some students can utilize on-campus dining locations, not all universities provide affordable meal plans [20,24]. Historically, research on college meal plans and dining options has focused on college students. As a result of limited research, similar rates among college athletes can be assumed.

4.3. Time

Although every student is responsible for time management, student-athletes face the additional challenge of managing their rigorous academic and athletic schedules and obligations, which has been shown to increase the rates of FI. Due to their commitment to athletics (e.g., practice, travel, and competitions), college athletes have less time for employment opportunities and mealtimes [4]. With these factors to consider, athletes must prioritize their mealtimes, which can be challenging, especially when many dining halls have limited hours of operation. Competition and practice times were often reported as interfering with dining hall hours, preventing athletes from accessing healthy meals on campus during appropriate mealtimes [4,7,8,11,19,20,25].

Many students struggle to find enough time in their schedules to prioritize grocery shopping, cooking, and eating because of their busy academic and athletic schedules [11]. Even though many athletes have a meal plan, they often report being too busy or too tired to cook for themselves [11]. Among a cohort of 787 student-athletes, 45.4% reported that practice hours interfered with dining hours and 22% reported that game times interfered with dining hours [8]. Student-athletes must obtain the appropriate number of calories to fuel their daily needs, including a demanding physical component. Even though athletes may understand their need to eat for sport, achieving those needs may be especially challenging due to their demanding schedules and the limited mealtimes provided by the institution.

4.4. Housing

The living environment of student-athletes also plays a significant role in the risk of FI. For those living off campus, the cost of rent in addition to other living expenses may increase the risk of FI. Living off campus with limited finances was reported as a major barrier to adequate food access for student-athletes [7]. Additionally, the increase in regional off-campus housing costs over the last few years may be related to the increased prevalence of FI among student-athletes [7]. Similarly, on-campus housing comes with an additional set of challenges. Dormitories and on-campus living quarters offer varying types of living arrangements and amenities which can influence students' food security status. Students living on campus at a public university in New England reported limited access to a kitchen as one of the many contributing factors to FI, as they must go out of their way to access resources associated with cooking and preparing meals [4,11]. Although some of the dorms offer amenities specific to cooking and preparing meals, this resource is not always guaranteed and is unique to each university.

Surrounding campus resources, such as grocery stores and eateries, should be considered when observing FI rates among student-athlete populations. A study assessing campus locations and the rates of FI found that the incidence of very low food security was two times greater in an urban compared to a rural setting [9]. Access to healthy food is also significantly impacted by the neighborhood and the surrounding environment. Food deserts are often located where there are smaller populations, elevated rates of abandonment or deserted homes, and residents with limited education, lower income, and higher levels of unemployment [31].

4.5. COVID-19

A lack of access to nutritious and readily available food was heightened as students navigated life during the COVID-19 pandemic. Among 2,018 college students, 15% were newly food insecure as a direct result of the pandemic [32]. The drastic lifestyle changes that occurred for Americans during the pandemic also contributed to major shifts in the day-to-day lives of college-athletes, potentially increasing the risk of FI. COVID-19 safety precautions led to the closure of athlete fueling stations, reducing access to free and healthy snacks [7]. Additionally, campus closures during the pandemic directly resulted in a decline in food production and access to healthy foods, which placed those already experiencing FI in a more vulnerable position [33]. In response to campus closures, students returned home, which may have negatively or positively impacted their access to food, depending on the existing factors at home. Although some students experienced lower rates of FI when moving back home, this was not the same situation for those living independently. For students living independently, FI rates increased along with stress levels, poor health status, and the number of hours worked [34]. The pandemic exacerbated the challenges that college student-athletes were already facing while navigating living independently and brought a level of awareness to the public regarding FI among this population. Post-pandemic findings identified the widespread impact of FI on students' overall health, wellness, and academic and athletic performance [7,8,11,19,20,25]. Given the connection between the pandemic and rates of FI, future studies may demonstrate the lasting impacts that the pandemic had on student-athletes' access to adequate nutrition.

4.6. Impact of FI among Student-Athletes

The impact of FI on student-athletes has not been thoroughly examined, yet previous research highlighting FI among college students in general provides some information. Approximately 66% of student-athletes agreed that access to food and snacks would increase overall academic and athletic performance [20]. A specific concern for student-athletes is REDs, a common issue among athletes who do not consume enough calories. Low energy consumption can contribute to hormonal and menstrual alterations, reduced physical performance, decreased concentration and coordination, depression, mood alterations, and injury [7]. Additionally, many student-athletes do not receive nutrition education from a qualified practitioner, such as a registered dietitian nutritionist (RDN), to help guide the types of foods that are appropriate for supporting and even enhancing their performance goals [35]. Subsequently, if athletes fail to meet their energy needs, they risk suboptimal performance and injury, which may result in less playing time and the potential loss of scholarship.

4.7. NCAA Feeding Regulations

It is important to note that the resources available to student-athletes differ based on NCAA division. The NCAA significantly influences food access for college athletes, particularly at NCAA institutions. In 2014, the NCAA approved a rule allowing unlimited meals and snacks for DI student-athletes, specifically addressing FI. Prior to this change, student-athletes received either three meals a day or a food stipend. However, this policy only benefits DI athletes, excluding over 122,000 and 195,000 students at DII and DIII institutions, respectively, from improved food security. Notably, DII institutions have the highest rate of first-generation students (20%) compared to DI and DIII, exacerbating FI for those already at risk [36–38]. In 2020, the NCAA introduced a new policy for DII and DIII athletes, allowing institutions to provide snacks and permissible nutritional supplements when participating in competition (bylaw 16.5.1. (e)) [39].

Additionally, the recent Name, Image, and Likeness (NIL) policy enables college athletes to secure endorsements, potentially reducing FI rates. Although NIL provides financial opportunities for athletes, it may also exacerbate disparities. Athletes in states with limited or no NIL guidance may experience an uneven distribution of resources. To comprehensively address FI, the NCAA must continue monitoring and adapting policies to support student-athletes' well-being.

4.8. Intervention Strategies

To better support student-athletes and diminish the prevalence of FI, campus interventions have been deemed an appropriate place to start. One basic primary step that team coaches can take is to screen for FI before athletes even arrive on campus. Coaches and staff can also use this screening as an opportunity to discuss the contributors to and risks of

FI and provide resources to aid those in need. Some campuses have introduced screening programs to detect FI to proactively address the situation, providing access to support staff who help with time management, thus providing options on where to eat and how to plan meals in response to their busy schedules [4].

In response to the growing concern about FI on college campuses, The College and University Food Bank Alliance created a Student Government Toolkit Guide to provide directions for running a campus-led food pantry. This resource provides directions on how to allocate needs surveys to students, advice on partnering with regional food banks, setting up a pantry, and tips on operating a pantry [40]. Although there is no simple solution to solving FI on college campuses, providing accessible student-focused interventions, such as the Student Government Toolkit Guide, which is a valuable resource to utilize when determining intervention strategies.

5. Conclusions

The overall findings from this scoping review demonstrate the significant prevalence of FI among college athletes. Among those experiencing FI, the primary contributors include limited financial resources, overwhelming time commitments, the location of resources, and housing arrangements. Lesser reported contributors include limited kitchen access and cooking skills, increased energy needs, a family history of FI, disordered eating, a lack of support from family members or the university, and the COVID-19 pandemic. Research in this realm is crucial, especially when advocating for policy change surrounding the needs of our collegiate athletes. Although athletes continue their college journey, there is a need for up-to-date solutions to prevent the climbing rates of FI among athletes. Athletic programs are advised to implement screening tools and assessments to gauge athletes' food security status and provide resources, such as fuel stations, created specifically for athletes.

Author Contributions: Conceptualization, B.E.S. and J.P.; methodology, B.E.S.; writing—original draft preparation, J.P.; writing—review and editing, J.P., B.E.S., E.K.L. and A.S. All authors have read and agreed to the published version of the manuscript.

Funding: This research received no external funding.

Data Availability Statement: The original contributions presented in this study are included in the article, further inquiries can be directed to the corresponding author.

Conflicts of Interest: The authors declare no conflicts of interest.

References

1. Rabbitt, M.P.; Hales, L.J.; Burke, M.P.; Coleman-Jensen, A. *Household Food Security in the United States in 2022*; U.S. Department of Agriculture, Economic Research Service: Washington, DC, USA, 2023.
2. Adamovic, E.; Newton, P.; House, V. Food Insecurity on a College Campus: Prevalence, Determinants, and Solutions. *J. Am. Coll. Health* **2022**, *70*, 58–64. [CrossRef] [PubMed]
3. Bruening, M.; Brennhofer, S.; van Woerden, I.; Todd, M.; Laska, M. Factors Related to the High Rates of Food Insecurity among Diverse, Urban College Freshmen. *J. Acad. Nutr. Diet.* **2016**, *116*, 1450–1457. [CrossRef] [PubMed]
4. Douglas, C.C.; Camel, S.P.; Mayeux, W. Food Insecurity among Female Collegiate Athletes Exists despite University Assistance. *J. Am. Coll. Health J. ACH* **2022**, 1–7. [CrossRef] [PubMed]
5. Larin, K. *Food Insecurity: Better Information Could Help Eligible College Students Access Federal Food Assistance Benefits*; US Government Accountability Office: Washington, DC, USA, 2018.
6. Loofbourrow, B.M.; Scherr, R.E. Food Insecurity in Higher Education: A Contemporary Review of Impacts and Explorations of Solutions. *Int. J. Environ. Res. Public Health* **2023**, *20*, 5884. [CrossRef] [PubMed]
7. Reader, J.; Gordon, B.; Christensen, N. Food Insecurity among a Cohort of Division I Student-Athletes. *Nutrients* **2022**, *14*, 4703. [CrossRef] [PubMed]
8. Brown, M.L.; Karpinski, C.; Bragdon, M.; Mackenzie, M.; Abbey, E. Prevalence of Food Insecurity in NCAA Division III Collegiate Athletes. *J. Am. Coll. Health J. ACH* **2023**, *71*, 1374–1380. [CrossRef] [PubMed]
9. Chimera, L.; Dellana, J.; Farris, A.; Wentz, L.; Harman, T.; Dommel, A.; Rushing, K.; Stowers, L.; Behrens, C., Jr. Food Insecurity Among College Student Athletes in the Southeastern Region: A Multi-Site Study. *Int. J. Exerc. Sci. Conf. Proc.* **2023**, *16*, 272.

10. Goldrick-Rab, S.; Richardson, B.; Baker-Smith, C. Hungry to Win: A First Look at Food and Housing Insecurity among Student-Athletes; 2020. Available online: https://www.luminafoundation.org/wp-content/uploads/2020/04/hungry-to-win.pdf (accessed on 26 April 2024).
11. Anziano, J.; Zigmont, V.A. Understanding Food Insecurity among College Athletes: A Qualitative Study at a Public University in New England. *J. Athl. Train.* **2024**, *59*, 410–418. [CrossRef] [PubMed]
12. Brauman, K.; Achen, R.; Barnes, J.L. The Five Most Significant Barriers to Healthy Eating in Collegiate Student-Athletes. *J. Am. Coll. Health J. ACH* **2023**, *71*, 578–583. [CrossRef] [PubMed]
13. Hickey, A.; Shields, D.; Henning, M. Perceived Hunger in College Students Related to Academic and Athletic Performance. *Educ. Sci.* **2019**, *9*, 242. [CrossRef]
14. Langhans, T. Food Insecurity in Collegiate Student-Athletes. *Train. Cond.* 2022. Available online: https://training-conditioning.com/article/food-insecurity-in-collegiate-student-athletes/ (accessed on 26 April 2024).
15. Chapter 11: Scoping Reviews. In *JBI Manual for Evidence Synthesis*; JBI: 2020; ISBN 978-0-648-84880-6. Available online: https://jbi-global-wiki.refined.site/space/MANUAL (accessed on 26 April 2024).
16. Daniels, E.; Hanson, J. Energy-Adjusted Dietary Intakes Are Associated with Perceived Barriers to Healthy Eating but Not Food Insecurity or Sports Nutrition Knowledge in a Pilot Study of ROTC Cadets. *Nutrients* **2021**, *13*, 3053. [CrossRef] [PubMed]
17. Poll, K.L.; Holben, D.H.; Valliant, M.; Joung, H.-W.D. Food Insecurity Is Associated with Disordered Eating Behaviors in NCAA Division 1 Male Collegiate Athletes. *J. Am. Coll. Health J ACH* **2020**, *68*, 105–109. [CrossRef] [PubMed]
18. Dellana, J.; Chimera, L.; Farris, A.; Nunnery, D.; Harman, T.; Dommel, A.; Rushing, K.; Stowers, L.; C Behrens, J. The Impact of Sexual Orientation on Food Insecurity Among Division 1 Student Athletes. *Int. J. Exerc. Sci. Conf. Proc.* **2023**, *16*, 271.
19. Gagnon, W.; Tingom, J.; Tredinnick, V.; Pfeiffer, S.; A Knab, F. Effect of Quarantine and Isolation on Nutrition and Food Insecurity in Student-Athletes. *Int. J. Exerc. Sci. Conf. Proc.* **2022**, *16*, 277.
20. Mayeux, W.; Camel, S.; Douglas, C. Prevalence of Food Insecurity in Collegiate Athletes Warrants Unique Solutions. *Curr. Dev. Nutr.* **2020**, *4*, nzaa043_090. [CrossRef]
21. Poll, K.; Valliant, M.; Joung, H.-W.D.; Holben, D.H. Food Insecurity and Food Behaviors of Male Collegiate Athletes. *FASEB J.* **2017**, *31*, 791.2. [CrossRef]
22. Anziano, J. Food Insecurity among College Athletes at a Public University in New England. Master's Thesis, Southern Connecticut State University, New Haven, CT, USA, 2020.
23. Bowman, T. Improving Health Programs for Seton Hill University First-Generation College Student-Athletes. Ph.D. Thesis, University of Pittsburgh, Pittsburgh, PA, USA, 2020.
24. Misener, P. Food Insecurity and College Athletes: A Study on Food Insecurity/Hunger among Division III Athletes. Ph.D. Thesis, State University, Binghamton, NY, USA, 2020.
25. Nilsson, K. Food Insecurity, Academic and Athletic Performance of Collegiate Athletes Survey Research Paper. Master's Thesis, New Mexico State University, Las Cruces, NM, USA, 2023.
26. Stowers, L.; Harman, T.; Pavela, G.; Fernandez, J.R. The Impact of Food Security Status on Body Composition Changes in Collegiate Football Players. *Int. J. Sports Exerc. Med.* **2022**, *8*, 238. [CrossRef]
27. USDA ERS-Survey Tools. Available online: https://www.ers.usda.gov/topics/food-nutrition-assistance/food-security-in-the-u-s/survey-tools/ (accessed on 13 December 2023).
28. Martinez, S.M.; Webb, K.; Frongillo, E.A.; Ritchie, L.D. Food Insecurity in California's Public University System: What Are the Risk Factors? *J. Hunger Environ. Nutr.* **2018**, *13*, 1–18. [CrossRef]
29. SNAP Eligibility | Food and Nutrition Service. Available online: https://www.fns.usda.gov/snap/recipient/eligibility (accessed on 7 November 2023).
30. Dubick, J.; Mathews, B.; Cady, C. Hunger on Campus: The Challenge of Food Insecurity for College Students. 2016. Available online: https://studentsagainsthunger.org/hunger-on-campus/ (accessed on 26 April 2024).
31. The Annie, E.; Casey Foundation. Exploring America's Food Deserts. Available online: https://www.aecf.org/blog/exploring-americas-food-deserts (accessed on 13 December 2023).
32. Hagedorn, R.L.; Walker, A.E.; Wattick, R.A.; Olfert, M.D. Newly Food-Insecure College Students in Appalachia during the COVID-19 Pandemic. *J. Nutr. Educ. Behav.* **2022**, *54*, 202–210. [CrossRef]
33. Pereira, M.; Oliveira, A.M. Poverty and Food Insecurity May Increase as the Threat of COVID-19 Spreads. *Public Health Nutr.* **2020**, *23*, 3236–3240. [CrossRef]
34. Davitt, E.D.; Heer, M.M.; Winham, D.M.; Knoblauch, S.T.; Shelley, M.C. Effects of COVID-19 on University Student Food Security. *Nutrients* **2021**, *13*, 1932. [CrossRef] [PubMed]
35. Eck, K.M.; Byrd-Bredbenner, C. Food Choice Decisions of Collegiate Division I Athletes: A Qualitative Exploratory Study. *Nutrients* **2021**, *13*, 2322. [CrossRef] [PubMed]
36. Our Division II Students. Available online: https://www.ncaa.org/sports/2021/4/21/our-division-ii-students.aspx (accessed on 25 April 2024).
37. Our Division III Students. Available online: https://www.ncaa.org/sports/2021/5/11/our-division-iii-students.aspx (accessed on 25 April 2024).
38. Our Division I Students. Available online: https://www.ncaa.org/sports/2021/5/11/our-division-i-students.aspx (accessed on 25 April 2024).

39. NCAA LSDBi Bylaw 16.5.1. Available online: https://web3.ncaa.org/lsdbi/search/bylawView?id=12180 (accessed on 27 October 2023).
40. Running an On-Campus Food Pantry. The Student PIRGs. Available online: https://studentpirgs.org/assets/uploads/2019/03/NSCAHH_Food_Pantry_Toolkit.pdf (accessed on 26 April 2024).

nutrients

MDPI

Review

The Role of Gut Microbiota, Nutrition, and Physical Activity in Depression and Obesity—Interdependent Mechanisms/Co-Occurrence

Klaudia Sochacka [1], Agata Kotowska [2] and Sabina Lachowicz-Wiśniewska [1,*]

1 Faculty of Medicine and Health Sciences, Calisia University, 62-800 Kalisz, Poland; k.sochacka@uniwersytetkaliski.edu.pl

2 Department of Social Policy, Institute of Sociological Sciences, College of Social Sciences, University of Rzeszow, 35-310 Rzeszow, Poland; akotowska@ur.edu.pl

* Correspondence: s.lachowicz-wisniewska@uniwersytetkaliski.edu.pl

Abstract: Obesity and depression are interdependent pathological disorders with strong inflammatory effects commonly found worldwide. They determine the health status of the population and cause key problems in terms of morbidity and mortality. The role of gut microbiota and its composition in the treatment of obesity and psychological factors is increasingly emphasized. Published research suggests that prebiotic, probiotic, or symbiotic preparations can effectively intervene in obesity treatment and mood-dysregulation alleviation. Thus, this literature review aims to highlight the role of intestinal microbiota in treating depression and obesity. An additional purpose is to indicate probiotics, including psychobiotics and prebiotics, potentially beneficial in supporting the treatment of these two diseases.

Keywords: probiotic microorganisms; nutrients; depression; obesity

1. Introduction

According to the latest data from the World Health Organization (WHO), as many as 300 million people are affected by mental disorders [1]. Approximately 800,000 suicides per year are attributed to depression, making it one of the most prevalent mental illnesses. [1]. It is characterized by persistent feelings of sadness; lowered self-esteem; feelings of uselessness; excessive and unwarranted feelings of guilt; a decreased ability to concentrate, pay attention, and remember; and a significant loss of previous interests. The American Psychiatric Association includes depressive disorders in the Diagnostic and Statistical Manual of Mental Disorders 5 (DSM-5), a classification used to diagnose or rule out psychiatric disorders [2]. According to the DSM-5, depressive disorders encompass various classifications, including major depressive disorder, persistent depressive disorder (dysthymia), premenstrual dysphoric disorder, substance- or drug-induced depressive disorder, and depressive disorder due to a general medical condition, among others [3]. A common feature of all depressive disorders is a chronic depressed mood and irritability, accompanied by co-occurring somatic and cognitive changes. Consequently, they significantly reduce a person's quality of life and daily functioning [2]. Depression is a significant risk factor for numerous metabolic diseases, including diabetes, obesity, and chronic heart disease. It is a fact that eating habits have a significant impact on mental health. Even single contingencies in a people's life can influence their dietary preferences and choices, thereby correlating with their overall nutritional status, which will consequently affect their overall mental state [1]. Consuming a high-fat diet has been demonstrated to cause inflammation and obesity throughout the body [4].

On the other hand, obesity, defined by an excessive accumulation of body fat, has long been classified as a disease by the WHO and is listed in the International Classification of

Diseases (ICD-10) as E66. It is determined by body mass index (BMI) and percentage of body fat. Furthermore, obesity poses a significant risk for several other diseases, including, but not limited to, cardiovascular disease, insulin resistance, neuropathy, and cancer. Age, gender, smoking, and chronic consumption of high-fat and highly processed diets, i.e., Western diets (WD), are the main predisposing factors for obesity. As an aside, it is worth noting that, despite the above classification, in the public perception, obesity is often treated solely as a consequence of an irresponsible lifestyle, and its control is not associated with the need for treatment, but only the demonstration of self-discipline by those affected. A stigmatizing and dismissive approach to obesity as an 'aesthetic affliction' can lead to the exacerbation of the pathological psychological conditions that accompany it in sufferers. It should be stressed that depression, anxiety disorders, and obesity very often co-exist and are interdependent. This is likely because these diseases share a common biological foundation. Depressive states often lead to heightened appetite and emotional regulation through food. When coupled with physical inactivity, this can result in a substantial weight gain. Moreover, due to the lack of sufficient public awareness of obesity, psychological problems often arise in people struggling with this condition, often leading to the emergence of depressive anxiety disorders. Numerous studies affirm a robust correlation between the simultaneous presence of obesity and depression [5]. Depression and obesity are considered to be among the biggest health problems in the world, both because of their prevalence and the high mortality rate from these diseases. The potential association between depression and obesity has been extensively studied and reported in the literature, although many relationships remain unclear. Both conditions pose an elevated risk of cardiovascular disease [6].

Recently, there has been a growing body of research aimed at comprehending the influence of the gut microbiota on energy storage and metabolism in the body. The microbiota exhibits significant differences between lean and obese individuals. In overweight individuals, it is characterized by a decrease in diversity and a significant reduction in commensal bacteria characterized by anti-inflammatory effects, while pathogenic microorganisms increase.

This leads to the manifestation of various metabolic pathways, which may be one of the etiological factors of obesity. Probiotic and prebiotic treatments are currently being used to restore the desired composition of the intestinal ecosystem [7].

Emotional stress is frequently experienced by obese patients, potentially resulting in mood disorders (MDs) such as depression and anxiety [8]. The risk of obesity was found to be 37% higher in patients with MD, while the risk of depression was 18% higher in obese patients, indicating that there may be a bidirectional relationship between obesity and MD [9]. A current review of *in vivo* studies on an animal model (mice) shows that obesity induced by a high-fat diet is responsible for the emergence of psychiatric conditions (anxiety and depression) [10]. Researchers are fascinated by the gut–brain axis because it plays a pivotal role in maintaining both physical and mental well-being. Disturbances in the gut microbiota's composition may affect the gut–brain axis, leading to alterations in the individual's mental and physical health [11].

Any abnormality in the composition of the gut microbiota, known as gut dysbiosis, can induce impaired energy utilization, leading to obesity, as the gut microbiota plays a crucial role in disposition and energy expenditure [12]. As mentioned earlier, the gut microbiota of lean and obese individuals differs significantly. Changes in the abundance of Bacteroidetes and Firmicutes suggest a significant role in mental health regulation [13]. Dysbiosis and gut inflammation have been associated with various mental illnesses, such as anxiety and depressive behavior, which are becoming increasingly prevalent in our society. Due to their ability to restore the proper balance of the gut microbiota, probiotics and psychobiotics might have a role in the treatment and prevention of anxiety and depression [14].

For moderate-to-severe depression, psychotherapy, including cognitive–behavioral therapy, meditation, and interpersonal psychotherapy, as well as pharmacological treatment, such as serotonin–norepinephrine reuptake inhibitors and selective serotonin reuptake inhibitors, are employed. There are several approved treatments, including antidepressants, atypical antidepressants, and tricyclic antidepressants [15]. Antidepressants, despite their proven efficacy, can cause problems due to significant weight increase. A cohort study with 294,719 participants indicated that antidepressants might contribute to a population-level weight gain of over 5% in the long term [16]. Alongside the therapies mentioned earlier, natural and alternative approaches like herbal medicine, physical activity, or meditation are also utilized [17]. A balanced diet following a rational eating pattern, stress reduction, and adequate sleep are also recommended [18]. Individuals grappling with depression exhibit decreased levels of vitamin B12 and D3 in contrast to those who are healthy [19]. Therefore, additional dietary supplementation is entirely warranted and may prove helpful in alleviating the symptoms of depression [20]. Innovative approaches to the treatment of depression, especially metabolic depression, suggest the administration of probiotics, including psychobiotics [15,21]. The gut microbiota may impact behavioral, physiological, and cognitive brain functions [22], suggesting that probiotics, including psychobiotics and their metabolites, could influence depression treatment [15]. Therefore, this review aims to underscore the role of intestinal microbiota in addressing depression and obesity. An additional purpose is to indicate that probiotics, including psychobiotics and prebiotics, are potentially beneficial in supporting the treatment of these two diseases.

2. The Role of Intestinal Microbiota

The human gastrointestinal tract hosts a complex ecosystem of microorganisms that profoundly affect the host and maintain overall organismal homeostasis. Several factors influence the development of human gut microbiota during infancy, with diet being the most significant, shaping its composition throughout life. Gut bacteria play crucial roles in maintaining immune and metabolic balance and defending against pathogens. Changes in gut bacteria composition (dysbiosis) are linked to various inflammatory diseases and infections [23]. A healthy human gut microbiota comprises a diverse microbial community of around 5000 species and 7000 strains, predominantly consisting of the bacterial clusters *Firmicutes, Bacteroidetes, Actinobacteria*, and *Proteobacteria* [24]. Recent studies highlight a close association between gut microbiota and the brain [25]. Probiotics, including psychobiotics, have emerged as potential treatments for psychiatric disorders and metabolic issues [26], suggesting their importance in mental disorder management [27,28]. Probiotics, consisting of live microorganisms offering health benefits to the host when consumed in adequate amounts, mainly belong to genera like *Lactobacillus*, *Bifidobacterium*, and *Saccharomyces* [29]. Psychobiotics, targeting mental health, are a subset of probiotics [30]. Probiotic microorganisms regulate the immune system, produce short-chain fatty acids (SCFAs), and bolster intestinal barrier integrity [27]. Various studies highlight the diversity and specificity of probiotic strains in influencing brain function. A meta-analysis by Miryam de Souza et al. [31] revealed that probiotics significantly alleviate depressive symptoms among individuals with depression [31]. Another study by Messaoudi et al. [32] found that consuming psychobiotics containing *Lactobacillus helveticus* R0052 and *Bifidobacterium longum* R0175 eased depression and anxiety symptoms compared to a placebo group [32]. Probiotics, including psychobiotics, can produce essential vitamins like B vitamins, crucial in depression etiology and treatment [28,29]. Moreover, probiotics serve as SCFA sources, which play vital roles in anti-inflammatory processes, insulin sensitivity enhancement, and fat accumulation reduction [33,34]. Probiotics, especially psychobiotics, are deemed significant adjunctive therapies for depression [26]. Skonieczna-Żydecka et al. [35] demonstrated that select probiotic strains directly activate neural pathways, regulate neurotrophic factors, and mitigate stress, including *Lactobacillus fermentum* NS8 and NS9, *Lactobacillus gasseri* OLL2809, and *Lactobacillus casei Shirota*, among others [35]. These strains significantly reduced depressive symptoms after four weeks of probiotic therapy [35]. In another study, patients consuming probiotics for eight weeks showed a greater improvement in well-being, as measured by a decrease in the Beck Depression Inventory scale [36]. Approximately 57% of gut microbiota composition is influenced by diet, while only 12% is due to genetic variation [37]. Probiotic interventions prevent and alleviate dysbiosis by enhancing the cytoskeletal structure, mucin secretion, and tight junction protein phosphorylation in the intestinal barrier, fostering improved gut microbiota variability and bacteriocin and organic acid production [38,39]. Probiotic and prebiotic preparations offer effective means to influence gut microbiota composition positively. Numerous types of bacteria, particularly psychobiotics, have been identified for their beneficial effects on mental health.

In a separate study, 40 patients received either a placebo or probiotics for 8 weeks, consisting of *Lactobacillus acidophilus* 2×10^9 CFU (colony-forming unit), *Bifidobacteria bifidum*, and *Lactobacillus casei* 2×10^9 CFU. The probiotic group exhibited a 5.7-point decrease on the Beck Depression Inventory scale (BDI scale), compared to a 1.5-point decrease in the placebo group, indicating a more significant improvement in well-being [36].

Approximately 57% of gut microbiota composition is influenced by diet, while only 12% is attributed to genetic variation [37]. Probiotic intervention has been shown in various studies to prevent and alleviate dysbiosis by enhancing the cytoskeletal structure, increasing mucin secretion through the activation of secretory proteins Mucin 2 and Mucin 3, and phosphorylating tight junction proteins in the intestinal barrier [38]. Improved dysbiosis is achieved through increased intestinal microbiota variability, and bacteriocin and organic acid production, creating an unfavorable environment for the colonization of pathogenic bacteria and their metabolites [39]. It is not only the composition of the intestinal microbiota that is essential but also the ability to alter it. This can be achieved with probiotic and prebiotic preparations. Research indicates that many types of bacteria, particularly psychobiotics, have a positive effect on mental health [40]. Their action influences the secretion of neuroactive substances such as GABA, also known as gamma-aminobutyric acid, a neurotransmitter with an inhibitory effect that moderates the stress response, and serotonin. Additionally, microbes have been shown to affect the HPA axis (hypothalamic–pituitary–adrenal axis), which exacerbates depressive symptoms and anxiety. Moreover, psychobiotics increase the concentration of oxytocin in the body, reducing the activity of the HPA axis and contributing to the regulation of the stress response and reduction of anxiety [41]. These include *Lactobacillus plantarum* strains 299V and PS128 (its long-term use has a beneficial effect on mood in depression (demonstrated by the Beck Depression Scale—BDI). On the other hand, *Bifidobacterium infantis* has a beneficial effect on regulating the HPA axis [42]. Gut microbes can produce a variety of neurotransmitters, acting both locally (in the gut) and affecting brain activity. *Bifidobacterium infantis* bacteria can increase plasma concentrations of tryptophan, which is a precursor of serotonin—a key neurotransmitter in regulating mood, appetite, and gastrointestinal function [39]. Strains such as *Lactobacillus brevis*, *Bifidobacterium dentium*, *Pseudomonas*, and *Escherichia coli* are capable of producing GABA; *Escheridia*, *Saccharomyces*, and *Bacillus* can manufacture norepinephrine; *Lactobacillus*—acetylcholine; *Enterococcus*, *Candida*, *Escheridia*, and *Streptococcus*—serotonin; and *Bacillus*—dopamine. The hypothesis that neurotransmitter deficiencies cause mood disorders, based on new data, may be linked to changes in microbial populations during intestinal dysbiosis [43,44].

The assessment of efficacy and the introduction of a new method to assist in the treatment of depression through probiotic and prebiotic therapy are promising, despite requiring numerous studies and meta-analyses for validation.

Among the most commonly studied strains are bacteria of the genus *Lactobacillus*. *In vivo* studies allow us to conclude that the application to rats subjected to the stress *L. helveticus* NS8 in an immobilization test resulted in a reduction in aggressive and depressive behavior. Blood corticosterone levels decreased, while serotonin and norepinephrine levels in the hippocampus increased [45]. A comparable research study was conducted by other authors [46], this time focusing on the effect of *L. reuteri* on mice exposed to chronic stress resulting from social failure. Improvements in depressive behavior were observed, potentially linked to an increase in 5-hydroxytryptamine (5-HT, or serotonin) [46]. Potential applications in the treatment of depression also include strains from the genus *Bifidobacteria*. One of the first studies was to test the effect of strain *B. infantis* 35,624 on depressive behavior induced by the swimming test in mice. The results showed that probiotic administration increased brainstem norepinephrine extent and decreased the manufacture of inflammatory cytokines—mainly IL-6 [47]. In another study, the administration of *B. infantis* led to an increased expression of tryptophan hydroxylase 1 (TPH1), resulting in the enhanced production of tryptophan, which serves as a precursor to serotonin. Others authors [48] developed a study demonstrating the synergistic antidepressant effects of bacteria from the above two genera. They investigated the effects of *L. mucosae* and *B. longum* on rats with stress-induced depression, and the findings indicated that the joint application of both strains led to a notable decrease in depressive symptoms, as evidenced by reductions in stress hormone levels, lipopolysaccharides, IL-6, and TNF-α [48]. A relatively new finding is the antidepressant and anti-anxiety effect of *Faecalibacterium prausnitzii* on chronically stressed mice. The research indicated that reduced levels of these bacteria in the gut microbiome correlated with increased depression severity and diminished mood. The positive impacts of this particular strain are facilitated by suppressing the nuclear factor NF-κB inflammatory pathway (a key factor in immune and inflammatory responses) through the release of anti-inflammatory microvesicles. Moreover, a decrease in inflammatory cytokine concentrations and fortification of the intestinal barrier (facilitated by butyrate, generated by the evaluated strain) were noted [49]. An antidepressant effect was also observed when treating *Clostridium butyricum* chronically stressed mice. The combination of this strain with antidepressants alleviates the symptoms of the disease in about 70% of cases [50].

Satisfactory results in animal models made it possible to conduct clinical trials in humans. In a psychiatric hospital in Switzerland, individuals diagnosed with depression were split into two cohorts. One group was administered a daily probiotic supplement comprising eight diverse bacterial strains, predominantly from the *Bifidobacteria* and *Lactobacillus* genera, while the other group received a placebo. Following a four-week period, the outcomes were assessed, revealing a notable enhancement in memory among patients consuming the probiotics. The deactivation of the hippocampus (the part of the brain that is primarily responsible for long-term and spatial memory), which is usually hyperactive in depressed patients, also had a beneficial effect on improving cognitive function. However, it should be mentioned that the study described here involved a small number of patients, due to the exclusion of cases with low compliance, thus requiring verification of the results in subsequent studies [51]. The effect of probiotics on depressive behavior proved to be of great interest, so a number of studies were conducted on different groups of people. The study group consisted of healthy patients and people with depressive symptoms, including elderly people and students, as well as patients with and without comorbidities. They received probiotic supplements with a variety of ingredients, but mainly from the genera *Bifidobacteria* and *Lactobacillus*. The efficacy of probiotics in mitigating the risk of severe depression has been broadly demonstrated, yet the findings remain inconclusive. In healthy individuals, no significant effect on emotion regulation was observed, making it difficult to confirm a beneficial effect of probiotics on mood disorders. Patient age also had a significant effect on the test results. A significant antidepressant effect was only observed in participants under 60 years of age. This shows that the composition of the probiotic used should be age appropriate. Importantly, studies presented that the use of a significant quantity of different strains is more effective than the use of a single strain [52]. Modulating the composition of the human microbiome cannot be achieved solely through probiotic supplementation. An approach involves fecal microbiota transplantation (FMT), where stool from a healthy donor is transferred into the gastrointestinal tract of an ailing recipient.

This method is often used for recurrent antibiotic-resistant *Clostridium difficile* infections. Research is currently being conducted into the use of fecal transplants to treat neurological conditions. In 2012, improvement after FMT was observed in 70% of patients with chronic fatigue syndrome, i.e., individuals diagnosed with irritable bowel syndrome (IBS). However, the number of ongoing studies is too small to conclusively confirm the beneficial effects of FMT on mood disorders [53].

Diseases of civilization, which include obesity, are currently a problem that we cannot cope with. Studies have highlighted the significance of probiotics and prebiotics in managing conditions like obesity. Research suggests that probiotics and synbiotics can have positive impacts on body mass index and fat mass in obese individuals, as well as for conditions such as insulin resistance, type 2 diabetes, and nonalcoholic fatty liver disease (NAFLD) [54].

Over the past decade, there has been a notable rise in the utilization of probiotics and synbiotics for both preventive and therapeutic purposes. These ingredients, commonly found in functional foods and nutraceuticals, offer health advantages by modulating the microbial ecosystem and enhancing gut barrier integrity. Obesity stands as a significant global health concern, impacting nations across the spectrum, from developed to emerging economies. Defined by an abnormal accumulation of white adipose tissue, it serves as a primary contributor to the onset of conditions such as diabetes, cardiovascular ailments, and cancer. In a study involving obese adolescents, the impact of *Lactobacillus salivarius* Ls-33 on gut microbiota, anthropometric parameters, inflammatory markers, and lipid and carbohydrate metabolism was examined. Following the administration of *L. salivarius* Ls-33, there was a notable increase in the ratio of bacteria from the *Bacteroides* and *Porphyromonas* groups compared to bacteria from the *Firmicutes* group, encompassing *Blautia coccoides*, *Clostridium* XIV, *Roseburia*, and the Eubacterium rectale group. However, no significant changes in body measurements or reduction in inflammation were observed [55,56]. In 2010, findings from a randomized clinical trial assessing the effectiveness of probiotics as a supplementary therapy for overweight and obesity were released. The impact of *L. gasseri* SBT2055 on alterations in anthropometric measurements was investigated in 43 individuals with a BMI ranging from 24.2 to 30.7 kg/m^2 and visceral obesity. Patients in the study group consumed kefir enriched with the bacterial strain described above for 12 weeks, while the control group consisted of 44 obese patients who did not consume probiotics in their diet. Observational findings suggest that probiotic supplementation leads to reductions in body weight, BMI, waist, and hip circumference, as well as visceral fat [57]. The effects of administering *L. acidophilus* La5, *L. casei* DN001, and *B. lactis* Bb12 were assessed in high-BMI individuals, who were randomly divided into three groups based on the respective intervention diets: one group consumed plain yoghurt with a low-calorie diet (RLCD), the second group consumed probiotic yoghurt with a low-calorie diet (PLCD), and the third group consumed probiotic yoghurt without a low-calorie diet (PWLCD) for approximately two months. A reduction in BMI, percentage body fat, and leptin levels was observed, with more pronounced effects in the groups following a weight-loss diet containing probiotic yoghurt. Additionally, after the 8-week intervention, a more significant reduction in serum CRP levels was observed in the PWLCD group compared to the PLCD and RLCD groups [58]. The impact of *L. rhamnosus* CGMCC1.3724 combined with oligo-fructose and inulin supplementation on weight loss and maintenance was investigated in obese men and women over 24 weeks. Women in the *L. rhamnosus* group experienced significantly greater weight loss after the first 12 weeks compared to those in the placebo group, while there was no significant difference in men between the two groups. Weight loss induced by *L. rhamnosus* in women was associated not only with a significant decrease in fat mass and circulating leptin levels (a hormone involved in regulating hunger and satiety) but also with changes in the relative abundance of bacteria from the *Lachnospiraceae* family in their stools—this family belongs to the *Firmicutes* phylum, which has previously been associated with obesity [59,60]. In recent years, there has been a growing focus on incorporating probiotics as a supplementary therapy for managing conditions such as obesity or type 2 diabetes. An interesting perspective is the so-called new-generation probiotics, i.e., probiotic preparations based on unique strains isolated from the human intestine, with high therapeutic potential. Their representative is the commensal bacterium *Akkermansia muciniphila*, whose numbers in the intestines of healthy people are significantly higher than those of patients with metabolic disorders. Scientific studies have shown that this bacterium has positive effects, including the ability to increase the intestinal barrier, stimulate the host immune system, suppress inflammation, or modify the metabolic response [61]. Obese mice and those on a high-fat diet (HFD) exhibited a notable decrease in the overall abundance of *A. muciniphila* compared to lean counterparts, with a negative correlation observed with fat mass [62]. Initial *in vivo* investigations in rodents provided evidence of the metabolic impacts of *A. muciniphila*. These findings highlighted a link between the microbial composition and the onset of obesity and type 2 diabetes, particularly noting a progressive decline in *A. muciniphila* levels in mice fed a high-fat diet [63]. Supplementation with *A. muciniphila* has been shown to reverse metabolic abnormalities caused by this diet, including fat gain, endotoxemia, and insulin resistance. Although *A. muciniphila* colonization did not alter serum cholesterol and triglyceride levels, it improved atherosclerosis [64,65].

Furthermore, *in vitro*, as well as *in vivo*, studies, while valuable for initial investigations, have limitations when extrapolating findings to human populations due to differences in physiology, metabolism, and genetic factors. Therefore, results observed in animal models may not always directly translate to humans. Furthermore, individual responses to probiotics can vary significantly due to factors such as age, gender, genetics, diet, gut microbiota composition, and overall health status. What works for one person may not necessarily work for another, making it challenging to predict the effectiveness of probiotics universally [66]. As a result, there is a critical need for further research to establish the efficacy of probiotics in humans through well-designed clinical trials. These trials should consider various factors, such as probiotic strain specificity, dosage, duration of treatment, and the target population's characteristics. Moreover, it is essential to recognize that probiotic interventions are not standalone solutions but should be considered within the context of overall dietary and lifestyle factors. Factors such as diet quality, physical activity, stress levels, and sleep patterns can influence gut health and microbial balance, affecting the effectiveness of probiotics [67]. Therefore, a holistic approach that integrates probiotic interventions with dietary modifications and lifestyle changes may yield more significant benefits for improving gut health and overall well-being. This underscores the importance of personalized and multifaceted approaches in leveraging the potential of probiotics for health promotion and disease prevention.

3. The Influence of Dietary Patterns on Mental Well-Being, Particularly in Alleviating Depressive Symptoms

The brain uses a significant proportion of the energy and nutrients it obtains. Its good nutrition requires an adequate supply of amino acids, fats, vitamins, minerals, and trace elements. The relationship between depression and dietary habits has been well documented [68]. An integral component among these is the antioxidant mechanism, which is crucial in the onset of mental disorders and reliant on the presence of nutrients inherent in our diet [69]. Likewise, the level of brain-derived neurotrophic factor (BDNF), vital for neuroplasticity and regeneration, hinges on nutrient intake [70]. Studies have revealed that adopting healthy dietary patterns correlates with reduced instances of depression and suicide. Clinical trials have explored the efficacy of dietary modifications as a therapeutic approach for depression [71]. Certain nutrient supplements may offer benefits in managing psychiatric conditions. These include compounds like S-adenosylmethionine; *N*-acetylcysteine; zinc; and B vitamins, including folic acid, as well as vitamin D. Omega-3 polyunsaturated fatty acids, in particular, have diverse effects, participating in synaptogenesis, modulating receptor activity, exerting anti-inflammatory properties, and impacting neurotransmitter regulation [72]. Zinc deficiency has been linked to heightened depressive symptoms, and zinc supplementation alongside antidepressant therapy aids in mood stabilization. Zinc also regulates cytokine function and influences neurogenesis by modulating BDNF levels. Vitamin B is essential for neural tissue function. Deficiency in folic acid (vitamin B9) has been associated with depressive symptoms and observed in individuals with suboptimal responses to antidepressants [73]. Low levels of vitamin D are linked to an increased risk of schizophrenia and depression [74].

Recognizing the pivotal role of diet in maintaining physical well-being is widespread, given the evident influence of dietary factors on cardiometabolic ailments, cancer, and premature death [75,76]. Yet, in addition to conventional food consumption, nutrients can also be ingested through supplements. Supplements are commonly utilized to do the following:

(a) Address dietary deficiencies or low measured plasma levels of specific nutrients to meet recommended intake levels;
(b) Provide specific nutrients at higher doses than typically found in a regular diet, aiming for potential physiological benefits;
(c) Offer nutrients in more readily absorbable forms for individuals with genetic variations or health conditions affecting nutrient absorption.

Supplements can be either artificially manufactured or derived directly from food sources, encompassing vitamins (e.g., folic acid and vitamin D); dietary minerals (e.g., zinc and magnesium); pre/probiotics (from specific gut-bacteria strains); polyunsaturated fatty acids (PUFAs), typically in the form of omega-3 fish oils; or amino acids (e.g., *N*-acetylcysteine and glycine). Presently, there is mounting academic and clinical interest in the utilization of nutrient supplements for managing various mental health disorders [77–79]. This burgeoning research interest partly stems from our evolving comprehension of the neurobiological foundations of mental illnesses, suggesting certain nutrients as potential supplementary treatments for several reasons [80]. Firstly, recent clinical investigations have revealed that many mental disorders coincide with heightened levels of oxidative stress and inflammation markers in both the central and peripheral systems [81–84]. Studies have indicated a correlation between the effectiveness of pharmacological and lifestyle interventions for mental illness and changes in these biomarkers [85,86]. Hence, the antioxidant and anti-inflammatory properties of certain nutrient supplements, such as *N*-acetylcysteine and omega-3 fish oils, suggest their potential efficacy in treating psychiatric conditions exacerbated by elevated inflammation and oxidative stress. Secondly, extensive data from large-scale studies indicate that psychotic and mood disorders are linked with significantly reduced serum levels of essential nutrients, including zinc, folate, and vitamin D [87–91]. Since these deficiencies appear to impact treatment response and clinical outcomes in affected populations, there is potential for nutrient supplementation to enhance outcomes [92,93]. Eicosapentaenoic acid (EPA) and docosahexaenoic acid (DHA) exert significant effects on the synthesis, release, receptor function, and storage of neurotransmitters during brain development and in neuropsychiatric disorders [94–97]. A national survey conducted in the United States found a notable association between EPA + DHA intake within the past 24 h and a 25% reduction in the prevalence of depressive symptoms among 10,480 adults [98]. A randomized controlled trial (RCT) by Rapaport et al. [99] demonstrated a positive impact of EPA in a subgroup of individuals with major depressive disorder (MDD) and elevated levels of inflammatory biomarkers. Another RCT involving depressed pregnant women showed that EPA supplementation, along with increased levels of estradiol during pregnancy, alleviated antenatal depression [100].

Studies examining serum magnesium levels in various mental disorders have been conducted, yet a definitive pathophysiological link between mental disorders and magnesium in patients has not been fully established. Some studies in animal models suggest a beneficial role of magnesium in reducing neuroinflammation [101,102]. The majority of studies in patients have primarily focused on depression, given magnesium's involvement in core mechanisms of depressive pathophysiology, including inflammation and oxidative stress [103]. Among other proposed mechanisms, magnesium may alleviate depression by blocking the NMDA receptor, which is implicated in depression pathology [104]. Further research is needed to elucidate the role of magnesium in the pathophysiology or treatment of bipolar disorder and obsessive–compulsive disorder (OCD).

Folate deficiency is prevalent in nearly 30% of severely depressed inpatients, often accompanied by increased plasma homocysteine levels [105]. Some RCTs suggest that folate and vitamin B12 supplementation could be beneficial for the long-term management of specific populations with depressive symptoms. However, meta-analyses by Almeida OP et al. [106] highlighted the limited number and heterogeneity of available studies, suggesting the need for additional investigations.

The role of alpha-tocopherol (vitamin E) in the brain has been explored in animal models with deficiencies in vitamins C and E, revealing increased expression of inflammatory-related genes and potential neuroinflammation [107]. *In vitro* and preclinical *in vivo* studies in animal models demonstrated that alpha-tocopherol supplementation decreased neuroinflammation and oxidative stress [108].

Overall, the reviewed research data suggest a favorable role for vitamin D, EPA, DHA, magnesium, alpha-tocopherol, and folic acid, either alone or in combination with medications, in maintaining normal brain function and mental well-being, partly through the modulation of neuroinflammation. Further clinical trials are warranted to validate the findings and gain deeper insights into the mechanisms of action and optimal dosage range of these nutrients in promoting mental health and well-being. Addressing these challenges will be crucial for advancing our understanding of nutrient supplementation as a potential therapeutic strategy for mental health disorders.

4. The Impact of Selected Diets on Depression and Obesity

Overall diets play a crucial role in both depression and obesity. Diets emphasizing whole foods, fiber-rich foods, lean proteins, and healthy fats, while limiting processed foods, sugar, and saturated fats, are recommended. These include the Mediterranean diet and the DASH (Dietary Approaches to Stop Hypertension) diet. These diets provide essential nutrients and antioxidants that support brain health and reduce inflammation, contributing to better mood regulation. Due to the escalating prevalence of individuals opting for a vegetarian diet, we have also chosen to assess its effects on obesity and depression.

4.1. Mediterranean Diet

A study conducted on 289 nursing students in Spain from October 2022 to March 2023, ranging in age from 17 to 30, revealed a robust connection between adherence to the Mediterranean diet (MD) and mental well-being. Those who followed the MD exhibited significantly lower levels of anxiety and depression compared to their counterparts who did not adhere to the diet. Researchers propose that the protective effect of the MD against depression may stem from a combination of factors, including an adequate intake of omega-3 fatty acids and other natural unsaturated fats, antioxidants from olive oil and nuts, flavonoids, and other antioxidant compounds from fruits and vegetables, as well as abundant natural folate and other B vitamins [109].

Similarly, a study by Hwang et al. [110], which examined the link between adherence to the Mediterranean diet and depression among a representative sample of South Korean adults, found a reduced risk of depression among those who adhered closely to the diet. This association was significant across both genders, with individuals adhering more to the Mediterranean diet showing a 42–73% lower risk of depression. These findings align with previous research indicating a 40–45% lower risk of depression among individuals with higher Mediterranean diet scores [111]. Obesity's adverse effects can be partially mitigated by significant weight loss, achievable through adherence to the Mediterranean diet (MD), particularly when coupled with a low-calorie approach and regular physical activity. Moreover, the MD's composition has been linked to a notable reduction in dyslipidemia and a positive modulation of the gut microbiota and immune system, leading to a significant decrease in inflammatory markers—a common trigger for various obesity-related disorders [112].

A study investigating the impact of calorie-restricted MD on weight loss in overweight and obese individuals over 12 months found that MD yielded slightly better results in weight reduction compared to low-fat diets [113]. In another intervention spanning 8 weeks, which involved a calorie-restricted and protein-enriched MD, obese men awaiting laparoscopic gastrectomy experienced significant reductions in body weight and visceral fat [114].

Similarly, another study conducted over a 6-week period revealed that a hypocaloric MD was more effective in reducing body weight and preserving fat-free body mass (FFM) compared to high-protein diets in young individuals with sedentary lifestyles. Maintaining FFM is crucial for sustaining both short- and long-term weight loss benefits, as FFM is associated with a lower basal metabolism and decreased risk of developing sarcopenic obesity [115]

4.2. Vegetarian Diet

Emerging research indicates a potential link between vegetarian and vegan diets and an increased risk of depression, a prevalent mental health condition affecting millions worldwide. This connection has garnered significant attention, particularly given the growing popularity of plant-based diets globally [116]. A vegetarian diet primarily consists of plant-derived foods, such as vegetables, whole grains, legumes, nuts, seeds, and fruits, with some including non-meat animal products, like dairy, eggs, or honey. There are various classifications of vegetarians, including lacto-vegetarians, ovovegetarians, and lactoovovegetarians, each with specific dietary restrictions regarding meat, poultry, seafood, eggs, and dairy. On the other hand, vegans strictly avoid all animal products, including honey, dairy, eggs, and any animal-derived ingredients in processed foods [117].

The potential risk of depression associated with vegetarian and vegan diets stems from their inherent deficiencies in essential nutrients, such as vitamin B12 and long-chain omega-3 polyunsaturated fats (PUFAs), that are crucial for optimal brain function [118]. However, these diets may also offer protective benefits against depression due to their higher intake of fruits and vegetables, rich in antioxidants like vitamin C, vitamin E, and beta-carotene, which can combat inflammation in the brain linked to depressive symptoms [119]. Additionally, vegetarian diets have shown positive effects on metabolic health, including improvements in blood lipid profiles and body weight [120].

A comprehensive meta-analysis exploring the relationship between vegetarian diets and mental health revealed intriguing findings. It indicated that individuals following vegan or vegetarian diets may face a heightened risk of depression and exhibit lower anxiety scores compared to their non-vegetarian counterparts. Particularly noteworthy was the observation that, among populations aged under 26 years, vegetarians and vegans exhibited a greater susceptibility to various mental disorders compared to those adhering to non-vegetarian diets [121]. However, contrasting perspectives emerged from another meta-analysis, which failed to establish a clear association between vegetarian dietary patterns and depression [122].

Adding depth to this discourse, a recent systematic review and meta-analysis delved into the intricate link between vegetarian diets and depression. This analysis, encompassing 16 observational studies, spotlighted a significant trend. Among the nine studies incorporated into the meta-analysis, adherence to a vegetarian diet was linked with a striking 53% higher risk of depression in comparison to diets incorporating meat. Despite these compelling insights, the researchers underscored the need for further observational studies to provide conclusive evidence in this domain [123]. In turn, in the study of Walsh et al. [124], a notable correlation emerges between the quality of diet and depressive symptoms across various dietary patterns, encompassing omnivore, vegetarian, and vegan regimens. The findings reveal that superior diet quality is inversely associated with depressive symptoms, with vegan diets exhibiting the highest quality and the most pronounced protective impact against depression. These results underscore the potential of diet quality, irrespective of its meat- or plant-based composition, as a modifiable lifestyle element to mitigate the risk of depressive symptoms.

In summary, some outcomes suggest higher rates of depression associated with vegetarian and vegan diets, while others indicate beneficial effects or no association. Therefore, the researchers underscored the need for further observational studies to provide conclusive evidence in this domain.

4.3. DASH Diet

Perez-Cornago et al. [125] provides further evidence supporting the notion that maintaining a healthy diet could serve as a potent shield against depressive symptoms. Their prospective cohort study, encompassing 14,051 participants, unveiled compelling insights. Over an eight-year follow-up period, individuals adhering to a diet closely resembling the Dietary Approaches to Stop Hypertension (DASH) regimen exhibited a significantly reduced risk of depression [126]. These findings echo similar sentiments echoed across various age demographics. For instance, research involving adolescent girls highlighted the protective effects of a DASH-like diet against depression when compared to diets less aligned with its principles. Moreover, recent investigations by Fresán et al. [127] underscore the potential efficacy of both the Mediterranean and DASH diets in staving off depressive symptoms. Further reinforcing these observations, a cross-sectional study conducted among Iranian girls aged 12-to-18 years shed light on the benefits of strict adherence to a DASH-style diet. Notably, a lower risk of depression was associated with such dietary patterns, despite a substantial proportion of participants experiencing depressive symptoms. However, intriguingly, no discernible link emerged between DASH-diet adherence and reduced aggression levels in this cohort.

In summary, adopting a dietary pattern akin to the DASH diet, characterized by abundant whole grains, fruits, and vegetables; a moderate consumption of legumes and nuts; and the limited intake of red meat, processed meat, and sodium, has been linked to a reduced risk of depression. Given the widespread prevalence of depression and the compelling findings of this investigation, it appears plausible to regard the DASH diet as a potential strategy for preventing or managing depressive disorders [126]. Research indicates that the DASH diet is not only effective in lowering high blood pressure but also shows promise in weight management. A meta-analysis involving 13 studies revealed that adults adhering to the traditional DASH diet experienced a notable decrease in weight over a 24-week period compared to those following a typical Western diet. Moreover, the low-calorie variant of the DASH diet resulted in even more substantial weight loss when compared to other low-carbohydrate diets [128].

5. The Impact of Physical Activity and Its Lack on Obesity and Depressive Disorders

Globally, there has been a noticeable decline in physical activity levels compared to previous decades. While research indicates that participation in sports and recreational activities has remained stable or slightly increased, these pursuits represent only a fraction of overall physical activity. The decline in physical activity is primarily attributed to shifts in work-related, household, and transportation activities, influenced by economic development, technological progress, and societal shifts. Its contribution to everyday life is influenced not only by advances in civilization or the way leisure time is managed. Its extent also depends on the social status of individuals. With increasing social polarization and pauperization of a huge part of the population of highly developed countries, physical activity in the form of an intentional recreational activity is becoming less and less available. The need to function on a multi-job basis limits the possibility of life hygiene in this respect. Engaging in physical activity boosts an individual's overall energy expenditure, aiding in maintaining energy balance and potentially leading to weight loss if calorie intake remains controlled. Additionally, regular physical activity is associated with decreased abdominal fat accumulation and overall body fat, which can help mitigate the progression of abdominal obesity. Moreover, participating in sports or exercise routines is linked to reduced feelings of depression and anxiety, with the resulting improved mood often serving as a motivating factor to sustain physical activity levels [129]. Aerobic exercise (AE), e.g., running, cycling, and rowing, are exercises that deplete oxygen in the muscles. Nevertheless, the oxygen consumption is sufficient to meet the energy requirements of the muscles and does not require energy to be obtained from another source. Aerobic exercise (AE) is a widely adopted approach for addressing obesity and overweight concerns. Numerous reviews and meta-analyses have scrutinized the impact of AE interventions on weight management. In a recent systematic review and meta-analysis conducted by Thorogood et al. [130], the efficacy of AE in individuals with obesity was assessed. Data from both 6-month and 12-month follow-ups were synthesized. The findings revealed that, after six months of exercise interventions, a modest weight loss of 1.6 kg was observed. Similarly, twelve-month AE interventions resulted in an average weight reduction of 1.7 kg and a decrease in waist circumference by 1.95 cm [130].

In Japan, a randomized controlled trial involving obese participants with at least two cardiovascular risk factors was conducted. The intervention group engaged in aerobic exercise 2–4 times per week for a duration of 6 months. Remarkably, this group exhibited significant reductions in body weight (−1.60 kg) and waist circumference (−1.8 cm), as well as improvements in triglyceride levels and C-reactive protein levels. Multiple studies suggested that aerobic exercise interventions lasting between 6 and 12 months, without calorie restriction, yield a 2–3% reduction in initial body weight. Notably, even a modest weight loss of less than 3%, attained through healthy lifestyle practices, including increased physical activity, offers health benefits comparable to more substantial weight loss without exercise [131]. Additionally, in 2009, Wu et al. [132] conducted a meta-analysis evaluating the impact of combined diet and exercise interventions lasting 6–12 months, compared to diet-only interventions, on weight loss among obese individuals. The findings indicated that combined diet and exercise interventions led to greater long-term weight loss compared to diet-only interventions [132].

Aerobic exercise stands out as a potent tool in combating obesity, known for its efficacy in improving overall fitness. It is advisable to engage in moderate-to-high-intensity aerobic activities that engage large muscle groups for optimal impact. To fully harness its benefits, aerobic exercise should be sustained over extended durations. Thus, aiming for at least 150-to-180 min of aerobic exercise per week can notably enhance fitness levels. Additionally, resistance exercise has demonstrated its effectiveness in contributing to weight management [133,134]. Kazmi et al. [135] conducted a study to assess the prevalence of obesity and overweight stemming from sedentary lifestyles in the urban slums of Lahore, Pakistan. Their research, involving 646 participants, spanned from September 2018 to September 2019. Results from the one-year follow-up revealed a noteworthy correlation between rising BMI and sedentary behavior, particularly among females who exhibited higher rates of overweight and obesity [135].

There is no denying that physical inactivity stands as the primary driver of the obesity epidemic, yet environmental factors can either exacerbate or mitigate this issue. A comprehensive meta-analysis involving 111,851 individuals revealed significant links between obesity, sedentary lifestyles, and a lack of physical activity [136].

Brandao et al. [137] demonstrated that physical activity can increase telomere length in obese individuals, independent of weight loss. Telomeres, protective protein complexes found at the ends of chromosomes, play a crucial role in limiting replication-induced chromosome shortening. Shortened telomeres have been associated with metabolic disorders, while maintaining and lengthening telomeres has been linked to longevity. In their study, Brandao et al. [137] worked with 13 premenopausal women with a BMI between 30 and 40 kg/m^2. These participants underwent an 8-week physical activity intervention program consisting of 55 min of combined aerobic exercise and resistance training three times a week. Although there were no significant changes in body weight or BMI after the training program ($p < 0.05$), the researchers observed a 6% increase in lean mass (kg) ($p < 0.05$), an 8% increase in VO2 max (maximal oxygen uptake) (mL/kg/min) ($p < 0.05$), and a 2% reduction in waist circumference [137].

Two studies investigated the impact of physical activity on brain health indicators, regardless of weight loss, among individuals with obesity, focusing on changes in sleep patterns and depressive symptoms. These studies implemented combined aerobic and resistance training regimens [137]. Mendham et al. [138] examined whether physical training influenced sleep quality and depressive symptoms in women with obesity from low-socioeconomic-status communities. Participants were randomly assigned to either an exercise or control group, with no initial differences between the groups. The exercise group underwent 12 weeks of combined resistance and aerobic training (40–60 min, 4 days per week), while the control group maintained their regular diet and activity levels. The effects of the exercise intervention on sleep quality, depressive symptoms, sleep characteristics, peak oxygen consumption, and glucose metabolism were evaluated over the 12-week period. The intervention led to improvements in sleep quality ($p < 0.001$), sleep efficiency ($p = 0.005$), and severity of depressive symptoms ($p = 0.002$). These improvements were also associated with increased peak oxygen consumption and reduced sedentary time. Notably, depressive symptoms were positively correlated with peak oxygen consumption ($p < 0.001$), while improved sleep was linked to decreased sitting time ($p = 0.018$) [139]. This systematic review underscores the diverse physiological benefits of increased physical activity for individuals with obesity, highlighting the importance of emphasizing these health improvements rather than solely focusing on weight loss. However, due to the lack of comprehensive research on optimal practices, further long-term investigations in this field are warranted. Research investigating the correlation between physical activity and mental well-being consistently indicates that increased physical exertion correlates with a reduced risk of depression-related symptoms, particularly among younger individuals [139]. Animal studies have further illuminated this relationship, demonstrating that regular physical activity acts as a protective factor against the adverse effects of chronic stress on the structure of the prefrontal cortex. Notably, aerobic training has been shown to exert a beneficial morphological influence on neurons within the prefrontal cortex of animals subjected to chronic stressors. These findings underscore the pivotal role of both pre- and post-pubertal exercise in safeguarding against neuronal and behavioral abnormalities arising from distress [140]. Multiple studies underscore the significant role of physical activity in the management of depressive disorders. One notable study observed a positive impact of 24 weeks of interval training on alleviating symptoms associated with mild depressive disorders, as measured by the Beck Depression Inventory, among a cohort of 36 women without concurrent somatic ailments. Additionally, reductions in anxiety levels were observed among the participants [141]. Other studies have corroborated the efficacy of both interval training and aerobic exercise in preventing depression, particularly among adults diagnosed with major depressive disorder. In one study, 50 participants were divided into two groups, each consisting of 25 individuals, and underwent 12 training sessions. While the first group engaged in interval training, the second group participated in aerobic exercise. Upon a comparative analysis, no significant differences were observed between the two groups regarding changes in exercise motivation, perceived mood, cardiorespiratory fitness, or depressive symptoms. These findings suggest that individuals with depression may benefit from the flexibility to choose between different forms of physical activity based on their preferences and needs regarding the type and intensity of exercise [142]. This flexibility is especially pertinent for men with depression, who typically exhibit lower motivation levels for engaging in activities aimed at alleviating depressive symptoms compared to women [143].

6. The Effects of Physical Activity on the Modulation of Gut Microbiota Composition

Hampton-Marcell et al. [144] and Durk et al. [145] conducted studies that revealed variations in the Firmicutes-to-Bacteroidetes (F/B) ratio in response to exercise. In the first study, a decrease (↓ F/B) was observed with a reduction in training volume, whereas the second study indicated an increase (↑ F/B) attributed to an enhancement in VO2 max [144,145]. Additionally, Scheiman et al. [146] conducted a 2-week study involving 15 runners, which demonstrated an increase in *Veillonella bacteria* [146]. Kern et al. [147], in a study involving 88 obese and overweight individuals, observed a 5% rise in the Shannon index of microbiota after three months of regular intense training [147].

Zhong et al. [148] investigated the impact of aerobic and resistance exercise on fourteen women, revealing an increase in bacteria associated with anti-inflammatory effects (e.g., *Verrucomicrobia*), alongside a decrease in pro-inflammatory bacteria (e.g., *Proteobacteria*) [148].

O'Donovan et al. [149] explored the differences between the effects of dynamic and static exercise on microbiota changes among 37 elite Irish athletes. Their findings highlighted a significant dominance of *Streptococcus suis, Clostridium bolteae, Lactobacillus phage* LfeInf, and *Anaerostipes* in the moderate dynamic sports groups. Conversely, individuals engaged in high dynamic sports exhibited a significant presence of *Bifidobacterium animalis, Lactobacillus acidophilus, Prevotella intermedia*, and *F. prausnitzii* [149].

Moreover, in mice undergoing moderate long-term exercise, an increase in immunoglobulin A (IgA) production and a reduction in B and T-CD4 cells in the intestines were observed compared to sedentary mice. These findings suggest that exercise may strengthen the commensal microbiota, aiding in the defense against intestinal pathogens [150,151]. However, some studies have noted a decrease in the genus *F. prausnitzii* in exercising mice, potentially linked to pathologies in the fatty intestine [152]. This suggests that an imbalance in dietary intake relative to the body's needs, coupled with exercise, could lead to alterations in the gut microbiota composition and barrier function of the intestinal mucosa [150,153].

These observations underscore the intricate relationship between nutritional status and exercise, particularly during early life, when the gut microbiota composition undergoes significant modifications. This shift is associated with appetite-related signaling, where serum leptin levels correlate positively with *Bifidobacterium* and *Lactobacillus populations* but negatively with *Bacteroides* spp. and *Prevotella* spp. levels. Conversely, ghrelin serum levels exert the opposite effects on these bacterial populations. Thus, early-life exercise may profoundly influence gut microbiota composition, fostering bacteria capable of inducing adaptive changes in host metabolism and optimizing brain function development [153,154].

7. Depression and Obesity and the Socio-Sociological Aspect

Depression and obesity represent significant public health challenges, as both have far-reaching implications for morbidity, mortality, and socioeconomic factors [150]. In the United States alone, the prevalence of major depressive disorder (MDD) approaches nearly 10% [155]. Depression stands as a leading cause of disability in developed nations. A recent review examining the impact of MDD revealed that individuals grappling with this condition experience functional impairment and a diminished quality of life comparable to, or even greater than, other prevalent chronic illnesses, such as diabetes, hypertension, and heart disease. Notably, effective treatment of depression yields comprehensive health enhancements encompassing mental, emotional, and social domains, along with an improved perception of health and quality of life [156,157]. Furthermore, depression correlates with increased absenteeism from work, amplifying the burden on workplaces. Conversely, alleviating depressive symptoms has been shown to enhance productivity in professional settings [157,158]. These findings underscore the multifaceted nature of depression's impact on individuals and society at large, underscoring the imperative for effective interventions and support mechanisms to address this pervasive health issue. Today's unprecedented prevalence of depression therefore carries serious social and systemic implications. The increased number of sufferers, with a significant proportion of young people, reduces their educational and occupational abilities. The consequences include untapped human potential, insufficient labor market participation, limited participation in public life, and the need to develop specialized medical services and reimbursement of medicines. Other consequences of the silent depression pandemic are reduced social mobility and negative demographic consequences, which are not insignificant for the maintenance of social security systems based on the principle of intergenerational solidarity.

Likewise, obesity stands as a pervasive global health challenge. In the United States, the prevalence of obesity hovers around 30%, a statistic that has shown a consistent upward trajectory in recent years [159]. This persistent rise in obesity rates underscores the urgency of addressing this issue on a societal level. Beyond its widely recognized medical complications, obesity also exerts profound psychiatric ramifications [160]. Moreover, it significantly diminishes quality of life, contributes to cognitive impairment, and is linked to premature mortality and reduced life expectancy. Particularly concerning for women, obesity can detrimentally affect reproductive health, serving as a confirmed factor in female infertility. Socially, individuals grappling with obesity encounter barriers in the job market, tend to retire earlier, and often rely more heavily on disability benefits due to increased absenteeism and decreased productivity [161]. Extensive epidemiological studies and meta-analyses have consistently underscored the association between depression and obesity as a prevalent comorbidity [162]. This intricate interplay between mental and physical health highlights the necessity for holistic approaches to address obesity and its multifaceted impacts on individuals and society.

8. Conclusions

The coexistence of obesity and depressive disorders represents a prevalent comorbidity, intertwining distinct yet interrelated pathophysiological pathways. Obesity exerts a direct and potentially toxic impact on brain function, exacerbating the complexity of mental health issues. This convergence of obesity and depressive disorders is tightly linked to detrimental health outcomes and subsequent social ramifications. Dysregulation in the composition of gut microbiota has been linked to mood disorders and depression, suggesting a potential therapeutic avenue through probiotic interventions. Incorporating strains with documented effects, alongside prebiotic substances and a balanced diet, holds promise for individuals grappling with such disorders. Encouraging findings from existing research underscore the need for robust clinical trials to evaluate the therapeutic potential of microbiota modulation, shedding light on the intricate mechanisms linking gut microbiota to mental well-being. Similarly, in the realm of obesity, mounting evidence underscores the detrimental impact of gut microbiota imbalance and compromised gut barrier function. Probiotics, encompassing psychobiotics and prebiotics, have emerged as valuable tools in mitigating metabolic dysregulation among overweight or obese individuals. Moreover, they exhibit potential in enhancing intestinal integrity, thereby reducing systemic inflammation risk. Notably, probiotics serve as a source of short-chain fatty acids (SCFAs), pivotal in orchestrating anti-inflammatory processes within the body. Strains that directly affect the activation of neural pathways, thereby reducing stress in the body, include strains such as *Lactobacillus casei Shirota*, *Lactobacillus fermentum* NS8 and NS9, *Lactobacillus rhamnosus* JB-1, *Lactobacillus gasseri* OLL2809, *Lactobacillus helveticus* Rosell-52, *Lactococcus lactis* W19 and W58, *Lactobacillus acidophilus* W37, *Lactobacillus brevis* W63, *Bifidobacterium longum* Rosell-175, *Bifidobacterium longum* 1714, *Bifidobacterium longum* NCC3001, *Bifidobacterium bifidum* W23, *Lactobacillus plantarum* 299v, and *Bifidobacterium lactis* W52.

Author Contributions: Conceptualization, S.L.-W. and K.S.; software, K.S.; validation, K.S.; formal analysis, K.S.; investigation, S.L.-W. and K.S.; resources, K.S.; writing—original draft preparation, K.S.; writing—review and editing, S.L.-W., A.K. and K.S.; visualization, S.L.-W., K.S. and A.K.; supervision, S.L.-W.; project administration, S.L.-W.; funding acquisition, S.L.-W. All authors have read and agreed to the published version of the manuscript.

Funding: This research was supported by National Science Centre (NCN), Poland (grant no. 2020/39/D/NZ9/01810). For the purpose of Open Access, the author has applied a CC-BY public copyright licence to any Author Accepted Manuscript (AAM) version arising from this submission.

Conflicts of Interest: The authors declare no conflicts of interest.

References

1. Ekinci, G.N.; Sanlier, N. The relationship between nutrition and depression in the life process: A mini-review. *Exp. Gerontol.* **2023**, *172*, 112072. [CrossRef]
2. Chand, S.P.; Arif, H. *Depression*; StatPearls Publishing: Treasure Island, FL, USA, 2024.
3. Heitzman, J. *Depressive Disorders–ICD-9-CM and ICD-10-CM Codes, Depressive Disorders: DSM-5®Selections*; Edra Urban&Partner; Amercian Psychiatric Association: Wrocław, Poland, 2016; pp. xiii–xiv.
4. Schachter, J.; Martel, J.; Lin, C.-S.; Chang, C.-J.; Wu, T.-R.; Lu, C.-C.; Ko, Y.-F.; Lai, H.-C.; Ojcius, D.M.; Young, J.D. Effects of obesity on depression: A role for inflammation and the gut microbiota. *Brain Behav. Immun.* **2018**, *69*, 1–8. [CrossRef] [PubMed]

5. Obara-Gołębiowska, M. Co-occurrence of depression, anxiety disorders, and obesity. Comparison of overweight and obese patients with patients with correct body weight in terms of expansion of depression-anxiety symptoms. *Nutr. Obes. Metab. Surg.* **2017**, *1*, 18–20. [CrossRef]
6. Blasco, B.V.; García-Jiménez, J.; Bodoano, I.; Gutiérrez-Rojas, L. Obesity and Depression: Its Prevalence and Influence as a Prognostic Factor: A Systematic Review. *Psychiatry Investig.* **2020**, *17*, 715–724. [CrossRef] [PubMed]
7. Ostrowska, L. The influence of intestinal microbiota on metabolic disorders and obesity. Internist's and dietetitian's view. *Clin. Gastroenterol.* **2016**, *8*, 62–73.
8. Sarwer, D.B.; Polonsky, H.M. The Psychosocial Burden of Obesity. *Endocrinol. Metab. Clin. N. Am.* **2016**, *45*, 677–688. [CrossRef]
9. Panda, S.S.; Nayak, A.; Shah, S.; Aich, P. A Systematic Review on the Association between Obesity and Mood Disorders and the Role of Gut Microbiota. *Metabolites* **2023**, *13*, 488. [CrossRef]
10. Li, Y.; Cheng, Y.; Zhou, Y.; Du, H.; Zhang, C.; Zhao, Z.; Chen, Y.; Zhou, Z.; Mei, J.; Wu, W.; et al. High fat diet-induced obesity leads to depressive and anxiety-like behaviors in mice via AMPK/mTOR-mediated autophagy. *Exp. Neurol.* **2022**, *348*, 113949. [CrossRef] [PubMed]
11. Kabouridis, P.S.; Pachnis, V. Emerging roles of gut microbiota and the immune system in the development of the enteric nervous system. *J. Clin. Investig.* **2015**, *125*, 956–964. [CrossRef]
12. Xiao, H.; Kang, S. The Role of the Gut Microbiome in Energy Balance With a Focus on the Gut-Adipose Tissue Axis. *Front. Genet.* **2020**, *11*, 297. [CrossRef]
13. Huang, Y.; Shi, X.; Li, Z.; Shen, Y.; Shi, X.; Wang, L.; Li, G.; Yuan, Y.; Wang, J.; Zhang, Y.; et al. Possible association of *Firmicutes* in the gut microbiota of patients with major depressive disorder. *Neuropsychiatr. Dis. Treat.* **2018**, *14*, 3329–3337. [CrossRef]
14. Clapp, M.; Aurora, N.; Herrera, L.; Bhatia, M.; Wilen, E.; Wakefield, S. Gut Microbiota's Effect on Mental Health: The Gut-Brain Axis. *Clin. Pract.* **2017**, *7*, 987. [CrossRef] [PubMed]
15. Huang, R.; Wang, K.; Hu, J. Effect of Probiotics on Depression: A Systematic Review and Meta-Analysis of Randomized Controlled Trials. *Nutrients* **2016**, *8*, 483. [CrossRef] [PubMed]
16. Gafoor, R.; Booth, H.P.; Gulliford, M.C. Antidepressant utilisation and incidence of weight gain during 10 years' follow-up: Population based cohort study. *BMJ* **2018**, *361*, k1951. [CrossRef] [PubMed]
17. Mörkl, S.; Butler, M.I.; Holl, A.; Cryan, J.F.; Dinan, T.G. Probiotics and the Microbiota-Gut-Brain Axis: Focus on Psychiatry. *Curr. Nutr. Rep.* **2020**, *9*, 171–182. [CrossRef] [PubMed]
18. Firth, J.; Marx, W.; Dash, S.; Carney, R.; Teasdale, S.B.; Solmi, M.; Stubbs, B.; Schuch, F.B.; Carvalho, A.F.; Jacka, F.; et al. The Effects of Dietary Improvement on Symptoms of Depression and Anxiety: A Meta-Analysis of Randomized Controlled Trials. *Psychosom. Med.* **2019**, *81*, 265–280. [CrossRef] [PubMed]
19. Cuomo, A.; Giordano, N.; Goracci, A.; Fagiolini, A. Depression and Vitamin D Deficiency: Causality, Assessment, and Clinical Practice Implications. *Neuropsychiatry* **2017**, *07*, 606–614. [CrossRef]
20. Naik, S.; Mahalle, N.; Bhide, V. Identification of vitamin B_{12} deficiency in vegetarian Indians. *Br. J. Nutr.* **2018**, *119*, 629–635. [CrossRef] [PubMed]
21. McEwen, B.J.; Fenasse, R. Probiotics and depression: The link between the microbiome gut-brain axis and digestive and mental health. *J. Aust. Tradit. -Med. Soc.* **2019**, *25*, 132.
22. David, L.A.; Maurice, C.F.; Carmody, R.N.; Gootenberg, D.B.; Button, J.E.; Wolfe, B.E.; Ling, A.V.; Devlin, A.S.; Varma, Y.; Fischbach, M.A.; et al. Diet rapidly and reproducibly alters the human gut microbiome. *Nature* **2014**, *505*, 559–563. [CrossRef]
23. Thursby, E.; Juge, N. Introduction to the human gut microbiota. *Biochem. J.* **2017**, *474*, 1823–1836. [CrossRef] [PubMed]
24. Liu, B.; He, Y.; Wang, M.; Liu, J.; Ju, Y.; Zhang, Y.; Liu, T.; Li, L.; Li, Q. Efficacy of probiotics on anxiety-A meta-analysis of randomized controlled trials. *Depress. Anxiety* **2018**, *35*, 935–945. [CrossRef] [PubMed]
25. Irum, N.; Afzal, T.; Hamid Faraz, M.; Aslam, Z.; Rasheed, F. The role of gut microbiota in depression: An analysis of the gut-brain axis. *Front. Behav. Neurosci.* **2023**, *17*, 1185522. [CrossRef] [PubMed]
26. Gawlik-Kotelnicka, O.; Strzelecki, D. Probiotics as a Treatment for "Metabolic Depression"? A Rationale for Future Studies. *Pharmaceuticals* **2021**, *14*, 384. [CrossRef] [PubMed]
27. Sanders, M.E.; Merenstein, D.J.; Reid, G.; Gibson, G.R.; Rastall, R.A. Probiotics and prebiotics in intestinal health and disease: From biology to the clinic. *Nat. Rev. Gastroenterol. Hepatol.* **2019**, *16*, 605–616. [CrossRef] [PubMed]
28. Trzeciak, P.; Herbet, M. Role of the Intestinal Microbiome, Intestinal Barrier and Psychobiotics in Depression. *Nutrients* **2021**, *13*, 927. [CrossRef] [PubMed]
29. Khalili, P.; Asbaghi, O.; Aghakhani, L.; Clark, C.C.T.; Haghighat, N. The effects of folic acid supplementation on depression in adults: A systematic review and meta-analysis of randomized controlled trials. *Nutr. Food Sci.* **2023**, *53*, 521–534. [CrossRef]
30. Del Toro-Barbosa, M.; Hurtado-Romero, A.; Garcia-Amezquita, L.E.; García-Cayuela, T. Psychobiotics: Mechanisms of Action, Evaluation Methods and Effectiveness in Applications with Food Products. *Nutrients* **2020**, *12*, 3896. [CrossRef] [PubMed]
31. Miryam de Souza, M.; Iasmim, M.; Raquel, S.-T. A systematic review of the effects of probiotics on depression and anxiety: An alternative therapy? *Ciênc. Saúde Coletiva* **2021**, *26*, 4087–4097.
32. Messaoudi, M.; Violle, N.; Bisson, J.-F.; Desor, D.; Javelot, H.; Rougeot, C. Beneficial psychological effects of a probiotic formulation (*Lactobacillus helveticus* R0052 and *Bifidobacterium longum* R0175) in healthy human volunteers. *Gut Microbes* **2011**, *2*, 256–261. [CrossRef]

33. Cristofori, F.; Dargenio, V.N.; Dargenio, C.; Miniello, V.L.; Barone, M.; Francavilla, R. Anti-Inflammatory and Immunomodulatory Effects of Probiotics in Gut Inflammation: A Door to the Body. *Front. Immunol.* **2021**, *12*, 578386. [CrossRef] [PubMed]
34. Wallace, C.J.K.; Milev, R. The effects of probiotics on depressive symptoms in humans: A systematic review. *Ann. Gen. Psychiatry* **2017**, *16*, 14. [CrossRef] [PubMed]
35. Skonieczna-Żydecka, K.; Marlicz, W.; Misera, A.; Koulaouzidis, A.; Łoniewski, I. Microbiome—The Missing Link in the Gut-Brain Axis: Focus on Its Role in Gastrointestinal and Mental Health. *J. Clin. Med.* **2018**, *7*, 521. [CrossRef] [PubMed]
36. Akkasheh, G.; Kashani-Poor, Z.; Tajabadi-Ebrahimi, M.; Jafari, P.; Akbari, H.; Taghizadeh, M.; Memarzadeh, M.R.; Asemi, Z.; Esmaillzadeh, A. Clinical and metabolic response to probiotic administration in patients with major depressive disorder: A randomized, double-blind, placebo-controlled trial. *Nutrition* **2016**, *32*, 315–320. [CrossRef] [PubMed]
37. Quigley, E.M.M. Microbiota-Brain-Gut Axis and Neurodegenerative Diseases. *Curr. Neurol. Neurosci. Rep.* **2017**, *17*, 94. [CrossRef]
38. La Fata, G.; Weber, P.; Mohajeri, M.H. Probiotics and the Gut Immune System: Indirect Regulation. *Probiotics Antimicrob. Proteins* **2018**, *10*, 11–21. [CrossRef]
39. Hegarty, J.W.; Guinane, C.M.; Ross, R.P.; Hill, C.; Cotter, P.D. Bacteriocin production: A relatively unharnessed probiotic trait? *F1000Research* **2016**, *5*, 2587. [CrossRef] [PubMed]
40. Dinan, T.G.; Cryan, J.F. The Microbiome-Gut-Brain Axis in Health and Disease. *Gastroenterol. Clin. N. Am.* **2017**, *46*, 77–89. [CrossRef] [PubMed]
41. Misra, S.; Mohanty, D. Psychobiotics: A new approach for treating mental illness? *Crit. Rev. Food Sci. Nutr.* **2019**, *59*, 1230–1236. [CrossRef]
42. Liu, W.-H.; Chuang, H.-L.; Huang, Y.-T.; Wu, C.-C.; Chou, G.-T.; Wang, S.; Tsai, Y.-C. Alteration of behavior and monoamine levels attributable to Lactobacillus plantarum PS128 in germ-free mice. *Behav. Brain Res.* **2016**, *298*, 202–209. [CrossRef]
43. Lombardi, V.C.; De Meirleir, K.L.; Subramanian, K.; Nourani, S.M.; Dagda, R.K.; Delaney, S.L.; Palotás, A. Nutritional modulation of the intestinal microbiota; future opportunities for the prevention and treatment of neuroimmune and neuroinflammatory disease. *J. Nutr. Biochem.* **2018**, *61*, 1–16. [CrossRef] [PubMed]
44. Lukić, I.; Getselter, D.; Koren, O.; Elliott, E. Role of Tryptophan in Microbiota-Induced Depressive-Like Behavior: Evidence From Tryptophan Depletion Study. *Front. Behav. Neurosci.* **2019**, *13*, 123. [CrossRef] [PubMed]
45. Skonieczna-Żydecka, K.; Łoniewski, I.; Marlicz, W. Intestinal microbiota as a potential cause of human emotional functioning disorders. *Med. Exp. Microbiol.* **2017**, *69*, 163–176.
46. Liang, S.; Wang, T.; Hu, X.; Luo, J.; Li, W.; Wu, X.; Duan, Y.; Jin, F. Administration of *Lactobacillus helveticus* NS8 improves behavioral, cognitive, and biochemical aberrations caused by chronic restraint stress. *Neuroscience* **2015**, *310*, 561–577. [CrossRef] [PubMed]
47. Abdrabou, A.M.; Osman, E.Y.; Aboubakr, O.A. Comparative therapeutic efficacy study of *Lactobacilli* probiotics and citalopram in treatment of acute stress-induced depression in lab murine models. *Hum. Microbiome J.* **2018**, *10*, 33–36. [CrossRef]
48. Tian, P.; Wang, G.; Zhao, J.; Zhang, H.; Chen, W. *Bifidobacterium* with the role of 5-hydroxytryptophan synthesis regulation alleviates the symptom of depression and related microbiota dysbiosis. *J. Nutr. Biochem.* **2019**, *66*, 43–51. [CrossRef] [PubMed]
49. Un-Nisa, A.; Khan, A.; Zakria, M.; Siraj, S.; Ullah, S.; Tipu, M.K.; Ikram, M.; Kim, M.O. Updates on the Role of Probiotics against Different Health Issues: Focus on *Lactobacillus*. *Int. J. Mol. Sci.* **2022**, *24*, 142. [CrossRef] [PubMed]
50. Hao, Z.; Wang, W.; Guo, R.; Liu, H. *Faecalibacterium prausnitzii* (ATCC 27766) has preventive and therapeutic effects on chronic unpredictable mild stress-induced depression-like and anxiety-like behavior in rats. *Psychoneuroendocrinology* **2019**, *104*, 132–142. [CrossRef] [PubMed]
51. Miyaoka, T.; Kanayama, M.; Wake, R.; Hashioka, S.; Hayashida, M.; Nagahama, M.; Okazaki, S.; Yamashita, S.; Miura, S.; Miki, H.; et al. *Clostridium butyricum* MIYAIRI 588 as Adjunctive Therapy for Treatment-Resistant Major Depressive Disorder: A Prospective Open-Label Trial. *Clin. Neuropharmacol.* **2018**, *41*, 151–155. [CrossRef]
52. Schneider, E.; Doll, J.P.K.; Schweinfurth, N.; Kettelhack, C.; Schaub, A.-C.; Yamanbaeva, G.; Varghese, N.; Mählmann, L.; Brand, S.; Eckert, A.; et al. Effect of short-term, high-dose probiotic supplementation on cognition, related brain functions and BDNF in patients with depression: A secondary analysis of a randomized controlled trial. *J. Psychiatry Neurosci.* **2023**, *48*, E23–E33. [CrossRef]
53. Surzenko, N.; Pjetri, E.; Munson, C.A.; Friday, W.B.; Hauser, J.; Mitchell, E.S. Prenatal exposure to the probiotic *Lactococcus lactis* decreases anxiety-like behavior and modulates cortical cytoarchitecture in a sex specific manner. *PLoS ONE* **2020**, *15*, e0223395. [CrossRef] [PubMed]
54. Sáez-Lara, M.; Robles-Sanchez, C.; Ruiz-Ojeda, F.; Plaza-Diaz, J.; Gil, A. Effects of Probiotics and Synbiotics on Obesity, Insulin Resistance Syndrome, Type 2 Diabetes and Non-Alcoholic Fatty Liver Disease: A Review of Human Clinical Trials. *Int. J. Mol. Sci.* **2016**, *17*, 928. [CrossRef]
55. Bass, R.; Eneli, I. Severe childhood obesity: An under-recognised and growing health problem. *Postgrad. Med. J.* **2015**, *91*, 639–645. [CrossRef] [PubMed]
56. Larsen, N.; Vogensen, F.K.; Gøbel, R.J.; Michaelsen, K.F.; Forssten, S.D.; Lahtinen, S.J.; Jakobsen, M. Effect of *Lactobacillus salivarius* Ls-33 on fecal microbiota in obese adolescents. *Clin. Nutr.* **2013**, *32*, 935–940. [CrossRef] [PubMed]
57. Kadooka, Y.; Sato, M.; Imaizumi, K.; Ogawa, A.; Ikuyama, K.; Akai, Y.; Okano, M.; Kagoshima, M.; Tsuchida, T. Regulation of abdominal adiposity by probiotics (*Lactobacillus gasseri* SBT2055) in adults with obese tendencies in a randomized controlled trial. *Eur. J. Clin. Nutr.* **2010**, *64*, 636–643. [CrossRef]

58. Zarrati, M.; Salehi, E.; Nourijelyani, K.; Mofid, V.; Zadeh, M.J.H.; Najafi, F.; Ghaflati, Z.; Bidad, K.; Chamari, M.; Karimi, M.; et al. Effects of Probiotic Yogurt on Fat Distribution and Gene Expression of Proinflammatory Factors in Peripheral Blood Mononuclear Cells in Overweight and Obese People with or without Weight-Loss Diet. *J. Am. Coll. Nutr.* **2014**, *33*, 417–425. [CrossRef] [PubMed]
59. Markowiak, P.; Śliżewska, K. Effects of Probiotics, Prebiotics, and Synbiotics on Human Health. *Nutrients* **2017**, *9*, 1021. [CrossRef]
60. Sanchez, M.; Darimont, C.; Drapeau, V.; Emady-Azar, S.; Lepage, M.; Rezzonico, E.; Ngom-Bru, C.; Berger, B.; Philippe, L.; Ammon-Zuffrey, C.; et al. Effect of *Lactobacillus rhamnosus* CGMCC1.3724 supplementation on weight loss and maintenance in obese men and women. *Br. J. Nutr.* **2014**, *111*, 1507–1519. [CrossRef] [PubMed]
61. Kobyliak, N.; Falalyeyeva, T.; Kyriachenko, Y.; Tseyslyer, Y.; Kovalchuk, O.; Hadiliia, O.; Eslami, M.; Yousefi, B.; Abenavoli, L.; Fagoonee, S.; et al. *Akkermansia muciniphila* as a novel powerful bacterial player in the treatment of metabolic disorders. *Minerva Endocrinol.* **2022**, *47*, 242–252. [CrossRef]
62. Yan, J.; Sheng, L.; Li, H. *Akkermansia muciniphila*: Is it the Holy Grail for ameliorating metabolic diseases? *Gut Microbes* **2021**, *13*, 1984104. [CrossRef]
63. Markowska, E.; Kiersztan, A. *Akkermansia muciniphila*—A promising candidate for a new generation probiotic. *Adv. Hyg. Exp. Med.* **2021**, *75*, 724–748. [CrossRef]
64. Hasani, A.; Ebrahimzadeh, S.; Hemmati, F.; Khabbaz, A.; Hasani, A.; Gholizadeh, P. The role of *Akkermansia muciniphila* in obesity, diabetes and atherosclerosis. *J. Med. Microbiol.* **2021**, *70*, 001435. [CrossRef] [PubMed]
65. Xu, Y.; Wang, N.; Tan, H.-Y.; Li, S.; Zhang, C.; Feng, Y. Function of *Akkermansia muciniphila* in Obesity: Interactions With Lipid Metabolism, Immune Response and Gut Systems. *Front. Microbiol.* **2020**, *11*, 219. [CrossRef]
66. Power, S.E.; O'Toole, P.W.; Stanton, C.; Ross, R.P.; Fitzgerald, G.F. Intestinal microbiota, diet and health. *Br. J. Nutr.* **2014**, *111*, 387–402. [CrossRef]
67. Wang, X.; Zhang, P.; Zhang, X. Probiotics regulate gut microbiota: An effective method to improve immunity. *Molecules* **2021**, *26*, 6076. [CrossRef]
68. Opie, R.S.; Itsiopoulos, C.; Parletta, N.; Sanchez-Villegas, A.; Akbaraly, T.N.; Ruusunen, A.; Jacka, F.N. Dietary recommendations for the prevention of depression. *Nutr. Neurosci.* **2017**, *20*, 161–171. [CrossRef] [PubMed]
69. Diniz, B.S.; Mendes-Silva, A.P.; Silva, L.B.; Bertola, L.; Vieira, M.C.; Ferreira, J.D.; Nicolau, M.; Bristot, G.; Da Rosa, E.D.; Teixeira, A.L.; et al. Oxidative stress markers imbalance in late-life depression. *J. Psychiatr. Res.* **2018**, *102*, 29–33. [CrossRef]
70. Guimarães, L.R.; Jacka, F.N.; Gama, C.S.; Berk, M.; Leitão-Azevedo, C.L.; Belmonte De Abreu, M.G.; Lobato, M.I.; Andreazza, A.C.; Ceresér, K.M.; Kapczinski, F.; et al. Serum levels of brain-derived neurotrophic factor in schizophrenia on a hypocaloric diet. *Prog. Neuro-Psychopharmacol. Biol. Psychiatry* **2008**, *32*, 1595–1598. [CrossRef] [PubMed]
71. Jacka, F.N.; O'Neil, A.; Opie, R.; Itsiopoulos, C.; Cotton, S.; Mohebbi, M.; Castle, D.; Dash, S.; Mihalopoulos, C.; Chatterton, M.L.; et al. A randomised controlled trial of dietary improvement for adults with major depression (the 'SMILES' trial). *BMC Med.* **2017**, *15*, 23. [CrossRef]
72. Mischoulon, D.; Freeman, M.P. Omega-3 Fatty Acids in Psychiatry. *Psychiatr. Clin. N. Am.* **2013**, *36*, 15–23. [CrossRef]
73. Lai, J.; Moxey, A.; Nowak, G.; Vashum, K.; Bailey, K.; McEvoy, M. The efficacy of zinc supplementation in depression: Systematic review of randomised controlled trials. *J. Affect. Disord.* **2012**, *136*, e31–e39. [CrossRef]
74. Eyles, D.W.; Burne, T.H.J.; McGrath, J.J. Vitamin D, effects on brain development, adult brain function and the links between low levels of vitamin D and neuropsychiatric disease. *Front. Neuroendocrinol.* **2013**, *34*, 47–64. [CrossRef] [PubMed]
75. Swinburn, B.A.; Kraak, V.I.; Allender, S. The global syndemic of obesity, undernutrition, and climate change: The Lancet Commission report. *Lancet* **2019**, *393*, 791–846. [CrossRef] [PubMed]
76. GBD. Diet Collaborators. Health effects of dietary risks in 195 countries, 1990-2017: A systematic analysis for the Global Burden of Disease Study. *Lancet* **2019**, *393*, 1958–1972. [CrossRef]
77. Sarris, J.; Logan, A.C.; Akbaraly, T.N. Medicine as mainstream in psychiatry. *Lancet Psychiatry* **2015**, *2*, 271–274. [CrossRef] [PubMed]
78. Sarris, J.; Logan, A.C.; Akbaraly, T.N. International Society for Nutritional Psychiatry Research consensus position statement: Nutritional medicine in modern psychiatry. *World Psychiatry* **2015**, *14*, 370–371. [CrossRef] [PubMed]
79. Fernstrom, J.D. Can nutrient supplements modify brain function? *Am. J. Clin. Nutr.* **2000**, *71*, 1669S–1673S. [CrossRef] [PubMed]
80. Berk, M.; Jacka, F.N. Diet and depression—From confirmation to implementation. *JAMA* **2019**, *321*, 842–843. [CrossRef] [PubMed]
81. Berk, M.; Williams, L.J.; Jacka, F.N. So depression is an inflammatory disease, but where does the inflammation come from? *BMC Med.* **2013**, *11*, 200. [CrossRef]
82. Miller, B.J.; Buckley, P.; Seabolt, W. Meta-analysis of cytokine alterations in schizophrenia: Clinical status and antipsychotic effects. *Biol. Psychiatry* **2011**, *70*, 663–671. [CrossRef]
83. Berk, M.; Kapczinski, F.; Andreazza, A. Pathways underlying neuroprogression in bipolar disorder: Focus on inflammation, oxidative stress and neurotrophic factors. *Neurosci. Biobehav. Rev.* **2011**, *35*, 804–817. [CrossRef] [PubMed]
84. Irwin, M.R.; Piber, D. Insomnia and inflammation: A two hit model of depression risk and prevention. *World Psychiatry* **2018**, *17*, 359–361. [CrossRef] [PubMed]
85. Köhler, C.A.; Freitas, T.H.; Stubbs, B. Peripheral alterations in cytokine and chemokine levels after antidepressant drug treatment for major depressive disorder: Systematic review and meta-analysis. *Mol. Neurobiol.* **2018**, *55*, 4195–4206. [CrossRef] [PubMed]

86. Schuch, F.B.; Deslandes, A.C.; Stubbs, B. Neurobiological effects of exercise on major depressive disorder: A systematic review. *Neurosci. Biobehav. Rev.* **2016**, *61*, 1–11. [CrossRef] [PubMed]
87. Swardfager, W.; Herrmann, N.; Mazereeuw, G. Zinc in depression: A meta-analysis. *Biol. Psychiatry* **2013**, *74*, 872–878. [CrossRef] [PubMed]
88. Joe, P.; Petrilli, M.; Malaspina, D. Zinc in schizophrenia: A meta-analysis. *Gen. Hosp. Psychiatry* **2018**, *53*, 19–24. [CrossRef]
89. Gilbody, S.; Lightfoot, T.; Sheldon, T. Is low folate a risk factor for depression? A meta-analysis and exploration of heterogeneity. *J. Epidemiol. Commun. Health* **2007**, *61*, 631–637. [CrossRef] [PubMed]
90. Belbasis, L.; Kohler, C.A.; Stefanis, N. Risk factors and peripheral biomarkers for schizophrenia spectrum disorders: An umbrella review of meta-analyses. *Acta Psychiatr. Scand.* **2018**, *137*, 88–97. [CrossRef]
91. Anglin, R.E.S.; Samaan, Z.; Walter, S.D. Vitamin D deficiency and depression in adults: Systematic review and meta-analysis. *Br. J. Psychiatry* **2013**, *202*, 100–107. [CrossRef]
92. Firth, J.; Carney, R.; Stubbs, B. Nutritional deficiencies and clinical correlates in first-episode psychosis: A systematic review and meta-analysis. *Schizophr. Bull.* **2018**, *44*, 1275–1292. [CrossRef]
93. Lally, J.; Ajnakina, O.; Singh, N. Vitamin D and clinical symptoms in first episode psychosis (FEP): A prospective cohort study. *Schizophr. Res.* **2019**, *204*, 381–388. [CrossRef]
94. Patrick, R.P.; Ames, B.N. Vitamin D and the omega-3 fatty acids control serotonin synthesis and action, part 2: Relevance for ADHD, bipolar disorder, schizophrenia, and impulsive behavior. *FASEB J.* **2015**, *29*, 2207–2222. [CrossRef]
95. Su, K.P. Biological mechanism of antidepressant effect of omega-3 fatty acids: How does fish oil act as a 'mind-body interface'? *Neurosignals.* **2009**, *17*, 144–152. [CrossRef]
96. Molfino, A.; Amabile, M.I.; Monti, M.; Muscaritoli, M. Omega-3 polyunsaturated fatty acids in critical illness: Anti-inflammatory, proresolving, or both? *Oxidative Med. Cell. Longev.* **2017**, *2017*, 5987082. [CrossRef] [PubMed]
97. Molfino, A.; Gioia, G.; Rossi Fanelli, F.; Muscaritoli, M. The role for dietary omega3 fatty acids supplementation in older adults. *Nutrients* **2014**, *6*, 4058–4073. [CrossRef]
98. Hoffmire, C.A.; Block, R.C.; Thevenet-Morrison, K.; van Wijngaarden, E. Associations between omega-3 poly-unsaturated fatty acids from fish consumption and severity of depressive symptoms: An analysis of the 2005–2008. *Natl. Health Nutr. Exam. Survey Prostaglandins Leukot. Essent. Fat. Acids* **2012**, *86*, 155–160. [CrossRef]
99. Rapaport, M.H.; Nierenberg, A.A.; Schettler, P.J.; Kinkead, B.; Cardoos, A.; Walker, R. Inflammation as a predictive biomarker for response to omega-3 fatty acids in major depressive disorder: A proof-of-concept study. *Mol. Psychiatry* **2016**, *21*, 71–79. [CrossRef] [PubMed]
100. Nishi, D.; Su, K.P.; Usuda, K.; Chang, J.P.; Hamazaki, K.; Ishima, T. Plasma estradiol levels and antidepressant effects of omega-3 fatty acids in pregnant women. *Brain Behav. Immun.* **2020**, *85*, 29–34. [CrossRef] [PubMed]
101. Johnson, A.C.; Tremble, S.M.; Chan, S.L.; Moseley, J.; LaMarca, B.; Nagle, K.J. Magnesium sulfate treatment reverses seizure susceptibility and decreases neuroinflammation in a rat model of severe preeclampsia. *PLoS ONE* **2014**, *9*, e113670. [CrossRef]
102. Wang, P.; Yu, X.; Guan, P.P.; Guo, J.W.; Wang, Y.; Zhang, Y. Magnesium ion influx reduces neuroinflammation in Aβ precursor protein/Presenilin 1 transgenic mice by suppressing the expression of interleukin-1β. *Cell. Mol. Immunol.* **2017**, *14*, 451–464. [CrossRef]
103. Botturi, A.; Ciappolino, V.; Delvecchio, G.; Boscutti, A.; Viscardi, B.; Brambilla, P. The role and the effect of magnesium in mental disorders: A systematic review. *Nutrients* **2020**, *12*, 1661. [CrossRef] [PubMed]
104. Pittenger, C.; Sanacora, G.; Krystal, J.H. The NMDA receptor as a therapeutic target in major depressive disorder. *CNS Neurol. Disord. Drug Targets* **2007**, *6*, 101–115. [CrossRef] [PubMed]
105. Bottiglieri, T.; Laundy, M.; Crellin, R.; Toone, B.K.; Carney, M.W.; Reynolds, E.H. Homocysteine, folate, methylation, and monoamine metabolism in depression. *J. Neurol. Neurosurg. Psychiatry* **2000**, *69*, 228–232. [CrossRef] [PubMed]
106. Almeida, O.P.; Ford, A.H.; Flicker, L. Systematic review and meta-analysis of randomized placebo-controlled trials of folate and vitamin B12 for depression. *Int. Psychogeriatr.* **2015**, *27*, 727–737. [CrossRef] [PubMed]
107. Takahashi, K.; Yanai, S.; Takisawa, S.; Kono, N.; Arai, H.; Nishida, Y. Vitamin C and vitamin E double-deficiency increased neuroinflammation and impaired conditioned fear memory. *Arch. Biochem. Biophys.* **2019**, *663*, 120–128. [CrossRef] [PubMed]
108. Elfakhri, K.H.; Abdallah, I.M.; Brannen, A.D.; Kaddoumi, A. Multi-faceted therapeutic strategy for treatment of Alzheimer's disease by concurrent administration of etodolac and α-tocopherol. *Neurobiol. Dis.* **2019**, *125*, 123–134. [CrossRef] [PubMed]
109. Ibáñez-del Valle, V.; Navarro-Martínez, R.; Cauli, O. Association between Depressive Symptoms and Adherence to the Mediterranean Diet in Nursing Students. *Nutrients* **2023**, *15*, 3158. [CrossRef] [PubMed]
110. Hwang, Y.-G.; Pae, C.; Lee, S.-H.; Yook, K.-H.; Park, C.I. Relationship between Mediterranean diet and depression in South Korea: The Korea National Health and Nutrition Examination Survey. *Front. Nutr.* **2023**, *10*, 1219743. [CrossRef] [PubMed]
111. Sadeghi, O.; Keshteli, A.H.; Afshar, H.; Esmaillzadeh, A.; Adibi, P. Adherence to Mediterranean dietary pattern is inversely associated with depression, anxiety and psychological distress. *Nutr. Neurosci.* **2021**, *24*, 248–259. [CrossRef]
112. Muscogiuri, G.; Verde, L.; Sulu, C.; Katsiki, N.; Hassapidou, M.; Frias-Toral, E.; Cucalón, G.; Pazderska, A.; Yumuk, V.D.; Colao, A.; et al. Mediterranean Diet and Obesity-related Disorders: What is the Evidence? *Curr. Obes. Rep.* **2022**, *11*, 287–304. [CrossRef]
113. Mancini, J.G.; Filion, K.B.; Atallah, R.; Eisenberg, M.J. Systematic Review of the Mediterranean Diet for Long-Term Weight Loss. *Am. J. Med.* **2016**, *129*, 407–415.e4. [CrossRef] [PubMed]

114. Schiavo, L.; Scalera, G.; Sergio, R.; De Sena, G.; Pilone, V.; Barbarisi, A. Clinical impact of Mediterranean-enriched-protein diet on liver size, visceral fat, fat mass, and fat-free mass in patients undergoing sleeve gastrectomy. *Surg. Obes. Relat. Dis.* **2015**, *11*, 1164–1170. [CrossRef] [PubMed]
115. Feidantsis, K.; Methenitis, S.; Ketselidi, K.; Vagianou, K.; Skepastianos, P.; Hatzitolios, A.; Mourouglakis, A.; Kaprara, A.; Hassapidou, M.; Nomikos, T.; et al. Comparison of short-term hypocaloric high-protein diets with a hypocaloric Mediterranean diet: Effect on body composition and health-related blood markers in overweight and sedentary young participants. *Nutrition* **2021**, *91–92*, 111365. [CrossRef] [PubMed]
116. Jain, R.; Larsuphrom, P.; Degremont, A.; Latunde-Dada, G.O.; Philippou, E. Association between vegetarian and vegan diets and depression: A systematic review. *Nutr. Bull.* **2022**, *47*, 27–49. [CrossRef] [PubMed]
117. Alcorta, A.; Porta, A.; Tárrega, A.; Alvarez, M.D.; Vaquero, M.P. Foods for Plant-Based Diets: Challenges and Innovations. *Foods* **2021**, *10*, 293. [CrossRef] [PubMed]
118. Clarys, P.; Deliens, T.; Huybrechts, I.; Deriemaeker, P.; Vanaelst, B.; De Keyzer, W.; Hebbelinck, M.; Mullie, P. Comparison of Nutritional Quality of the Vegan, Vegetarian, Semi-Vegetarian, Pesco-Vegetarian and Omnivorous Diet. *Nutrients* **2014**, *6*, 1318–1332. [CrossRef] [PubMed]
119. Orlich, M.J.; Jaceldo-Siegl, K.; Sabaté, J.; Fan, J.; Singh, P.N.; Fraser, G.E. Patterns of food consumption among vegetarians and non-vegetarians. *Br. J. Nutr.* **2014**, *112*, 1644–1653. [CrossRef] [PubMed]
120. Oussalah, A.; Levy, J.; Berthezène, C.; Alpers, D.H.; Guéant, J.-L. Health outcomes associated with vegetarian diets: An umbrella review of systematic reviews and meta-analyses. *Clin. Nutr.* **2020**, *39*, 3283–3307. [CrossRef]
121. Iguacel, I.; Huybrechts, I.; Moreno, L.A.; Michels, N. Vegetarianism and veganism compared with mental health and cognitive outcomes: A systematic review and meta-analysis. *Nutr. Rev.* **2021**, *79*, 361–381. [CrossRef]
122. Askari, M.; Daneshzad, E.; Darooghegi Mofrad, M.; Bellissimo, N.; Suitor, K.; Azadbakht, L. Vegetarian diet and the risk of depression, anxiety, and stress symptoms: A systematic review and meta-analysis of observational studies. *Crit. Rev. Food Sci. Nutr.* **2022**, *62*, 261–271. [CrossRef]
123. Fazelian, S.; Sadeghi, E.; Firouzi, S.; Haghighatdoost, F. Adherence to the vegetarian diet may increase the risk of depression: A systematic review and meta-analysis of observational studies. *Nutr. Rev.* **2022**, *80*, 242–254. [CrossRef] [PubMed]
124. Walsh, H.; Lee, M.; Best, T. The association between vegan, vegetarian, and omnivore diet quality and depressive symptoms in adults: A cross-sectional study. *Int. J. Environ. Res. Public Health* **2023**, *20*, 3258. [CrossRef] [PubMed]
125. Perez-Cornago, A.; Sanchez-Villegas, A.; Bes-Rastrollo, M.; Gea, A.; Molero, P.; Lahortiga-Ramos, F.; Martinez-Gonzalez, M.Á. Relationship between adherence to Dietary Approaches to Stop Hypertension (DASH) diet indices and incidence of depression during up to 8 years of follow-up. *Public Health Nutr.* **2017**, *20*, 2383–2392. [CrossRef] [PubMed]
126. Khayyatzadeh, S.S.; Mehramiz, M.; Mirmousavi, S.J.; Mazidi, M.; Ziaee, A.; Kazemi-Bajestani, S.M.R.; Ferns, G.A.; Moharreri, F.; Ghayour-mobarhan, M. Adherence to a Dash-style diet in relation to depression and aggression in adolescent girls. *Psychiatry Res.* **2018**, *259*, 104–109. [CrossRef] [PubMed]
127. Fresán, U.; Bes-Rastrollo, M.; Segovia-Siapco, G.; Sanchez-Villegas, A.; Lahortiga, F.; De La Rosa, P.-A.; Martínez-Gonzalez, M.-A. Does the MIND diet decrease depression risk? A comparison with Mediterranean diet in the SUN cohort. *Eur. J. Nutr.* **2019**, *58*, 1271–1282. [CrossRef] [PubMed]
128. Soltani, S.; Shirani, F.; Chitsazi, M.J.; Salehi-Abargouei, A. The effect of dietary approaches to stop hypertension (DASH) diet on weight and body composition in adults: A systematic review and meta-analysis of randomized controlled clinical trials. *Obes. Rev.* **2016**, *17*, 442–454. [CrossRef] [PubMed]
129. Hu, F. *Physical Activity, Sedentary Behaviors, and Obesity, in: Obesity Epidemiology*; Oxford University Press: New York, NY, USA, 2008; pp. 301–319. [CrossRef]
130. Thorogood, A.; Mottillo, S.; Shimony, A.; Filion, K.B.; Joseph, L.; Genest, J.; Pilote, L.; Poirier, P.; Schiffrin, E.L.; Eisenberg, M.J. Isolated Aerobic Exercise and Weight Loss: A Systematic Review and Meta-Analysis of Randomized Controlled Trials. *Am. J. Med.* **2011**, *124*, 747–755. [CrossRef] [PubMed]
131. Ross, R.; Blair, S.; De Lannoy, L.; Després, J.-P.; Lavie, C.J. Changing the Endpoints for Determining Effective Obesity Management. *Prog. Cardiovasc. Dis.* **2015**, *57*, 330–336. [CrossRef] [PubMed]
132. Wu, T.; Gao, X.; Chen, M.; Van Dam, R.M. Long-term effectiveness of diet-plus-exercise interventions vs. diet-only interventions for weight loss: A meta-analysis. *Obes. Rev.* **2009**, *10*, 313–323. [CrossRef]
133. Bray, G.A.; Heisel, W.E.; Afshin, A.; Jensen, M.D.; Dietz, W.H.; Long, M.; Kushner, R.F.; Daniels, S.R.; Wadden, T.A.; Tsai, A.G.; et al. The Science of Obesity Management: An Endocrine Society Scientific Statement. *Endocr. Rev.* **2018**, *39*, 79–132. [CrossRef]
134. Ruban, A.; Stoenchev, K.; Ashrafian, H.; Teare, J. Current treatments for obesity. *Clin. Med.* **2019**, *19*, 205–212. [CrossRef] [PubMed]
135. Kazmi, T.; Nagi, L.F.; Iqbal, S.P.; Razzak, S.; Hassnain, S.; Khan, S.; Shahid, N. Relationship Between Physical Inactivity and Obesity in the Urban Slums of Lahore. *Cureus* **2022**, *14*, e23719. [CrossRef] [PubMed]
136. Silveira, E.A.; Mendonça, C.R.; Delpino, F.M.; Elias Souza, G.V.; Pereira De Souza Rosa, L.; De Oliveira, C.; Noll, M. Sedentary behavior, physical inactivity, abdominal obesity and obesity in adults and older adults: A systematic review and meta-analysis. *Clin. Nutr. ESPEN* **2022**, *50*, 63–73. [CrossRef]
137. Brandao, C.F.C.; Nonino, C.B.; De Carvalho, F.G.; Nicoletti, C.F.; Noronha, N.Y.; San Martin, R.; De Freitas, E.C.; Junqueira-Franco, M.V.M.; Marchini, J.S. The effects of short-term combined exercise training on telomere length in obese women: A prospective, interventional study. *Sports Med. Open* **2020**, *6*, 5. [CrossRef]

138. Mendham, A.E.; Goedecke, J.H.; Fortuin-de Smidt, M.C.; Phiri, L.; Clamp, L.; Swart, J.; Lipinska, G.; Rae, D.E. Improved Sleep Quality and Depressive Symptoms With Exercise Training in Obese Women From a Low Socioeconomic Community: A Randomized Controlled Trial. *J. Phys. Act. Health* **2021**, *18*, 440–449. [CrossRef] [PubMed]
139. Gorham, L.S.; Jernigan, T.; Hudziak, J.; Barch, D.M. Involvement in Sports, Hippocampal Volume, and Depressive Symptoms in Children. *Biol. Psychiatry Cogn. Neurosci. Neuroimaging* **2019**, *4*, 484–492. [CrossRef] [PubMed]
140. Ghalandari-Shamami, M.; Nourizade, S.; Yousefi, B.; Vafaei, A.A.; Pakdel, R.; Rashidy-Pour, A. Beneficial Effects of Physical Activity and Crocin Against Adolescent Stress Induced Anxiety or Depressive-Like Symptoms and Dendritic Morphology Remodeling in Prefrontal Cortex in Adult Male Rats. *Neurochem. Res.* **2019**, *44*, 917–929. [CrossRef]
141. Viana, R.B.; Gentil, P.; Naves, J.P.A.; Rebelo, A.C.S.; Santos, D.A.T.; Braga, M.A.O.; De Lira, C.A.B. Interval Training Improves Depressive Symptoms But Not Anxious Symptoms in Healthy Women. *Front. Psychiatry* **2019**, *10*, 661. [CrossRef]
142. Gerber, M.; Minghetti, A.; Beck, J.; Zahner, L.; Donath, L. Sprint Interval Training and Continuous Aerobic Exercise Training Have Similar Effects on Exercise Motivation and Affective Responses to Exercise in Patients With Major Depressive Disorders: A Randomized Controlled Trial. *Front. Psychiatry* **2018**, *9*, 694. [CrossRef]
143. Smail-Crevier, R.; Powers, G.; Noel, C.; Wang, J. Health-Related Internet Usage and Design Feature Preference for E-Mental Health Programs Among Men and Women. *J. Med. Internet Res.* **2019**, *21*, e11224. [CrossRef]
144. Hampton-Marcell, J.T.; Eshoo, T.W.; Cook, M.D.; Gilbert, J.A.; Horswill, C.A.; Poretsky, R. Comparative analysis of gut microbiota following changes in training volume among swimmers. *Int. J. Sports Med.* **2020**, *41*, 292–299. [CrossRef] [PubMed]
145. Durk, R.P.; Castillo, E.; Márquez-Magaña, L.; Grosicki, G.J.; Bolter, N.D.; Lee, C.M.; Bagley, J.R. Gut Microbiota composition is related to cardiorespiratory fitness in healthy young adults. *Int. J. Sport Nutr. Exerc. Metab.* **2019**, *29*, 249–253. [CrossRef] [PubMed]
146. Scheiman, J.; Luber, J.M.; Chavkin, T.A.; MacDonald, T.; Tung, A.; Pham, L.D.; Wibowo, M.C.; Wurth, R.C.; Punthambaker, S.; Tierney, B.T.; et al. Meta-omics analysis of elite athletes identities a performance-enhancing microbe that functions via lactate metabolism. *Nat. Med.* **2019**, *25*, 1104–1109. [CrossRef] [PubMed]
147. Kern, T.; Blond, M.B.; Hansen, T.H.; Rosenkilde, M.; Quist, J.S.; Gram, A.S.; Ekstrøm, C.T.; Hansen, T.; Stallknecht, B. Structured exercise alters the gut microbiota in humans with overweight and obesity—A randomized controlled trial. *Int. J. Obes.* **2020**, *44*, 125–135. [CrossRef] [PubMed]
148. Zhong, F.; Wen, X.; Yang, M.; Lai, H.Y.; Momma, H.; Cheng, L.; Sun, X.; Nagatomi, R.; Huang, C. Effect of an 8-week exercise training on gut microbiota in physically inactive older women. *Int. J. Sports Med.* **2021**, *42*, 610–623. [CrossRef] [PubMed]
149. O'Donovan, C.M.; Madigan, S.M.; Garcia-Perez, I.; Rankin, A.; O' Sullivan, O.; Cotter, P.D. Distinct microbiome composition and metabolome exists across subgroups of elite Irish athletes. *J. Sci. Med. Sport* **2020**, *23*, 63–68. [CrossRef] [PubMed]
150. Matsumoto, M.; Inoue, R.; Tsukahara, T.; Ushida, K.; Chiji, H.; Matsubara, N.; Hara, H. Voluntary running exercise alters microbiota composition and increases n-butyrate concentration in the rat cecum. *Biosci. Biotechnol. Biochem.* **2008**, *72*, 572–576. [CrossRef] [PubMed]
151. Pant, K.; Peixoto, E.; Richard, S.; Gradilone, S.A. Role of histone deacetylases in carcinogenesis: Potential role in cholangiocarcinoma. *Cells* **2020**, *9*, 780. [CrossRef]
152. Campbell, S.C. *Faecalibacterium prausnitzii* abundance in mouse and human gut can predict metabolism of oat avenanthramides. *J. Nutr.* **2021**, *151*, 1369–1370. [CrossRef]
153. Mailing, L.J.; Allen, J.M.; Buford, T.W.; Fields, C.J.; Woods, J.A. Exercise and the gut microbiome: A review of the evidence, potential mechanisms, and implications for human health. *Exerc. Sport Sci. Rev.* **2019**, *47*, 75–85. [CrossRef]
154. Singh, R.K.; Chang, H.W.; Yan, D.; Lee, K.M.; Ucmak, D.; Wong, K.; Abrouk, M.; Farahnik, B.; Nakamura, M.; Zhu, T.H.; et al. Influence of diet on the gut microbiome and implications for human health. *J. Transl. Med.* **2017**, *15*, 73. [CrossRef] [PubMed]
155. Mohr, A.E.; Jäger, R.; Carpenter, K.C.; Kerksick, C.M.; Purpura, M.; Townsend, J.R.; West, N.P.; Black, K.; Gleeson, M.; Pyne, D.B.; et al. The athletic gut microbiota. *J. Int. Soc. Sports Nutr.* **2020**, *17*, 1–33. [CrossRef] [PubMed]
156. Mika, A.; Fleshner, M. Early-life exercise may promote lasting brain and metabolic health through gut bacterial metabolites. *Immunol. Cell Biol.* **2016**, *94*, 151–157. [CrossRef] [PubMed]
157. Evans, D.L.; Charney, D.S. Mood disorders and medical illness: A major public health problem. *Biol. Psychiatry* **2003**, *54*, 177–180. [CrossRef] [PubMed]
158. Simon, G.E. Social and economic burden of mood disorders. *Biol. Psychiatry* **2003**, *54*, 208–215. [CrossRef] [PubMed]
159. Chrostowska, M.; Szyndler, A.; Hoffmann, M.; Narkiewicz, K. Impact of obesity on cardiovascular health. *Best Pract. Res. Clin. Endocrinol. Metab.* **2013**, *27*, 147–156. [CrossRef] [PubMed]
160. Allison, D.B.; Newcomer, J.W.; Dunn, A.L.; Blumenthal, J.A.; Fabricatore, A.N.; Daumit, G.L.; Cope, M.B.; Riley, W.T.; Vreeland, B.; Hibbeln, J.R.; et al. Obesity Among Those with Mental Disorders. *Am. J. Prev. Med.* **2009**, *36*, 341–350. [CrossRef] [PubMed]
161. Miller, A.H.; Maletic, V.; Raison, C.L. Inflammation and Its Discontents: The Role of Cytokines in the Pathophysiology of Major Depression. *Biol. Psychiatry* **2009**, *65*, 732–741. [CrossRef]
162. Kloiber, S.; Ising, M.; Reppermund, S.; Horstmann, S.; Dose, T.; Majer, M.; Zihl, J.; Pfister, H.; Unschuld, P.G.; Holsboer, F.; et al. Overweight and Obesity Affect Treatment Response in Major Depression. *Biol. Psychiatry* **2007**, *62*, 321–326. [CrossRef]

nutrients

MDPI

Review

Improving Eating Habits at the Office: An Umbrella Review of Nutritional Interventions

Aleksandra Hyży, Mariusz Jaworski, Ilona Cieślak, Joanna Gotlib-Małkowska and Mariusz Panczyk *

Department of Education and Research in Health Sciences, Faculty of Health Science, Medical University of Warsaw, 00-581 Warsaw, Poland; aleksandra.hyzy@wum.edu.pl (A.H.); mariusz.jaworski@wum.edu.pl (M.J.); ilona.cieslak@wum.edu.pl (I.C.); joanna.gotlib@wum.edu.pl (J.G.-M.)

* Correspondence: mariusz.panczyk@wum.edu.pl

Abstract: (1) Workplace nutrition interventions have garnered attention as a pivotal component of employee well-being and organisational productivity. However, the effectiveness of various intervention types remains inconclusive. This review aims to systematically evaluate the efficacy of cognitive, behavioural, and mixed nutrition interventions in the workplace, considering the nuances of intervention design, setting, and target demographics. (2) A comprehensive umbrella review was conducted, categorising the existing literature into person-oriented and environmental strategies. This review was prepared in line with the Joanna Briggs Institute methodology for umbrella reviews and the preferred reporting items for systematic reviews and meta-analyses reporting standard. (3) The analysis revealed a lack of definitive evidence supporting the universal effectiveness of any single intervention type. Nonetheless, behavioural and mixed interventions demonstrated more favourable outcomes as compared to purely cognitive strategies. Factors such as intervention design, workplace setting, and target group characteristics were identified as significant determinants of the intervention success. (4) The review emphasises the imperative for additional investigations that utilise evidence-based approaches to formulate sound guidelines for efficacious nutrition interventions in occupational settings. This review functions as a foundational framework for guiding both scholarly research and the pragmatic execution of nutrition programs in the workplace.

Keywords: workplace nutrition; behavioural interventions; cognitive interventions; employee well-being; organisational productivity

1. Introduction

The concept of well-being comprises health, happiness, and prosperity, including feeling mentally well, being satisfied with life, having a sense of purpose, and managing stress effectively [1]. Proper nutrition and a healthy diet are fundamental to good health and well-being. A balanced diet provides the necessary energy for daily activity as well as essential nutrients for growth and repair, promoting strength and health. It also facilitates the prevention of diet-related illnesses. An increasing body of research indicates that diet and nutrition have a substantial impact on mood and mental well-being, as well as on work performance [2]. This is of particular interest to employers, employees, and the public health sector, with well-being as an aspect of public health. The World Health Organisation collaborates with its member states and partners to promote the concept of well-being in global health and to achieve the 17 Sustainable Development Goals adopted by the United Nations [3].

Workplace well-being activities have a long history. Formal corporate well-being programs date back to the 1950s [4,5] and have observed rapid growth since the 1970s, mainly in the United States. Employers, wishing to reduce losses due to sickness absence, presenteeism (attendance at work despite illness) [6] or compensations, introduced preventive measures in the workplace. These measures resulted from the peculiarities of the US healthcare system, which does not entail public health insurance coverage; thus, healthcare costs are passed on to citizens and employers [7]. Initially, the implementation of well-being and health programs (e.g., as part of Employee Assistance Programs) aimed to prevent work-related illness and accidents. Over time, they also began to shape an employer-focused corporate culture oriented towards health promotion, enhancing the company's brand and market position [8]. This became important in order to attract employees, whose expectations are constantly increasing; to create a company brand that is perceived as responsible and supportive of the employee; or to position the company through the awards given to top employers. This is also a result of the growing popularity of CSR (corporate social responsibility) and ESG (environment, social responsibility, and corporate governance). Over time, such an approach became recognised world-wide, and well-being initiatives have become a permanent part of the corporate culture of many companies [9–11].

Due to increased global health needs (staff shortages, challenges in obtaining healthcare services, aging population), for several years now, the World Health Organisation has identified the workplace setting as crucial for health promotion. The average employee spends one-third of the day in the workplace; thus, measures taken just in this environment seem reasonable and relatively easy to implement [12,13]. Currently, health-related benefits such as private health insurance, fitness perks, fruit and vegetable delivery to the office or lunch subsidies are among the most frequently offered, and their scope is steadily increasing. The reason for this is both the employers' aspirations to distinguish themselves and the steadily rising employee expectations [9,11]. In addition, the workplace is also a space for socializing, sharing ideas and making friends and acquaintances, which can further contribute to the development of healthy eating habits [9,11].

When undertaking activities to promote health in the workplace, it is necessary to clearly define the target group, as well as the purpose and form of the activities (interventions) to be undertaken. Office workers are one of the most frequently addressed group of employee-directed health-related activities [10]. This is due to a number of factors that facilitate the design, implementation and evaluation of such interventions, e.g., a fixed pattern of work—work at similar times of the day and for a comparable amount of time, making most employees available at roughly the same place and time; or a similar range of duties—typically sedentary work that does not require the extra effort associated with, for example, having to stand for long periods of time or carrying objects. In addition, office workers in most cases are not shift workers, which has a huge impact on their circadian rhythm, meal times, eating habits and associated health risks. In addition, their privileged social position, higher education and higher earnings, and thus higher overall health competence, may be a major factor in the more frequent provision of well-being programs to this group of employees. All this makes it easier to establish a fairly homogeneous study group, allowing for the assessment of intervention effectiveness [10,11,14].

Another important step is to determine the purpose and form of the intervention. Overall, interventions can be divided into three main categories. The first category comprises cognitive interventions, which aim to increase nutritional knowledge and awareness of the impact of nutrition on health, e.g., through education, training or lectures. The second category comprises behavioural interventions, which are skill-giving interventions, i.e., interventions that focus on the recipient (e.g., through workshops or prevention programs) or that implement the changes needed to alter eating behaviour, as well as environmental interventions that focus on changes in access to or labelling of foods, e.g., providing fruit in the office or the colour-coding of cafeteria meals based on their nutritional value. The third category comprises mixed interventions, which combine cognitive and behavioural interventions. The cognitive interventions group may include, e.g., lectures (onsite and online) and e-learning courses. Behavioural interventions include, e.g., changing the availability of certain foods (limiting sweets in vending machines or providing fresh fruit and vegetables to the office), labelling healthy meals in the employee cafeteria with colours or symbols [15,16] or financial incentives for choosing healthy products [17]. Mixed interventions involve both components and may consist of workshops with a health care professional (doctor, nurse, nutritionist, public health specialist health educator, etc.), well-being programs combining lectures, workshops, exercise and dietary change, or, for example, diabetes prevention programs targeting the prevention and treatment of a particular disease [18–20].

The evaluation of the effectiveness of workplace nutrition interventions is a crucial component of their implementation [21]. Effectiveness can be measured using various indicators and methods. Cognitive interventions often involve pre- and post-intervention knowledge tests. The effectiveness of behavioural and mixed interventions can be assessed using work environment and economic indicators (e.g., absenteeism, presenteeism, costs) or health-related indicators (e.g., BMI, glucose levels, cholesterol levels, disease exacerbation, consumption of specific food groups). These indicators may be combined to provide a more comprehensive evaluation of the impact of interventions.

Currently, there is a notable lack of consensus on well-defined guidelines or recommendations for the design and implementation of workplace nutrition interventions. The proliferation of systematic reviews and meta-analyses on this subject presents a challenge in terms of consolidating the evidence and arriving at definitive conclusions. An umbrella review was determined to be the most appropriate approach to effectively collect and analyze existing data on nutritional interventions among office workers [22]. This method provides an overview of the evidence presented in available systematic reviews and meta-analyses, allowing for their comparison and evaluation. The umbrella review is optimal for exploring existing data, as it facilitates the discussion of various types of interventions, enabling conclusions to be drawn and gaps in the current state of knowledge to be identified.

Aim and Research Question

The aim of this study was to synthesise the available scientific evidence regarding the effectiveness of various workplace-based nutrition interventions for office workers, as reported in secondary studies. An umbrella review was conducted to answer the following research questions:

- What kind of nutrition interventions are used in the office setting?
- What workplace nutrition interventions are effective for office workers?
- What are the factors contributing to the effectiveness of workplace nutrition interventions?

2. Materials and Methods

This review was prepared in line with the Joanna Briggs Institute (JBI) methodology for umbrella reviews [23] and the preferred reporting items for systematic reviews and meta-analyses (PRISMA) reporting standard [24].

2.1. Search Strategy

The overall search strategy was developed using the PICOS framework [25]:

- Population: office workers of all ages and genders;
- Interventions: dietary interventions, counselling, nutrition programs;
- Comparisons: not applicable;
- Outcomes: nutritional knowledge, economic indicators (e.g., absenteeism, presenteeism, costs) or health-related indicators (e.g., BMI, glucose levels, cholesterol levels, disease exacerbation, consumption of specific food groups);

In order to expand the scope of the search outcomes, no restrictions were imposed on the publication date. The literature search was carried out in November 2022, utilizing the PubMed/Medline, Embase, ProQuest, Scopus, and Web of Science Core Collection databases. Keywords were obtained through an initial search of articles on PubMed/Medline and the use of medical subject heading (MeSH) terms. The search strategies employed for each database are provided in Supplementary S1.

2.2. Eligibility Criteria

The inclusion criteria were as follows:

- Type of study: meta-analysis or systematic reviews that covered quantitative, qualitative, or mixed method studies that were peer reviewed.
- Type of participants: office workers.
- Type of controls: not applicable.
- Type of outcomes: nutritional knowledge, economic or health-related indicators.
- Language: papers written in English.

The following exclusion criteria were applied:

- Studies that included grey literature or professional guidelines.
- Studies that focused on groups of workers other than the target population.
- Studies that aimed to analyze the relationship between physical activity participation/adherence and the effects of nutrition interventions.
- Studies published in languages other than English.

2.3. Selection Process

All search results were imported into EndNote ver. 20 (Clarivate™, London, UK), i.e., reference management software. Duplicate entries were removed, and two researchers (AH, MP) independently screened the remaining articles based on their titles and abstracts using the Rayyan platform, an intelligent research collaboration tool for systematic literature reviews [26]. Discrepancies were resolved upon discussion, and if a consensus could not be reached, a third researcher was consulted. The full texts of the selected studies were then evaluated for inclusion in the study.

2.4. Data Collection Process

Data from the included reviews were extracted by both reviewers using a standardised data extraction sheet (Supplementary S2). The researchers divided the reviews for data extraction and subsequently checked 90% of each other's extractions for accuracy. In cases of disagreement, a third reviewer was consulted. Information such as the title, authors, journal, publication year, review type (meta-analysis or systematic review), type of study (randomised controlled trials, quasi-experimental or observational studies), type of intervention(s) in the review (cognitive, behavioural or mixed), number of reviews included, total number of participants of primary studies included in the review, and data sources were extracted by one researcher and verified by the other.

2.5. Review Risk of Bias Assessment

The methodological quality of systematic reviews or meta-analysis of interventional studies was evaluated with the Assessing the Methodological Quality of Systematic Reviews 2 (AMSTAR 2) measurement tool [27]. Two reviewers independently rated the risk of bias and discrepancies were discussed with the third reviewer, if needed. The AMSTAR 2 measurement tool comprises seven critical domains, including: prospective registration of the protocol, search strategy, justification for the exclusion of particular studies, quality assessment of included studies, appropriateness of the analysis method, consideration of quality when interpreting results, and the presence of publication bias. In addition, there are nine non-critical domains. Each item is scored yes/partially yes/no/, and the overall methodological quality is classified as high (only $\leq$1 item in a non-critical domain rated as "yes"), moderate (>1 item in a non-critical domain rated as "yes"), low (1 item in a critical domain rated as "yes" regardless of the ratings in the non-critical domains), or critically low (>1 item in a critical domain rated as "yes" regardless of ratings in non-critical domains) (Supplementary S3).

2.6. *Effect Measures*

Given the broad scope of the review questions and the anticipated diversity, specific effect measures were intentionally left unspecified. The diverse nature of interventions, varying in scope and methodology across studies, necessitated an approach where specific effect measures were not pre-defined. This choice aligns with the practices in umbrella reviews where heterogeneity in study designs is a common challenge. Despite the unspecified effect measures, the methodological rigor of our approach ensures quality. We employed stringent selection criteria and comprehensive data analysis techniques to provide a robust synthesis of the available literature, preserving the integrity and applicability of our findings.

2.7. *Synthesis Methods*

Data were synthesised using a Microsoft Excel matrix. Information on the nutrition interventions in each of the included studies was extracted and categorisoned into three groups: cognitive, behavioural and mixed interventions. Within each of the defined groups, data were drawn on results, outcomes and final conclusions. Based on content analysis, the syntheses were summarised in a narrative format for each type of intervention [28].

3. Results

3.1. *Search Process*

Based on specific keywords, 969 articles were identified from PubMed (Medline), Web of Science Core Collection, ProQuest, Scopus and Embase databases. After removing duplicates, 721 articles were screened for titles and abstract content. Subsequently, following the exclusion of 670 articles that did not meet the criteria, 51 were further subjected to full-text analysis. Ultimately, 16 systematic reviews (including four with meta-analysis) qualified for review. The remaining 35 reviews were rejected because the study group was different from that assumed in the inclusion criteria, there was no dietary intervention in the study, the review was not a systematic one (scoping or narrative review/overview), the intervention was in a setting other than the workplace, or it was a conference abstract (Figure 1).

3.2. *Description of Included Systematic Reviews*

The umbrella review comprised sixteen systematic reviews published from 2009 to 2022. These secondary studies included a total of 205 primary studies (after duplicate removal). The primary studies included in the reviews were published from 1976 to 2020. The results of the primary studies were mostly from the United States (116), Japan (12), Denmark (9), Germany (6), Australia (8), UK (8) and the Netherlands (11). Other studies were conducted in India, Tunisia, Singapore, Brazil, Sweden and Finland. There was only one primary international multicentre study.

The total number of primary study participants in those 16 systematic reviews exceeded 261,000, with the 5 largest studies involving more than 10,000 participants (57%). In some studies, data for analysis were obtained, e.g., from vending machines or cafeterias, hence the number of study participants was not determined. The characteristics of the 16 secondary studies included in this analysis are detailed in Table 1.

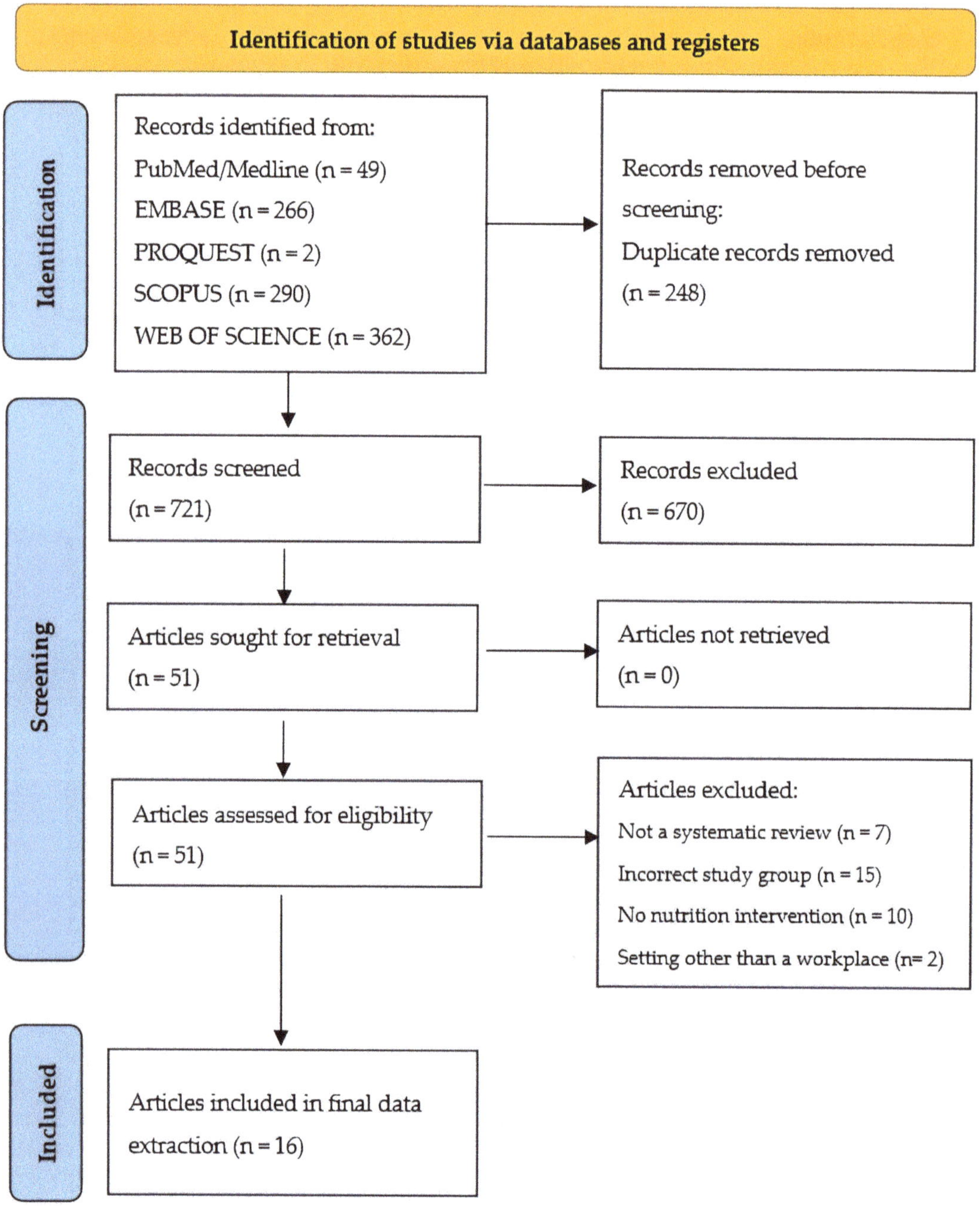

Figure 1. PRISMA flowchart of the systematic search and the selection process.

Table 1. Secondary studies included in the umbrella review.

Author (Year)	Number of Primary Surveys	Number of Participants	Type of Primary Research	Type of Intervention	Type of Review	Quality Assessment of Primary Research (Yes/No; Name of Tool)	AMSTAR2 Evaluation
Allan et al. (2017) [15]	22	N/A *	RCTs, Quasi-experiments	Behavioural	Systematic review	Cochrane Risk of Bias Tool	Low
Anderson et al. (2009) [29]	47	76,941 **	RCTs, Quasi-experiments, Observational studies	Mixed	Systematic review and meta-analysis	Community Guide	Moderate
Brown et al. (2018) [30]	22	35,197	RCTs, Quasi-experiments, Observational studies	Behavioural	Systematic review	Cochrane criteria	Low
Cabrera et al. (2021) [18]	13	5423	RCTs, Quasi-experiments	Mixed	Systematic review and meta-analysis	Not specified	Low
Fitzpatrick-Lewis et al. (2022) [31]	5	1494	RCTs, Observational studies	Mixed	Systematic review and meta-analysis	Cochrane Risk of Bias 1 tool	Low
Geaney et al. (2013) [16]	6	N/A *	RCTs, Quasi-experiments	Behavioural	Systematic review	Cochrane Collaboration's risk of bias tool	Low
Ghobadi et al. (2022) [32]	8	1797	RCTs	Mixed	Systematic review	Cochrane Collaboration's risk of bias tool	Low
Groeneveld et al. (2010) [33]	31	16,013	RCTs, Quasi-experiments	Mixed	Systematic review	Delhi list based tool	Low
Gudzune et al. (2013) [34]	9	76,465 **	RCTs, Quasi-experiments	Mixed	Systematic review	Downs and Black methodological quality assessment checklist	Low
Hendren et al. (2017) [19]	18	37,744	RCTs	Mixed	Systematic review	Quality characteristics and bias criteria were adapted from two previously published systematic reviews	Low
Lee et al. (2022) [20]	11	13,233	RCTs	Mixed	Systematic review	The Joanna Briggs Institute Critical Appraisal Checklist for Randomised Controlled Trials	Low
Madden et al. (2020) [35]	20	3311	RCTs, Quasi-experiments	Mixed	Systematic review	Cochrane Risk of Bias, ROBINS-I (risk of bias in non-randomised studies of interventions)	Low
Ni Mhurchu et al. (2010) [36]	16	N/A *	RCTs, Quasi-experiments	Mixed	Systematic review	A checklist adapted from a previous review	Low
Park et al. (2019) [37]	7	2854	RCTs	Behavioural	Systematic review and meta-analysis	Cochrane's Risk of Bias	Low

Table 1. *Cont.*

Author (Year)	Number of Primary Surveys	Number of Participants	Type of Primary Research	Type of Intervention	Type of Review	Quality Assessment of Primary Research (Yes/No; Name of Tool)	AMSTAR2 Evaluation
Sandercock et al. (2018) [38]	23	41,867	RCTs, Quasi-experiments, Observational studies	Mixed	Systematic review	Quality Criteria Checklist from the Academy of Nutrition and Dietetics (AND) Evidence Analysis Manual	Low
Sawada et al. (2019) [17]	3	3013	RCTs	Behavioural	Systematic review	GRADE (Grading of Recommendations, Assessment, Development and Evaluation)	Low

N/A—Not Applicable; RCTs—Randomised Controlled Trials; AMSTAR2—Assessment of Multiple Systematic Reviews (version 2). * In some studies, the number of participants is not given, as the study was conducted in cafeterias; the intervention involved a change in products offered in vending machines, making it significantly difficult or impossible to determine the number of participants; or the number of participants is not given **—WHO review.

3.3. Reviews on Cognitive Interventions

It is important to note that, although none of the systematic reviews included in the analysis focused exclusively on the systematic evaluation of cognitive interventions, these reviews include seven primary studies with this type of intervention. The most common interventions were one-on-one counselling (in person or via electronic means of communication such as email or telephone) or lectures on nutrition education. Two studies involved enhanced nutritional education [39,40], of which one placed special emphasis on cultural differences (a study involving African-American women). The results of these studies are inconclusive—some emphasise the need to supplement cognitive intervention with behaviour change components [41,42], while others show the effectiveness of lectures or education alone, especially if personalised [43,44]. Secondary studies describing mixed interventions have shown that cognitive interventions alone, while more frequent, easier and cheaper to implement, are not effective unless supplemented with elements of support and behaviour change [18].

3.4. Behavioural Intervention Reviews

Behavioural interventions were discussed in five systematic reviews. The most common were: facilitating access to healthy foods (most commonly fruit and vegetables) or modifying diets [15,16,37], e.g., making fruit and healthy snacks (nuts, whole-grain cereals, vegetable and fruit snacks) available in the workplace; modifying the composition of meals (less fat, more vegetables in meals) available in the employee canteen or restaurant; modifying the size of the portions available; financial benefits or discounts based on the choice of specific products; labelling products with, e.g., colours, based on to the composition of a particular meal [17]; or multi-component programs aimed at changing eating habits in patients with diabetes or prediabetes [30]. Although the available studies demonstrate low strength of evidence, interventions aimed at changing the intake of some of the products available in vending machines or employee cafeterias (POP—point of purchase) or those increasing the availability of fresh fruit and vegetables appear as the most effective in terms of modifying employee diets. A detailed description of systematic reviews regarding behavioural interventions is presented in Table 2. To provide more specificity, this review includes an overview of common effect measures observed in the studies, such as changes in nutritional knowledge, dietary patterns, BMI, and productivity-related outcomes, offering insights into the varied nature of intervention impacts.

Table 2. Secondary studies with behavioural interventions included in the umbrella review.

Author (Year)	Description of the Intervention	Results	Implications
Allan et al. (2016) [15]	Environmental intervention (environmental intervention) affecting eating habits	For behavioural endpoints, 13 of 22 studies showed a significant effect on primary endpoints. For physical endpoints, some studies showed no difference in BMI or body weight, while others confirmed it.	The current state of knowledge does not allow for clear recommendations for introducing environmental interventions to change eating habits in the workplace.
Brown et al. (2017) [30]	Workplace well-being programs to prevent or treat diabetes (nutrition—cooking workshops, individual dietary consultations, dietary changes; physical activity pedometers, workout plans; smoking cessation; usually in combination)	The study demonstrated a steady improvement in health in biological measures, self-reported behavioural adherence measures, and psychosocial variables. The authors presented data that showed improvement in most cases.	Workplace diabetes prevention programs can be useful in reducing disease occurrence and progression, but better design of interventions is needed. Employer education and further research in this area are crucial.
Geaney et al. (2013) [16]	Change in the composition of meals available at work, change in portion sizes (usually reduction), changes in access to healthy products for employees.	All of the included studies showed changes in fruits and vegetables intake, but none showed an effect size greater than a half-portion increase in fruit and vegetables consumption.	Modification of workers' meals may increase fruit and vegetables intake, but the strength of evidence is low.
Park et al. (2019) [37]	A nutritional intervention that limits the intake of energy and certain nutrients (carbohydrates or fats) or a balanced diet that ensures a normal supply of all nutrients	Employees' body weight decreased significantly: WMD of −4.37 kg (95% CI −6.54 to −2.20; Z = 3.95, $p < 0.001$), so did BMI: WMD of −1.26 (95% CI −1.98 to −0.55) kg/m^2, but it was statistically significant (Z = 3.47, $p = 0.001$), blood cholesterol and blood pressure values also declined—but the problem is the duration of the study and the quality of the data.	It is challenging to definitely state the effectiveness of interventions, but it is a good start for further research.
Sawada et al. (2019) [17]	Discounts on healthy food products or for a smaller portion ordered in the employee cafeteria, colour-coding of dishes (yellow, green and red),	No significant changes in BMI, blood cholesterol levels or changes in diet	Link between the intervention and the outcomes cannot be established; poor quality of evidence; a need for further research in this area.

CI—confidence interval; *p*—probability value; WMD—weighted mean difference; BMI—body mass index; Z—z-score statistics.

The most common endpoints evaluating the effectiveness of the intervention were: change in body weight or composition, consumption of specific products, or the results of biochemical tests (e.g., glucose, total cholesterol, LDL, HDL). The findings have been inconclusive and do not allow us to make clear recommendations for workplace interventions. The situation is particularly challenging due to the variety of factors such as age, gender, place of residence, type of work, and cultural aspects. Moreover, the significance of longer follow-up periods is emphasised, as it is not always possible to observe the effects of interventions, not because of their absence, but because of their emergence towards the end of the follow-up period. Depending on the study, there have been one-time interventions (with no follow-up period) and interventions with a short follow-up period (up to three months), for to up to two years of the follow-up. To address this, it is necessary to conduct further well-designed, methodologically sound studies capable of producing high quality results. It is also important to educate employers about the importance of such studies, for the sake of future research and interventions with measurable effectiveness.

3.5. Reviews on Mixed Interventions

The umbrella review comprised 11 systematic reviews of studies with mixed interventions, both cognitive and behavioural. The most common endpoints evaluating the effectiveness of the interventions were, as with behavioural interventions, the change in body weight or composition, consumption of specific foods, or the results of biochemical tests (e.g., glucose, total cholesterol, LDL, HDL). The interventions encompassed comprehensive programs including lectures or workshops, individual consultations with a specialist, coaching (cognitive interventions) and environmental interventions (changing the menu in the employee cafeteria, labelling products, changing the composition of products available in vending machines and access to fresh fruit and vegetables in the workplace), exercise programs, financial benefits (discounts on healthier products or a certain amount of money for reaching a goal set in the study), self-management interventions and other behavioural interventions. The interventions described applied to both the general population of office workers (7 reviews) and specific groups of employees: women [35], overweight and obese individuals [20,38], individuals at risk for type II diabetes [31] and individuals at risk for the metabolic syndrome [18]. A detailed description of reviews focused on mixed interventions is presented in Table 3.

Table 3. Secondary studies with cognitive and behavioural interventions included in the umbrella review.

Author (Year)	Description of the Intervention	Results	Implications
Anderson et al. (2009) [29]	Environmental, educational or behavioural interventions to achieve and/or maintain a healthy body weight	There is evidence of a modest reduction in body weight as a result of workplace health promotion programs aimed at improving nutrition, physical activity or both. Program effects are consistent, with a net loss of 2.8 pounds (95% CI −4.63, −0.96) among workers at 6–12-month follow-up, based on the meta-analysis of nine RCTs. In terms of BMI, a net loss of 0.47 BMI (95% CI −1.02, −0.2) at 6–12 months was observed in six RCTs.	There is strong evidence of a consistent, although small, effect (weight loss), in both men and women. The research quality is lacking and indicates the need and room for more research.
Cabrera et al. (2021) [18]	Basic nutrition education and general nutrition counselling, implementation of a specific diet, or dietary changes, motivational changes and/or coaching, physical activity and stress and/or sleep quality management. Most of the interventions studied were partially or fully delivered online using online platforms and/or social media	The effects of nutritional interventions: reduction in waist circumference (−4.9 cm, 95% CI −8.0 to −1.7), systolic blood pressure (−6.5 mmHg, 95% CI −10.7 to −2.3), diastolic blood pressure (−1.9 mmHg, 95% CI −3.6 to −0.2), triglycerides (SMD −0.46, 95% CI −0.88 to −0.04) fasting glucose (SMD −0.68, 95% CI −1.20 to −0.15).	Nutrition interventions in the workplace are beneficial for employees with the metabolic syndrome in terms of preventing the disease and also improving health parameters. Interventions that affect health-related behaviours and attitudes, as well as employee motivation, are the most effective—purely educational interventions are the most common but do not yield the anticipated outcomes.

Table 3. *Cont.*

Author (Year)	Description of the Intervention	Results	Implications
Fitzpatrick-Lewis et al. (2022) [31]	A diabetes prevention program or a program with 3 components of diabetes prevention (nutrition educator/coach, focus on nutrition and increased physical activity)	Participants in diabetes prevention programs were 3.85 times more likely to lose weight $\geq$ 5% (4 RCTs; RR = 3.85; 95% CI, 1.58 to 9.38; $p < 0.05$) and had a 9.36-fold greater chance of weight loss $\geq$ 7% (2 RCTs; RR = 9.36; 95% CI, 2.31 to 37.97; $p < 0.05$), a significant reduction in BMI was observed (5 RCTs; MD = −0.86; 95% CI, −1.37 to −0.34; $p < 0.05$). Interventions based on diabetes prevention programs were 2.12 times more effective in increasing physical activity compared to the control group (RR = 2.12; 95% CI, 1.06 to 4.25; $p < 0.05$).	The quality of these data are low to average. Due to doubts about the quality of the data and its limited availability, further research is needed in this area.
Ghobadi et al. (2022) [32]	Nutrition interventions: educational, counseling and environmental	Improvements in lipid indices (HDL, LDL) were observed. Available data say that while dietary interventions are effective in improving the cholesterol profile, they do not affect other variables.	More high-quality primary research is needed to confirm these relationships.
Gudzune et al. (2013) [34]	Self-management, dietary, physical activity and/or environmental intervention	There were no statistically significant changes in body weight and BMI in either women or men. However, those in the group with a higher BMI at baseline who received the intervention lost weight, while those in the control group gained weight (a statistically significant relationship).	There is weak to moderate evidence that self-management, dietary, physical activity and/or environmental interventions prevent weight gain in workers.
Groeneveld et al. (2010) [33]	Lifestyle or health promotion intervention with emphasis on nutrition and physical activity	There is no evidence that interventions of this type have a positive effect on body weight, blood pressure values, lipid profile or glucose levels. In contrast, there is strong evidence of their effect on fat reduction.	The effectiveness of interventions depends on whether the patients included in the study were at CVD risk or not, with interventions working better for those at risk.
Hendren et al. (2017) [19]	Greater availability of fruit and vegetables, subsidies for healthy produce, changing menus/portion sizes, education at point of purchase, combination of education and community intervention	It showed an increase in fruit and vegetables intake which was statistically significant in 13 out of 14 studies ($p < 0.05$). Only one study showed a statistically significant decrease ($p = 0.007$). Three studies produced mixed results. One study showed a significant increase in vegetable intake ($p = 0.002$) but no change in fruit intake ($p = 0.78$). Another study showed a significant increase in fruit consumption ($p = 0.001$) but no change in salad sales ($p = 0.139$).	Environmental interventions conducted at the employee cafeteria/canteen can increase fruit and vegetable consumption, but the lack of consistency in the available literature limits the development of specific recommendations.

Table 3. *Cont.*

Author (Year)	Description of the Intervention	Results	Implications
Lee et al. (2022) [20]	Weight loss interventions carried out using electronic devices such as computers, tablets, smartphones, apps and personal electronic assistants	Video consultations appear to be more effective than face-to-face appointments, while wearable devices (telemedicine devices, smartwatches and smart phones) and apps have proven to be the most effective.	As technology advances, the form of the message has to be updated. Also, these interventions lack a theoretical foundation—indicating the potential for future research.
Madden et al. (2020) [35]	Lifestyle programs to improve diet, physical activity and weight-related factors	In mixed activities (diet + physical activity), interventions that were not led by a health worker (possibly a healthcare worker and someone who is not—at the same time) were more effective. Emphasis was placed on how the interventions were delivered and on responding to the needs of female employees.	Proper social support and the right choice of interventions are key to the effectiveness of interventions with female employees.
Ni Mhurchu et al. (2010) [36]	A weight loss or healthy eating intervention in the workplace, lasting a minimum of 8 weeks	None of the studies showed measurable effects on presenteeism, productivity and/or health care costs. Overall, the effects of dietary interventions were positive, but the self-reported nature of dietary assessment poses a high risk of error.	Nutrition interventions in the workplace have a positive, though small, effect on employees' eating habits.
Sandercock et al. (2018) [38]	Physical activity and nutrition education	The results of some studies have shown statistically significant changes in body composition (lower BMI, body fat percentage and waist circumference). Even though changes in body composition have been confirmed in other studies, the results are not statistically significant. Six interventions showed no change, and one showed an increase in BMI.	Interventions affect the body composition of the study participants, but the strength of evidence is low. More studies with better endpoint determination are needed—the authors suggest, e.g., BIA.

CI—confidence interval, *p*—probability value, RCTSs—randomized controlled trials, BMI—body mass index, SMD—standardized mean difference, RR—relative risk, MD—mean difference, HDL—high-density lipoprotein, LDL—low-density lipoprotein, CVD—cardiovascular disease, BIA—bio-electrical Impedance Analysis.

Studies and interventions involving only women, emphasised the role of social factors, the methodology of intervention, and intervention tailoring to the needs of the specific group, all of which have an influence on intervention effectiveness [35]. For employees at risk of type II diabetes, the health benefits of implementing Diabetes Prevention Programs could be observed, but since the quality of evidence is low, emphasis is put on the need for further research and education in this area [30,31]. Research on overweight and obese employee populations points to the need for further, better quality studies [38] and the need to adapt the intervention delivery method to changing living conditions; advancing technologies, such as social media and virtual assistants Lee et al. (2022) [20], among office workers at risk for the metabolic syndrome, mixed or behavioural interventions appear to be more effective than cognitive interventions [18]. Other studies show little effect or low strength of evidence for the effectiveness of interventions. The authors highlight the small number of available studies or errors in their design and conduct (e.g., lack of consideration of the needs of a specific group, insufficient follow-up period). As with behavioural interventions, the difficulty in evaluating the effectiveness of interventions lies in the multiplicity of factors such as age, gender, place of residence, type of work, cultural factors or comorbidity (which run differently in everyone) conditioning inclusion in the intervention. Interventions in employee canteens or dietary changes combined with counselling and nutrition education appear to be the most effective, although what is highlighted is the need for further research to confirm the evidence as well as the introduction of longer follow-up periods, as those assumed in particular studies may not have been sufficient to observe the effects of the interventions, which does not necessarily mean that they did not occur at all. There is also emphasis on the importance of personalised interventions (e.g., in terms of the topic or selection of the intervention provider) and on the development of new technologies and the opportunities they offer for nutrition intervention and education.

4. Discussion

This is the first umbrella review which discusses the effectiveness of workplace nutrition interventions. There are more and more employee well-being initiatives introduced by employers. They embrace a wide range of health- and wellness-related aspects, e.g., physical activity, mental health, substance abuse prevention, and guidelines for proper nutrition. The issue is increasingly important and interventions are expected to be undertaken, especially for office workers (white-collar professionals). Nevertheless, public health specialists and practitioners implementing them face a substantial challenge to design them in such way so that they are effective, evidence-based and cost-effective/cost-efficient.

The narrative synthesis has demonstrated that behavioural and mixed (cognitive-behavioural) interventions are more effective rather than solely cognitive ones. Therefore, it seems reasonable to promote those interventions that involve comprehensive well-being programs, personalised consultations and environmental interventions, such as menu modifications or improving access to healthy snacks at the workplace. A properly designed intervention needs to account for the needs and characteristics of its future participants. When designing workplace nutrition interventions, it is also important to consider employee diversity. Factors such as employee sex, religion, economic or social status, among others, may influence the overall participation and effectiveness. The analysis of employee needs and abilities should also be taken into consideration when designing interventions so that they are prepared 'with' the employees instead of just 'for' them.

Apart from the employees, employers also should be engaged into designing interventions as well. After all, they are the ones who make the final decision and provide financial coverage for the intervention which may offer better access to healthy products or improve consumption patterns of the employees. This may further improve employee health and limit the costs of healthcare providers as well as build better workplace organisational culture. Then, either as a continuation or a separate intervention, it may be beneficial to reduce access to snacks such as sweets, crisps and sweetened beverages found in vending machines or canteens, and replace them with fruit and vegetables for the employees.

In recent years, an increase in overweight and obesity rates has been observed, especially after the COVID-19 pandemic [45]. This is particularly noticeable among office workers with sedentary jobs which may contribute to the development of diseases of affluence such as diabetes or the metabolic syndrome. Therefore, the implementation of disease prevention programs in the workplace may improve employee health. As it was observed, these programs featured comprehensive approaches to those diseases and combined the aspects of nutrition, physical activity and counselling [18,30,31]. They are considered to be slightly effective but with no major improvement. Nevertheless, the obtained results are still insufficient to properly assess the effectiveness, as flaws can be found both in the design of the interventions themselves as well as in data quality.

Though no systematic reviews discussing only cognitive interventions were included in the umbrella review, there are some primary studies available that describe the effectiveness of this type of intervention. As cognitive interventions mainly include education in the form of lectures or individual consultations, they are not considered effective if they do not involve behavioural change [41,42]. This is because dietary choices are determined by a number of factors, rather than just knowledge, and include environmental factors (e.g., availability of food, social and cultural practices, price and advertising of food), intrapersonal factors (e.g., beliefs, attitudes), interpersonal factors such as friends and family relations, experience with food, and biologically determined behavioural predispositions [46]. Therefore, it is difficult to imagine that solely offering knowledge will profoundly alter one's dietary choices. Cognitive interventions are very often cost-effective, easier to organise and implement. Moreover, they do not require special tools, buying and transporting food to the workplace, and there are also fewer people involved in the execution of such an intervention. In most cases, it is enough to involve one employee and one speaker to run the lecture or consultations. Nonetheless, it has been suggested that for cognitive interventions to be more effective, they should be a part of comprehensive solutions and not performed on their own [18].

In order to properly evaluate the effectiveness of behavioural interventions, they should be categorised into person-oriented and environmental interventions. The first group comprises individual counselling, workshops, behavioural prevention programs or financial incentives. As for workshops and counselling, there is no sufficient data to fully confirm their effectiveness [17,30]. This is because the effects may vary from person to person, as each employee has different needs and meeting them all may be challenging. The intervention should be performed by a specialist who understands the basics of nutritional education and counselling not only in the field of nutrition, but also in the field of social psychology, health education, anthropology and economics [46]. Financial incentives such as lower prices for healthy food or discounts for healthy snacks are relatively new and less commonly used interventions, as they require considerable financial coverage by the employer. Therefore, there is limited information to assess their effectiveness [17]. Nonetheless, they may be promising in the following years, especially when, with more and more employees underscoring the financial aspect of shaping their nutritional habits and benefits at the workplace that would satisfy them, as well as the fact that prices of healthy food are much higher compared to unhealthy food, this possibly becomes a significant barrier for the employees to buy healthy food themselves [47,48].

Environmental interventions are employed when aiming to induce behavioural changes and focus on food accessibility, e.g., more access to healthy foods such as fruit and vegetables and less access to unhealthy snacks in canteens or vending machines; food labelling, e.g., using colours to highlight nutritional value and encourage healthier choices; or collecting something, e.g., like stamps or points, to document health-promoting behaviours. Offering a special diet in the workplace (e.g., ready-to-consume meals, changing the menu in the canteen) may be effective, but has its limits. After all, employees do not spend their entire day at work and their nutritional habits are shaped in other settings as well. Still, there is not enough evidence to fully confirm or deny the effectiveness of these interventions [16]. The same principle applies to providing fruit and vegetables in the workplace. Their consumption may increase on-site, but not elsewhere. Thus, ensuring access to healthy snacks may be even more important with the steadily growing costs of food [48]. There is more research needed in this area, with special attention placed on intervention design and employer education [15,30].

As for mixed interventions, many components bear resemblance to those in cognitive and behavioural interventions. Nonetheless, mixed interventions also focused on some issues that may bring new light to workplace interventions, i.e., the use of technology in self-control and self-regulation health interventions in the workplace as well as focus on specific groups of employees.

Technological advancements and possibility of their implementation, e.g., in the form of video-consultations, wearable devices (e.g., smart watches, smart phones, sensors) or nutrition apps, draw from the self-control intervention model which facilitates the change of dietary habits. Wearables and apps appear to be effective tools, as one can always have them close; however, there is no collective agreement or guidelines on this matter. Nonetheless, this could pose a challenge, especially to employees with little or no digital competence, such as the elderly employees near retirement or other employees vulnerable to digital exclusion. This field being relatively novel, there is little theoretical research addressing such issues, which makes it worth exploring, especially with the growing popularity of end-user apps and devices [20,49].

Another action that may form a part of complex interventions is addressing the specific needs of particular groups of employees. As it turns out, in female-only groups addressing their specific needs and offering social support are more important than the focus on the intervention itself. Furthermore, the interpersonal and teaching skills of the instructor are key factors determining the effectiveness of the intervention. What has also been highlighted in the review is that the most effective interventions were not those run by a healthcare professional (or alternatively by someone outside the healthcare system who was only supported by a healthcare professional) [35]. This may serve as a warning sign for healthcare professionals, as it became evident that the effective communication and delivery of the intervention are equally or more important than qualifications of the instructor. This is particularly concerning at the present time, with the rising number of influencers discussing health issues. Therefore, it seems vital to prepare healthcare professionals to conduct interventions and wisely use social media to promote health-related matters [50,51]. Healthcare professionals should be well-prepared to implement interventions and learn the necessary know-how that will enable them to function not only as experts, but also as successful educators.

All that being said, most factors contributing to the effectiveness of nutrition interventions can be categorised into three aspects: the setting, the design and the group. The setting is mainly the place where the intervention is about to take place, with all of the tools needed to implement it. Starting from the office, the office kitchen or open space, it is important to adapt the surroundings to the needs of the employees and plans of the instructor. The requirements for the intervention should be taken into account, e.g., a laptop and a projector for the lecture, labels for the meals in the canteen, or a complete kitchen and supplies for cooking. It appears that the most effective settings are the ones nearest to the employees, e.g., wearables and apps, the canteen and the office, where they spend most of their working hours [16,20,29].

Intervention design should consider the type of intervention (cognitive, behavioural or mixed), timeframe and anticipated budget. As previously stated, behavioural and mixed interventions are considered more effective than just cognitive ones [18]. The assumed timeframe should enable the employees to benefit from the intervention fully; that is, the interventions should not be planned in summer months when most employees are on vacation or during important, e.g., national events. Also, the form (onsite, online) should be adjusted to the type of work in a particular office. Longer prevention programs might be more effective due to their extended length and increased availability [18,31]. The budget should be tailored to the employer's financial resources and their specific needs. When there is sufficient funding for such interventions, it is considerably easier to design complex programs with many activities. However, low-cost and effective interventions can be found, such as food-labelling or changing the menu available in the canteen [17].

Focus on the background and specific needs of the target group is another crucial factor which may strongly influence the effectiveness of workplace nutrition interventions. The nutritional education model accounts for factors determining the motivation for change and action, i.e., past behaviours, demographics and the cultural context, food preferences and prior experience with food, personality, moods and emotions, media exposure, and other individual differences. All of these factors should be carefully considered and used for the proper design of the intervention to ensure its maximum effectiveness [46,52].

Limitations

The main limitation of this umbrella review is the lack of good quality and full evidence studies confirming or denying the effectiveness of workplace nutritional interventions. Most reviews scored "low" on the AMSTAR2 scale, which suggests the need for further research and better-quality evidence.

5. Conclusions

With the limitations in mind, it is important to note that the interventions discussed lack sufficient evidence from high-quality studies. Therefore, there is a need for further, comprehensive research to be conducted using evidence-based methods and tools, to enable the comparison of study results.

The insights from this review might help in further research needed to establish the guidelines for effective future interventions. This paper serves as a foundation for further scientific research, but it also offers guidance for practitioners responsible for implementing workplace programs and interventions.

The researchers should take into account both the type of intervention (behavioural or mixed, rather than just cognitive) and the factors (demographic, economic, social and health) that may influence intervention effectiveness in a given study group. This will result in interventions which are better suited for the needs of employees and, as such, will produce better outcomes. The main challenge is to seek innovative interventions grounded in strong evidence-based practices, as well as theoretical frameworks, including psychological and learning factors.

For practitioners, this will also enhance the quality of interventions and will help to achieve the optimal cost-effectiveness and cost-efficiency, making it easier to design customised intervention programs from which employees genuinely benefit. It should also be emphasised that when designing or implementing interventions, practitioners should make more use of research or studies accessible for reference, e.g., standardised tools to compare intervention effectiveness. Future research with standardised effect measures is recommended to facilitate direct comparisons and meta-analyses. For workplace interventions to become truly evidence-based, practitioners should integrate the previously mentioned employees' needs and values, their own experience and expertise, as well as research evidence provided in this review, with all of these factors being of equal importance.

Supplementary Materials: The following supporting information can be downloaded at: https://www.mdpi.com/article/10.3390/nu15245072/s1, Supplementary S1: search strategies (MeSH); Supplementary S2: data extraction sheet; Supplementary S3: Detailed assessment of multiple systematic reviews.

Author Contributions: Conceptualisation: M.J. and M.P.; Data curation: A.H.; Formal analysis: A.H.; Investigation: A.H.; Methodology: M.J. and M.P.; Project administration: M.J. and M.P.; Resources: A.H.; Software: A.H. and M.P.; Supervision: M.J. and M.P.; Writing—original draft: A.H., M.J., I.C., J.G.-M. and M.P.; Writing—review and editing: A.H., I.C. and J.G.-M. All authors have read and agreed to the published version of the manuscript.

Funding: This research received no external funding.

Institutional Review Board Statement: Not applicable.

Informed Consent Statement: Not applicable.

Data Availability Statement: The datasets generated for this study are available on request to the corresponding author.

Acknowledgments: We would like to express our deepest gratitude to Maria Chojnacka for her invaluable assistance in the translation and linguistic correction of the manuscript.

Conflicts of Interest: The authors declare no conflict of interest.

References

1. World Health Organisation. *Health Promotion Glossary of Terms*; World Health Organisation: Geneva, Switzerland, 2021.
2. Muscaritoli, M. The Impact of Nutrients on Mental Health and Well-Being: Insights from the Literature. *Front. Nutr.* **2021**, *8*, 656290. [CrossRef] [PubMed]
3. World Health Organisation. Available online: https://www.who.int/europe/about-us/our-work/core-priorities/promoting-health-and-well-being (accessed on 23 March 2023).
4. Nielsen, K.N.M.; Ogbonnaya, C.; Känsälä, M.; Saari, E.; Isaksson, K. Workplace resources to improve both employee well-being and performance: A systematic review and meta-analysis. *Work Stress* **2017**, *31*, 101–120. [CrossRef]
5. Adams, J.M. The Value of Worker Well-Being. *Public Health Rep.* **2019**, *134*, 583–586. [CrossRef] [PubMed]
6. Koopman, C.; Pelletier, K.R.; Murray, J.F.; Sharda, C.E.; Berger, M.L.; Turpin, R.S.; Hackleman, P.; Gibson, P.; Holmes, D.M.; Bendel, T. Stanford presenteeism scale: Health status and employee productivity. *J. Occup. Environ. Med.* **2002**, *44*, 14–20. [CrossRef]
7. Rice, T.; Rosenau, P.; Unruh, L.Y.; Barnes, A.J. United States: Health System Review. *Health Syst. Transit.* **2020**, *22*, 1–441.
8. Reardon, J. The history and impact of worksite wellness. *Nurs. Econ.* **1998**, *16*, 117–121. [PubMed]
9. Top Employers Institute. *HR Trends Report 2021—Priorities and Practices of the World's Top Employers*; Top Employers Institute: Amsterdam, The Netherlands, 2021.
10. Grant Thornton. *Medicover 2019. Zdrowy Pracownik, Zdrowy Pracodawca. Jak w Dobie Walki o Talenty Polscy Pracodawcy Dbają o Zdrowie Swoich Kadr*; Grant Thornton: Chicago, IL, USA, 2019.
11. Korzeniowska, E.; Puchalski, K. *Co Firmy Powinny Wiedzieć, by Skutecznie Promować Zdrowe Odżywianie i Aktywność Fizyczną Pracowników? Raport z Wyników Reprezentatywnego Badania 1000 Pracowników Średnich i Dużych Firm w Polsce*; Ministerstwo Zdrowia: Warsaw, Poland, 2019.
12. World Health Organisation. Available online: https://www.who.int/southeastasia/activities/healthy-workplace (accessed on 23 March 2023).
13. World Health Organisation. *Healthy Workplaces: A Model for Action for Employers, Workers, Policy-Makers and Practitioners*; World Health Organisation: Geneva, Switzerland, 2010.
14. Puchalski, K.; Korzeniowska, E.; Goszczyńska, E.; Petrykowska, A. *Kto Wymaga Szczególnej Uwagi w Promocji Zdrowego Odżywiania i Aktywności Fizycznej w Firmach?* Krajowe Centrum Promocji Zdrowia w Miejscu Pracy: Łódź, Poland, 2020.
15. Allan, J.; Querstret, D.; Banas, K.; de Bruin, M. Environmental interventions for altering eating behaviours of employees in the workplace: A systematic review. *Obes. Rev.* **2017**, *18*, 214–226. [CrossRef]
16. Geaney, F.; Kelly, C.; Greiner, B.A.; Harrington, J.M.; Perry, I.J.; Beirne, P. The effectiveness of workplace dietary modification interventions: A systematic review. *Prev. Med.* **2013**, *57*, 438–447. [CrossRef]
17. Sawada, K.; Wada, K.; Shahrook, S.; Ota, E.; Takemi, Y.; Mori, R. Social marketing including financial incentive programs at worksite cafeterias for preventing obesity: A systematic review. *Syst. Rev.* **2019**, *8*, 66. [CrossRef]
18. Gea Cabrera, A.; Caballero, P.; Wanden-Berghe, C.; Sanz-Lorente, M.; López-Pintor, E. Effectiveness of Workplace-Based Diet and Lifestyle Interventions on Risk Factors in Workers with Metabolic Syndrome: A Systematic Review, Meta-Analysis and Meta-Regression. *Nutrients* **2021**, *13*, 4560. [CrossRef]
19. Hendren, S.L.J. Impact of worksite cafeteria interventions on fruit and vegetable consumption in adults: A systematic review. *Int. J. Workplace Health Manag.* **2017**, *10*, 134–152. [CrossRef]
20. Lee, Y.; Lee, N.Y.; Lim, H.J.; Sung, S. Weight Reduction Interventions Using Digital Health for Employees with Obesity: A Systematic Review. *Diabetes Metab. Syndr. Obes.* **2022**, *15*, 3121–3131. [CrossRef]
21. Rachmah, Q.; Martiana, T.; Mulyono, M.; Paskarini, I.; Dwiyanti, E.; Widajati, N.; Ernawati, M.; Ardyanto, Y.D.; Tualeka, A.R.; Haqi, D.N.; et al. The effectiveness of nutrition and health intervention in workplace setting: A systematic review. *J. Public Health Res.* **2021**, *11*, 2312. [CrossRef] [PubMed]
22. Papatheodorou, S.I.; Evangelou, E. Umbrella Reviews: What They Are and Why We Need Them. *Methods Mol. Biol.* **2022**, *2345*, 135–146. [CrossRef] [PubMed]
23. Aromataris, E.; Fernandez, R.; Godfrey, C.M.; Holly, C.; Khalil, H.; Tungpunkom, P. Summarizing systematic reviews: Methodological development, conduct and reporting of an umbrella review approach. *Int. J. Evid. Based Healthc.* **2015**, *13*, 132–140. [CrossRef] [PubMed]
24. Page, M.J.; McKenzie, J.E.; Bossuyt, P.M.; Boutron, I.; Hoffmann, T.C.; Mulrow, C.D.; Shamseer, L.; Tetzlaff, J.M.; Akl, E.A.; Brennan, S.E.; et al. The PRISMA 2020 statement: An updated guideline for reporting systematic reviews. *BMJ* **2021**, *372*, n71. [CrossRef] [PubMed]
25. Frandsen, T.F.; Bruun Nielsen, M.F.; Lindhardt, C.L.; Eriksen, M.B. Using the full PICO model as a search tool for systematic reviews resulted in lower recall for some PICO elements. *J. Clin. Epidemiol.* **2020**, *127*, 69–75. [CrossRef] [PubMed]
26. Ouzzani, M.; Hammady, H.; Fedorowicz, Z.; Elmagarmid, A. Rayyan-a web and mobile app for systematic reviews. *Syst. Rev.* **2016**, *5*, 210. [CrossRef]

27. Shea, B.J.; Reeves, B.C.; Wells, G.; Thuku, M.; Hamel, C.; Moran, J.; Moher, D.; Tugwell, P.; Welch, V.; Kristjansson, E.; et al. AMSTAR 2: A critical appraisal tool for systematic reviews that include randomised or non-randomised studies of healthcare interventions, or both. *BMJ* **2017**, *358*, j4008. [CrossRef]
28. Cooper, H.; Hedges, L.V.; Valentine, J.C. (Eds.) *The Handbook of Research Synthesis and Meta-Analysis*; Russell Sage Foundation: New York, NY, USA, 2019.
29. Anderson, L.M.; Quinn, T.A.; Glanz, K.; Ramirez, G.; Kahwati, L.C.; Johnson, D.B.; Buchanan, L.R.; Archer, W.R.; Chattopadhyay, S.; Kalra, G.P.; et al. The effectiveness of worksite nutrition and physical activity interventions for controlling employee overweight and obesity: A systematic review. *Am. J. Prev. Med.* **2009**, *37*, 340–357. [CrossRef]
30. Brown, S.A.; García, A.A.; Zuñiga, J.A.; Lewis, K.A. Effectiveness of workplace diabetes prevention programs: A systematic review of the evidence. *Patient Educ. Couns.* **2018**, *101*, 1036–1050. [CrossRef]
31. Fitzpatrick-Lewis, D.; Ali, M.U.; Horvath, S.; Nagpal, S.; Ghanem, S.; Sherifali, D. Effectiveness of Workplace Interventions to Reduce the Risk for Type 2 Diabetes: A Systematic Review and Meta-Analysis. *Can. J. Diabetes* **2022**, *46*, 84–98. [CrossRef]
32. Ghobadi, K.; Eslami, A.; Pirzadeh, A.; Mazloomi, S.M.; Hosseini, F. Effects of the nutritional interventions in improving employee's cardiometabolic risk factors in the workplace: A systematic review. *Clin. Nutr. Open Sci.* **2022**, *42*, 73–83. [CrossRef]
33. Groeneveld, I.F.; Proper, K.I.; van der Beek, A.J.; Hildebrandt, V.H.; van Mechelen, W. Lifestyle-focused interventions at the workplace to reduce the risk of cardiovascular disease--a systematic review. *Scand. J. Work Environ. Health* **2010**, *36*, 202–215. [CrossRef]
34. Gudzune, K.; Hutfless, S.; Maruthur, N.; Wilson, R.; Segal, J. Strategies to prevent weight gain in workplace and college settings: A systematic review. *Prev. Med.* **2013**, *57*, 268–277. [CrossRef]
35. Madden, S.K.; Cordon, E.L.; Bailey, C.; Skouteris, H.; Ahuja, K.; Hills, A.P.; Hill, B. The effect of workplace lifestyle programmes on diet, physical activity, and weight-related outcomes for working women: A systematic review using the TIDieR checklist. *Obes. Rev.* **2020**, *21*, e13027. [CrossRef]
36. Ni Mhurchu, C.; Aston, L.M.; Jebb, S.A. Effects of worksite health promotion interventions on employee diets: A systematic review. *BMC Public Health* **2010**, *10*, 62. [CrossRef]
37. Park, S.H.; Kim, S.Y. Effectiveness of worksite-based dietary interventions on employees' obesity: A systematic review and meta-analysis. *Nutr. Res. Pract.* **2019**, *13*, 399–409. [CrossRef]
38. Sandercock, V.; Andrade, J. Evaluation of Worksite Wellness Nutrition and Physical Activity Programs and Their Subsequent Impact on Participants' Body Composition. *J. Obes.* **2018**, *2018*, 1035871. [CrossRef]
39. Anderson, J.; Dusenbury, L. Worksite cholesterol and nutrition: An intervention project in Colorado. *Aaohn. J.* **1999**, *47*, 99–106. [CrossRef]
40. Ard, J.D.; Cox, T.L.; Zunker, C.; Wingo, B.C.; Jefferson, W.K.; Brakhage, C. A study of a culturally enhanced EatRight dietary intervention in a predominately African American workplace. *J. Public Health Manag. Pract.* **2010**, *16*, E1–E8. [CrossRef]
41. Byers, T.; Mullis, R.; Anderson, J.; Dusenbury, L.; Gorsky, R.; Kimber, C.; Krueger, K.; Kuester, S.; Mokdad, A.; Perry, G. The costs and effects of a nutritional education program following work-site cholesterol screening. *Am. J. Public Health* **1995**, *85*, 650–655. [CrossRef]
42. Edye, B.V.; Mandryk, J.A.; Frommer, M.S.; Healey, S.; Ferguson, D.A. Evaluation of a worksite programme for the modification of cardiovascular risk factors. *Med. J. Aust.* **1989**, *150*, 574, 576–578, 581. [CrossRef]
43. Baer, J.T. Improved plasma cholesterol levels in men after a nutrition education program at the worksite. *J. Am. Diet Assoc.* **1993**, *93*, 658–663. [CrossRef]
44. Briley, M.E.; Montgomery, D.H.; Blewett, J. Worksite nutrition education can lower total cholesterol levels and promote weight loss among police department employees. *J. Am. Diet Assoc.* **1992**, *92*, 1382–1384. [CrossRef]
45. Daily Fruits. *Raport—Wpływ Pracy Zdalnej na Nawyki Żywieniowe Polaków*; Daily Fruits: Marlboro, MA, USA, 2021.
46. Contento, I.R. Nutrition education: Linking research, theory, and practice. *Asia Pac. J. Clin. Nutr.* **2008**, 17 (Suppl. S1), 176–179.
47. ICAN Institute. *Raport "Benefity Przyszłości"*; ICAN Institute: Albuquerque, NM, USA, 2023.
48. Goudie, S. *The Broken Plate 2023. The state of the Nation's Food System*; The Food Foundation: London, UK, 2023.
49. Milne-Ives, M.; Lam, C.; De Cock, C.; Van Velthoven, M.H.; Meinert, E. Mobile Apps for Health Behavior Change in Physical Activity, Diet, Drug and Alcohol Use, and Mental Health: Systematic Review. *JMIR mHealth uHealth* **2020**, *8*, e17046. [CrossRef]
50. Pilgrim, K.; Bohnet-Joschko, S. Selling health and happiness how influencers communicate on Instagram about dieting and exercise: Mixed methods research. *BMC Public Health* **2019**, *19*, 1054. [CrossRef]
51. Rogers, A.; Wilkinson, S.; Downie, O.; Truby, H. Communication of nutrition information by influencers on social media: A scoping review. *Health Promot. J. Austr.* **2022**, *33*, 657–676. [CrossRef]
52. Contento, I.R. *Edukacja Żywieniowa*, 1st ed.; PWN: Warszawa, Poland, 2018; ISBN 978-83-01-19857-2.

nutrients

Article

Effects of mHealth Practice Patterns on Improving Metabolic Syndrome Using the Information–Motivation–Behavioral Skills Model †

Na-Young Park [1] and Sarang Jang [2,*]

1 Korea Institute for Health and Social Affairs, Sejong 30147, Republic of Korea; dudsky04@kihasa.re.kr
2 Department of Public Health, Sahmyook University, Seoul 01795, Republic of Korea
* Correspondence: srjang@syu.ac.kr
† This article was derived from Na-Young Park's doctoral dissertation.

Abstract: Chronic diseases contribute to 68% of global mortality, highlighting the importance of early detection and management of conditions such as metabolic syndrome. Effective lifestyle interventions, particularly through mobile health (mHealth), have shown potential in promoting health and reducing cardiometabolic risk. This study utilized mobile health data from public health centers in South Korea, targeting adults with risk factors for metabolic syndrome. The Intervention-Motivation-Behavioral skills (IMB) theoretical model was applied to categorize participants' practice patterns over time using the Group-Based Trend Model (GBTM). And the Generalized Estimating Equations (GEE) methodology was applied to confirm the effective practice patterns for improving metabolic syndrome. Data were collected over 24 weeks. The dataset encompasses life-log data capable of capturing changes in intervention, self-report surveys, and clinical measurements, all linked to personal identification keys and thereby integrated. Participants demonstrated improved health behaviors, with the healthy eating score increasing from 5.0 to 6.4 and physical activity rates rising from 41.5% to 59%. Health risk factors decreased significantly, with the mean number of risk factors dropping from 2.4 to 1.4. The percentage of subjects with three or more metabolic syndrome components decreased from 42.3% in the initial period to 19.2% in the final period. Practice patterns by IMB components were classified into three categories: continuous type, late decline type, and early decline type. Improvements in health behavior and metabolic syndrome were observed in the continuous type of each IMB component. The mHealth interventions were confirmed to be positively associated with improved health behavior and management of metabolic syndrome in the continuous practice patterns of IMB.

Keywords: mHealth; IMB model; metabolic syndrome; chronic disease; health promotion; GBTM; GEE

1. Introduction

1.1. Background

The importance of preventing chronic diseases is emphasized as 68% of global mortality is due to chronic diseases [1,2]. Chronic diseases related to metabolic syndrome include cardiovascular disease, diabetes, hypertension, obesity, and dyslipidemia [3–8]. Management of metabolic syndrome plays a central role in the prevention of chronic diseases. Therefore, early detection and management of metabolic syndrome are crucial in preventing the development of chronic diseases [7,9,10].

Metabolic syndrome is a condition in which three or more health risk factors, such as high blood pressure, high blood glucose, abdominal obesity, hypertriglyceridemia, and low high-density lipoprotein (HDL) cholesterol level, are clustered together. In clinical practice, the modified National Cholesterol Education Program Adult Treatment Panel III (ATP III) [4] and the International Diabetes Federation (IDF) [11] definitions have become the most widely utilized. And in relation to abdominal obesity, application standards differing by ethnicity and country were agreed upon. In South Korea, the NCEP-ATP III standard is used to determine the health risk factors for metabolic syndrome. High blood pressure is defined as systolic blood pressure of 130 mmHg or more, or diastolic blood pressure of 85 mmHg or more. High blood sugar is defined as fasting blood glucose of 100 mg/dL or more. Hypertriglyceridemia is defined as triglycerides of 150 mg/dL or more. Reduced HDL cholesterol is defined as less than 40 mg/dL for males and less than 50 mg/dL for females. Abdominal obesity refers to the Asian standards presented by the IDF, applying a clinical standard of waist circumference of 90 cm or more for males and 85 cm or more for females as the criteria for abdominal obesity in adults.

The prevalence of metabolic syndrome presents considerable measurement challenges, resulting in a scarcity of comprehensive global data [9]. According to a recent meta-analysis of global data, the prevalence of metabolic syndrome varied from 12.5% to 31.4% by region, but predominantly tended to increase in line with the country's income level [12]. As reported by the IDF Diabetes Atlas [13], the global prevalence of diabetes was 8.8% (415 million individuals) in 2015, with projections indicating an increase to 10.4% (642 million individuals) by 2040. Given that metabolic syndrome is estimated to be approximately three times more common than diabetes, it is plausible to infer that metabolic syndrome affects roughly one-quarter of the global population, equating to over one billion individuals currently afflicted by metabolic syndrome worldwide [9]. In South Korea, 21.3% of individuals undergoing a health checkup in 2021, accounting for approximately 17 million people, were identified as having metabolic syndrome. Consequently, early detection and management of metabolic syndrome are crucial for preventing the onset of chronic diseases [14].

However, metabolic syndrome can worsen into a disease state due to the combined effects of multiple risk factors influenced by poor lifestyle habits. Metabolic syndrome can be managed through improvements in lifestyle [5,11,15,16]. Therefore, upon identifying abnormal findings for one or more health risk factors, individuals should actively evaluate and improve their lifestyle habits, including smoking cessation, moderating alcohol consumption, adopting healthier dietary patterns, weight management, and regular physical activity [1,9,17,18].

Mobile health (mHealth) was introduced as a behavioral intervention strategy to enhance healthcare delivery, addressing the constraints of in-person services and resources. In particular, the exponential growth of health management applications (apps) from a preventive standpoint and the evolution of interconnected devices have heightened the demand for health promotion programs aimed at managing lifestyle habits, such as diet, physical activity, and sleep, among healthy individuals, thereby accelerating innovation in health management services. The European Commission indicated that mHealth functions as a valuable tool for fostering behavioral change. According to the report, mHealth assists patients in transitioning from passive to active engagement, enabling patients to manage their health through apps and adhere to dietary and medication routines [19]. Indeed, mHealth has significant potential for promoting a healthy lifestyle [8,20].

Health behavior interventions aimed at improving lifestyle habits should utilize multiple intervention methods, simultaneously [21]. By facilitating the implementation of multiple behavioral interventions beyond conventional face-to-face services, mHealth offers opportunities for education, information dissemination, establishing personalized goals, monitoring, individualized counseling, motivational app prompts, incentives, gamification, and peer communication. This enables comprehensive integration of various behavior change techniques (BCTs). Technological advances not only reinforce the promotion and maintenance of patient behavior through mHealth but also enhance the interaction between service providers and recipients, resulting in improved service quality through restorative feedback and a positive influence on health outcomes [22,23]. mHealth behavioral interventions exhibit higher service completion rates than control groups, with an average completion rate of 83.3% in one study [24] and 79.6% in a review [25]. Furthermore, multiple studies have indicated that health management utilizing mHealth not only impacts healthy eating and physical activity but also leads to other alterations in health behaviors [8,16,20,21,26–29].

However, studies investigating the impact of mHealth based on theoretical frameworks of practice patterns are limited. Therefore, this study applied a theoretical health promotion model to evaluate the collective health promotion effect of metabolic syndrome healthcare services utilizing mHealth by categorizing the quantified practice patterns of users for each BCT.

1.2. Theoretical Framework

Numerous theories have been proposed to elucidate health behavior changes, among which the Information–Motivation–Behavioral Skills (IMB) model is notable. This model conceptualizes the integration of information, motivation, and behavioral skills necessary to modify and sustain health-risk behaviors (Figure 1).

According to the IMB model, individuals experience promoted behavior change and its maintenance, as well as positive health outcomes when they attain adequate health information, exhibit motivation for behavior change, and cultivate the requisite behavioral skills [30]. Information encompasses knowledge and essential technical details concerning the etiology, symptoms, treatment protocols, and actionable measures related to the symptom or disease. Motivation comprises an individual's inclination to engage in health behaviors, the social support they receive, and subjective norms regarding health behaviors from their social environment, all of which exert significant influence on health behavior performance. Behavioral skills pertain to an individual's tangible abilities and self-efficacy required for executing health-related actions. Thus, the IMB model enables the design and assessment of diverse intervention strategies and proves effective in health promotion and chronic disease management [31].

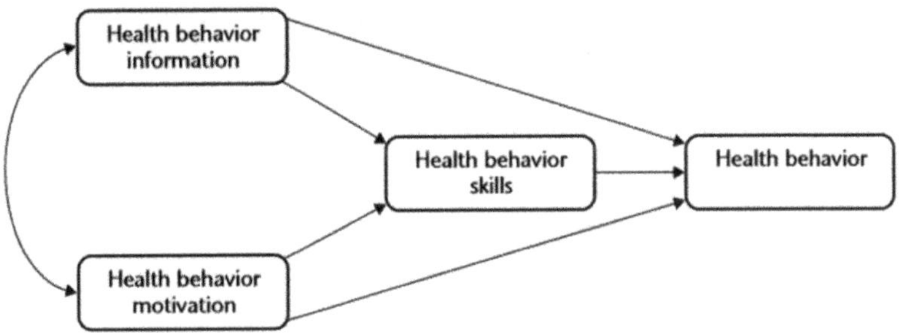

Figure 1. The Information–Motivation–Behavioral Skills model. Source: Fisher et al., 2003 [31].

1.3. Objectives

This study classifies various mHealth interventions according to the IMB theoretical model and categorizes participants' practice patterns over time using the Group-Based Trend Model (GBTM). Additionally, this study aims to identify meaningful types of health-improvement effects from these categorized practice patterns. Furthermore, this study proposes an efficacious behavioral intervention method utilizing mHealth behavior change techniques (BCTs) for the management of metabolic syndrome.

2. Materials and Methods

2.1. Study Participants

This study utilized mHealth data from the public health centers of the Korea Health Promotion Institute to target adults with risk factors for metabolic syndrome. Launched as a pilot in 2016 and expanded annually, the program employed mobile phone apps and devices administered by a team of healthcare professionals to deliver tailored health services. This study analyzed mHealth data from 35 public health centers collected over 24 weeks from 15 May to 19 November 2017.

2.2. Contents of mHealth Intervention

The service aimed to facilitate health-promoting activities such as walking and self-recording nutrition and exercise using a mobile phone app (Figure 2). The program entailed a six-month service designed to monitor health using mobile apps and devices (activity meter, body composition meter, blood sugar meter, blood pressure meter). Personal health behavior information was collected using pictures and graphs on a daily, weekly, and monthly basis. The expressed figures could be checked on the mobile dashboard. Prior to the commencement of the service, an evaluation was conducted, and tailored health goals were set for each participant to encourage healthy behaviors. The program emphasized nutrition and exercise and offered monthly counseling sessions. The system was designed to carry out missions in accordance with set goals and enabled self-recognition by applying an alarm (push) technique if implementation was not carried out well. Weekly health information was provided through the mobile app, and monthly health reports were provided by comprehensively analyzing individual health status and health behavior information. To sustain participation, various and engaging game techniques such as unexpected missions and commenting were included. Health points were accumulated according to the level of participation, and rewards were given based on the accumulated rank. In the community, participants could support each other through writing and sharing information. After three months, participants revisited the public health center for a follow-up checkup, where goals were reassessed and counseling was adjusted based on changes in measurements. This process was repeated for an additional three months. At the end of six months (24 weeks), a final evaluation was conducted, and the program was concluded.

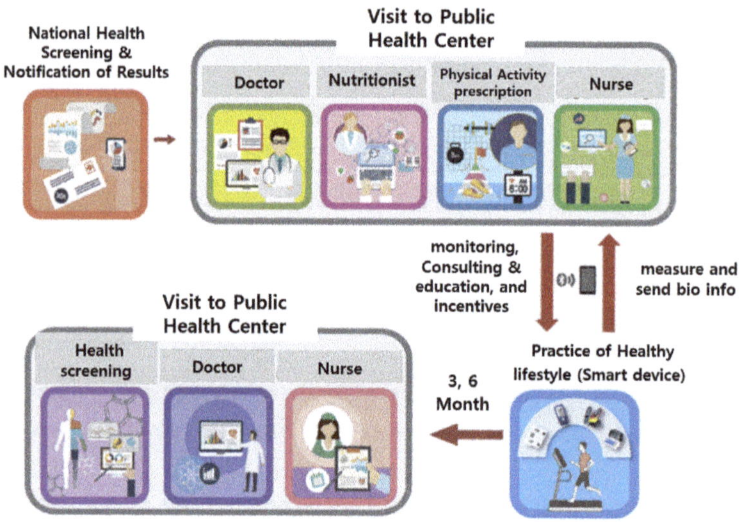

Figure 2. mHealth service process. Source: Korea Health Promotion Institute, 2016 [32].

2.3. Analysis Model and Variables

The analytical model of this study was designed by integrating the IMB model of health behavior, as modified in various studies [30,33,34]. The model was constructed to partition the independent and dependent variables of mHealth BCTs based on constructs, in accordance with the theoretical framework (Figure 3).

The dataset encompasses life-log data capable of capturing changes in intervention service behavior, detailed activity logs from a mobile phone app, self-report surveys, and clinical measurements, all linked to personal identification keys and thereby integrated. At this time, the questions in the survey were applied to large-scale national surveys and examinations such as the Korea National Health and Nutrition Examination Survey [35], Community Health Survey [36], and National Dietary Guidelines for Koreans [37].

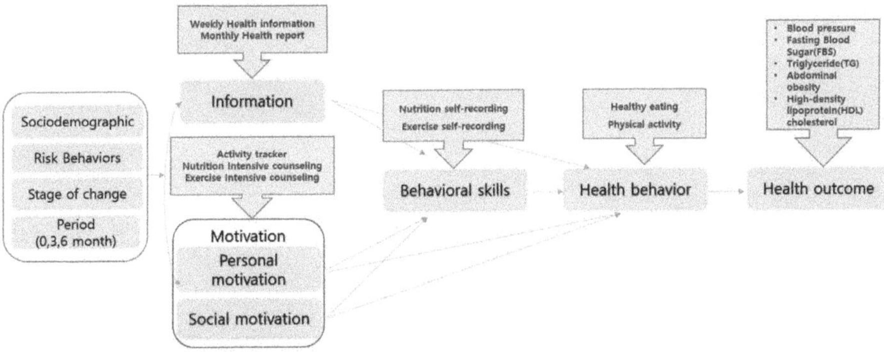

Figure 3. Modified Information–Motivation–Behavioral Skills model of health behavior.

2.3.1. Dependent Variables

This study examined changes in the number of health risk factors as outcome variables to assess the effect of metabolic syndrome on health improvement. Next, health behaviors were examined, focusing on healthy eating and physical activity. The healthy eating lifestyle practice score ranges from 1 to 9 points, with 1 point assigned for each "Yes" response and 0 points for each "No" response, for the nine items (grain intake, vegetable intake, fruit intake, dairy product intake, balanced meal consumption, breakfast consumption, abstention from animal oil intake, abstention from high-calorie sugar intake such as fried foods, and abstention from salt intake), practiced more than five times in the previous week. The physical activity rate evaluated whether walking or moderate exercise was performed for more than five days in the previous week and was treated as a continuous variable, taking into consideration the duration and intensity of walking and moderate exercise. The data were based on a survey and clinical measurements conducted by mHealth participants over a total of three public health center visits.

2.3.2. Independent Variables Related to mHealth Intervention

Information encompasses knowledge regarding disease etiology, symptoms, treatment procedures, and behavioral practices, as well as technical details enabling the independent acquisition of necessary information [31]. Weekly health information provided through this service included disease-specific insights vital for participants with risk factors for metabolic syndrome, guidance on appropriate physical activities, exercise videos, low-sodium diet cooking tutorials, dietary guidelines, and interpretation of nutritional information. A continuous variable was employed to determine the frequency of checking the weekly health information sent to the participant (1 to 24 times). Subsequently, a monthly report on health status trends (blood pressure, blood glucose, and body fat) and health behavior patterns (achievement rate of goals, exercise duration, cumulative distance traveled, and calorie intake), accompanied by expert opinions, was received for six months. The frequency of utilization (ranging from one to six times) constituted an information variable.

Motivation refers to an individual's inclination to adopt recommended health behaviors and social support for behavior modification [31]. In this study, the mean number of weekly link days (ranging from zero to seven) was designated as an activity tracker, serving as an indicator of personal motivation by tracking the prescribed exercise regimen. The variables reflecting social motivation included the number of intensive exercise counseling sessions and intensive nutrition sessions conducted by experts (ranging from 0 to 12 sessions).

Behavioral skill is a critical concept that assesses the ability of a highly motivated individual to effectively engage in health behaviors by considering the individual's objective capacity and self-efficacy in performing a given health-related behavior [31]. In this study, the repetitive completion of food diaries and exercise logs over several days was operationally defined as enhanced behavioral skills, with the average number of recording days per week (ranging from zero to seven) used as a variable.

The control variables included sex, age, education, occupation, city type, presence of national health insurance, smoking status, alcohol consumption status, and behavior change stage, which assessed the readiness of the participant to engage in services. Additionally, longitudinal data comprising the initial, intermediate, and final time variables were employed to observe changes over time.

2.4. Statistical Analysis

All intervention items were aligned with the IMB framework. The degree of practice for each construct was then classified through the application of a Group-Based Trajectory Model (GBTM), which constitutes a statistical approach adept at tracing the longitudinal practice patterns of participants, spanning from inception to the conclusion of reiterated, distinct longitudinal datasets. This serves as a valuable tool for characterizing each pattern encounter [38].

The methodology was developed in previous studies [38,39] and is used to model unique trends in the analyzed groups. It categorizes behavior types into groups, over time, and estimates the shape of the trends, for each group. This assumes that over time, mHealth participants will split into different groups that exhibit different types of practices during their time in service. The process of determining the number of practice-type groups has been extensively discussed in prior publications, often involving the selection of an appropriate model using the Bayesian Information Criterion (BIC) [38,39]. A lower BIC value indicates a better-fitting model, and the model with the most negative BIC value is selected. Simultaneously, Akaike's Information Criteria (AIC) were considered, and the smallest value was prioritized for selection. Nonetheless, it is important to acknowledge that selecting a model with the minimum value may lead to the identification of an undifferentiated group, making it challenging to discern a specific pattern owing to excessive differentiation. In such instances, discretionary judgment assumes significance [40–42].

Next, Generalized Estimating Equations (GEE) analysis was conducted. This was employed to estimate causal models across or within panel data. Specifically, it is an analytical method that uses a Generalized Linear Model (GLM) for multivariate variables that do not conform to a normal distribution. The GEE can effectively manage repeated measurement time-series data, which are challenging to handle using a GLM [43,44]. All analyses were conducted using Stata version 16.

3. Results

3.1. General Characteristics

In this study, mHealth participants who completed all surveys and clinical measurements during three visits to public health centers were included. Of the 4080 initial participants, 3505 (85.9%) were included in the analysis, after accounting for dropouts and missing data (Figure 4).

Among them, 44.6% were male and 55.4% were female (Table 1). The highest proportion of participants belonged to the 40s age group (36.0%), followed by the 50s age group (29.4%) and the 30s age group (24.3%). A significant majority (72.0%) of the participants had a college degree or higher education level. The largest occupational category was office workers (30.5%), followed by homemakers/unemployed (23.0%) and managers/professionals (22.5%). Most health insurance subscribers were employed. Regarding municipalities, 40.8% resided in a large city, 42.6% in a small- to medium-sized city, and 16.6% in a rural area. The prevalence of smoking was 12.6%, and the monthly alcohol consumption rate was 59.7%. Prior to participation in the service, it was crucial to assess the willingness of participants to engage. Of the participants, 25.2% were already practitioners (action and maintenance) in the healthy eating change stage, 59.6% were in the preparation stage to commence within one month, and 15.2% were in the pre-preparation stage. Regarding the exercise change stage, 42.1% were already practicing (action and maintenance), 44.2% were in the preparation stage and aimed to initiate within one month, and 13.7% were in the pre-preparation stage. In addition, 57.7% of subjects had one or two health risks, and 42.3% had three or more metabolic symptoms.

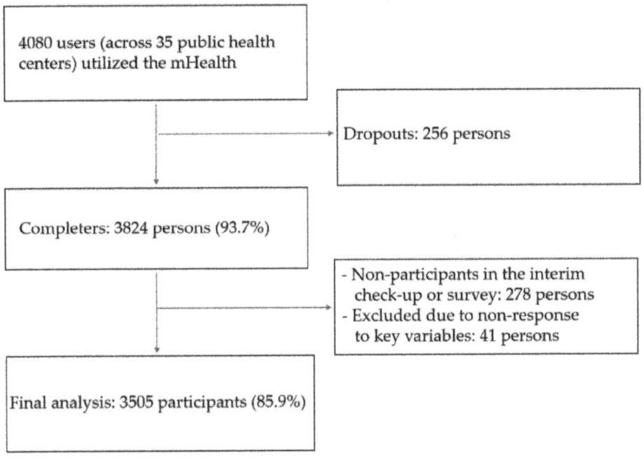

Figure 4. Flowchart of the study participants for this research.

Table 1. Characteristics of the study participants (No. of individuals: 3505).

Analyzed Variables		N	%	Analyzed Variables		N	%
Sex	Male	1562	44.6	Smoking	Yes	442	12.6
	Female	1943	55.4		No	3063	87.4
Age group	20s	161	4.6	Alcohol consumption (monthly)	Yes	2092	59.7
	30s	853	24.3		No	1413	40.3
	40s	1263	36	Stages of change in healthy eating	Precontemplation	97	2.8
	50s	1031	29.4		Contemplation	435	12.4
	60s	197	5.6		Preparation	2088	59.6
Education level	High school graduate or less	981	28		Action	352	10
	College degree or higher	2524	72		Maintenance	533	15.2
Occupation	Managers/professionals	788	22.5	Stages of change in exercise	Precontemplation	155	4.4
	Office workers	1070	30.5		Contemplation	325	9.3
	Service/sales workers	492	14		Preparation	1549	44.2
	Other workers	349	10		Action	707	20.2
	Homemakers/unemployed	806	23		Maintenance	769	21.9
Municipality	Large city	1430	40.8	No. of health risk factors	Mean (standard deviation)	2.4 (1.1)	
	Small- to medium-sized city	1492	42.6		One	950	27.1
	Rural area	583	16.6		Two	1072	30.6
					Three	835	23.8
					Four	508	14.5
					Five	140	4

3.2. Practice Patterns of mHealth Intervention

The usage trends of each intervention among mHealth recipients over the six-month (24-week) period were as follows (Figure 5): The health information usage rate was 94.1% in week 1 but decreased to 86.0% in the 12th week and 74.4% in the 24th week. The monthly report rate was maintained from 87.6% at one month to 82.6% at three months but decreased to 68.9% at six months. Next, the weekly frequency of accessing the goal screen, which tracks various activity metrics (such as steps, calories burned, exercise time, and moderate exercise), was examined. It decreased slightly from 76.3 times at week 1 to 55.8 times at week 12 and then to 74 times at week 13 and to 44.4 times at week 24. The number of days linked to the activity tracker remained at 6.4 days at week 1 and 6.1 days at week 12 but decreased to 6.1 days at week 23 and 5.8 days at week 24. Participation in intensive nutrition counseling, held once a month, decreased to 86% at one month, 84.9% at three months, and 78.1% at six months. Participation in intensive exercise counseling was 92.1% at one month, 88.2% at three months, and 84.8% at six months. Meanwhile, examining nutrition self-recording and exercise self-recording, nutrition self-recording was 3.1 days at week 1, 2.8 days at week 2, 1.8 days at week 12, 1.2 days at week 23, and tended to decrease to 0.8 days at week 24. Exercise self-recording gradually decreased to 1.6 days at week 1, 1.2 days at week 12, and 1.0 days at week 19 and then decreased to 0.8 days at week 23 and 0.6 days at week 24.

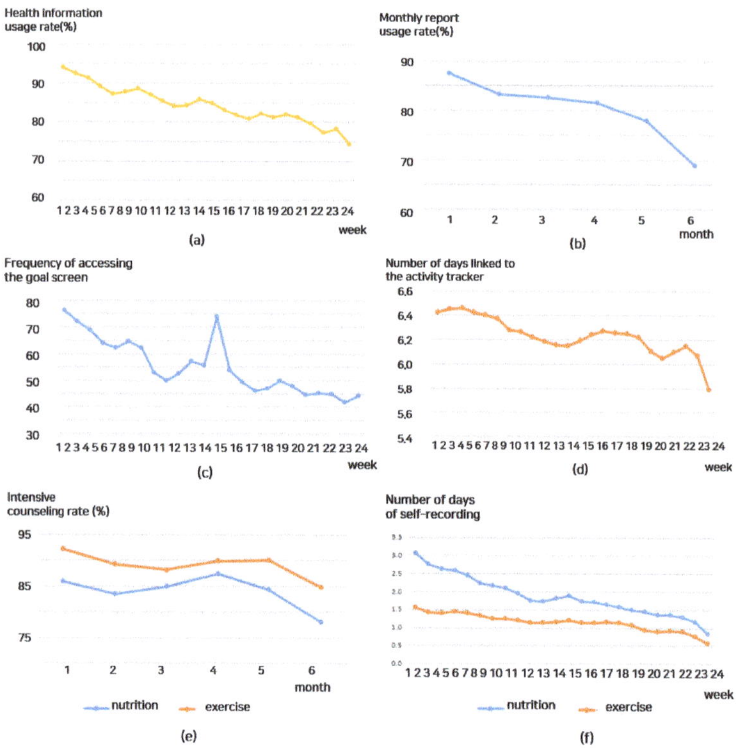

Figure 5. Usage patterns of mHealth interventions over 24 weeks by subject: (**a**) weekly health information utilization rate; (**b**) monthly report utilization rate; (**c**) weekly goal screen access frequency; (**d**) weekly activity tracker access count; (**e**) monthly intensive counseling rate; (**f**) weekly self-recording days.

3.3. Validation of the Analytical Model and Practice Patterns

The GBTM categorizes longitudinal behavioral patterns over time, using repeated measurements. Following the examination of the BIC and AIC values, two group classifications were deemed most appropriate. However, to investigate additional differentiation patterns through the application of the GBTM, the number of groups was expanded to a level where the disparity in the BIC size was minimal. Simultaneously, a secondary assessment was conducted to ascertain the presence of statistical differences between the groups using mean difference tests (T-test, analysis of variance) and regression analysis.

Finally, a fitting model for each IMB construct was selected and classified into three categories: information, motivation, and behavioral skills (Table 2).

Table 2. BIC and AIC values for each component concept.

Analyzed Variables		Group	BIC † (N = 3505)	AIC (N = 3505)	Group1 (%)	Group2 (%)	Group3 (%)
Information	Multi-information	Two	−24,516.42	−24,464.04	74.1	25.9	
		Three	−2206.72	−21,986.62	69.7	16.3	14.0
Motivation	Activity tracker	Two	−125,497.55	−125,466.74	75.7	24.3	
		Three	−122,140.39	−122,094.18	66.4	23.9	9.8
	Integrated intensive counseling	Two	−11,009.87	−10,957.50	69.3	30.7	
		Three	−9910.26	−9830.16	16.9	71.4	11.7
Behavior Skills	Integrated self-recording	Two	−198,589.07	−198,530.53	34.3	65.6	
		Three	−188,488.45	−188,402.19	18.3	33.3	48.4

† Based on the minimum BIC value, two groups are deemed appropriate. However, to explore differentiation comprehensively, significant differences between groups were determined based on practice type for each constituent concept, ultimately resulting in the division into three groups.

3.4. Practice Patterns by IMB Components

3.4.1. Information

Health information and monthly reports were categorized into three types (Figure 6). The types of health information checking are as follows: the continuous type, 71.6%; the late decline type, 12.6%; and the early decline type, 15.7%. The monthly report showed the continuous type, 75.7%; the late decline type, 7.4%; and the early decline type 16.9%.

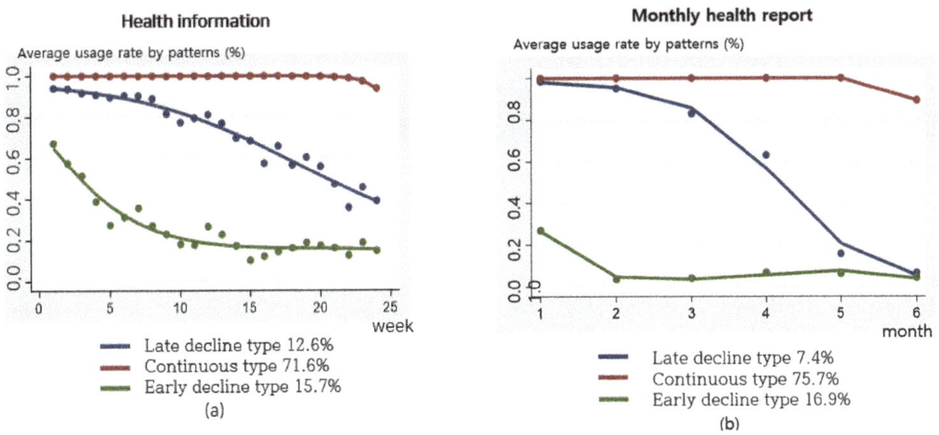

Figure 6. Practice patterns for health information and monthly reports: (**a**) weekly health information usage rate by practice patterns; (**b**) monthly report usage rate by practice patterns.

3.4.2. Motivation

(1) Personal motivation

The mHealth service recommends linking with the activity tracker mobile phone app at least five times a week (Figure 7). From the results of categorizing weekly interlocking practices, 66.4% were the continuous type, linking an average of seven times a week; 23.9% were the late decline type, practicing an average of five times per week and then gradually decline; and 9.8% were the early decline type.

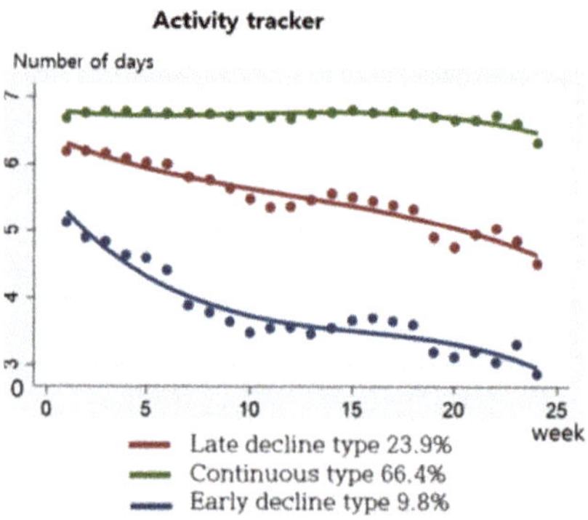

Figure 7. Practice patterns for activity tracker.

(2) Social motivation

Nutrition intensive counseling and exercise intensive counseling were provided once a month (Figure 8). The distribution of nutrition intensive counseling practice was as follows: 65.6% for the continuous type, 15.5% for the late decline type, and 18.9% for the early decline type. For exercise intensive counseling, the distribution was 72.0% for the continuous type, 17.0% for the late decline type, and 11.0% for the early decline type. For the practice patterns of intensive counseling, the late decline type started to decline at five months. For the early decline type, practice remained low for two to three months. For the early decline type, practice remained low for two to three months, and after intermediate face-to-face counseling (three months), intensive counseling increased at four to five months and then decreased again.

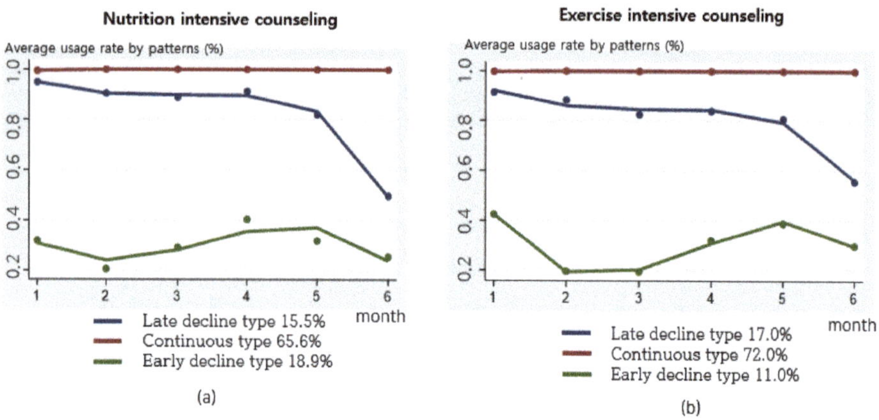

Figure 8. Practice patterns for nutrition and exercise intensive counseling: (**a**) monthly nutrition intensive counseling rate by practice patterns; (**b**) monthly exercise intensive counseling rate by practice patterns.

3.4.3. Behavior Skills

Behavior skills were assessed using weekly nutrition self-recording and exercise self-recording (Figure 9). Nutrition self-recording was 18.4% for the continuous type, 30.6% for the late decline type, and 51.0% for the early decline type. Exercise self-recording was 13.2% for the continuous type, 29.2% for the late decline type, and 57.5% for the early decline type. Compared to other practices, the early decline type was the highest, followed by the late decline type and the continuous type.

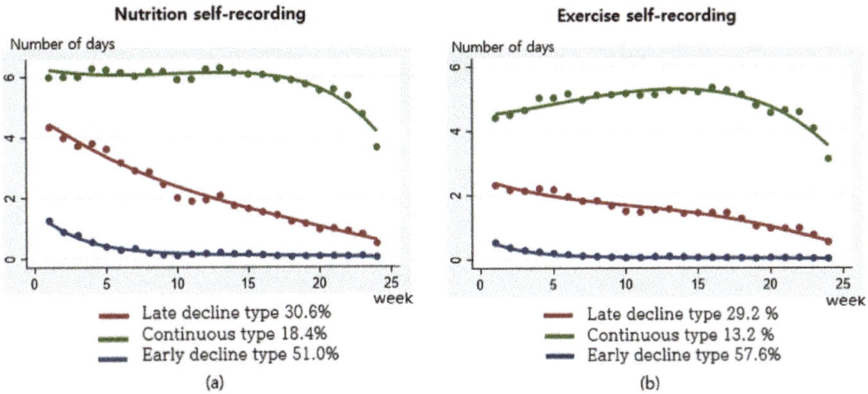

Figure 9. Practice patterns for nutrition and exercise self-recording: (**a**) weekly nutrition self-recoding rate by practice patterns; (**b**) weekly exercise self-recoding rate by practice patterns.

3.5. Health Risk Factors and Health Behavior

To examine changes in health risks and health behaviors, mHealth participants were analyzed based on clinical information and self-reported questionnaires measured during initial, mid-term, and final visits to public health centers (Table 3). Examining changes in health risk factors, the initial mean decreased from 2.4 to a mid-term mean of 1.7 and subsequently to a final mean of 1.4. The proportion of subjects with three or more metabolic syndrome risk factors declined from 42.3% in the initial period to 27.2% in the mid-term and further to 19.2% in the final period. Additionally, by the end of this study, 24.5% of the subjects exhibited no health risk factors. Furthermore, the analysis of health behaviors revealed improvements in healthy eating and physical activity. The healthy eating lifestyle practice score increased from an initial 5.0 points to 6.4 points by the final measurement. The physical activity rate also showed significant improvement, rising from 41.5% at the beginning of this study to 59% at its conclusion.

3.6. Health Promotion Effects by Practice Patterns of mHealth

A multi-GBTM methodology was applied. Interventions were integrated by construct (information, motivation, and behavioral skills) to distinguish the quantified practice patterns of participants. In addition, the effect on improving healthy living practices and health outcomes according to the three practice types of information–motivation–behavioral skills (the continuous type, the late decline type, and the early decline type) was examined. The analysis was conducted using the GEE of panel regression analysis that considers the correlation of response variables resulting from three repeated measurements: before, during, and after. The control variables included sex, age, education, occupation, city type, risky behaviors (smoking and alcohol consumption), stage of behavior change (continuous variable), and service participation period (Table 4).

Table 3. Changes in health risk factors and health behavior according to participation period (No. of individuals: 3505).

Variable		**Initial**		**Intermediate (3 Months)**		**Final (6 Months)**		**Intermediate Change (%p)**	**Final Change (%p)**	**F**
		N	%	N	%	N	%			
No. of health risk factors	Mean (standard deviation)	2.4 (1.1)		1.7 (1.3)		1.4 (1.2)		−0.7	−1	557.77 *
	None	-	-	644	18.4	859	24.5	18.4	24.5	
	One	950	27.1	1009	28.8	1134	32.4	1.7	5.3	
	Two	1072	30.6	898	25.6	840	24	−5	−6.6	
	Three	835	23.8	593	16.9	476	13.6	−6.9	−10.2	
	Four	508	14.5	298	8.5	174	5	−6	−9.5	
	Five	140	4	63	1.8	22	0.6	−2.2	−3.4	
Healthy eating score † Mean (standard deviation)		5.0 (2.1)		6.0 (1.9)		6.4 (1.9)		1	1.4	448.22 *
Physical activity rate ††	walking and moderate exercise	324	9.2	421	12	493	14.1	2.8	4.9	91.91 *
	moderate exercise	76	2.2	49	1.4	42	1.2	−0.8	−1	
	walking	1056	30.1	1439	41.1	1532	43.7	11	13.6	
	do nothing	2049	58.5	1596	45.5	1438	41	−13	−17.5	

* $p < 0.001$. † Healthy eating score is divided into 9 items consumed at least 5 times a week (frequency of grain intake, frequency of vegetable intake, frequency of fruit intake, frequency of dairy product intake, frequency of balanced meals, frequency of breakfast, non-consumption frequency of animal oil, non-consumption frequency of high-calorie foods such as fried foods, non-consumption frequency of salt) added together. †† Physical activity rate means walking for more than 10 min five times a week or engaging in moderate-intensity exercise for more than 10 min.

Table 4. Impact on health behavior and health risk factors by practice patterns of mHealth (No. of observations: 10,515; No. of individuals: 3505).

	Analyzed Variables		Model 1		Model 2		Model 3		Model 4	
			Practice Patterns of I,M,B → Healthy Eating		Practice Patterns of I,M,B → Physical Activity		Health Behavior → Health Risk Factors		All → Health Risk Factors	
			β	S.E	β	S.E	β	S.E	β	S.E
Sociodemographic characteristics	Sex (ref = Male)									
		Female	0.250 ***	−0.053	−0.040 *	−0.017	−0.475 ***	−0.04	−0.482 ***	−0.04
	Age Group (ref = 20s)									
		30s	0.286 **	−0.11	−0.122 ***	−0.035	0.242 **	−0.084	0.259 **	−0.084
		40s	0.775 ***	−0.109	−0.201 ***	−0.035	0.358 ***	−0.082	0.394 ***	−0.083
		50s	1.147 ***	−0.111	−0.142 ***	−0.036	0.452***	−0.084	0.492 ***	−0.085
		60s	1.634 ***	−0.141	−0.032	−0.045	0.454 ***	−0.106	0.503 ***	−0.107
	Education (ref = High school graduate or less)									
		College degree or higher	0.057	−0.054	−0.049 **	−0.017	−0.118 **	−0.041	−0.113 **	−0.041
	Occupation (ref = managers/professionals)									
		Office workers	−0.139 *	−0.06	−0.055 **	−0.019	−0.068	−0.046	−0.063	−0.046
		Service/sales workers	−0.211 **	−0.075	−0.004	−0.024	0.091	−0.057	0.086	−0.057
		Other workers	−0.190 *	−0.085	0.032	−0.027	−0.084	−0.065	−0.065	−0.065
		Housewives/unemployed	−0.155 *	−0.07	−0.024	−0.022	0.073	−0.053	0.09	−0.053
	Municipality (ref = Bic city)									
		Small- to medium-sized city	−0.02	−0.048	−0.056 ***	−0.015	−0.04	−0.036	−0.028	−0.036
		Rural area	−0.104	−0.063	−0.167 ***	−0.02	0.003	−0.048	0.008	−0.048
Risk behaviors	Smoking (ref = No) Yes		−0.336 ***	−0.066	0.023	−0.022	0.159 ***	−0.047	0.147 **	−0.047
	Monthly alcohol consumption (ref = No) Yes		−0.208 ***	−0.041	−0.067 ***	−0.014	−0.016	−0.028	−0.017	−0.028
Stages of behavior change	Stages of change in Healthy eating (Precontemplation = 1, continuous variable)		0.612 ***	−0.017	0.035 ***	−0.006	−0.034 **	−0.011	−0.045 ***	−0.011
	Stages of change in exercise (Precontemplation = 1, continuous variable)		0.080 ***	−0.017	0.133 ***	−0.006	−0.049 ***	−0.011	−0.034 **	−0.011

Table 4. *Cont.*

Analyzed Variables			Model 1		Model 2		Model 3		Model 4	
			Practice Patterns of I,M,B → Healthy Eating		Practice Patterns of I,M,B → Physical Activity		Health Behavior → Health Risk Factors		All → Health Risk Factors	
			β	S.E	β	S.E	β	S.E	β	S.E
Participation period		(ref = Initial)								
		Intermediate (3 months)	0.727 ***	−0.032	0.091 ***	−0.011	−0.585 ***	−0.02	−0.588 ***	−0.02
		Final (6 months)	0.976 ***	−0.032	0.120 ***	−0.012	−0.856 ***	−0.021	−0.860 ***	−0.021
Integrated information		(ref = Early decline type)								
		Late decline type	0.089	−0.083	0.037	−0.027			0.064	−0.063
		Continuous type	0.217 *	−0.085	0.021	−0.027			−0.034	−0.065
Motivation	Personal	Activity tracker (ref = Early decline type)								
		Late decline type	0.055	−0.083	0.004	−0.026			−0.029	−0.063
		Continuous type	0.156 *	−0.08	0.043	−0.025			−0.097	−0.06
	Social	Integrated Intensive counseling (ref = Early decline type)								
		Late decline type	−0.063	−0.088	−0.049	−0.028			0.016	−0.067
		Continuous type	−0.105	−0.094	−0.013	−0.03			0.021	−0.071
Behavior skills		Integrated Self-recording (ref = Early decline type)								
		Late decline type	0.015	−0.051	0.011	−0.016			−0.023	−0.039
		Continuous type	0.156 *	−0.066	0.165 ***	−0.021			−0.116 *	−0.05
Health behavior		Healthy eating					−0.021 **	−0.006	−0.019 **	−0.006
		Physical activity					−0.072 ***	−0.018	−0.067 ***	−0.018
Intercept			1.919 ***	−0.165	0.115 *	−0.053	2.767 ***	−0.11	2.800 ***	−0.122

* $p < 0.05$, ** $p < 0.01$, *** $p < 0.001$

In Model 1, the results showed that the continuous type of information ($\beta = 0.217$, $p < 0.001$), the continuous type of personal motivation ($\beta = 0.156$, $p < 0.001$), and the continuous type of behavioral skills ($\beta = 0.156$, $p < 0.001$) all significantly influenced the adoption of healthy eating. In Model 2, when analyzing the effects of information, motivation, and behavioral skills on physical activity, it was found that there was a significant impact from the continuous type of behavioral skills ($\beta = 0.165$, $p < 0.001$). Model 3 examined the effect of health-related behavior practice (healthy eating and physical activity) on health risk factors. The results showed that the higher the healthy eating score ($\beta = -0.021$, $p < 0.001$), the more physical activity significantly reduced health risk factors ($\beta = -0.072$, $p < 0.001$). Model 4 examined the impact of changes in the number of health risk factors by considering all variables of information, motivation, behavioral skills, and health behavior. The results showed that health risk factors decreased as the continuous type of behavioral skills ($\beta = -0.116$, $p < 0.001$) and health behavior practice (healthy eating, $\beta = -0.019$; physical activity, $\beta = -0.067$) increased.

The other control variables showed that compared to males, females engaged in less physical activity but were better at practicing healthy eating. As age increased, healthy eating improved. The physical activity rate was high in those in their 20s and 60s, with the lowest physical activity rate found in those in their 40s. Smoking and alcohol consumption had a negative effect on healthy eating. Alcohol consumption reduced physical activity, and smoking had a negative effect on health risk factors. The higher the stage of behavior change and the longer the period of participation (three months → six months), the more positive the influence on health outcomes; however, the number of health risks increased with age.

4. Discussion

4.1. Principal Findings

The IMB model can be effectively utilized to design and evaluate various interventions by incorporating strategies related to information, motivation, and behavior skills within each construct. Interventions based on IMB theory aimed at improving medication compliance, self-management, and risk prevention behavior have demonstrated strong efficacy [31,33,34,45–47]. This study applied the IMB theory to mHealth intervention services to improve the risk factors for metabolic syndrome and examined its effects and influencing factors. Among the IMB components, the higher the continuity of behavioral skills and rate of health behavior practice, the more positive the influence on improving health. This finding is consistent with those of systematic reviews and meta-analyses that have shown that physical activity and lifestyle interventions based on mHealth technology are effective in reducing cardiometabolic risk [8].

Although not presented in Table 4, an examination of the relationship between IMB components reveals that the late decline type and continuous types of information and motivation influence behavioral skills and health behavior, aligning with existing research [31]. In Model 1, healthy eating habits were implemented in all continuous types of IMB other than social motivation. A separate detailed analysis showed that social motivation had an effect on healthy eating habits, but its influence was smaller than that of information or personal motivation. Nevertheless, the participants were already receiving social support, such as receiving information from experts, and the difference here can be seen that participants with high personal motivation who continuously put into practice the information provided were practicing healthy eating well. In Model 2, it was confirmed that only continuous types of behavioral skills affect physical activity. It can be assumed that IMB practice needs to be strengthened more to change physical activity than to change healthy eating. Next, in a separate detailed analysis, it was confirmed that IMB affects health behavior, but in Models 3 and 4, only health behavior (healthy eating, physical activity) was confirmed to be significant for health outcomes (reduction in health risk factors). This appears to have canceled out the individual effects of IMB when considering all variables.

However, it is important to consider all components because IMB must be performed well for health behavior to continue.

In this study, participants learned about the activities and methods necessary for health management through mHealth services, and their self-monitoring and goal management abilities improved with the use of an activity tracker. Counseling that assists in changing behavior through social motivation may positively affect behavioral skills. Moreover, the continuous application of behavioral skills has a decisive influence on the performance of health behaviors. Behavioral skills are a critical concept that assesses whether a motivated individual can proficiently execute health behaviors using available health information. They center on an individual's objective capability and self-efficacy in performing specific health-related behaviors. The behavioral skills in this study involved repeated self-recording of nutrition and exercise, which are difficult to practice. As seen in the practice pattern of weekly nutrition and exercise self-recording in Figure 9, the percentage of the continuous type in behavioral skills was lower than that of other behavioral change techniques (BCTs), with more than 50% showing an early decline type. In other words, practicing behavioral skills was more difficult than other interventions, but those who practiced them well had a strong willingness to continue participating in mHealth services, which appeared to have a positive effect on health outcomes.

According to a qualitative study on change in health behavior and app use experience [48], the act of recording behavior via apps engenders a sense of control, indicating proficient self-management of health. This self-awareness in effectively managing health facilitates the implementation of health behavior changes. This finding aligns with the results indicating that participants initiate self-management by actively acknowledging their attitudes and behaviors towards health through self-monitoring and behavioral feedback techniques. Furthermore, self-management skills were enhanced through persistent repetition, as evidenced in previous studies [48,49].

In this study, in addition to the IMB composition, it was difficult to quantitatively examine changes in daily life expected to result from positive behavioral changes, such as purchasing healthy food, joining an exercise group, learning a new sport, and purchasing exercise equipment. However, in focus group interviews that analyzed the experiences of mHealth participants in a prior study [50], participants who had health improvement effects continued to make choices that were beneficial to their health. In other words, practicing health behaviors and experiencing health improvements would have increased self-efficacy to continue health-seeking behaviors in daily life.

However, mHealth faces challenges in the management of metabolic syndrome. Although mHealth has shown health improvement effects in individuals with risk factors for metabolic syndrome, it also has limitations owing to the lack of compulsion in non-face-to-face interactions. Mobile phone apps operate non-face-to-face, where users transmit practice information, and counseling and management are conducted based on the degree of participation. Therefore, if inactive participants do not input their practice information, counselors find it difficult to understand their behavior and can only provide general and simplistic information. Consequently, inactive participants lose interest in mobile phone apps and do not engage in health practices, creating a vicious cycle. Another study [51] points out that non-users of mobile phone apps avoid them because the mobile phone platform does not fit their lifestyle patterns or because the activity of manually entering health practices is cumbersome. This suggests that although mobile phone platforms have several advantages in a non-face-to-face environment, face-to-face or similar interventions are still needed.

Future studies should compare and analyze the sociodemographic characteristics between continuous-type and non-continuous-type subjects. Additionally, interventions incorporating behavioral economic factors using nudges should be developed and tailored to subjects through the design of an automated algorithm.

4.2. Limitations and Implications

This study had several limitations, but it has implications nonetheless. First, the lack of a comparison group made it impossible to control for external variables, thereby limiting causal inferences. In the evaluation of program interventions, randomized controlled trials or studies using quasi-experimental methodologies are typically conducted to compare an experimental group with a control group and explain the causal effects. A previous study used quasi-experimental methods, such as propensity score matching analysis and difference-in-differences analysis, to compare the effectiveness of the mHealth intervention with a control group. The results indicated that the mHealth intervention group was more effective than the control group [52]. Second, although the aim was to examine various practice types using GBTM, participants maintained a similarly high adherence rate because of personalized management. Therefore, the practice types were not diverse, posing limitations in explaining the full spectrum of practice changes over time. Nonetheless, unlike most intervention studies that derive causal results through before–after cross-sectional analysis at two or three time points, this study is meaningful in quantifying individual practice patterns over time according to the concepts of health behavior theory. This can be utilized as a basis for determining the selection of intervention elements and frequency of interventions in future mHealth services. Third, when selecting subjects, there is a possibility that the majority of users will participate voluntarily rather than in an experimental setting for research, resulting in selective bias. This can reduce internal validity in revealing the causal relationship between services. Nevertheless, looking at the characteristics of the subjects analyzed in this study, compared to the voluntary use of public health center users, 58.7% of users who received follow-up health care services due to abnormal findings after the national health checkup were randomly included, which can be explained by data minimizing user selection bias.

Despite the limitations noted above, this study employed large-scale mHealth empirical data to categorize practice types according to health behavior theory and evaluate their health promotion effects. Unlike typical intervention studies that rely on self-report surveys and clinical measurements for assessing behavioral changes, this study utilized life-log data to capture nuanced behavioral patterns over time. This methodological approach enhances the depth and reliability of our findings.

5. Conclusions

Based on our comprehensive analysis using a multi-GBTM methodology, integrated interventions focusing on information, motivation, and behavioral skills delineated distinct practice patterns among participants. Our study identified significant influences from continuous types of these constructs, notably enhancing the adoption of healthy eating and physical activity. These findings underscore the critical role of targeted interventions in promoting healthier lifestyles and reducing health risk factors associated with metabolic syndrome.

Author Contributions: Conceptualization, N.-Y.P.; methodology, N.-Y.P. and S.J.; software, S.J.; validation, N.-Y.P. and S.J.; formal analysis, N.-Y.P.; investigation, N.-Y.P.; resources, N.-Y.P. and S.J.; data curation, S.J.; writing—original draft preparation, N.-Y.P.; writing—review and editing, N.-Y.P. and S.J.; visualization, N.-Y.P. and S.J.; supervision, N.-Y.P. and S.J.; project administration, S.J.; funding acquisition, N.-Y.P. and S.J. All authors have read and agreed to the published version of the manuscript.

Funding: This research was supported by the Health Fellowship Foundation, the Smart Healthcare Network Foundation, and the National Research Foundation of Korea (NRF) grant funded by the Korean government (MSIT) (No. RS-2023-00213294).

Institutional Review Board Statement: This study was conducted in accordance with the Declaration of Helsinki and approved by the Institutional Review Board of Seoul National University (1912/001-008), Approval date: 10 June 2019.

Informed Consent Statement: Informed consent was obtained from all the participants involved in this study.

Data Availability Statement: We kindly request that any inquiries regarding the data used in this study be directed to the corresponding author. The datasets used in this study are available upon request.

Conflicts of Interest: The authors declare no conflicts of interest.

References

1. OECD. Health at a Glance 2019. Available online: https://www.oecd.org/health/health-at-a-glance (accessed on 26 February 2024).
2. World Health Organization. Available online: https://www.who.int/ncds/en/ (accessed on 20 May 2020).
3. Borch-Johnsen, K. The Metabolic Syndrome in a Global Perspective. The Public Health Impact--Secondary Publication. *Dan. Med. Bull.* **2007**, *54*, 157–159. [PubMed]
4. Grundy, S.M.; Cleeman, J.I.; Daniels, S.R.; Donato, K.A.; Eckel, R.H.; Franklin, B.A.; Gordon, D.J.; Krauss, R.M.; Savage, P.J.; Smith, S.C.; et al. Diagnosis and Management of the Metabolic Syndrome. *Circulation* **2005**, *112*, 2735–2752. [CrossRef] [PubMed]
5. Grundy, S.M. Metabolic Syndrome Update. *Trends Cardiovasc. Med.* **2016**, *26*, 364–373. [CrossRef] [PubMed]
6. Nilsson, P.M.; Tuomilehto, J.; Rydén, L. The Metabolic Syndrome–What Is It and How Should It Be Managed? *Eur. J. Prev. Cardiol.* **2019**, *26*, 33–46. [CrossRef] [PubMed]
7. Rao, D.P.; Dai, S.; Lagace, C.; Krewski, D. Metabolic syndrome and chronic disease. *Health Promot. Chronic Dis. Prev. Can.* **2014**, *34*, 36–45. [CrossRef]
8. Sequi-Dominguez, I.; Alvarez-Bueno, C.; Martinez-Vizcaino, V.; Fernandez-Rodriguez, R.; del Saz Lara, A.; Cavero-Redondo, I. Effectiveness of Mobile Health Interventions Promoting Physical Activity and Lifestyle Interventions to Reduce Cardiovascular Risk Among Individuals with Metabolic Syndrome: Systematic Review and Meta-Analysis. *J. Med. Internet Res.* **2020**, *22*, e17790. [CrossRef] [PubMed]
9. Saklayen, M.G. The global epidemic of the metabolic syndrome. *Curr. Hypertens. Rep.* **2018**, *20*, 12. [CrossRef] [PubMed]
10. Ahima, R.S. Overview of metabolic syndrome. In *Metabolic Syndrome: A Comprehensive Textbook*; Springer International Publishing: Cham, Switzerland, 2024; pp. 3–14.
11. Alberti, K.G.M.M.; Zimmet, P.; Shaw, J. Metabolic Syndrome—A New Worldwide Definition. A Consensus Statement from the International Diabetes Federation. *Diabet. Med.* **2006**, *23*, 469–480. [CrossRef] [PubMed]
12. Noubiap, J.J.; Nansseu, J.R.; Lontchi-Yimagou, E.; Nkeck, J.R.; Nyaga, U.F.; Ngouo, A.T.; Bigna, J.J. Geographic distribution of metabolic syndrome and its components in the general adult population: A meta-analysis of global data from 28 million individuals. Diabetes Res. *Clin. Pract.* **2022**, *188*, 109924. [CrossRef]
13. Ogurtsova, K.; da Rocha Fernandes, J.D.; Huang, Y.; Linnenkamp, U.; Guariguata, L.; Cho, N.H.; Cavan, D.; Shaw, J.E.; Makaroff, L.E. IDF Diabetes Atlas: Global Estimates for the Prevalence of Diabetes for 2015 and 2040. *Diabetes Res. Clin. Pract.* **2017**, *128*, 40–50. [CrossRef]
14. Health Insurance Review and Assessment Service & National Health Insurance Service. *2021 National Health Insurance Statistical Yearbook*. Approval number 920006. 2022. ISSN 1738-8945. Available online: https://www.hira.or.kr/bbsDummy.do?pgmid=HIRAJ030000007001&brdScnBltNo=4&brdBltNo=6&pageIndex=1&pageIndex2=1 (accessed on 28 April 2024).
15. Heo, G.-B. *Metabolic Syndrome*, 2nd ed.; Jin Planning: Seoul, Republic of Korea, 2009.
16. Świątkiewicz, I.; Nuszkiewicz, J.; Wróblewska, J.; Nartowicz, M.; Sokołowski, K.; Sutkowy, P.; Woźniak, A. Feasibility and Cardiometabolic Effects of Time-Restricted Eating in Patients with Metabolic Syndrome. *Nutrients* **2024**, *16*, 1802. [CrossRef] [PubMed]
17. National Cholesterol Education Program (NCEP) Expert Panel on Detection, Evaluation, and Treatment of High Blood Cholesterol in Adults (Adults Treatment Panel III). Third report of the national cholesterol education program (NCEP) Expert Panel on detection, evaluation, and treatment of high blood cholesterol in adults (Adults Treatment Panel III) final report. *Circulation* **2002**, *106*, 3143–3421. [CrossRef]
18. Shim, J.-Y.; Kang, H.-T.; Kim, S.-Y.; Kim, J.-S.; Kim, J.-W.; Kim, J.-Y.; Park, H.-A.; Shin, J.-Y.; Cho, S.-H.; Choi, Y.-E. Prevention and Treatment of Metabolic Syndrome in Korean Adults. *Korean J. Fam. Pract.* **2015**, *5*, 375–420.
19. European Commission. *Green Paper on Mobile Health*; European Commission: Brussels, Belgium, 2014.
20. Daud, M.H.; Yusoff, F.H.; Ramli, A.S. The Effect of Mobile Health (mHealth) Interventions on Clinical Outcomes and Self-Management Behaviours in Individuals with Metabolic Syndrome: A Narrative Review of Evidence. *J. Clin. Health Sci.* **2023**, *8*, 6–33. [CrossRef]
21. Schoeppe, S.; Alley, S.; Van Lippevelde, W.; Bray, N.A.; Williams, S.L.; Duncan, M.J.; Vandelanotte, C. Efficacy of interventions that use apps to improve diet, physical activity and sedentary behaviour: A systematic review. *Int. J. Behav. Nutr. Phys. Act.* **2016**, *13*, 127. [CrossRef] [PubMed]
22. Silva, B.M.C.; Rodrigues, J.J.P.C.; Díez, I.T.; Coronado, M.L.; Saleem, K. Mobile-health: A review of current state in 2015. *J. Biomed. Inform.* **2015**, *56*, 265–272. [CrossRef] [PubMed]
23. Fedele, D.A.; Cushing, C.C.; Fritz, A.; Amaro, C.M.; Ortega, A. Mobile health interventions for improving health outcomes in youth: A meta-analysis. *JAMA Pediatr.* **2017**, *171*, 461–469. [CrossRef] [PubMed]

24. Milne-Ives, M.; Lam, C.; De Cock, C.; Van Velthoven, M.H.; Meinert, E. Mobile Apps for Health Behavior Change in Physical Activity, Diet, Drug and Alcohol Use, and Mental Health: Systematic Review. *JMIR Mhealth Uhealth* **2020**, *8*, e17046. [CrossRef] [PubMed]
25. Payne, H.E.; Lister, C.; West, J.H.; Bernhardt, J.M. Behavioral functionality of mobile apps in health interventions: A systematic review of the literature. *JMIR Mhealth Uhealth* **2015**, *3*, e20. [CrossRef] [PubMed]
26. Cavero-Redondo, I.; Martinez-Vizcaino, V.; Fernandez-Rodriguez, R.; Saz-Lara, A.; Pascual-Morena, C.; Álvarez-Bueno, C. Effect of behavioral weight management interventions using lifestyle mHealth self-monitoring on weight loss: A systematic review and meta-analysis. *Nutrients* **2020**, *12*, 1977. [CrossRef]
27. Wang, L.; Langlais, C.S.; Kenfield, S.A.; Chan, J.M.; Graff, R.E.; Allen, I.E.; Van Blarigan, E.L. mHealth interventions to promote a healthy diet and physical activity among cancer survivors: A systematic review of randomized controlled trials. *Cancers* **2022**, *14*, 3816. [CrossRef] [PubMed]
28. Kim, H.J.; Lee, K.H.; Lee, J.H.; Youk, H.; Lee, H.Y. The Effect of a Mobile and Wearable Device Intervention on Increased Physical Activity to Prevent Metabolic Syndrome: Observational Study. *JMIR mHealth uHealth* **2022**, *10*, e34059. [CrossRef] [PubMed]
29. Lugones-Sanchez, C.; Recio-Rodriguez, J.I.; Agudo-Conde, C.; Repiso-Gento, I.; Adalia, E.G.; Ramirez-Manent, J.I.; EVIDENT 3 Investigators. Long-Term Effectiveness of a Smartphone App Combined with a Smart Band on Weight Loss, Physical Activity, and Caloric Intake in a Population with Overweight and Obesity (EVIDENT 3 Study): Randomized Controlled Trial. *J. Med. Internet Res.* **2022**, *24*, e30416. [CrossRef] [PubMed]
30. Fisher, W.A.; Fisher, J.D.; Harman, J. The information-motivation-behavioral skills model: A general social psychological approach to understanding and promoting health behavior. In *Social Psychological Foundations of Health and Illness*; John Wiley & Sons: Hoboken, NJ, USA, 2003; pp. 82–106.
31. Fisher, J.D.; Fisher, W.A. Changing AIDS-risk behavior. *Psychol. Bull.* **1992**, *111*, 455. [CrossRef] [PubMed]
32. Korea Health Promotion Institute. *Mobile Healthcare Pilot Project Guide*; Korea Health Promotion Institute: Seoul, Republic of Korea, 2016.
33. Mayberry, L.S.; Osborn, C.Y. Empirical validation of the information–motivation–behavioral skills model of diabetes medication adherence: A framework for intervention. *Diabetes Care* **2014**, *37*, 1246–1253. [CrossRef] [PubMed]
34. Bian, C.; Xu, S.; Wang, H.; Li, N.; Wu, J.; Zhao, Y.; Lu, H. A study on the application of the information-motivation-behavioral skills (IMB) model on rational drug use behavior among second-level hospital outpatients in Anhui, China. *PLoS ONE* **2015**, *10*, e0135782.
35. Korea National Health and Nutrition Examination Survey. 2015. Available online: https://knhanes.kdca.go.kr/knhanes/main.do (accessed on 15 June 2016).
36. Community Health Survey. 2015. Available online: https://chs.kdca.go.kr/chs/index.do (accessed on 17 June 2016).
37. Ministry of Health and Welfare. *National Dietary Guidelines for Koreans*; Ministry of Health and Welfare: Sejong, Republic of Korea, 2016.
38. Nagin, D.S.; Odgers, C.L. Group-based trajectory modeling in clinical research. *Annu. Rev. Clin. Psychol.* **2010**, *6*, 109–138. [CrossRef] [PubMed]
39. Nagin, D.S. *Group-based Modeling of Development*; Harvard University Press: Cambridge, MA, USA, 2005.
40. Hong, B.-I.; Kim, H.-Y. A Study on the Type of Retirement Processes and Its Determinants for the Aged. *Korean J. Soc. Policy* **2010**, *17*, 291–319.
41. Min, H.-J. Mothers' Employment Experience Surrounding a First Childbirth in South Korea: An Application of Group-Based Trajectory Model. *Korean J. Sociol.* **2012**, *46*, 61–87.
42. Yeo, H.-S. Analysis of Retirement Patterns Depending on Resignation Voluntariness at Middle and Senior Age. Master's Thesis, Seoul National University, Department of Social Welfare, Seoul, Republic of Korea, 2014.
43. Liang, K.-Y.; Zeger, S.L. Longitudinal data analysis using generalized linear models. *Biometrika* **1986**, *73*, 13–22. [CrossRef]
44. Min, I.-S.; Choi, P.-S. *STATA Advanced Statistical Analysis*; Jipil Media: Gyeonggi, Republic of Korea, 2019.
45. Chang, S.J.; Choi, S.; Kim, S.-A.; Song, M. Intervention strategies based on information-motivation-behavioral skills model for health behavior change: A systematic review. *Asian Nurs. Res.* **2014**, *8*, 172–181. [CrossRef]
46. Jeon, E.-J. Development and Effectiveness Evaluation of Diabetes Self-Management Mobile App Based on IMB Model. Ph.D. Thesis, Seoul National University Graduate School, Seoul, Republic of Korea, 2017.
47. Lee, S.-H.; Kim, H.-R. Predictive Model of Self-Management Implementation and Quality of Life in Elderly Diabetic Patients Using a Community Health Promotion Room. *J. Korean Acad. Nurs.* **2017**, *47*, 514–525. [CrossRef] [PubMed]
48. Ha, M.-Y.; Lee, Y.-J.; Kwon, S.-J.; Kim, J.-W. The Impact of Health Behavior Recording on Health Behavior Change in Healthcare Application Users: Based on Grounded Theory. In Proceedings of the Korean HCI Conference, Seoul, Republic of Korea, 22–26 October 2018; pp. 444–448.
49. McKay, F.H.; Slykerman, S.; Dunn, M. The App Behavior Change Scale: Creation of a scale to assess the potential of apps to promote behavior change. *JMIR Mhealth Uhealth* **2019**, *7*, e11130. [CrossRef]
50. Park, N.Y.; Hwang, J.H.; Choi, Y.-K.; Park, S.-H.; Lee, Y.K. A study on the experience of mHealth based on health belief model: Focus group interview. *Korean J. Health Educ. Promot.* **2019**, *36*, 97–111. [CrossRef]

51. Yong, J.; Bae, B.-J. An Analysis of Non-users of Mobile Healthcare Applications: Based on Diffusion of Innovations Theory. *J. Korean Soc. Inf. Manag.* **2017**, *34*, 135–154.
52. Park, N.Y.; Lee, Y.K.; Kim, D.J.; Kim, M.S.; Cho, B.H. Evaluation of Health Improvement Effect of M-Health Project in Public Sector Using ICT: Propensity Score Matching Method and Difference in Differences with Comparison Groups. *Health Soc. Sci.* **2018**, *49*, 169–197. [CrossRef]

nutrients

MDPI

Article

Intermittent Fasting: Socio-Economic Profile of Spanish Citizens Who Practice It and the Influence of This Dietary Pattern on the Health and Lifestyle Habits of the Population

Elena Sandri [1,2], Daniele Borghesi [3], Eva Cantín Larumbe [4], Germán Cerdá Olmedo [1], María Jesús Vega-Bello [1,*] and Vicente Bernalte Martí [5]

1 Faculty of Medicine and Health Sciences, Catholic University of Valencia San Vicente Mártir, c/Quevedo, 2, 46001 Valencia, Spain; elena.sandri@ucv.es (E.S.); german.cerda@ucv.es (G.C.O.)
2 Doctoral School, Catholic University of Valencia San Vicente Mártir, c/Quevedo 2, 46001 Valencia, Spain
3 Master's Degree in Data Science and Business Informatics, University of Pisa, Lungarno Pacinotti 43, 56126 Pisa, Italy; d.borghesi@studenti.unipi.it
4 Degree in Data Science, Polytechnical University of Valencia, Camí de Vera, s/n, 46022 Valencia, Spain; evacantinlarumbe@gmail.com
5 Predepartmental Nursing Unit, Faculty of Health Sciences, Jaume I University, Avda. Sos Baynat, s/n, 12071 Castellón, Spain; bernalte@uji.es
* Correspondence: mj.vega@ucv.es

Abstract: Intermittent fasting (IF) is a dietary approach that has gained popularity in recent years. More and more Spanish people are following this eating pattern, which consists of alternating periods of fasting with periods of food intake. Its benefits include improved metabolic and vascular health and weight loss. Objectives: 1. To study the prevalence of IF among the Spanish population. 2. To explore how demographic factors influence the choice to adopt this dietary approach. Methods: A descriptive cross-sectional study was conducted on the Spanish population using the NutSo-HH questionnaire, which was constructed, validated, and disseminated by the research team through a non-probabilistic snowball sampling approach, collecting socio-demographic data and nutritional, social and lifestyle habits of the population. Results and conclusions: A valid sample of 22,181 people participated, of whom 4.59% (n = 1018) said they practiced IF. The data show that more middle-aged men than women practice IF. In addition, individuals who follow IF methods are less likely to have no control over their food intake, are less scared to gain weight and have a higher body image, but no differences were found related to unhealthy food and nights out. There were also no significant differences in terms of the level of education, income, size of municipality, or region of residence. In conclusion, a person who practices IF seems to have adopted a healthier lifestyle and social habits.

Keywords: intermittent fasting; Mediterranean diet; healthy lifestyle; survey; Spain

1. Introduction

Intermittent fasting (IF) is an eating pattern that alternates between fasting and eating periods [1]. There are several approaches to IF; for example, the two most common ones are alternating fasting days with non-fasting days and daily fasting by eating in a specific time frame. The first one is based on changes between days with no food consumption for 24 h and non-fasting days with normal food intake; for example, with the 5:2 method, where individuals fast for 24 h twice a week and consume a very-low-calorie diet for the remaining 5 days. Fasting can occur on consecutive or non-consecutive days. The second method is time-restricted eating, where the time during which food can be eaten is limited. Typically, eating is allowed during a 6 h period per day, with breakfast in the morning and lunch before 3 p.m. This allows for a fasting period of 14–18 h per day [2,3].

Fasting is not a new practice; it has always been around in different communities and for various reasons [4], including cultural and religious reasons [5]. However, in recent years, the IF diet has become a scientifically studied dietary pattern followed by millions of people worldwide.

The benefits of IF include weight loss [6] due to limiting the eating time, so that the opportunity to consume food is reduced, which can help control caloric intake. It is also known to improve insulin sensitivity and blood sugar regulation [7]. By alternating between periods of fasting and eating, blood insulin levels can be reduced, which can help prevent insulin resistance and type 2 diabetes. Moreover, studies have shown that it promotes cardiovascular health by lowering cardiovascular risk factors such as blood pressure, cholesterol levels and markers of inflammation [8]. Practicing IF has also been shown to have positive effects on brain function, including improving neuronal plasticity, protecting against oxidative stress and reducing the risk of some neurodegenerative diseases [9]. Some animal research suggests that intermittent fasting may be associated with increased longevity and reduced risk of age-related diseases [10]. Lastly, not only can time-restricted fasting induce autophagy and provide similar health benefits to a low-calorie diet, but it is also a suitable alternative for elite athletes who require a high caloric intake. Integrating periods of fasting can optimize metabolic health, improve recovery and maintain high performance without compromising the required energy intake [11].

Despite having several potential health benefits, intermittent fasting can also have negative side effects. Some of the most common are hypoglycemia [12], dizziness and weakness [13], which can be particularly serious if combined with the use of medication [12]. Fasting without an adequate protein replacement can also cause muscle wasting [14]. This is why IF is not suitable for everyone and it is particularly contraindicated for sensitive population groups [15], such as pregnant or breastfeeding women, people with eating disorders [16] or the elderly [17].

It has been demonstrated that socio-demographic factors play an important role in the prevalence and adoption of different dietary patterns [18–20]. While there are numerous studies focused on investigating the benefits of IF, there are currently just a few studies specifically investigating the socio-demographic determinants that guide the uptake of this type of dietary practice and none of them focuses on the Spanish population. A recent study explored the benefits, side effects, quality of life and knowledge of the Saudi population practicing IF and related those to socio-demographic variables of the population studied [21]. Another recent study, again conducted on the Saudi population, aimed to describe the practice of IF outside of Ramadan [22]. A third study, conducted on the Swedish population, aimed to determine the socio-demographic factors associated with adherence to a specific diet and attempts to lose weight. However, this study did not focus specifically on IF [23]. There are other studies in the literature that explore socio-demographic factors and intermittent fasting, but they focus on specific population groups; to be more specific, on the pediatric population [24], on the elderly population [25], on people with eating disorders [26] or on people with mental health disorders or pathologies [27].

Further knowledge about the prevalence of IF in the population and its socio-demographic determinants is certainly of scientific and, above all, public health interest. Understanding how the practice of IF varies according to factors such as gender, age, educational level, socio-economic status or area of residence can help to identify health disparities and develop targeted interventions for vulnerable groups. This can contribute to reducing health inequalities and promoting equitable access to beneficial health practices. Also, as this dietary practice has been associated with a range of health benefits and disease prevention [6–10], understanding the prevalence of the dietary practice and its determinants can help to identify population groups at risk of diet-related health problems and develop appropriate interventions. Finally, data on the prevalence and determinants of IF can influence the development of public health policies and the creation of programs aimed at promoting healthy lifestyles and improving the health of the general population. This could include educational initiatives, awareness campaigns and community intervention programs.

Also, it is well known that the habits a person develops throughout their life have a significant impact on their health [28–30]. When someone adopts a specific diet, such as IF, their habits can undergo significant changes [31]. It is crucial to understand in detail how these changes occur to determine both the potential benefits and the adverse effects that this dietary practice may have on a person's health.

Study Aim and Scope

For all the above reasons, this study focuses on analyzing a large sample of Spanish citizens living in Spain with the following objectives:

1. Analyze the prevalence of intermittent fasting in the Spanish population,
2. Explore the socio-demographic variables that influence the practice of this type of dietary style,
3. Investigate the relationship between the influence of intermittent fasting on the nutritional, social and lifestyle habits adopted by the population and their impact on health.

2. Materials and Methods

2.1. Type of Study and Sampling

A cross-sectional investigation was conducted to examine the adult population of Spain, focusing on individuals aged 18 and above. Those with chronic illnesses or temporary conditions that might affect their diet (such as hospitalization, a stay in a penitentiary or living in a community) were excluded from the study.

2.2. Ethical Approval

Ethical guidelines set forth in the Declaration of Helsinki [32] were followed, and approval was obtained from the Research Ethics Committee of the Catholic University of Valencia (approval code UCV/2019-2020/152, date of approval, 18 June 2020). Prior to their involvement, all the participants provided informed consent.

2.3. Instrument

The data collection tool used in this research was a questionnaire explicitly created for this study, encompassing several sections. In the first part, participants provided anthropometric data such as weight, height, and socio-demographic variables. Subsequent sections delved into the frequency of consumption of various food groups, drinking habits, and sports and lifestyle behaviors associated with health.

The questionnaire, named the NutSo-HH Scale, was developed and validated according to rigorous methodological standards and psychometric tests were carried out [33]. To ensure the questionnaire's validity and reliability, the validation procedures involved several steps. First, a pilot group of 53 individuals with characteristics akin to the studied population provided feedback on the questionnaire. Second, a nominal group consisting of seven health experts, including a nutritionist, two family doctors, two psychologists, a social educator, and a communication expert, participated in the validation process.

Finally, to assess the construct validity, Confirmatory Factor Analysis (CFA) was conducted using the weighted least squares robust method (WLS-MV). The model fit was evaluated using several indices: the Chi-square test (χ^2), Root Mean Square Error of Approximation (RMSEA), Comparative Fit Index (CFI), Tucker and Lewis Index (TLI), Standardized Root Mean Square Index of Approximation (SRMSEA), and Standardized Root Mean Square Residual (SRMR). A good fit was indicated by RMSEA values ≤ 0.05, CFI and TLI values ≥ 0.95, SRMSEA values ≤ 0.95, and SRMR values ≤ 0.08.

2.4. Data Collection

The questionnaire was hosted on Google Forms and a non-probabilistic snowball sampling method [34] was used to distribute it, mainly through social networks. The leading platform was Instagram, where the @elretonutricional account was created, and the survey was disseminated to a varied audience with the help of various professionals, influencers, and supporters. In addition, the researchers used their personal networks, LinkedIn, Twitter, WhatsApp and Facebook, to promote the dissemination.

In addition to virtual dissemination, a significant effort was made to physically disseminate the questionnaire to ensure that it also reached those respondents who were less familiar with and active on social networks. This was conducted in collaboration with establishments throughout Spain, selected for their diverse clientele (e.g., pharmacies or tobacconists). These establishments were told about the research project, and those who wanted to join were provided with posters to display on their premises. By scanning the QR code on the poster, customers could access the questionnaire and fill it out if they wished. Data collection covered the period from August 2020 to November 2021.

2.5. Variables

The questionnaire covers a broad spectrum of socio-demographic and anthropometric health factors, including gender, age, birthplace, residence, occupation, education, income, weight, height, self-perceived health, diet-affecting conditions, and signs of eating disorders. Furthermore, it explores dietary patterns, frequency of food consumption, sedentary behaviors, participation in physical activity, and health-related social habits like sleep patterns, smoking, and alcohol consumption.

Most variables are qualitative, offering respondents multiple options to select. However, some variables are quantitatively continuous, including self-reported age, weight, height, and the number of minutes spent on sports per week. Additionally, discrete quantitative variables, such as self-reported health levels, follow the Likert scale format.

2.6. Categorization of Variables

In order to analyze the data, the responses collected for the different variables were categorized, following the criteria explained below.

For the age variable, three groups were selected: young (18–30 years), adult (31–50 years), and middle-aged and elderly (≥51 years). For the level of income, two categories were distinguished: low income (<EUR 2200/month per household) and medium–high income (≥EUR 2200/month). For the level of education, two categories were established: basic education (comprising the responses of no education, primary, secondary, high school, and vocational training) and higher education (bachelor, master and doctorate).

The nutritional variables and health habit variables were categorized on a Likert scale ranging from 1 to 4 points (as shown in Table 1), except the symptoms of eating disorders, which utilized a scale ranging from 1 to 6. This categorization offers a structured evaluation of these health-related behaviors, enabling a detailed understanding of the participants' habits in these specific domains.

Table 1. Categorization of the health and lifestyle variables.

Variable	Category	Score
Sleeping hours	<6 h	1
	6 h–7 h	2
	7 h–8 h	3
	>8 h	4
Getting up rested	Never	1
	Very seldom and sometimes	2
	Frequently and almost always	3
	Always	4
Sleep quality	0 and 1	1
	2	2
	3	3
	4 and 5	4

Table 1. *Cont.*

Variable	Category	Score
Water	Never and very rarely (2 max. per month) or 1–2 glasses/cups per week	1
	2 glasses/cups or less every day	2
	3 to 5 glasses every day	3
	More than 5 glasses every day	4
Sugary soft drinks, coffee and energy drinks, juice	Never and very rarely (2 glasses max. per month)	4
	One glass per week and 2 or more glasses per week	3
	2 glasses or less every day	2
	3 to 5 glasses and more than 5 glasses every day	1
Consumption of fast food, fried food and ultra-processed dishes	Never	1
	Very seldom (2 times a month maximum)	2
	Once a week	3
	Several times a week	4
Getting drunk	Never or less than once a month	1
	Monthly	2
	Weekly	3
	Daily or almost daily	4
Alcohol consumption	Never or once a month	1
	2–4 times a month	2
	2–3 times a week	3
	4–5 times a week or every day	4
Smoking	Non-smoker	1
	Light smoker (less than 5 cigarettes per day)	2
	Moderate smoker (6–15 cigarettes per day)	3
	Severe smoker (more than 16 cigarettes per day)	4
Night outings	Never and sporadically	1
	Between a and 2 night a week	2
	More than 3 times a week	3
	Every day	4
Daily sedentary lifestyle	Less than 7 h	1
	Between 7 and 9 h	2
	Between 9 and 11 h	3
	More than 11 h	4
Obesophobia, no control, body image	Always	6
	Very frequently	5
	Frequently	4
	Occasionally	3
	Rarely	2
	Never	1

2.7. *Healthy Eating Index for the Spanish Population (IASE)*

The results of the food frequency variables were utilized to calculate the IASE (Healthy Eating Index for the Spanish population). Based on a condensed version validated by Norte and Ortiz [35], this index includes variables such as fruits, vegetables, meat, dairy, cereals, pulses, and soft drinks. It assesses the frequency of consumption of foods recommended for daily, weekly, and occasional intake, as well as dietary variety, a vital aspect of a healthy diet. Behaviors aligning with the recommendations of the Spanish Society of Community Nutrition (SENC) [36] received a score of 10, with the maximum index score being 73. Based on the IASE score obtained, the population's nutritional habits can be categorized into three groups: "Healthy" (58.4 < IASE < 73), "Needs changes" (36.5 < IASE < 58.4), and "Unhealthy" (IASE < 36.5).

2.8. Data Analysis

Socio-demographic categorical variables are shown as absolute values and percentages. Continuous variables are presented as the mean and standard deviation. For the analysis of the continuous variables, the nonparametric Mann–Whitney test was used when comparing two groups or the Kruskal–Wallis test with Hochberg correction when comparing three groups [37]. A p-value < 0.05 was considered statistically significant. Data were analyzed using Python version 3.9.13.

Principal Component Analysis (PCA) [38] was performed in R Studio version 4.3.0 [39]. PCA is an unsupervised machine-learning model that reduces the dimensionality of a dataset by transforming a large set of variables into a smaller set of principal components, which still preserves most of the data's variance. These principal components are new variables constructed as linear combinations or mixtures of the original variables. PCA enables the identification of the variables that best characterize Spanish IF followers and elucidates the relationships between the variables under study.

3. Results

A valid sample of n = 22,181 Spanish citizens was recruited by disseminating the questionnaire. Of the respondents, 80.84% were women compared to 19.16% men, and the average age of the participants was 34.86 years. Detailed data can be found in Table 2.

Table 2. Sample and their socio-demographic characteristics (n = 22,181).

	Mean ± SD or *n* (%)
Male	4251 (19.16%)
Female	17,930 (80.84%)
Age (years)	34.86 ± 11.70
Male Age (years)	34.47 ± 11.22
Female Age (years)	36.50 ± 13.41
	Total
Education level	
Basic education	15,154 (68.32%)
Higher education	7027 (31.68%)
Income level	
Low	9727 (43.85%)
Medium–high	10,616 (47.86%)
Don't know–no answer	1838 (8.29%)
Municipality	
<2000	1014 (4.57%)
2000–10,000	3587 (16.17%)
>10,000	17,580 (79.26%)

Of all the respondents, 79.22% (n = 17,573) claimed not to follow any diet, the other 16.19% (n = 3590) were divided between different dietary styles (vegetarian, vegan, raw, Weight Watchers, ketogenic, paleo, and others). Moreover, 4.59% (n = 1018) claimed to practice intermittent fasting.

The socio-demographic characteristics of the group practicing IF are shown in detail in Table 3. Out of this group, 235 respondents were men (23.08%) compared to 783 women (76.92%); the average age of those who practice IF was 36.78 years.

Table 3. Sample and their socio-demographic characteristics (n = 1018).

	Mean ± SD or n (%)
Men	235 (23.08%)
Women	783 (76.92%)
Age (years)	36.78 ± 10.71
Age men (years)	37.10 ± 10.79
Age women (years)	35.73 ± 10.38
	Total
Education level	
Basic education	724 (71.12%)
Higher education	294 (28.88%)
Income level	
Low	510 (50.10%)
Medium–high	446 (43.81%)
Don't know–no answer	62 (6.09%)
Municipality	
<2000	41 (4.06%)
2000–10,000	169 (16.74%)
>10,000	808 (80.00%)
BMI (Kg/m^2) (WHO *)	
Underweight (<18.5)	11 (1.08%)
Normal range (18.5–24.9)	687 (67.49%)
Overweight (25–29.9)	218 (21.41%)
Obesity (≥30)	102 (10.02%)

* World Health Organization.

Focusing on the intermittent fasters (n = 1018), a Principal Component Analysis (PCA) was conducted to reduce the dimensionality of the variables. The selection of the number of proper principal components is supported by the scree plot (Figure 1), which represents the percentage of explained variance alongside the number of dimensions and by the diagrams in Figure 2a,b which indicate the contribution of the variables in each of the dimensions. It is essential to comment that the dashed red line is the average of the explained variance of all the dimensions. In this study, we chose two components, explaining the 23.7% of the data variance, following the elbow method [40].

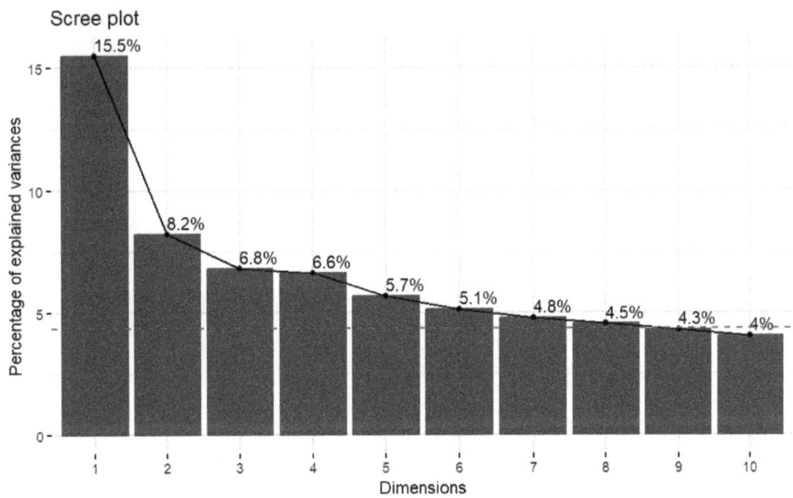

Figure 1. Scree plot of the PCA model.

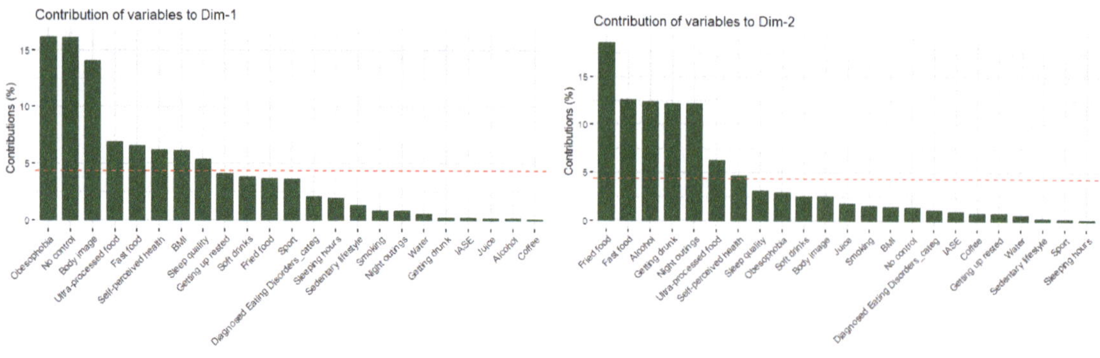

(a) **(b)**

Figure 2. (**a**) Contribution of the variables to the first dimension of the PCA model. Note: The red line indicates the average percentage of contribution if all the dimensions contribute the same. (**b**) Contribution of the variables to the second dimension of the PCA model. Note: The red line indicates the average percentage of contribution if all the dimensions contribute the same.

The variables that contribute the most to the PCA model are Obesophobia, No control and Body Image, for the first dimension (a), and Fried food and Fast food for the second dimension (b). This can also be observed in Figure 3, where these variables have a more reddish color than the rest of the variables.

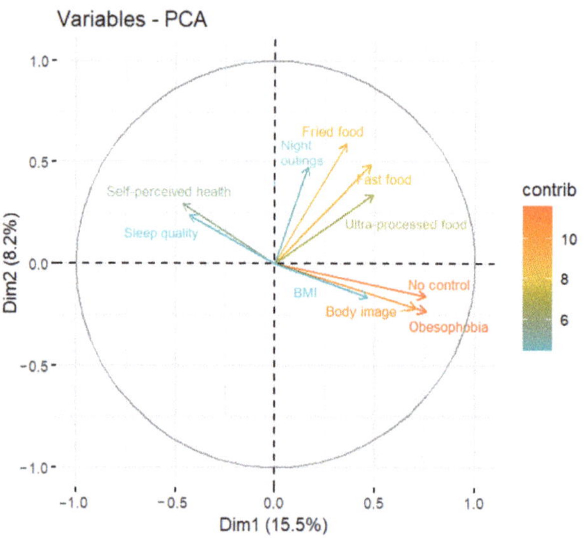

Figure 3. Variables plot of the PCA model. (Note: only the top ten variables contributing the most to the PCA model are represented.).

It is important to state that No control, Obesophobia, Body Image and BMI are highly correlated (the arrows are at 0°). Moreover, the first three variables contribute highly to the first dimension (the ones next to the horizontal line), which indicates that they capture most of the variance of the dataset. Therefore, the differences between individuals following IF are found in No control, Obesophobia, and Body Image. On the other hand, we could not observe any correlation between these variables and Fried food, Fast food or Night outings because the arrows are at a 90° angle. However, in our data, these three variables are positively correlated, indicating that respondents who usually consume fried and fast food are prone to go out at night. Finally, it was found that No control, Obesophobia, Body Image and BMI are negatively correlated with Sleep quality and Self-perceived health (the arrows are at a 180° angle). In other words, the participants with obesophobia, no control over their food intake or with body image concerns have worse self-perceived health or sleep quality than the ones who do not have these types of feelings.

If we represent the individuals who practice IF in the two dimensions of the PCA and color them by the different socio-demographic variables, we obtain the plots shown in Figures 4–6. Figure 4 shows the distribution of individuals divided into three age groups: young people (18–30 years old) in green, middle-aged adults (31–50 years old) in red and adults over 50 years old in blue.

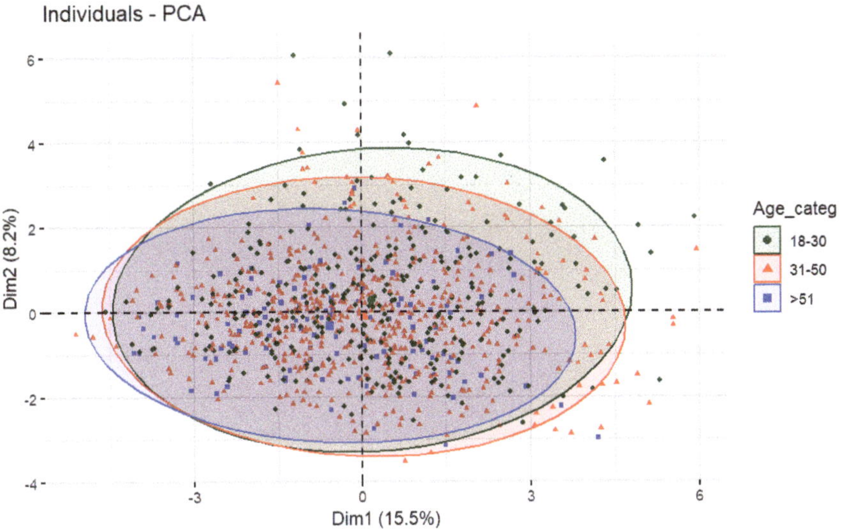

Figure 4. Individuals plot of the PCA model depending on age.

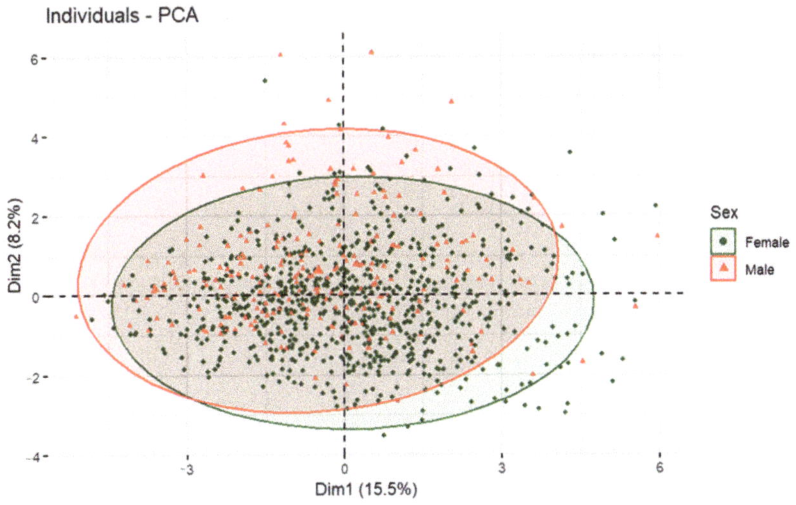

Figure 5. Individuals plot of the PCA model depending on sex.

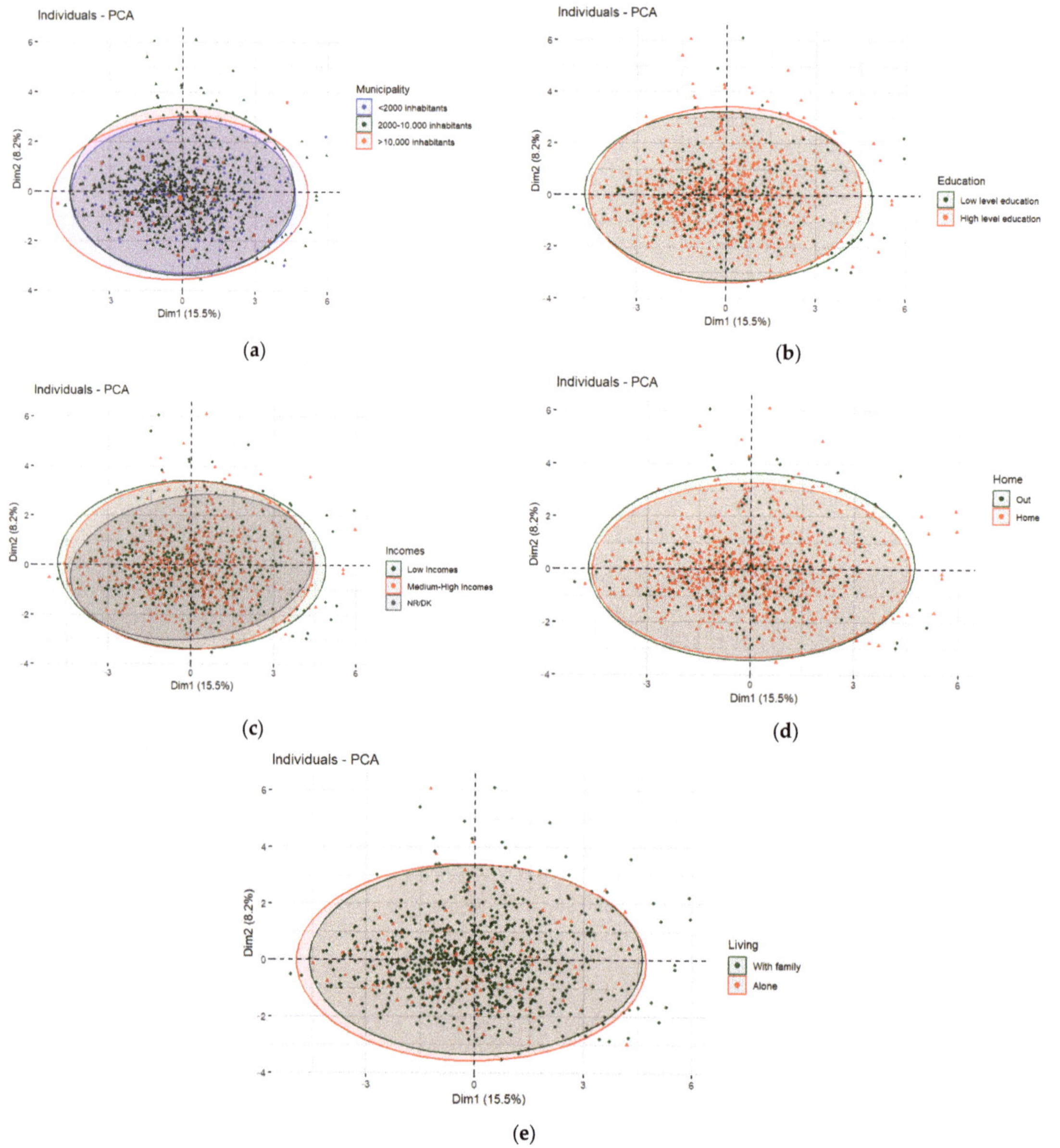

Figure 6. (**a**) Individuals plot of the PCA model depending on municipality. (**b**) Individuals plot of the PCA model depending on education. (**c**) Individuals plot of the PCA model depending on incomes. (**d**) Individuals plot of the PCA model depending on home. (**e**) Individuals plot of the PCA model depending on living.

In Figure 4, the ellipse representing young adults is displaced to the upper right side compared to the rest of the age groups. By overlapping Figures 3 and 4, we can determine that young adults tend to consume more fast, fried, and ultra-processed food and that they tend go out at night more frequently. Furthermore, as the blue ellipse (>51 years) presents less displacement on the lower right side, older adults might have fewer body image concerns and obesophobia and more control over their food intake.

This also can be observed in Table 4, which represents the health and lifestyle habits of the IF practitioners divided into the three age groups. Statistically significant differences can be seen in the frequency of weekly consumption of fried food between young and middle-aged people (2.06 vs. 1.93; $p = 0.03$) and between young and old people (2.06 vs. 1.78; $p < 0.001$). The same trend is observed for the consumption of fast food (Y = 2.28 vs. M = 2.18 and L = 1.74; *p*-value Y-L: <0.001; *p*-value M-L: <0.001), for the consumption of ultra-processed products (Y = 2.25 vs. M = 2.03 and L = 1.70; *p*-value Y-M: <0.001; *p*-value Y-L: <0.001; *p*-value M-L: <0.001) and for nightlife (Y = 1.28 vs. M = 1.09 and L = 1.07; *p*-value Y-L: <0.001; *p*-value M-L: <0.001).

Table 4. Health and lifestyle habits of the three age groups of the respondents who practice intermittent fasting.

Habits Variable	Young Adults (18–30 Years) Mean ± SD	Middle-Aged Adults (31–50 Years) Mean ± SD	Older Adults (>51 Years) Mean ± SD	*p*-Value **
BMI	23.51 ± 3.52	24.50 ± 4.37	24.29 ± 4.61	<0.001 Y-M: <0.001
Fried food	2.06 ± 0.76	1.93 ± 0.75	1.78 ± 0.71	<0.001 Y-M: 0.03 Y-L: 0.001
Fast food	2.28 ± 0.70	2.18 ± 0.75	1.74 ± 0.64	<0.001 Y-L: <0.001 M-L: <0.001
Ultra-processed food	2.25 ± 0.87	2.03 ± 0.88	1.70 ± 0.82	<0.001 Y-M: <0.001 Y-L: <0.001 M-L: <0.001
Self-perceived health	3.91 ± 0.74	3.85 ± 0.88	3.88 ± 0.85	0.84
Sleep quality	3.54 ± 0.92	3.41 ± 0.99	3.29 ± 0.90	0.03 Y-L: 0.04
Night outings	1.28 ± 0.49	1.09 ± 0.31	1.07 ± 0.28	<0.001 Y-L: <0.001 M-L: <0.001
Obesophobia	3.79 ± 1.51	3.68 ± 1.44	3.35 ± 1.42	0.02 Y-L: 0.02
No control	2.97 ± 1.31	2.96 ± 1.25	2.65 ± 1.12	0.05
Body image	4.01 ± 1.33	3.77 ± 1.31	3.54 ± 1.26	<0.001 Y-M: 0.02 Y-L: 0.001

** Kruskal–Wallis test with Hochberg correction.

Figure 5 shows the sample divided into men and women and colored accordingly. It is observed that the ellipse created by the answers of the masculine contestants (in red) is displaced to the upper left side, where Self-perceived health and Sleep quality are found. Therefore, we can conclude that men assigned themselves a higher self-perceived health punctuation and a better sleep quality than women. On the other hand, the ellipse created by the answers of the feminine contestants (in green) is displaced to the lower right side, where Obesophobia, No control, and Body Image are located (Figure 3). In a nutshell, females tend to have more concerns about their body image, gaining weight, and not having control over their food intake than men.

In Table 5, these results are expressed numerically, and the described relationships are confirmed by calculating the *p*-values using the Mann–Whitney test for the indicated variables.

Table 5. Health and lifestyle habits by sex of the respondents who practice intermittent fasting.

Numerical Variable	Woman Mean ± SD	Man Mean ± SD	*p*-Value ***
BMI	23.76 ± 4.19	25.41 ± 3.78	<0.001
Fried food	1.92 ± 0.75	2.06 ± 0.77	0.01
Fast food	2.12 ± 0.74	2.31 ± 0.74	<0.001
Ultra-processed food	2.07 ± 0.89	2.03 ± 0.87	0.52
Self-perceived health	3.80 ± 0.85	4.11 ± 0.72	<0.001
Sleep quality	3.39 ± 0.85	3.58 ± 0.72	0.004
Night outings	1.15 ± 0.39	1.16 ± 0.40	0.56
Obesophobia	3.89 ± 1.43	2.98 ± 1.38	<0.001
No control	3.07 ± 1.26	2.47 ± 1.15	<0.001
Body image	3.94 ± 1.29	3.44 ± 1.35	<0.001

*** Mann–Whitney test.

Figure 6 (a) shows the distribution of people following IF according to the size of the municipality of residence (blue < 2000 inhabitants; green 2000–10,000 inhabitants; red > 10,000 inhabitants), (b) according to the level of education (green: basic level of education; red: higher education), (c) by income level (green: low income; red: upper-middle income; gray: don't know–no answer), (d) by whether a person lives with (red) or without family (green) and (e) by whether the respondent lives alone (red) or not (green). The data indicate that none of these socio-demographic variables show any statistically significant differences in terms of the analyzed social and lifestyle habits.

Finally, Figure 7 shows the percentage of people practicing IF in each autonomous Spanish community. To find out between which regions statistically significant differences occur, Dunn's test was carried out, the results of which can be found in detail in Figure A1 of Appendix A. It was found that the practice of IF was highest in the region of Murcia and lowest in La Rioja.

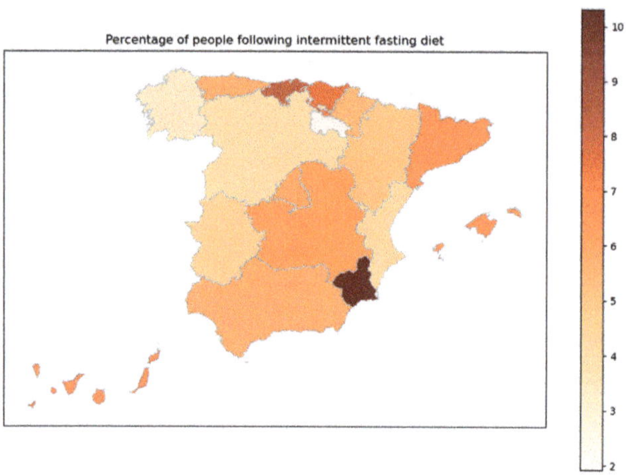

Figure 7. Percentage of people practicing intermittent fasting for each autonomous community in Spain.

4. Discussion

In our study, we explore lifestyle habits as well as health perceptions among a sample of Spanish adults following an IF diet to better understand the practice of this dietary approach. IF, as a highly intriguing clinical nutritional approach, is more and more recognized in our society not only for its health benefits [22,41–43] but also for the convenience of practicing it [44,45]. A growing popularity has been noticed as well as an increasing interest among the Spanish population, decreasing the interest in the Mediterranean diet [46]. Therefore, IF is currently postulated as a public health tool to prevent diseases and to improve quality of life.

First, it is essential to highlight the high level of people's engagement observed in this study. Participants exhibited remarkable interest toward the central topic, "nutritional and social habits". Of particular note is the predominance of female participants, who provide 80.84% (n = 17,930) of the data of the sample. This fact leads to an imbalance between the number of men and women who reported following an IF diet, with 783 women (76.92%) out of the total 1018 IF practitioners in our sample. This gender distribution may reflect either a heightened interest among women in diet interventions [17] or that men are less likely to participate in surveys [22,42,47]. An exception is presented in a study conducted on the Saudi population, which showed a slightly higher participation of men compared to women [21].

The results obtained from the PCA indicate that individuals who feel they lack control over the amount of food they consume, experience guilt, show fear of gaining weight, or who are concerned about their body shape are more likely to engage in intermittent fasting. Various studies have demonstrated that the concepts of guilt or control related to food impact consumers' eating behavior and, therefore, the choice of a specific diet and lifestyle [48,49]. Perceptions of guilt have the potential to lead consumers to seek healthier and more sustainable food solutions by positively influencing their food choices, eating behavior, purchasing decisions, and lifestyle [50]. Several authors have investigated the personal, social, and/or cultural motivations behind a consumer's choice of one diet over another; for example, in Finland [51], Australia [52], Germany [53] or in the USA [54], concluding that understanding the effect of control or guilt on food choices and eating behaviors could be significant in promoting healthy eating behaviors.

Furthermore, it has been observed that individuals experiencing obesophobia also exhibit concerns regarding their body image and opt for intermittent fasting as a dietary approach. Recent studies, such as the one carried out in Australia by Sutin et al. [55], indicate that people with a fear of gaining weight may experience weight-based discrimination, which can lead to unhealthy eating behaviors or dietary choices [56–58]. In this last case, IF is not advisable and would be contraindicated [16].

Regarding body image and its relationship with IF, a greater concern about body image is associated with a higher likelihood of engaging in IF behaviors. To explain this relationship, it is necessary to consider that body image is a complex and subjective construct that incorporates perceptions of size, satisfaction with appearance, attractiveness evaluation, and body control practices [59,60]. Available research conducted on a sample of Australian men and women suggests that a more tolerant and positive attitude toward body shape and size is associated with a lower likelihood of engaging in intermittent fasting behaviors [61], and individuals display less concern about weight changes and adopt positive health behaviors, as we see in studies with respondents from a variety of countries [62,63] or in one from with participants from Brazil [64]. The findings of other studies from the USA [65,66] or Spain [67] also indicate that concern about body weight control significantly influences a person's perception of their own body, as evidenced in this study.

Another important finding of the PCA is that fried and fast food consumption is not related to the behavioral variables Control, Obesophobia and Body Image, and vice versa. This means, for example, that the increase or decrease in fast food consumption of an IF practitioner does not provide information about the fear of gaining weight. Integrating fried or fast food into an IF diet is not advisable due to them typically containing high amounts of calories, fats, and refined sugars [68]. Regular consumption of these types of food can contribute to a variety of negative health outcomes, including cardiovascular diseases, type 2 diabetes, increased risk of obesity, and certain types of cancer, which is backed up by studies conducted both worldwide [69] and focusing on just one nation, such as Spain [70], Colombia [71] or the USA [72].

Hence, there is a need to address not only the nutritional implications but also the broader health consequences associated with these types of alimentation, making it necessary to identify the best strategy to reduce any negative impact their consumption may have on public health [73].

One final observation drawn from the PCA is that participants with a higher body weight report poorer self-perceived health and worse sleep quality than those with a normal weight. Our data indicate that 31.43% ($n = 320$) of the population practicing IF is overweight or obese, which implies, in addition to poorer self-perceived health, a greater fear of gaining weight [56] as well as poorer sleep quality, with reduced sleep hours, insomnia, sleep apnea, and daytime sleepiness. Evidence on this topic can be found in Brazil [74], the USA [75], Japan [76] and Greece [77]. However, as indicated in a Dutch clinical trial, IF can improve sleep through interfering with circadian rhythms [78] or by reducing body weight, as shown in some studies carried out in the USA [79–81].

Regarding age, it is known that younger individuals have a lower BMI than older adults, a trend also observed in studies from other countries; for example, in the USA [82,83] or Norway [84]. However, losing and maintaining a healthy weight is a primary concern for people of all age groups [42], as evidenced in our study by observing that the mean BMI in all the age groups is lower than 25, which indicates a healthy weight. On the other hand, older adults report lower consumption of fried food, fast food, and ultra-processed food than young adults or middle-aged adults. Age is a factor that can influence food choices [85,86], but it is not the only one. There is a great body of evidence indicating that food preferences change throughout life due to various factors such as sensory characteristics (texture, taste, smell) and perceptual features (color, size, quality) of foods [87–90], social environment [91], psychological characteristics [92] physiological needs [93], habits [94], and cognitive factors (nutrition knowledge, skills, attitudes, tastes, and preferences) [95].

Young people who practice IF report better sleep quality than older adults. In a study by McStay et al. [96] in the USA, it is indicated that the effects of IF on sleep quality are uncertain because it is necessary to consider whether there is an underlying problem such as sleep apnea or insomnia. However, existing evidence from Italy indicates that aging influences in the structure and quality of sleep [97].

Lastly, regarding age, it is interesting to mention that the fear of gaining weight or the concern about body shapes affects young people who practice IF significantly more. The literature shows that these concerns can occur in any age group [98]. However, in young adults, social pressure, beauty standards, and the influence of the media can contribute to a greater concern about body image and fear of gaining weight [99,100], potentially leading to restrictive diets or excessive exercise. Conversely, in older adults, although concern about body image may still be relevant, priorities shift with ageing, with health and overall well-being becoming more important [17].

If we reflect on the health and lifestyle habits by gender of the surveyed individuals practicing IF, in our study, women have a lower BMI, consume fewer fried and fast foods, report poorer sleep quality, and also perceive their health as poorer. In contrast, men feel as if they have less control over the amount of food they consume, less fear of gaining weight, and are less concerned about their body image. According to data from the Informe Anual del Sistema Nacional de Salud 2022 [101], men (79.3%) report a better health status than women (71.9%), a pattern observed in our study of the IF practitioners, too. The same report states that obesity in Spain affects 16.0% of the population aged 18 and over (16.5% men and 15.5% women). In the existing literature, overweight or obese individuals experience more fear of gaining weight than underweight or normal weight participants [56], with women again reporting more fear of gaining weight, which indicates more concern about weight [102].

Regarding sleep problems, Spanish women report greater difficulties falling asleep and waking up multiple times at night [103]. Moreover, some studies worldwide [104,105] have found that men are significantly less dissatisfied with their bodies compared to women. Others, on the contrary, such as the study by Millstein et al. in the USA [106], inform that an important percentage of women are satisfied with their appearance and have a positive judgement of excess weight.

In this study, the size of the municipality of residence, the level of education, the income level, if the individual is living with family or not and if the individual is living alone or with other people were not found to have a significant association with the habits followed by those who practice IF. However, we discovered the following observations in other papers. In rural areas with smaller populations, there are indications of certain problems with optimal dietary intake or reports of barriers to accessing certain foods [107]. Individuals with higher income levels can access healthier food and maintain better nutrition [108]. They also have a lower BMI, according to the Encuesta Nacional de Salud de España [109]. This same survey also indicates that a higher level of education is associated with a lower BMI, implying greater awareness of the importance of a balanced diet and the potential health risks associated with incorrect or inadequate nutrition [108]. Moreover, it has been observed that living alone or in an arrangement without family connections influences some nutritional patterns and health habits [110], with individuals living with family having a higher BMI than those living elsewhere [111].

Regarding the percentage of people practicing intermittent fasting for each autonomous community in Spain, the results seem to indicate that there is no clear pattern. A higher adherence to this type of diet is observed in the region of Murcia and, on the contrary, a lower use of the diet is observed among the population of La Rioja, but this difference is not statically significant, it just marks a slight trend. Nevertheless, a possible explanation for this, as indicated in the Informe del Consumo Alimentario en España 2021 [112], is that in the northern regions of the country such as the northwest and north center, meals are more often consumed outside of the individual's own living space compared to the national average, while the Levante region has a higher number of meals consumed at home. The report also indicates that the region of Murcia exceeds the national average of the per capita consumption of meals outside of home by the end of 2021. Conversely, La Rioja is the autonomous community with the lowest per capita consumption. In La Rioja, more olive oil, wine, meat, fish, milk and derivatives, and bread are consumed than in Murcia. On the other hand, in Murcia, more rice (with consumption higher than the national average), cereals, fresh fruits and vegetables, eggs, and legumes are consumed. The more frequent consumption of olive oil, wine, meat, fish, milk and derivatives, as well as bread, could be influenced by the local gastronomic tradition in La Rioja, as well as by the natural resources available there, such as olive groves and vineyards.

In contrast, the greater consumption of rice, cereals, fresh fruits and vegetables, eggs, and legumes in Murcia suggests a more varied diet in terms of agricultural products. Murcia is known for its intensive agriculture and its climate benefits the cultivation of a wide variety of fruits, vegetables, and cereals, which may influence the dietary preferences of the population. All these presented statements about regional food consumption may not only be influenced by local preferences but also by the climatic conditions and the availability of products in each region. Therefore, we can see how cultural, geographical, and economic factors might influence the dietary habits of a community.

Statistically significant differences in the IF practitioners are observed when comparing the regions of Valencian Community and Catalonia, Valencian Community and Murcia, Castile/León and Murcia, and Galicia and Murcia. According to the latest data published by the Instituto Nacional de Estadística in 2024 [113], the highest percentage of young adults and middle-aged adults in these autonomous communities is found in the region of Murcia, with 18.88% and 36.96% respectively. In contrast, the lowest percentage of the older adult population is also found in the Region de Murcia, with 44.16%. These official data are consistent with the results obtained in this study, where we can observe that those communities with a higher proportion of young individuals show a greater interest in the IF model.

Strengths and Limitations

The main strength of this study is that we could verify the influence of lifestyle and health habits on the population practicing the IF model, which can aid in the creation of public health programs that support and promote the controlled use of this type of diet to ensure the physical and psychological well-being of the population, avoiding harmful eating habits and sedentary lifestyles. Another undeniable strength of this study is the extensive sample size, encompassing diverse demographics in terms of age, education, and income levels. Furthermore, geographical representation across all the regions of Spain ensures a comprehensive understanding of the health status, as well as nutritional and lifestyle habits, of the entire Spanish population. This breadth of diversity enhances the reliability and robustness of the study's findings.

One limitation of the study is that we investigated people who practice IF and the relationship with lifestyle and health habits, but we did not study the type of IF or duration and frequency of IF. Future research could explore these dimensions, including both the length and regularity of IF behaviors, to achieve a more comprehensive understanding of this phenomenon.

Another limitation to highlight is that the data collection was based on self-reported data to evaluate the association between IF and lifestyle and health habits. Consequently, these data cannot be independently verified, so we cannot totally exclude biases such as selective memory, exaggeration, or attribution. Future research should consider the use of objective measurement tools to validate the research results, thus promoting the accuracy of the results.

The last weakness of this study is attributed to the sampling method employed, primarily utilizing snowball sampling and prevalent dissemination through social media. While snowball sampling facilitates reaching a wide array of responses, it carries the risk of self-selection bias, as the sample composition depends on initial participants recommending additional participants. In social networks, influencers play a significant role in disseminating content related to specific topics, attracting followers who often share similar interests and behaviors. It is plausible that the survey reached some of these communities through influencers, potentially also influencing respondents' behaviors and preferences. To minimize this bias, a major effort has been made to also disseminate the questionnaire outside the social networks, as described above.

5. Conclusions

The intermittent fasting diet offers a wide array of health benefits for various conditions, like obesity, diabetes mellitus, cardiovascular diseases, cancer, and neurological disorders. However, it is essential to note that this dietary approach is not suitable for all individuals. It is necessary to individualize it to obtain better health results without suffering unnecessary risks.

Therefore, it is important to understand how intermittent fasting relates to other determinants such as a person's lifestyle and their socio-demographic variables.

In the present study, the PCA highlights that the main variables in which the individuals following an intermittent diet are different from each other are Lack of Control, Obesophobia, and Body Image. Additionally, respondents with obesophobia, lack of control over food intake, or concerns about body image reported worse self-perceived health and sleep quality compared to those without such concerns.

Regarding age, younger individuals tend to consume more fast food, fried foods, and ultra-processed foods, and they go out at night more frequently. In contrast, older adults seem to have fewer body image concerns, less obesophobia, and more control over their food intake.

As for gender, men reported a higher self-perceived health scores and better sleep quality than women. Women tend to have more concerns about their body image, weight gain, and lack of control over food intake.

Socio-demographic variables such as the size of the municipality of residence, education level, income level, living alone or with others, and living with family or independently did not show statistically significant differences concerning the habits followed.

Finally, regarding the geographic region of residence, it was found that the practice of intermittent fasting was more common in the region of Murcia and less common in La Rioja.

The results obtained are a starting point for understanding the interaction between intermittent fasting, lifestyle habits and socio-demographic variables in the Spanish population. Although this information needs to be further expanded and extrapolated to other populations, this understanding may help to design more effective public health and preventive strategies.

Author Contributions: E.S.: Conceptualization, data curation, investigation, methodology, validation, writing—original draft, writing—review and editing. D.B.: Data curation, formal analysis, writing—review and editing. E.C.L.: Data curation, formal analysis, visualization, writing—review and editing. G.C.O.: Conceptualization, investigation, methodology, writing—review and editing. M.J.V.-B.: Writing—review and editing. V.B.M.: Writing—original draft, writing—review and editing. All authors approved the final manuscript. All authors have read and agreed to the published version of the manuscript.

Funding: This research work has been funded by the Catholic University of Valencia San Vicente Martir.

Institutional Review Board Statement: This research strictly followed ethical principles outlined in the Declaration of Helsinki and received approval from the Ethics Research Committee of the Catholic University of Valencia (approval code UCV/2019-2020/152, date of approval, 18 June 2020). Prior to participating, explicit informed consent was obtained from all individuals, ensuring they were fully informed about the study's objectives, procedures, and potential risks, and emphasizing the voluntary nature of their participation.

Informed Consent Statement: Informed consent was obtained from all the subjects involved in the study.

Data Availability Statement: The data presented in this study are available upon reasonable request from the corresponding author. The data are not publicly available due to privacy.

Acknowledgments: The authors sincerely appreciate the collaboration of all the individuals who contributed to this research. Special thanks to those who played a role in sharing the questionnaire and to those who devoted their time to participate in and provide responses to the survey. The authors would also like to thank the Universidad Católica de Valencia San Vicente Martir for the support in paying for publication in the open-access journal.

Conflicts of Interest: None of the authors had any financial, personal or professional conflicts of interest in relation to the results of this study.

Appendix A

Figure A1 shows the results of the Dunn's test performed for each region of Spain with respect to the percentage of people following the intermittent fasting diet. The p-values < 0.001 indicate that statistically significant differences in the practice of this type of diet are found between these two regions of Spain.

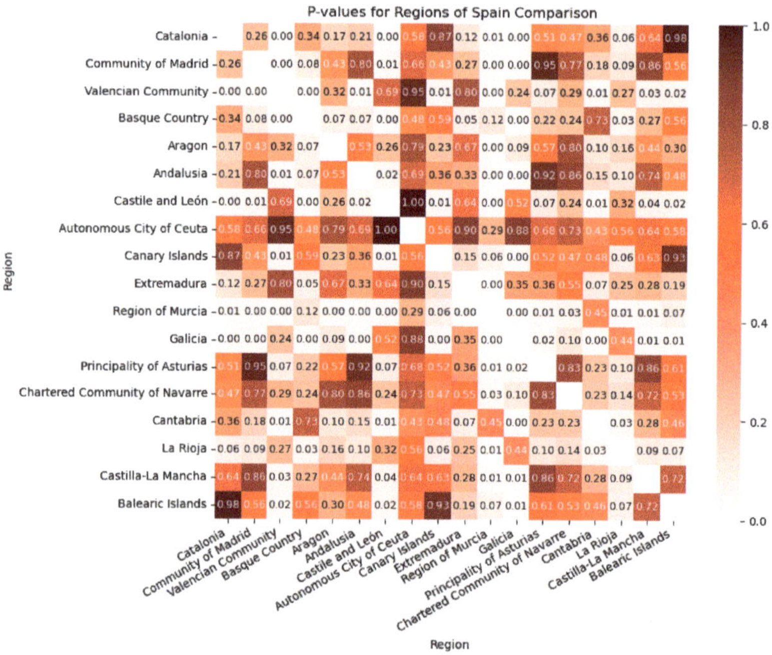

Figure A1. Dunn's test of the percentage of intermittent fasting practice for each region of Spain.

References

1. Patterson, R.E.; Sears, D.D. Metabolic effects of intermittent fasting. *Annu. Rev. Nutr.* **2017**, *37*, 371–393. [CrossRef]
2. Nowosad, K.; Sujka, M. Effect of Various Types of Intermittent Fasting (IF) on Weight Loss and Improvement of Diabetic Parameters in Human. *Curr. Nutr. Rep.* **2021**, *10*, 146–154. [CrossRef]
3. Anton, S.D.; Moehl, K.; Donahoo, W.T.; Marosi, K.; Lee, S.A.; Mainous, A.G.; Leeuwenburgh, C.; Mattson, M.P. Flipping the Metabolic Switch: Understanding and Applying the Health Benefits of Fasting. *Obesity* **2018**, *26*, 254–268. [CrossRef]
4. Vasim, I.; Majeed, C.N.; DeBoer, M.D. Intermittent Fasting and Metabolic Health. *Nutrients* **2022**, *14*, 631. [CrossRef]
5. Kerndt, P.R.; Naughton, J.L.; Driscoll, C.E.; Loxterkamp, D.A. Fasting: The history, pathophysiology and complications. *West. J. Med.* **1982**, *137*, 379–399.
6. Welton, S.; Minty, R.; O'Driscoll, T.; Willms, H.; Poirier, D.; Madden, S.; Kelly, L. Intermittent fasting and weight loss: Systematic review. *Can. Fam. Physician* **2020**, *66*, 117–125.
7. Yuan, X.; Wang, J.; Yang, S.; Gao, M.; Cao, L.; Li, X.; Hong, D.; Tian, S.; Sun, C. Effect of Intermittent Fasting Diet on Glucose and Lipid Metabolism and Insulin Resistance in Patients with Impaired Glucose and Lipid Metabolism: A Systematic Review and Meta-Analysis. *Int. J. Endocrinol.* **2022**, *2022*, 6999907. [CrossRef] [PubMed]
8. Varady, K.A.; Cienfuegos, S.; Ezpeleta, M.; Gabel, K. Cardiometabolic Benefits of Intermittent Fasting. *Annu. Rev. Nutr.* **2021**, *41*, 333–361. [CrossRef] [PubMed]
9. Gudden, J.; Arias Vasquez, A.; Bloemendaal, M. The Effects of Intermittent Fasting on Brain and Cognitive Function. *Nutrients* **2021**, *13*, 3166. [CrossRef]
10. Longo, V.D.; Di Tano, M.; Mattson, M.P.; Guidi, N. Intermittent and periodic fasting, longevity and disease. *Nat. Aging* **2021**, *1*, 47–59. [CrossRef]
11. Kaufman, M.; Nguyen, C.; Shetty, M.; Oppezzo, M.; Barrack, M.; Fredericson, M. Popular Dietary Trends' Impact on Athletic Performance: A Critical Analysis Review. *Nutrients* **2023**, *15*, 3511. [CrossRef] [PubMed]
12. Beshyah, S.A.; Hassanein, M.; Ahmedani, M.Y.; Shaikh, S.; Ba-Essa, E.M.; Megallaa, M.H.; Afandi, B.; Ibrahim, F.; Al-Muzaffar, T. Diabetic hypoglycaemia during Ramadan fasting: A trans-national observational real-world study. *Diabetes Res. Clin. Pract.* **2019**, *150*, 315–321. [CrossRef] [PubMed]
13. Dardano, A.; Penno, G.; Del Prato, S.; Miccoli, R. Optimal therapy of type 2 diabetes: A controversial challenge. *Aging* **2014**, *6*, 187–206. [CrossRef] [PubMed]
14. de Cabo, R.; Mattson, M.P. Effects of Intermittent Fasting on Health, Aging, and Disease. *N. Engl. J. Med.* **2019**, *381*, 2541–2551. [CrossRef]

15. Soliman, G.A. Intermittent fasting and time-restricted eating role in dietary interventions and precision nutrition. *Front. Public Health* **2022**, *10*, 1017254. [CrossRef]
16. Blumberg, J.; Hahn, S.L.; Bakke, J. Intermittent fasting: Consider the risks of disordered eating for your patient. *Clin. Diabetes Endocrinol.* **2023**, *9*, 4. [CrossRef] [PubMed]
17. Anton, S.; Ezzati, A.; Witt, D.; McLaren, C.; Vial, P. The effects of intermittent fasting regimens in middle-age and older adults: Current state of evidence. *Exp. Gerontol.* **2021**, *156*, 111617. [CrossRef]
18. Oviedo-Solís, C.I.; Hernández-Alcaraz, C.; Sánchez-Ortíz, N.A.; López-Olmedo, N.; Jáuregui, A.; Barquera, S. Association of sociodemographic and lifestyle factors with dietary patterns among men and women living in Mexico City: A cross-sectional study. *Front. Public Health* **2022**, *10*, 859132. [CrossRef]
19. de Juras, A.R.; Hsu, W.C.; Hu, S.C. Dietary Patterns and Their Association with Sociodemographic and Lifestyle Factors in Filipino Adults. *Nutrients* **2022**, *14*, 886. [CrossRef]
20. Beck, K.L.; Jones, B.; Ullah, I.; McNaughton, S.A.; Haslett, S.J.; Stonehouse, W. Associations between dietary patterns, socio-demographic factors and anthropometric measurements in adult New Zealanders: An analysis of data from the 2008/09 New Zealand Adult Nutrition Survey. *Eur. J. Nutr.* **2018**, *57*, 1421–1433. [CrossRef]
21. Shalabi, H.; Hassan, A.S., IV; Al-Zahrani, F.A.; Alarbeidi, A.H.; Mesawa, M.; Rizk, H.; Aljubayri, A.A. Intermittent Fasting: Benefits, Side Effects, Quality of Life, and Knowledge of the Saudi Population. *Cureus* **2023**, *15*, e34722. [CrossRef] [PubMed]
22. Alnasser, A.; Almutairi, M. Considering intermittent fasting among Saudis: Insights into practices. *BMC Public Health* **2022**, *22*, 592. [CrossRef] [PubMed]
23. Bärebring, L.; Winkvist, A.; Augustin, H. Sociodemographic factors associated with reported attempts at weight loss and specific dietary regimens in Sweden: The SWEDIET-2017 study. *PLoS ONE* **2018**, *13*, e0197099. [CrossRef] [PubMed]
24. Tucker, J.M.; Siegel, R.; Murray, P.J.; Han, J.C.; Boyer, K.; Reed, N.; Allenby, T.; Novick, M. Acceptability of Time-Limited Eating in Pediatric Weight Management. *Front. Endocrinol.* **2022**, *13*, 811489. [CrossRef] [PubMed]
25. Ooi, T.C.; Meramat, A.; Rajab, N.F.; Shahar, S.; Ismail, I.S.; Azam, A.A.; Sharif, R. Intermittent Fasting Enhanced the Cognitive Function in Older Adults with Mild Cognitive Impairment by Inducing Biochemical and Metabolic changes: A 3-Year Progressive Study. *Nutrients* **2020**, *12*, 2644. [CrossRef] [PubMed]
26. Cuccolo, K.; Kramer, R.; Petros, T.; Thoennes, M. Intermittent fasting implementation and association with eating disorder symptomatology. *Eat. Disord.* **2022**, *30*, 471–491. [CrossRef]
27. Murta, L.; Seixas, D.; Harada, L.; Damiano, R.F.; Zanetti, M. Intermittent Fasting as a Potential Therapeutic Instrument for Major Depression Disorder: A Systematic Review of Clinical and Preclinical Studies. *Int. J. Mol. Sci.* **2023**, *24*, 15551. [CrossRef]
28. Farhud, D.D. Impact of Lifestyle on Health. *Iran. J. Public Health* **2015**, *44*, 1442–1444.
29. Kinoshita, S.; Hirooka, N.; Kusano, T.; Saito, K.; Nakamoto, H. Does Improvement in Health-Related Lifestyle Habits Increase Purpose in Life among a Health Literate Cohort? *Int. J. Environ. Res. Public Health* **2020**, *17*, 8878. [CrossRef]
30. Mizia, S.; Felińczak, A.; Włodarek, D.; Syrkiewicz-Świtała, M. Evaluation of Eating Habits and Their Impact on Health among Adolescents and Young Adults: A Cross-Sectional Study. *Int. J. Environ. Res. Public Health* **2021**, *18*, 3996. [CrossRef]
31. Gherasim, A.; Arhire, L.I.; Niță, O.; Popa, A.D.; Graur, M.; Mihalache, L. The relationship between lifestyle components and dietary patterns. *Proc. Nutr. Soc.* **2020**, *79*, 311–323. [CrossRef] [PubMed]
32. World Medical Association Declaration of Helsinki. Ethical Principles for Medical Research Involving Human Subjects. *JAMA* **2013**, *310*, 2191–2194. [CrossRef] [PubMed]
33. Sandri, E.; Piredda, M.; De Maria, M.; Mancin, S.; Sguanci, M.; Cabo, A.; Olmedo, G.C. Development and psychometric testing of the nutritional and social health habits scale (NutSo-HH): A methodological review of existing tools. *MethodsX* **2024**, *12*, 102768. [CrossRef] [PubMed]
34. Biernacki, P.; Waldorf, D. Snowball Sampling: Problems and Techniques of Chain Referral Sampling. *Sociol. Methods Res.* **1981**, *10*, 141–163. [CrossRef]
35. Norte Navarro, A.I.; Ortiz Moncada, R. Spanish diet quality according to the healthy eating index. *Nutr. Hosp.* **2011**, *26*, 330–336. [PubMed]
36. Grupo Colaborativo de la Sociedad Española de Nutrición Comunitaria (SENC). Guías alimentarias para la población española; la nueva pirámide de la alimentación saludable. *Nutr. Hosp.* **2016**, *33*, 1–48.
37. Benjamini, Y.; Hochberg, Y. Controlling the False Discovery Rate: A Practical and Powerful Approach to Multiple Testing. *J. R. Stat. Soc. B* **1995**, *57*, 289–300. [CrossRef]
38. Pearson, K. LIII. On lines and planes of closest fit to systems of points in space. *Lond. Edinb. Dublin Philos. J. Sci.* **1901**, *2*, 559–572. [CrossRef]
39. RStudio Team. RStudio: Integrated development for R. In *RStudio*; PBC: Boston, MA, USA, 2020.
40. Thorndike, R.L. Who belongs in the family? *Psychometrika* **1953**, *18*, 267–276. [CrossRef]
41. Wilhelmi de Toledo, F.; Grundler, F.; Sirtori, C.R.; Ruscica, M. Unravelling the health effects of fasting: A long road from obesity treatment to healthy life span increase and improved cognition. *Ann. Med.* **2020**, *52*, 147–161. [CrossRef]
42. Dairi, G.; Alafghani, R.; Ghafouri, K.; Noorwali, E. Effect of Intermittent Fasting on Body Image Satisfaction and Appreciation Among Saudi Adults. *Cureus* **2023**, *15*, e33468. [CrossRef]

43. Catenacci, V.A.; Pan, Z.; Ostendorf, D.; Brannon, S.; Gozansky, W.S.; Mattson, M.P.; Martin, B.; MacLean, P.S.; Melanson, E.L.; Troy Donahoo, W. A randomized pilot study comparing zero-calorie alternate-day fasting to daily caloric restriction in adults with obesity. *Obesity* **2016**, *24*, 1874–1883. [CrossRef]
44. Martínez-Pina, P.P. *Ayuno intermitente. Revisión bibliográfica sobre su efecto en la salud cardiometabólica y en la pérdida de peso*; Revista Univ Oberta Catalunya: Barcelona, Spain, 2019.
45. Horne, B.D.; Muhlestein, J.B.; Anderson, J.L. Health effects of intermittent fasting: Hormesis or harm? A systematic review. *Am. J. Clin. Nutr.* **2015**, *102*, 464–470. [CrossRef]
46. Modrego-Pardo, I.; Solá-Izquierdo, E.; Morillas-Ariño, C. Spanish population trends in Internet searches for information on different diets. *Endocrinol. Diabetes Nutr. (Engl. Ed.)* **2020**, *67*, 431–437. [CrossRef]
47. Singer, E.; Van Hoewyk, J.; Maher, M.P. Experiments with incentives in telephone surveys. *Public Opin. Q.* **2000**, *64*, 171–188. [CrossRef] [PubMed]
48. Gibson, E.L. Emotional influences on food choice: Sensory, physiological and psychological pathways. *Physiol. Behav.* **2006**, *89*, 53–61. [CrossRef] [PubMed]
49. Köster, E.P. Diversity in the determinants of food choice: A psychological perspective. *Food Qual. Prefer.* **2009**, *20*, 70–82. [CrossRef]
50. Yu, H.; Chambers, E.I.V.; Koppel, K. Exploration of the food-related guilt concept. *J. Sens. Stud.* **2021**, *36*, e12622. [CrossRef]
51. Lindeman, M.; Väänänen, M. Measurement of ethical food choice motives. *Appetite* **2000**, *34*, 55–59. [CrossRef] [PubMed]
52. Hardcastle, S.J.; Thøgersen-Ntoumani, C.; Chatzisarantis, N.L. Food Choice and Nutrition: A Social Psychological Perspective. *Nutrients* **2015**, *7*, 8712–8715. [CrossRef] [PubMed]
53. Renner, B.; Sproesser, G.; Strohbach, S.; Schupp, H.T. Why we eat what we eat. The Eating Motivation Survey (TEMS). *Appetite* **2012**, *59*, 117–128. [CrossRef] [PubMed]
54. Phan, U.T.X.; Chambers, E., IV. Application of An Eating Motivation Survey to Study Eating Occasions. *J. Sens. Stud.* **2016**, *31*, 114–123. [CrossRef]
55. Sutin, A.R.; Stephan, Y.; Robinson, E.; Daly, M.; Terracciano, A. Body-related discrimination and dieting and substance use behaviors in adolescence. *Appetite* **2020**, *151*, 104689. [CrossRef] [PubMed]
56. Macho, S.; Andrés, A.; Saldaña, C. Anti-fat attitudes among Spanish general population: Psychometric properties of the anti-fat attitudes scale. *Clin. Obes.* **2022**, *12*, e12543. [CrossRef] [PubMed]
57. Puhl, R.; Suh, Y. Health Consequences of Weight Stigma: Implications for Obesity Prevention and Treatment. *Curr. Obes. Rep.* **2015**, *4*, 182–190. [CrossRef]
58. Wott, C.B.; Carels, R.A. Overt weight stigma, psychological distress and weight loss treatment outcomes. *J. Health Psychol.* **2010**, *15*, 608–614. [CrossRef] [PubMed]
59. Cash, T.; Smolak, L. *Body Image: A Handbook of Science, Practice, and Prevention*, 2nd ed.; Guilford Press: New York, NY, USA, 2011.
60. Grogan, S. *Body Image: Understanding Body Dissatisfaction in Men, Women, and Children*, 3rd ed.; Routledge: London, UK, 2017.
61. Lonergan, A.R.; Bussey, K.; Mond, J.; Brown, O.; Griffiths, S.; Murray, S.B.; Mitchison, D. Me, my selfie, and I: The relationship between editing and posting selfies and body dissatisfaction in men and women. *Body Image* **2019**, *28*, 39–43. [CrossRef] [PubMed]
62. Rynders, C.A.; Thomas, E.A.; Zaman, A.; Pan, Z.; Catenacci, V.A.; Melanson, E.L. Effectiveness of Intermittent Fasting and Time-Restricted Feeding Compared to Continuous Energy Restriction for Weight Loss. *Nutrients* **2019**, *11*, 2442. [CrossRef] [PubMed]
63. Stockman, M.C.; Thomas, D.; Burke, J.; Apovian, C.M. Intermittent Fasting: Is the Wait Worth the Weight? *Curr. Obes. Rep.* **2018**, *7*, 172–185. [CrossRef]
64. Santos, H.O.; Macedo, R.C.O. Impact of intermittent fasting on the lipid profile: Assessment associated with diet and weight loss. *Clin. Nutr. ESPEN.* **2018**, *24*, 14–21. [CrossRef]
65. Wu, Y.K.; Berry, D.C. Impact of weight stigma on physiological and psychological health outcomes for overweight and obese adults: A systematic review. *J. Adv. Nurs.* **2018**, *74*, 1030–1042. [CrossRef] [PubMed]
66. Friedman, K.E.; Reichmann, S.K.; Costanzo, P.R.; Zelli, A.; Ashmore, J.A.; Musante, G.J. Weight stigmatization and ideological beliefs: Relation to psychological functioning in obese adults. *Obes. Res.* **2005**, *13*, 907–916. [CrossRef] [PubMed]
67. Godoy-Izquierdo, D.; González-Hernández, J.; Lara, R.; Rodríguez-Tadeo, A.; Ramírez, M.J.; Navarrón, E.; Ogallar-Blanco, A.; López-Mora, C.; Arbinaga, F. Considering BMI, Body Image and Desired Weight Change for Suitable Obesity Management Options. *Span. J. Psychol.* **2020**, *23*, e35. [CrossRef] [PubMed]
68. Maldonado-Pereira, L.; Barnaba, C.; de Los Campos, G.; Medina-Meza, I.G. Evaluation of the Nutritional Quality of Ultra-Processed Foods (Ready to Eat + Fast Food): Fatty Acids, Sugar, and Sodium. *J. Food Sci.* **2022**, *87*, 3659–3676. [CrossRef] [PubMed]
69. Sandri, E.; Cantín Larumbe, E.; Cerdá Olmedo, G. The Influence of Socio-Economic Factors on Diet and Active Lifestyle in the Spanish Female Population. *Nutrients* **2023**, *15*, 3319. [CrossRef] [PubMed]
70. GBD 2017 Risk Factor Collaborators. Global, regional, and national comparative risk assessment of 84 behavioural, environmental and occupational, and metabolic risks or clusters of risks for 195 countries and territories, 1990–2017: A systematic analysis for the Global Burden of Disease Study 2017. *Lancet* **2018**, *392*, 1923–1994.
71. Pardo Escallón, J.C.; Pardo Beltrán, S.A. Evaluación nutricional del menú infantil ofrecido en servicios de comida rápida mediante análisis cuantitativo: Un estudio de corte transversal. *Rev. Nutr. Clín. Metab.* **2021**, *4*, 4–14. [CrossRef]

72. Oliva Chávez, O.H.; Fragoso Díaz, S. Consumo de comida rápida y obesidad, el poder de la buena alimentación en la salud. *RIDE Rev. Iberoam. Para Investig. Desarro. Educ.* **2015**, *4*, 176. [CrossRef]
73. Bauer, K.W.; Hearst, M.O.; Earnest, A.A.; French, S.A.; Oakes, J.M.; Harnack, L.J. Energy content of U.S. fast-food restaurant offerings: 14-year trends. *Am. J. Prev. Med.* **2012**, *43*, 490–497. [CrossRef]
74. Zimberg, I.Z.; Dâmaso, A.; Del Re, M.; Carneiro, A.M.; de Sá Souza, H.; de Lira, F.S.; Tufik, S.; de Mello, M.T. Short sleep duration and obesity: Mechanisms and future perspectives. *Cell Biochem. Funct.* **2012**, *30*, 524–529. [CrossRef]
75. Hoddy, K.K.; Potts, K.S.; Bazzano, L.A.; Kirwan, J.P. Sleep Extension: A Potential Target for Obesity Treatment. *Curr. Diabetes Rep.* **2020**, *20*, 81. [CrossRef] [PubMed]
76. Sawamoto, R.; Nozaki, T.; Furukawa, T.; Tanahashi, T.; Morita, C.; Hata, T.; Komaki, G.; Sudo, N. Higher sleep fragmentation predicts a lower magnitude of weight loss in overweight and obese women participating in a weight-loss intervention. *Nutr. Diabetes* **2014**, *4*, e144. [CrossRef] [PubMed]
77. Yannakoulia, M.; Anastasiou, C.A.; Karfopoulou, E.; Pehlivanidis, A.; Panagiotakos, D.B.; Vgontzas, A. Sleep quality is associated with weight loss maintenance status: The MedWeight study. *Sleep Med.* **2017**, *34*, 242–245. [CrossRef] [PubMed]
78. Verhoef, S.P.; Camps, S.G.; Gonnissen, H.K.; Westerterp, K.R.; Westerterp-Plantenga, M.S. Concomitant changes in sleep duration and body weight and body composition during weight loss and 3-mo weight maintenance. *Am. J. Clin. Nutr.* **2013**, *98*, 25–31. [CrossRef] [PubMed]
79. Martin, C.K.; Bhapkar, M.; Pittas, A.G.; Pieper, C.F.; Das, S.K.; Williamson, D.A.; Scott, T.; Redman, L.M.; Stein, R.; Gilhooly, C.H.; et al. Effect of Calorie Restriction on Mood, Quality of Life, Sleep, and Sexual Function in Healthy Nonobese Adults: The CALERIE 2 Randomized Clinical Trial. *JAMA Intern. Med.* **2016**, *176*, 743–752. [CrossRef] [PubMed]
80. St-Onge, M.P.; Shechter, A. Sleep disturbances, body fat distribution, food intake and/or energy expenditure: Pathophysiological aspects. *Horm. Mol. Biol. Clin. Investig.* **2014**, *17*, 29–37. [CrossRef] [PubMed]
81. Alfaris, N.; Wadden, T.A.; Sarwer, D.B.; Diwald, L.; Volger, S.; Hong, P.; Baxely, A.; Minnick, A.M.; Vetter, M.L.; Berkowitz, R.I.; et al. Effects of a 2-year behavioral weight loss intervention on sleep and mood in obese individuals treated in primary care practice. *Obesity* **2015**, *23*, 558–564. [CrossRef]
82. Hales, C.M.; Carroll, M.D.; Fryar, C.D.; Ogden, C.L. Prevalence of Obesity and Severe Obesity Among Adults: United States, 2017–2018. *NCHS Data Brief* **2020**, *360*, 1–8.
83. Yang, Y.C.; Walsh, C.E.; Johnson, M.P.; Belsky, D.W.; Reason, M.; Curran, P.; Aiello, A.E.; Chanti-Ketterl, M.; Harris, K.M. Life-course trajectories of body mass index from adolescence to old age: Racial and educational disparities. *Proc. Natl. Acad. Sci. USA* **2021**, *118*, e2020167118. [CrossRef]
84. Horn, J.W.; Feng, T.; Mørkedal, B.; Aune, D.; Strand, L.B.; Horn, J.; Mukamal, K.J.; Janszky, I. Body Mass Index Measured Repeatedly over 42 Years as a Risk Factor for Ischemic Stroke: The HUNT Study. *Nutrients* **2023**, *15*, 1232. [CrossRef]
85. Symmank, C.; Mai, R.; Ho_mann, S.; Stok, F.M.; Renner, B.; Lien, N.; Rohm, H. Predictors of food decisión making: A systematic interdisciplinary mapping (SIM) review. *Appetite* **2017**, *110*, 25–35. [CrossRef] [PubMed]
86. Hoek, A.; Pearson, D.; James, S.; Lawrence, M.; Friel, S. Healthy and environmentally sustainable food choices: Consumer responses to point-of-purchase actions. *Food Qual. Prefer.* **2017**, *58*, 94–106. [CrossRef]
87. McCrickerd, K.; Forde, C.G. Sensory influences on food intake control: Moving beyond palatability. *Obes. Rev.* **2016**, *17*, 18–29. [CrossRef] [PubMed]
88. Boesveldt, S.; de Graaf, K. The differential role of smell and taste for eating behavior. *Perception* **2017**, *46*, 307–319. [CrossRef] [PubMed]
89. Hansen, T.; Sørensen, M.I.; Eriksen, M.-L.R. How the interplay between consumer motivations and values influences organic food identity and behavior. *Food Policy* **2018**, *74*, 39–52. [CrossRef]
90. Asioli, D.; Aschemann-Witzel, J.; Caputo, V.; Vecchio, R.; Annunziata, A.; Næs, T.; Varela, P. Making sense of the "clean label" trends: A review of consumer food choice behavior and discussion of industry implications. *Food Res. Int.* **2017**, *99*, 58–71. [CrossRef] [PubMed]
91. Larson, N.; Story, M. A review of environmental influences on food choices. *Ann. Behav. Med.* **2009**, *38*, 56–73. [CrossRef] [PubMed]
92. Gutjar, S.; de Graaf, C.; Kooijman, V.; de Wijk, R.A.; Nys, A.; Ter Horst, G.J.; Jager, G. The role of emotions in food choice and liking. *Food Res. Int.* **2015**, *76*, 216–223. [CrossRef]
93. Leng, G.; Adan, R.A.; Belot, M.; Brunstrom, J.M.; de Graaf, K.; Dickson, S.L.; Hare, T.; Maier, S.; Menzies, J.; Preissl, H. The determinants of food choice. *Proc. Nutr. Soc.* **2017**, *76*, 316–327. [CrossRef]
94. McCarthy, M.B.; Collins, A.M.; Flaherty, S.J.; McCarthy, S.N. Healthy eating habit: A role for goals, identity, and self-control? *Psychol. Mark.* **2017**, *34*, 772–785. [CrossRef]
95. Trendel, O.; Werle, C.O. Distinguishing the affective and cognitive bases of implicit attitudes to improve prediction of food choices. *Appetite* **2016**, *104*, 33–43. [CrossRef] [PubMed]
96. McStay, M.; Gabel, K.; Cienfuegos, S.; Ezpeleta, M.; Lin, S.; Varady, K.A. Intermittent Fasting and Sleep: A Review of Human Trials. *Nutrients* **2021**, *13*, 3489. [CrossRef] [PubMed]
97. Casagrande, M.; Forte, G.; Favieri, F.; Corbo, I. Sleep Quality and Aging: A Systematic Review on Healthy Older People, Mild Cognitive Impairment and Alzheimer's Disease. *Int. J. Environ. Res. Public Health* **2022**, *19*, 8457. [CrossRef] [PubMed]

98. Slof-Op't Landt, M.C.T.; van Furth, E.F.; van Beijsterveldt, C.E.M.; Bartels, M.; Willemsen, G.; de Geus, E.J.; Ligthart, L.; Boomsma, D.I. Prevalence of dieting and fear of weight gain across ages: A community sample from adolescents to the elderly. *Int. J. Public Health* **2017**, *62*, 911–919. [CrossRef] [PubMed]
99. Cook, K.; Wilson, C.L. Representations of fatness in Parents magazine: A critical discourse analysis. *Fat Stud.* **2019**, *8*, 320–333. [CrossRef]
100. Ata, R.N.; Thompson, J.K. Weight bias in the media: A review of recent research. *Obes. Facts* **2010**, *3*, 41–46. [CrossRef] [PubMed]
101. Ministerio de Sanidad. *Informe Anual de Sistema Nacional de Salud 2022*; Disponible en: [Informe Anual 2022]; Ministerio de Sanidad: Madrid, Spain, 2022. Available online: https://www.sanidad.gob.es/estadEstudios/estadisticas/sisInfSanSNS/tablasEstadisticas/InfAnualSNS2022/INFORME_ANUAL_2022.pdf (accessed on 19 May 2024).
102. Rodgers, R.F.; Fischer, L.E.; Murray, S.B.; Franko, D.L. Integrating fear of fatness into sociocultural models of body image and eating concerns. *Eat. Behav.* **2022**, *46*, 101653. [CrossRef] [PubMed]
103. INEbase. *Estilos de Vida y Prácticas Preventivas. Cifras Relativas*; Disponible en: [INEbase]; Instituto Nacional de Estadística: Madrid, Spain, 2024. Available online: https://www.ine.es/jaxi/Tabla.htm?path=/t15/p419/a2006/p07/l0/&file=03056.px&L=0 (accessed on 19 May 2024).
104. Silva, D.; Ferriani, L.; Viana, M.C. Depression, anthropometric parameters, and body image in adults: A systematic review. *Rev. Assoc. Med. Bras.* **2019**, *65*, 731–738. [CrossRef] [PubMed]
105. Seijo, M.; Minckas, N.; Cormick, G.; Comandé, D.; Ciapponi, A.; BelizÁn, J.M. Comparison of self-reported and directly measured weight and height among women of reproductive age: A systematic review and meta-analysis. *Acta Obs. Gynecol. Scand.* **2018**, *97*, 429–439. [CrossRef]
106. Millstein, R.A.; Carlson, S.A.; Fulton, J.E.; Galuska, D.A.; Zhang, J.; Blanck, H.M.; Ainsworth, B.E. Relationships between body size satisfaction and weight control practices among US adults. *Medscape J. Med.* **2008**, *10*, 119. [PubMed] [PubMed Central]
107. Rivero-Jiménez, B.; Conde-Caballero, D.; Mariano-Juárez, L. Health and Nutritional Beliefs and Practices among Rural Elderly Population: An Ethnographic Study in Western Spain. *Int. J. Environ. Res. Public Health* **2020**, *17*, 5923. [CrossRef] [PubMed]
108. Sandri, E.; Cantín Larumbe, E.; Part-Ferrer, R.; Ferrer-Torregrosa, J.; Fernández-Ehrling, N. Diet and Lifestyle in the Spanish Population and Their Relationship with Sociodemographic Variables: A Descriptive Study. *Foods* **2023**, *12*, 3409. [CrossRef] [PubMed]
109. *Encuesta Nacional de Salud de España 2017*; Disponible en: [Encuesta Nacional de Salud 2017]; Ministerio de Sanidad: Madrid, Spain, 2024. Available online: https://www.sanidad.gob.es/estadEstudios/estadisticas/encuestaNacional/encuesta2017.htm (accessed on 19 May 2024).
110. Sandri, E.; Modesto IAlapont, V.; Cantín Larumbe, E.; Cerdá Olmedo, G. Analysis of the Influence of Socio-Demographic Variables and Some Nutrition and Lifestyle Habits on Beverage Consumption in the Spanish Population. *Foods* **2023**, *12*, 4310. [CrossRef]
111. Sandri, E.; Pérez-Bermejo, M.; Cabo, A.; Cerdá-Olmedo, G. Living Alone: Associations with Diet and Health in the Spanish Young Adult Population. *Nutrients* **2023**, *15*, 2516. [CrossRef]
112. *Informe del Consumo Alimentario en España 2021*; Ministerio de Agricultura, Pesca y Alimentación: Madrid, Spain, 2021. Available online: https://www.mapa.gob.es/es/alimentacion/temas/consumo-tendencias/informe-consumo-alimentario-2021-baja-res_tcm30-624017.pdf (accessed on 19 May 2024).
113. INEbase. *Estadística Continua de Población. Últimos Datos*; Disponible en: [INEbase]; Instituto Nacional de Estadística: Madrid, Spain, 2024. Available online: https://www.ine.es/dyngs/INEbase/es/operacion.htm?c=Estadistica_C&cid=1254736177095&menu=ultiDatos&idp=1254735572981 (accessed on 19 May 2024).

nutrients

MDPI

Article

Does Dietary Supplement Use Increase Micronutrient Intake Adequacy in Healthy Adults with Habitual Omnivorous, Vegetarian, Vegan, and Low-Carbohydrate High-Fat Diets?

Nives Bogataj Jontez, Karin Šik Novak, Zala Jenko Pražnikar, Ana Petelin, Saša Kenig and Nina Mohorko *

University of Primorska, Faculty of Health Sciences, 6310 Izola, Slovenia; 97200376@student.upr.si (N.B.J.); karin.novak@fvz.upr.si (K.Š.N.); zala.praznikar@fvz.upr.si (Z.J.P.); ana.petelin@fvz.upr.si (A.P.); sasa.kenig@fvz.upr.si (S.K.)

* Correspondence: nina.mohorko@fvz.upr.si; Tel.: +386-566-35818

Abstract: Diets omitting whole food groups pose a risk for micronutrient insufficiencies, but there are no data as to whether those are suitably attenuated with dietary supplements (DS). Micronutrient intakes with food and DSs were analyzed in 130 healthy adults: 32 vegans, 37 vegetarians, 24 following low-carbohydrate high-fat diet (LCHF), and 37 omnivores. A total of 63% used DS (84% of vegans, 75% of LCHF, 54% of vegetarians, and 46% of omnivores); however, a DS did not always tackle dietary insufficiencies. Vitamin B_{12} was often supplemented in vegans in doses substantially higher than recommended, but it was supplemented less often in vegetarians, despite the low prevalence of sufficient intake. Only 43% of participants supplemented vitamin D in wintertime, 23% of them with an insufficient dose. Supplementation of potassium, calcium, and iodine was rare, despite low intake adequacy with food alone in all groups. Some micronutrients were supplemented unnecessarily, such as vitamin K, riboflavin, biotin, and iron. Multimicronutrient DSs were used often; they increased intake adequacy of group B vitamins but failed to sufficiently supplement vitamin D, potassium, calcium, and iodine. Although DS use increased micronutrient intake sufficiency when used properly, the knowledge on micronutrient inadequacy in all dietary patterns should be increased and the public should be educated on the proper use of DSs. Multimicronutrient DSs should be reformulated to tackle the insufficiencies.

Keywords: vitamin D; vitamin B_{12}; potassium; calcium; multimicronutrient dietary supplement

1. Introduction

The popularity of nutritional patterns excluding whole food groups such as vegetarian, vegan, and low-carbohydrate high-fat (LCHF) diets are rising in areas where the traditional diet has been omnivorous [1], such as Europe, including Slovenia [2]. The vegetarian diet excludes meat, meat products, and often fish, while the vegan diet excludes all foods from animal origin such as milk and milk products, eggs, as well as animal products like honey. The LCHF diet excludes all starchy foods and foods containing sugar. Micronutrients are present in different amounts in different foods and food groups and omitting a whole food group raises the risk of low intake of micronutrients that are abundant in the omitted food group, and consequent micronutrient deficiency [3]. Adequate micronutrient intake is crucial to avoid diseases caused by malnutrition, such as anemia, osteoporosis, rickets, and others [4]. Furthermore, micronutrient adequacy is also important for optimal immune system function [5] and for preventing chronic noncommunicable diseases, such as thyroid deficiency, cardiovascular diseases, and cancer [6]. The literature identifies different micronutrient insufficiencies in different dietary patterns [7,8]. Very few data are available on the habitual LCHF diet practiced without supervision. The most commonly reported deficiency in the vegan diet is vitamin B_{12} deficiency, which can occur also in vegetarians, as vitamin B_{12} is present only in foods from animal origin [9]. Vitamin D intake is generally very low across the population, with especially low intakes in vegans and vegetarians [7,10]. Additionally, in Slovenia, there is a high prevalence of vitamin D deficiency, especially in the winter months when the endogenous production of vitamin D is insufficient due to the angle of the sun [11]. In those practicing LCHF diets, low vitamin C intake was reported [8]. The highest vitamin C intake was previously shown in the vegan group, followed by vegetarians and was lowest in the omnivorous group, but the study did not have a LCHF group [7]. The highest intake of folate was reported in vegans, followed by vegetarians and omnivores [7]. Slovenian national data showed low intakes of folate in 58% of the adult population (mostly omnivores) and folate deficiency in 7.6% of adults [12]. A Swedish study on real-life LCHF diet showed sufficient folate intake in the LCHF group [8]. Low calcium intake was observed in vegans [7,10] and the LCHF diet [13]. Magnesium intake was the highest in the vegan group [7], but usually vegan diets also contain the highest amounts of phytic acid, which inhibits its absorption. The LCHF diet was shown to have low magnesium intake [8,14], and low intakes of iron and potassium were also reported [8].

Nutritional deficiencies can be corrected with dietary supplements (DS), concentrated forms of nutrients or other substances with physiological value [15]. DS use is rising worldwide [16–18] and it is assessed that about half to two-thirds of people in Western countries take at least one DS [18,19]. In the USA, multimicronutrient DS (MMN DS) are the most common among DS users, followed by vitamin C [19]. DS users are more likely to adopt positive health-related habits and are often interested in nutrition and its health benefits [19]. It was shown that DS use increases with age, income, and education, it is also known that women are more likely to take DSs [17,19]. People with higher diet quality are more likely DS users [17], but little is known about DS use in different dietary groups such as vegans, vegetarians, and people practicing the LCHF diet.

The aim of this study was to compare micronutrient intake adequacy and DS intake in three habitual nutritional patterns excluding whole food groups and the omnivorous (traditional) dietary pattern in healthy lean adults with matching body mass index (BMI).

2. Materials and Methods

2.1. Study Design and Participants

A total of 130 participants (97 females), highly interested in healthy nutrition, that self-classified in four dietary groups (omnivorous, vegan, vegetarian, and LCHF) participated in this cross-sectional study. They were included based on the following inclusion criteria: BMI between 18.5 and 30 kg/m^2, 20–60 years old, and at least six-months adherence to one of the four eligible dietary patterns. Exclusion criteria included change in body mass (more than 3 kg in the preceding 3 months), any chronic disease, taking medications (except contraception) and being pregnant or lactating. All participants were healthy adults, without any chronic diseases.

This study was approved by the Slovenian National Medical Ethics Committee (No. 0120–557/2017/4) and registered at ClinicalTrials.gov, accessed on 8 August 2023. (NCT04347213). Recruitment and protocol have been described in detail previously [2].

2.2. Dietary Assessment

Diet was recorded in detail with three-day food diary (two weekdays and one weekend day) and validated food frequency questionnaire (FFQ, [20]). The participants weighed and recorded all foods and beverages immediately before eating and weighed all leftovers. Labels and recipes for mixed dishes were included. Dietitian checked all three-day food diaries and FFQs and any vagueness or questions were clarified on the day the participants came to the Faculty of Health Sciences for measurements in the same week. Three-day food diaries and FFQ were analyzed with the Open Platform for Clinical Nutrition (OPEN, http://opkp.si/, accessed on 20 March 2024). OPEN includes data on micronutrient content from the Slovenian food composition database [21], Souci Fachmann Kraut database [22], and United States National Nutrient Database for Standard Reference [23]. Analysis returned energy intake and energy density, macronutrient intake, and micronutrient intake.

All DSs were recorded in detail, the dose taken was provided. DS data were manually analyzed from the labels and data provided by the manufacturers. For the purpose of this study, the term multimicronutrient DS (MMN DS) will be used for DSs containing three or more vitamins and/or minerals. Number of DS taken, and dose and frequency of intake were determined for all participants.

For the report of each micronutrient intake, the participants were further subdivided within the groups into DS users and nonusers. Intakes of each micronutrient with food alone and with food plus DS are reported in Results Section 3.3.

Prevalence of adequate micronutrient intake was calculated for each dietary group and further for nonusers and DS users, with food alone and with added DS. Slovenian recommendations for micronutrient intake were used as reference values [24].

Healthy eating index (HEI) was calculated from three-day food diaries for diet quality assessment, as described before [2].

2.3. *Lifestyle Assessment*

Body mass was measured, after an overnight fast of at least 12 h, in light clothing and without shoes with bioelectric impedance analyzer Tanita BC 418MA (Tanita Corporation, Arlington Heights, IL, USA). Height was measured and BMI was calculated.

Participants completed Lifestyle Questionnaire, International Physical Activity Questionnaire (IPAQ), and Socio-Economic Questionnaire, as described before [2].

2.4. *Statistical Analysis*

Statistical analysis was performed using IBM SPSS Statistics 26.0 (IBM, Armonk, NY, USA). Means and standard deviations were calculated. The prevalence of participants with adequate intakes was calculated. The normality of data distribution was evaluated with the Shapiro–Wilk test. On the basis of the data normality distribution, ANOVA and the Kruskal–Wallis' test were used to compare groups, and Student's *t*-test and the Mann–Whitney test were used to compare two groups. Pearson's and Spearman's correlation were used to evaluate associations between parameters. p-values < 0.05 were considered statistically significant.

3. Results

3.1. *Participants' Characteristics*

The participants were divided into four groups based on nutritional pattern: omnivorous, vegan, vegetarian, and LCHF groups (Table 1). The groups were comparable in BMI and energy intake, while macronutrient distribution significantly differed among groups [2] (Table 1). The vegan group reached the highest proportion of recommended intake of carbohydrates, followed by vegetarians and omnivores (84.4%, 54.1%, and 21.6%, respectively). Fat intake below the highest recommended value (RV) was also seen in the highest prevalence in vegans (53.1%), followed by vegetarians and omnivores (21.6% and 18.9%, respectively). On the contrary, all participants in the LCHF group reached the recommended protein intake, while 8.1% of omnivores, 31.2% of vegans, and 35.1% of vegetarians did not reach the RV for protein. The highest intake of dietary fibers was seen in vegans, where 71.9% reached the RV, followed by vegetarians, omnivores, and the LCHF group, where 43.2%, 35.1%, and 8.3% reached the RV [2].

Table 1. Study participants' characteristics.

Variable (Unit)	All	Omnivorous	Vegan	Vegetarian	LCHF
N (Female)	130 (97)	37 (25)	32 (23)	37 (30)	24 (19)
Age (years) *	37 ± 10	36 ± 12 [c]	34 ± 10 [e]	37 ± 11 [f]	41 ± 6
Body mass (kg)	65 ± 11	66 ± 13	63 ± 8	65 ± 10	68 ± 13
BMI (kg/m^2)	22.5 ± 2.8	22.6 ± 3.0	21.8 ± 2.1	22.4 ± 2.6	23.4 ± 3.1
Nutritional intakes					
Energy (kcal)	2060 ± 630	2160 ± 670	2070 ± 650	1960 ± 630	2030 ± 530
Protein (g) *	80 ± 37	91 ± 42 [a,b,c]	65 ± 31 [e]	65 ± 23 [f]	108 ± 35
CHO (g) *	230 ± 130	250 ± 110 [a,c]	310 ± 120 [d,e]	250 ± 110 [f]	51 ± 35
Fat (g) *	88 ± 42	81 ± 20 [a,c]	64 ± 27 [d,e]	76 ± 27 [f]	151 ± 46
Fibers (g) *	32 ± 28	27 ± 15 [a,c]	50 ± 43 [d,e]	32 ± 15 [f]	18 ± 21

LCHF—low-carbohydrate high-fat; N—numerus; BMI—body mass index; CHO—carbohydrate. All data are provided as means ± standard deviation except for the numerus. *—$p < 0.05$, Kruskal–Wallis H test; [a–f]—$p < 0.05$, Mann–Whitney test between [a]—omnivorous and vegan group; [b]—omnivorous and vegetarian group; [c]—omnivorous and LCHF group; [d]—vegan and vegetarian group; [e]—vegan and LCHF group; [f]—vegetarian and LCHF group.

3.2. Dietary Supplement Use

Almost two-thirds of participants were taking at least one DS. The four most frequently used DSs were vitamin B_{12}, vitamin D, vitamin C, and MMN DS. The highest prevalence of DS use (Figure 1) was in the vegan group (84.4%), followed by the LCHF (75.0%), vegetarian (54.1%), and omnivorous group (45.9%), with a significant difference between groups ($p = 0.004$). One DS was taken by 27.7% of participants, two by 19.2%, three by 9.2% and four or more DSs by 7.0% of participants. The highest prevalence of four or more DSs being used at the same time was reported in the vegan and LCHF group, while no participants from the omnivorous group took four or more DSs (Figure 1). The LCHF group also had the highest prevalence of use of three DSs. The choice of micronutrients that were supplemented differed among the groups (Table 2).

In addition to DSs including one or more micronutrients, 36.9% of participants were taking other DSs. The most common 'other' supplements were probiotics, maca (*Lepidium meyenii*), methylsulfonylmethane (MSM), collagen, immunobiotics, and creatine. We will only consider micronutrient DSs in this article.

The prevalence of participants taking DSs did not differ between genders (M 51.5%, F 67.0%; $p = 0.141$). There was no significant difference between DS users and nonusers in age ($Z = -0.490$; $p = 0.624$), physical activity assessed with IPAQ ($Z = -0.440$; $p = 0.660$), smoking prevalence ($Z = -0.309$; $p = 0.757$), alcohol consumption ($Z = -0.963$; $p = 0.334$), education ($Z = -0.986$; $p = 0.324$), fruit intake ($Z = -0.014$; $p = 0.988$), vegetable intake ($Z = -1.112$; $p = 0.266$), diet quality determined with HEI ($Z = -0.757$; $p = 0.449$), income ($Z = -0.006$; $p = 0.995$), self-assessed health status ($Z = -0.325$; $p = 0.745$) and self-assessed health self-care ($Z = 1.236$; $p = 0.216$).

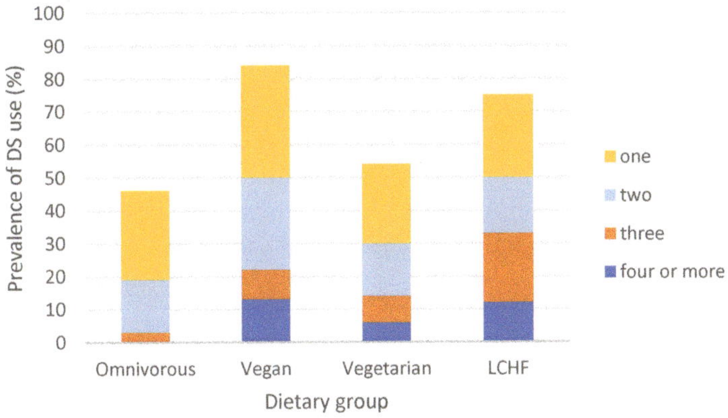

Figure 1. Prevalence (%) of micronutrient dietary supplement use and number of DS used at the same time by participants in a dietary group. DS—dietary supplement; LCHF—low-carbohydrate high-fat.

3.3. Micronutrient Intake Adequacy

Micronutrient intake is shown by dietary groups (white), with the groups further subdivided into DS users (dark grey) and nonusers (light grey). For clearer representation, data was divided in multiple tables: vitamins A and D (Table 2), vitamins E, K and C (Table 3), thiamin, riboflavin and niacin (Table 4), pantothenic acid, pyridoxine and biotin (Table 5), folate, Vitamin B12 and potassium (Table 6), calcium, phosphorus and iron (Table 7), magnesium, iodine and zinc (Table 8), selenium, copper and manganese (Table 9) and chromium, molybdenum, sodium and chloride (Table 10). The intake with food alone is presented for DS nonusers, while for the DS users, the intake with food alone (middle grey) and intake with food plus DS (dark grey) is shown (Tables 2–10). Vitamin D is shown in two parts (Table 2); the first part shows all participants and the second just the participants who were measured in wintertime. We analyzed wintertime participants separately because Slovenia is on a latitude where sun exposure from October to March is not sufficient for endogenous synthesis of vitamin D, due to the angle of the sun, and therefore vitamin D supplementation is recommended.

Between-group differences in micronutrient intake with food alone of all participants from a dietary group (DS nonusers and DS users) were analyzed and the prevalence of intake adequacy of each micronutrient is shown (Tables 2–10). Participants from all dietary groups had a low prevalence of adequate micronutrient intake with food alone for vitamin D, iodine, potassium, molybdenum, pantothenic acid, and calcium. Many participants did not reach the recommended intake for numerous micronutrients, despite the adequate mean intake of the group. For example, mean vitamin A intake in the vegan group was 1.2 mg and in the LCHF group it was 1.0 mg, but only 53% of vegans and 54% of the LCHF group met the vitamin A RV, which is 1.0 mg [24]. Furthermore, mean pantothenic acid intake in the LCHF group was 7 mg, but only half of the group met the RV of 6 mg [24]. Vegans had the highest mean intake of potassium, with 4100 mg (the RV in Slovenia is 4000 mg [24]), but only 38% met the RV.

Differences in the prevalence of DS users between dietary groups were analyzed (Tables 2–10). The statistical difference between DS users and nonusers was observed in the vegetarian group for calcium intake, where DS users had higher calcium intake with food alone than nonusers ($Z = -2.310$; $p = 0.021$). Despite no significant difference in mean intake, a higher prevalence of adequate intake with food alone was seen in vegetarian DS users for vitamin E ($Z = -2.203$; $p = 0.028$). Other differences between DS users and nonusers in intakes with food alone were not observed.

Table 2. Vitamins A and D intake and prevalence (%) of participants with adequate intake with food alone and with inclusion of dietary supplements.

Variable (Unit)			All (M ± SD)	Omnivorous (M ± SD)	Vegan (M ± SD)	Vegetarian (M ± SD)	LCHF (M ± SD)	RV [1]
Vitamin A (mg)	All *	Food sources	0.9 ± 0.8	0.8 ± 0.4 [c]	1.2 ± 1.4 [d]	0.8 ± 0.4 [f]	1.0 ± 0.4	1.0
		Adequate intake (%)	41.5%	29.7%	53.1%	35.1%	54.2%	
	Nonusers	Food sources	0.9 ± 0.8	0.8 ± 0.4	1.2 ± 1.5	0.7 ± 0.3	1.1 ± 0.5	
		Adequate intake (%)	41.2%	27.8%	55.2%	30.3%	68.8%	
			12.3% (N = 16)	2.7% (N = 1) [c]	9.4% (N = 3) [e]	10.8% (N = 4) [f]	33.3% (N = 8)	
		Food sources	0.9 ± 0.5	1.3	0.7 ± 0.3	1.3 ± 0.8	0.8 ± 0.1	
		Adequate intake (%)	43.8%	100%	33.3%	75%	25%	
		Food sources + DS	1.6 ± 0.5	1.7	1.4 ± 0.6	1.7 ± 0.8	1.6 ± 0.4	
		Adequate intake (%)	87.5%	100%	66.7%	75%	100%	
Vitamin D (μg)	All *	Food sources	4 ± 4	5 ± 4 [a,b,c]	2 ± 2 [d,e]	3 ± 3 [f]	7 ± 4	20
		Adequate intake (%)	0%	0%	0%	0%	0%	
	Nonusers	Food sources	4 ± 4	5 ± 4	2 ± 2	3 ± 3	8 ± 4	
		Adequate intake (%)	0%	0%	0%	0%	0%	
	DS users		33.8% (N = 44)	18.9% (N = 7)	43.8% (N = 14)	35.1% (N = 13)	41.7% (N = 10)	
		Food sources	3 ± 4	6 ± 5	1 ± 1	3 ± 3	5 ± 2	
		Adequate intake (%)	0%	0%	0%	0%	0%	
		Food sources + DS	41 ± 41	39 ± 24	38 ± 22	58 ± 67	22 ± 15	
		Adequate intake (%)	68.2%	71.4%	85.7%	69.2%	40.0%	
Vitamin D (μg)—winter	All *	Food sources	3 ± 3	4 ± 3 [a]	1 ± 2 [e]	3 ± 4 [f]	5 ± 2	20
	N = 51	Adequate intake (%)	0%	0%	0%	0%	0%	
	Nonusers		56.9% (N = 29)	88.9% (N = 16)	36.4% (N = 4)	47.1% (N = 8)	20.0% (N = 1)	
		Food sources	3 ± 3	3 ± 2	2 ± 2	4 ± 4	7	
		Adequate intake (%)	0%	0%	0%	0%	0%	
	DS users +		43.1% (N = 22)	11.1% (N = 2) [a,b,c]	63.6% (N = 7)	52.9% (N = 9)	80.0% (N = 4)	
		Food sources	3 ± 4	8 ± 6	1 ± 1	3 ± 3	5 ± 2	
		Adequate intake (%)	0%	0%	0%	0%	0%	
		Food sources + DS	46 ± 53	16 ± 6	37 ± 13	69 ± 78	26 ± 10	
		Adequate intake (%)	77.3%	50.0%	100%	66.7%	75.0%	

LCHF—low-carbohydrate high-fat; DS—dietary supplement; RV—Reference Values for Slovene population. * $p < 0.05$, Kruskal-Wallis H test of micronutrient intake with food alone for all participants between dietary groups; + $p < 0.05$, Kruskal-Wallis H test of DS use prevalence between dietary groups; [a–f]—$p < 0.05$, Mann-Whitney test between: [a]—omnivorous and vegan group; [b]—omnivorous and vegetarian group; [c]—omnivorous and LCHF group; [d]—vegan and vegetarian group; [e]—vegan and LCHF group; [f]—vegetarian and LCHF group. [1]—[24].

Table 3. Vitamins E, K and C intake and prevalence (%) of participants with adequate intake with food alone and with inclusion of dietary supplements.

Variable (Unit)			All (M ± SD)	Omnivorous (M ± SD)	Vegan (M ± SD)	Vegetarian (M ± SD)	LCHF (M ± SD)	RV [1]
Vitamin E (mg)	All *	Food sources	13 ± 7	12 ± 7 [c]	13 ± 5	13 ± 8	16 ± 7	13–15
		Adequate intake (%)	45.4%	37.8%	50.0%	35.1%	66.7%	
	Nonusers	Food sources	13 ± 7	12 ± 8	13 ± 5	13 ± 8	17 ± 8	
		Adequate intake (%)	41.0%	37.1%	50.0%	26.7%	66.7%	
	DS users +		19.2% (N = 25)	5.4% (N = 2) [c]	12.5% (N = 4) [e]	18.9% (N = 7) [f]	50.0% (N = 12)	
		Food sources	14 ± 5	12 ± 2	13 ± 5	15 ± 4	14 ± 6	
		Adequate intake (%)	64.0%	50.0%	50.0%	71.4%	66.7%	
		Food sources + DS	37 ± 54	27 ± 17	90 ± 140	24 ± 7	28 ± 11	
		Adequate intake (%)	96.0%	100%	100%	100%	91.7%	
Vitamin K (μg)	All *	Food sources	200 ± 170	200 ± 160	280 ± 240 [d,e]	160 ± 80	160 ± 150	70–80
		Adequate intake (%)	85.4%	81.1%	93.8%	94.6%	66.7%	
	Nonusers	Food sources	190 ± 170	180 ± 130	290 ± 260	150 ± 80	160 ±160	
		Adequate intake (%)	85.2%	80.6%	96.3%	93.8%	65%	
	DS users		11.5% (N = 15)	2.7% (N = 1)	15.6% (N = 5)	13.5% (N = 5)	16.7% (N = 4)	
		Food sources	250 ± 180	774	250 ± 150	220 ± 80	140 ± 90	
		Adequate intake (%)	86.7%	100%	80.0%	100%	75.0%	
		Food sources + DS	280 ± 180	789	280 ± 160	280 ± 60	170 ± 100	
		Adequate intake (%)	100%	100%	100%	100%	100%	
Vitamin C (mg)	All *	Food sources	140 ± 120	100 ± 60 [a,b]	200 ± 180 [d,e]	150 ± 100	110 ± 70	110
		Adequate intake (%)	58.5%	40.5%	78.1%	64.9%	50.0%	
	Nonusers	Food sources	130 ± 80	90 ± 50	180 ± 90	140 ± 100	130 ± 70	
		Adequate intake (%)	57.9%	36.7%	78.3%	63.3%	58.3%	
	DS users +		26.9% (N = 35)	18.9% (N = 7) [c]	28.1% (N = 9)	18.9% (N = 7) [f]	50.0% (N = 12)	
		Food sources	160 ± 180	150 ± 100	260 ± 320	160 ± 110	90 ± 50	
		Adequate intake (%)	60.0%	57.1%	77.8%	71.4%	41.7%	
		Food sources + DS	520 ± 860	280 ± 120	900 ± 1600	520 ± 460	370 ± 320	
		Adequate intake (%)	91.4%	100%	100%	85.7%	83.3%	

LCHF—low-carbohydrate high-fat; DS—dietary supplement; RV—Reference Values for Slovene population. * $p < 0.05$, Kruskal-Wallis H test of micronutrient intake with food alone for all participants between dietary groups; + $p < 0.05$, Kruskal-Wallis H test of DS use prevalence between dietary groups; [a–f]—$p < 0.05$, Mann-Whitney test between: [a]—omnivorous and vegan group; [b]—omnivorous and vegetarian group; [c]—omnivorous and LCHF group; [d]—vegan and vegetarian group; [e]—vegan and LCHF group; [f]—vegetarian and LCHF group. [1]—[24].

Table 4. Thiamin, riboflavin and niacin intake and prevalence (%) of participants with adequate intake with food alone and with inclusion of dietary supplements.

Variable (Unit)			All (M ± SD)	Omnivorous (M ± SD)	Vegan (M ± SD)	Vegetarian (M ± SD)	LCHF (M ± SD)	RV [1]
Thiamin (mg)	All *	Food sources	1.3 ± 0.7	1.3 ± 0.5 [c]	1.6 ± 0.9 [d,e]	1.3 ± 0.6	1.0 ± 0.6	1.2–1.3
		Adequate intake (%)	60.8%	67.6%	71.9%	59.5%	37.5%	
	Nonusers	Food sources	1.4 ± 0.7	1.3 ± 0.4	1.7 ± 1.0	1.3 ± 0.6	1.0 ± 0.6	
		Adequate intake (%)	62.4%	68.6%	70.8%	58.6%	38.5%	
	DS users +		22.3% (N = 29)	5.4% (N = 2) [a,b,c]	25.0% (N = 8)	21.6% (N = 8) [f]	45.8% (N = 11)	
		Food sources	1.3 ± 0.5	1.9 ± 1.4	1.4 ± 0.4	1.2 ± 0.4	1.1 ± 0.5	
		Adequate intake (%)	55.2%	50.0%	75.0%	62.5%	36.4%	
		Food sources + DS	4.7 ± 6.0	3.7 ± 0.3	3.3 ± 1.3	3.8 ± 1.9	6.5 ± 9.5	
		Adequate intake (%)	96.6%	100%	100%	100%	90.9%	
Riboflavin (mg)	All *	Food sources	1.6 ± 0.7	1.7 ± 0.6 [a,b,c]	1.4 ± 0.6 [e]	1.4 ± 0.7 [f]	2.0 ± 0.7	1.3–1.4
		Adequate intake (%)	82.3%	91.9%	65.5%	75.7%	100%	
	Nonusers	Food sources	1.6 ± 0.7	1.7 ± 0.5	1.4 ± 0.7	1.4 ± 0.7	2.1 ± 0.8	
		Adequate intake (%)	80.0%	91.4%	62.5%	71.4%	100%	
	DS users +		23.1% (N = 30)	5.4% (N = 2) [a,b,c]	25.0% (N = 8)	24.3% (N = 9)	45.8% (N = 11)	
		Food sources	1.6 ± 0.6	2.3 ± 1.3	1.3 ± 0.5	1.6 ± 0.8	1.8 ± 0.4	
		Adequate intake (%)	90.0%	100%	75.0%	88.9%	100%	
		Food sources + DS	5.1 ± 6.0	4.5 ± 0.7	3.4 ± 1.5	4.5 ± 2.3	7.0 ± 9.5	
		Adequate intake (%)	100%	100%	100%	100%	100%	
Niacin (mg)	All *	Food sources	18 ± 9	24 ± 10 [a,b,c]	15 ± 7	17 ± 7	15 ± 7	15–16
		Adequate intake (%)	70.8%	91.9%	59.4%	75.7%	45.8%	
	Nonusers	Food sources	18 ± 9	23 ± 9	15 ± 8	17 ± 8	14 ± 7	
		Adequate intake (%)	73.8%	91.4%	58.3%	80.0%	42.9%	
	DS users +		20.8% (N = 27)	5.4% (N = 2) [a,c]	25.0% (N = 8)	18.9% (N = 7)	41.7% (N = 10)	
		Food sources	17 ± 11	47 ± 11	14 ± 5	17 ± 8	15 ± 7	
		Adequate intake (%)	59.3%	100%	62.5%	57.1%	50.0%	
		Food sources + DS	35 ± 14	67 ± 4	30 ± 9	30 ± 15	37 ± 10	
		Adequate intake (%)	100%	100%	100%	100%	100%	

LCHF—low-carbohydrate high-fat; DS—dietary supplement; RV—Reference Values for Slovene population. * $p < 0.05$, Kruskal-Wallis H test of micronutrient intake with food alone for all participants between dietary groups; + $p < 0.05$, Kruskal-Wallis H test of DS use prevalence between dietary groups; [a–f]—$p < 0.05$, Mann-Whitney test between: [a]—omnivorous and vegan group; [b]—omnivorous and vegetarian group; [c]—omnivorous and LCHF group; [d]—vegan and vegetarian group; [e]—vegan and LCHF group; [f]—vegetarian and LCHF group. [1]—[24].

Table 5. Pantothenic acid, pyridoxine and biotin intake and prevalence (%) of participants with adequate intake with food alone and with inclusion of dietary supplements.

Variable (Unit)			All (M ± SD)	Omnivorous (M ± SD)	Vegan (M ± SD)	Vegetarian (M ± SD)	LCHF (M ± SD)	RV [1]
Pantothenic acid (mg)	All *	Food sources	5 ± 3	5 ± 2 [c]	6 ± 4 [e]	5 ± 2 [f]	7 ± 3	6
		Adequate intake (%)	30.8%	21.6%	28.1%	29.7%	50.0%	
	Nonusers	Food sources	5 ± 3	5 ± 2	5 ± 3	5 ± 3	7 ± 3	
		Adequate intake (%)	30.8%	20.0%	26.9%	34.5%	57.1%	
	DS users +		20.0% (N = 26)	5.4% (N = 2) [b,c]	18.8% (N = 6)	21.6% (N = 8)	41.7% (N = 10)	
		Food sources	6 ± 5	8 ± 4	8 ± 8	4 ± 2	6 ± 2	
		Adequate intake (%)	30.8%	50.0%	33.3%	12.5%	40.0%	
		Food sources + DS	14 ± 8	17 ± 5	13 ± 9	12 ± 8	16 ± 9	
		Adequate intake (%)	92.3%	100%	100%	75.0%	100%	
Pyridoxine (mg)	All	Food sources	2.3 ± 2.3	2.3 ± 1.7	2.4 ± 1.8	2.5 ± 3.6	1.7 ± 0.7	1.6
		Adequate intake (%)	68.5%	70.3%	81.3%	62.2%	58.3%	
	Nonusers	Food sources	2.2 ± 1.6	2.0 ± 1.0	2.7 ± 2.0	2.1 ± 2.0	2.0 ± 0.8	
		Adequate intake (%)	69.3%	68.6%	87.0%	60.0%	61.5%	
	DS users +		22.3% (N = 29)	5.4 (N = 2) [a,c]	28.1% (N = 9)	18.9% (N = 7) [f]	45.8% (N = 11)	
		Food sources	2.6 ± 4.0	7.1 ± 4.4	1.8 ± 0.7	4.4 ± 7.4	1.3 ± 0.5	
		Adequate intake (%)	65.5%	100%	66.7%	71.4%	54.5%	
		Food sources + DS	10.0 ± 19.7	9.7 ± 6.6	15.9 ± 33.4	7.9 ± 8.9	6.5 ± 9.6	
		Adequate intake (%)	100%	100%	100%	100%	100%	
Biotin (μg)	All *	Food sources	40 ± 26	37 ± 16 [a,c]	30 ± 25 [e]	32 ± 17 [f]	70 ± 29	30–60
		Adequate intake (%)	55.4%	56.8%	28.1%	48.6%	100%	
	Nonusers	Food sources	41 ± 27	37 ± 15	32 ± 28	32 ± 17	82 ± 33	
		Adequate intake (%)	54.9%	55.9%	37.5%	46.7%	100%	
	DS users +		21.5% (N = 28)	8.1% (N = 3) [c]	25.0% (N = 8)	18.9% (N = 7)	41.7% (N = 10)	
		Food sources	39 ± 19	47 ± 24	23 ± 7	33 ± 18	54 ± 13	
		Adequate intake (%)	57.1%	66.7%	0%	57.1%	100%	
		Food sources + DS	120 ± 110	320 ± 180	68 ± 34	120 ± 120	100 ± 4	
		Adequate intake (%)	92.9%	100%	75.0%	100%	100%	

LCHF—low-carbohydrate high-fat; DS—dietary supplement; RV—Reference Values for Slovene population. * $p < 0.05$, Kruskal-Wallis H test of micronutrient intake with food alone for all participants between dietary groups; + $p < 0.05$, Kruskal-Wallis H test of DS use prevalence between dietary groups; [a–c,e,f]—$p < 0.05$, Mann-Whitney test between: [a]—omnivorous and vegan group; [b]—omnivorous and vegetarian group; [c]—omnivorous and LCHF group; [e]—vegan and LCHF group; [f]—vegetarian and LCHF group. [1]—[24].

Table 6. Folate, Vitamin B_{12} and potassium intake and prevalence (%) of participants with adequate intake with food alone and with inclusion of dietary supplements.

Variable (Unit)			All (M ± SD)	Omnivorous (M ± SD)	Vegan (M ± SD)	Vegetarian (M ± SD)	LCHF (M ± SD)	RV [1]
Folate (μg)	All *	Food sources	380 ± 260	340 ± 130 [a]	530 ± 430 [d,e]	360 ± 150	290 ± 120	300
		Adequate intake (%)	58.5%	51.4%	81.3%	56.8%	41.7%	
	Nonusers	Food sources	400 ± 280	340 ± 120	580 ± 490	370 ± 160	330 ± 130	
		Adequate intake (%)	62.4%	52.9%	87.0%	55.2%	60.0%	
	DS users [+]		22.3% (N = 29)	8.1% (N = 3) [a,c]	28.1% (N = 9)	21.6% (N = 8)	37.5% (N = 9)	
		Food sources	330 ± 160	330 ± 260	430 ± 180	330 ± 90	240 ± 100	
		Adequate intake (%)	44.8%	33.3%	66.7%	62.5%	11.1%	
		Food sources + DS	610 ± 260	540 ± 200	730 ± 300	610 ± 330	510 ± 160	
		Adequate intake (%)	100%	100%	100%	100%	100%	
Vitamin B_{12} (μg)	All *	Food sources	10 ± 73	4.3 ± 2.9 [a,b,c]	27 ± 147 [d,e]	3.2 ± 4.2 [f]	7.0 ± 6.3	4.0
		Adequate intake (%)	33.8%	43.2%	6.3%	16.2%	83.3%	
	Nonusers	Food sources	4.1 ± 4.3	4.0 ± 2.6	0.8 ± 0.9	2.8 ± 2.9	8.1 ± 7.4	
		Adequate intake (%)	37.8%	40.0%	0%	15.4%	92.9%	
	DS users [+]		36.9% (N = 48)	5.4% (N = 2) [a,b,c]	78.1% (N = 25) [d,e]	29.7% (N = 11)	41.7% (N = 10)	
		Food sources	20 ± 120	9.5 ± 3.2	35 ± 170	4.3 ± 6.3	5.6 ± 4.0	
		Adequate intake (%)	27.1%	100%	8.0%	18.2%	70.0%	
		Food sources + DS	420 ± 830	14.3 ± 9.2	670 ± 1050	250 ± 540	90 ± 160	
		Adequate intake (%)	89.6%	100%	84.0%	90.9%	100%	
Potassium (mg)	All *	Food sources	3200 ± 1800	3200 ± 1100 [c]	4100 ± 2900 [e]	3100 ± 1100 [f]	2500 ± 700	4000
		Adequate intake (%)	22.3%	18.9%	37.5%	21.6%	8.3%	
	Nonusers	Food sources	3200 ± 1800	3100 ± 1000	4100 ± 2900	3100 ± 1100	2400 ± 700	
		Adequate intake (%)	22.0%	16.7%	37.5%	21.6%	9.1%	
	DS users		2.3% (N = 3)	2.7% (N = 1)	0%	0%	8.3% (N = 2)	
		Food sources	4300 ± 2100	6600	/	/	3100 ± 700	
		Adequate intake (%)	33.3%	100%	/	/	0%	
		Food sources + DS	4300 ± 2100	6700	/	/	3100 ± 700	
		Adequate intake (%)	33.3%	100%	/	/	0%	

LCHF—low-carbohydrate high-fat; DS—dietary supplement; RV—Reference Values for Slovene population. * $p < 0.05$, Kruskal-Wallis H test of micronutrient intake with food alone for all participants between dietary groups; [+] $p < 0.05$, Kruskal-Wallis H test of DS use prevalence between dietary groups; [a–f]—$p < 0.05$, Mann-Whitney test between: [a]—omnivorous and vegan group; [b]—omnivorous and vegetarian group; [c]—omnivorous and LCHF group; [d]—vegan and vegetarian group; [e]—vegan and LCHF group; [f]—vegetarian and LCHF group. [1]—[24].

Table 7. Calcium, phosphorus and iron intake and prevalence (%) of participants with adequate intake with food alone and with inclusion of dietary supplements.

Variable (Unit)			All (M ± SD)	Omnivorous (M ± SD)	Vegan (M ± SD)	Vegetarian (M ± SD)	LCHF (M ± SD)	RV [1]
Calcium (mg)	All	Food sources	840 ± 380	960 ± 370	730 ± 310	810 ± 350	870 ± 480	1000
		Adequate intake (%)	26.9%	43.2%	12.5%	24.3%	25.0%	
	Nonusers	Food sources	820 ± 380	940 ± 360	740 ± 310	750 ± 300	870 ± 550	
		Adequate intake (%)	23.9%	41.7%	12.9%	15.9%	22.1%	
	DS users $^{+}$		10.0% (N = 13)	2.7% (N = 1) ^{c}	3.1% (N = 1) ^{e}	13.5% (N = 5)	25.0% (N = 6)	
		Food sources	1020 ± 380	1570	590	1200 ± 420	850 ± 210	
		Adequate intake (%)	53.8%	100%	0%	80.0%	33.2%	
		Food sources + DS	1200 ± 410	1630	640	1390 ± 380	1070 ± 350	
		Adequate intake (%)	61.5%	100%	0%	80.0%	50.0%	
Phosphorus (mg)	All *	Food sources	1230 ± 470	1350 ± 440 ^{a,b}	1120 ± 560 ^{e}	1100 ± 370 ^{f}	1430 ± 450	700
		Adequate intake (%)	90.0%	94.6%	78.1%	89.2%	100%	
	Nonusers	Food sources	1230 ± 460	1310 ± 390	1130 ± 560	1110 ± 370	1440 ± 480	
		Adequate intake (%)	89.3%	94.4%	77.4%	88.6%	100%	
	DS users		6.2% (N = 8)	2.7% (N = 1)	3.1% (N = 1)	5.4% (N = 2)	16.7% (N = 4)	
		Food sources	1320 ± 600	2580	750	900 ± 240	1360 ± 270	
		Adequate intake (%)	100%	100%	100%	100%	100%	
		Food sources + DS	1450 ± 620	2640	780	1020 ± 220	1540 ± 370	
		Adequate intake (%)	100%	100%	100%	100%	100%	
Iron (mg) [2]	All *	Food sources	17 ± 10	16 ± 6 ^{a}	22 ± 15 ^{d,e}	16 ± 7	14 ± 5	10
		Adequate intake (%)	90.0%	91.9%	96.9%	83.8%	87.5%	
	Nonusers	Food sources	17 ± 10	16 ± 6	23 ± 16	16 ± 7	14 ± 6	
		Adequate intake (%)	89.3%	91.2%	96.6%	83.9%	83.3%	
	DS users		13.8% (N = 18)	8.1% (N = 3)	9.4% (N = 3)	16.2% (N = 6)	25.0% (N = 6)	
		Food sources	17 ± 6	17 ± 11	20 ± 6	18 ± 5	15 ± 3	
		Adequate intake (%)	94.4%	100%	100%	83.3%	100%	
		Food sources + DS	29 ± 12	23 ± 9	34 ± 22	28 ± 8	31 ± 13	
		Adequate intake (%)	100%	100%	100%	100%	100%	

LCHF—low-carbohydrate high-fat; DS—dietary supplement; RV—Reference Values for Slovene population. * $p < 0.05$, Kruskal-Wallis H test of micronutrient intake with food alone for all participants between dietary groups; $^{+}$ $p < 0.05$, Kruskal-Wallis H test of DS use prevalence between dietary groups; $^{a-f}$—$p < 0.05$, Mann-Whitney test between: ^{a}—omnivorous and vegan group; ^{b}—omnivorous and vegetarian group; ^{c}—omnivorous and LCHF group; ^{d}—vegan and vegetarian group; ^{e}—vegan and LCHF group; ^{f}—vegetarian and LCHF group. [1]—[24]. [2] The amount of iron intake was not corrected for lower bioavailability for those on a plant-based diet.

Table 8. Magnesium, iodine and zinc intake and prevalence (%) of participants with adequate intake with food alone and with inclusion of dietary supplements.

Variable (Unit)			All (M ± SD)	Omnivorous (M ± SD)	Vegan (M ± SD)	Vegetarian (M ± SD)	LCHF (M ± SD)	RV [1]
Magnesium (mg)	All *	Food sources	420 ± 270	390 ± 180 [a]	560 ± 390 [d,e]	410 ± 230	290 ± 130	350–400
		Adequate intake (%)	61.5%	54.1%	81.3%	64.9%	41.7%	
	Nonusers	Food sources	440 ± 290	370 ± 160	590 ± 420	440 ± 250	280 ± 140	
		Adequate intake (%)	62.6%	50.0%	85.7%	66.7%	33.3%	
	DS users +		23.8% (N = 31)	13.5% (N = 5) [c]	12.5% (N = 4) [e]	27.0% (N = 10)	50.0% (N = 12)	
		Food sources	360 ± 170	520 ± 240	400 ± 140	340 ± 140	290 ± 120	
		Adequate intake (%)	58.1%	80.0%	50.0%	60.0%	50.0%	
		Food sources + DS	710 ± 540	1300 ± 1200	670 ± 260	570 ± 160	590 ± 250	
		Adequate intake (%)	93.5%	100%	100%	90.0%	91.7%	
Iodine (µg)	All *	Food sources	80 ± 50	90 ± 40	70 ± 50 [e]	80 ± 40	100 ± 60	180–200
		Adequate intake (%)	3.1%	2.7%	3.1%	0%	8.3%	
	Nonusers	Food sources	80 ± 50	90 ± 40	70 ± 50	70 ± 40	100 ± 60	
		Adequate intake (%)	3.4%	2.8%	3.1%	0%	11.1%	
	DS users +		8.5 % (N = 11)	2.7 % (N = 1) [c]	0% (N = 0) [e]	10.8% (N = 4)	25.0% (N = 6)	
		Food sources	100 ± 40	160	/	110 ± 40	90 ± 40	
		Adequate intake (%)	0%	0%	/	0%	0%	
		Food sources + DS	190 ± 50	190	/	180 ± 60	190 ± 60	
		Adequate intake (%)	63.6%	100%	/	50.0%	66.7%	
Zinc (mg)	All *	Food sources	10 ± 5	11 ± 5 [b]	10 ± 6 [e]	9 ± 5 [f]	11 ± 4	11–16
		Adequate intake (%)	62.3%	70.3%	59.4%	45.9%	79.2%	
	Nonusers	Food sources	10 ± 5	11 ± 4	9 ± 5	9 ± 4	11 ± 4	
		Adequate intake (%)	62.2%	71.4%	60.7%	48.5%	73.3%	
	DS users +		14.6% (N = 19)	5.4% (N = 2) [c]	12.5% (N = 4) [e]	10.8% (N = 4) [f]	37.5% (N = 9)	
		Food sources	12 ± 7	12 ± 9	14 ± 10	13 ± 12	11 ± 3	
		Adequate intake (%)	63.2%	50.0%	50.0%	25.0%	88.9%	
		Food sources + DS	24 ± 15	14 ± 9	33 ± 27	19 ± 11	25 ± 11	
		Adequate intake (%)	94.7%	100%	75.0%	100%	100%	

LCHF—low-carbohydrate high-fat; DS—dietary supplement; RV—Reference Values for Slovene population. * $p < 0.05$, Kruskal-Wallis H test of micronutrient intake with food alone for all participants between dietary groups; + $p < 0.05$, Kruskal-Wallis H test of DS use prevalence between dietary groups; a–f—$p < 0.05$, Mann-Whitney test between: a—omnivorous and vegan group; b—omnivorous and vegetarian group; c—omnivorous and LCHF group; d—vegan and vegetarian group; e—vegan and LCHF group; f—vegetarian and LCHF group. 1—[24].

Table 9. Selenium, copper and manganese intake and prevalence (%) of participants with adequate intake with food alone and with inclusion of dietary supplements.

Variable (Unit)			All (M ± SD)	Omnivorous (M ± SD)	Vegan (M ± SD)	Vegetarian (M ± SD)	LCHF (M ± SD)	RV [1]
Selenium (μg)	All *	Food sources	90 ± 80	110 ± 120 [a,b]	60 ± 30 [e]	75 ± 60 [f]	120 ± 60	M: 70
		Adequate intake (%)	61.5%	75.7%	37.5%	48.6%	91.7%	F: 60
	Nonusers	Food sources	90 ± 80	110 ± 110	60 ± 40	70 ± 60	120 ± 60	
		Adequate intake (%)	59.0%	75.0%	35.5%	47.1%	93.8%	
	DS users [+]		10.0% (N = 13)	2.7% (N = 1) [c]	3.1% (N = 1) [e]	8.1% (N = 3) [f]	33.3% (N = 8)	
		Food sources	120 ± 80	310	70	90 ± 40	110 ± 60	
		Adequate intake (%)	84.6%	100%	100%	66.7%	87.5%	
		Food sources + DS	140 ± 70	330	80	110 ± 50	135 ± 50	
		Adequate intake (%)	100%	100%	100%	100%	100%	
Copper (mg)	All *	Food sources	2.0 ± 1.1	1.9 ± 0.7 [a,c]	2.7 ± 1.7 [d,e]	1.9 ± 0.8 [f]	1.4 ± 0.7	1.0–1.5
		Adequate intake (%)	90.0%	91.9%	100%	94.6%	66.7%	
	Nonusers	Food sources	2.0 ± 1.1	1.8 ± 0.7	2.7 ± 1.7	1.9 ± 0.8	1.3 ± 0.6	
		Adequate intake (%)	90.1%	91.7%	100%	94.1%	65.0%	
	DS users		6.9% (N = 9)	2.7% (N = 1)	3.1% (N = 1)	8.1% (N = 3)	16.7% (N = 4)	
		Food sources	2.1 ± 0.9	3.5	2.0	2.3 ± 0.6	1.7 ± 1.0	
		Adequate intake (%)	88.9%	100%	100%	100%	75.0%	
		Food sources + DS	2.7 ± 0.9	4.0	2.2	2.8 ± 0.5	2.5 ± 1.2	
		Adequate intake (%)	100%	100%	100%	100%	100%	
Manganese (mg)	All *	Food sources	5.4 ± 3.8	5.0 ± 3.1 [a,c]	7.7 ± 4.5 [d,e]	5.6 ± 3.4 [f]	2.4 ± 1.4	2.0–5.0
		Adequate intake (%)	89.2%	94.6%	100%	97.3%	54.2%	
	Nonusers	Food sources	5.5 ± 3.8	4.9 ± 3.1	7.8 ± 4.6	5.7 ± 3.4	2.3 ± 1.1	
		Adequate intake (%)	90.8%	94.4%	100%	97.1%	55.6%	
	DS users [+]		7.7% (N = 10)	2.7% (N = 1) [c]	3.1% (N = 1) [e]	5.4% (N = 2) [f]	25.0% (N = 6)	
		Food sources	4.0 ± 2.6	8.3	6.3	4.3 ± 2.6	2.8 ± 2.1	
		Adequate intake (%)	70.0%	100%	100%	100%	50.0%	
		Food sources + DS	6.1 ± 2.2	8.8	6.3	5.1 ± 2.4	5.9 ± 2.4	
		Adequate intake (%)	90.0%	100%	100%	100%	83.3%	

LCHF—low-carbohydrate high-fat; DS—dietary supplement; RV—Reference Values for Slovene population. * $p < 0.05$, Kruskal-Wallis H test of micronutrient intake with food alone for all participants between dietary groups; [+] $p < 0.05$, Kruskal-Wallis H test of DS use prevalence between dietary groups; [a–f]—$p < 0.05$, Mann-Whitney test between: [a]—omnivorous and vegan group; [b]—omnivorous and vegetarian group; [c]—omnivorous and LCHF group; [d]—vegan and vegetarian group; [e]—vegan and LCHF group; [f]—vegetarian and LCHF group. [1]—[24].

Table 10. Chromium, molybdenum, sodium and chloride intake and prevalence (%) of participants with adequate intake with food alone and with inclusion of dietary supplements.

Variable (Unit)			All (M ± SD)	Omnivorous (M ± SD)	Vegan (M ± SD)	Vegetarian (M ± SD)	LCHF (M ± SD)	RV [1]
Chromium (μg)	All	Food sources	40 ± 50	50 ± 70	40 ± 50	40 ± 40	30 ± 30	30–100
		Adequate intake (%)	50.0%	56.8%	37.5%	54.1%	50.0%	
	Nonusers	Food sources	40 ± 50	50 ± 70	40 ± 50	40 ± 40	30 ± 20	
		Adequate intake (%)	49.1%	55.6%	41.4%	52.9%	58.8%	
	DS users [+]		10.8% (N = 14)	2.7% (N = 1) [c]	9.4% (N = 3)	8.1% (N = 3) [f]	29.2% (N = 7)	
		Food sources	60 ± 60	240	20 ± 10	50 ± 50	40 ± 30	
		Adequate intake (%)	57.1%	100%	0%	66.7%	71.4%	
		Food sources + DS	80 ± 60	250	50 ± 20	70 ± 50	70 ± 30	
		Adequate intake (%)	85.7%	100%	66.7%	100%	85.7%	
Molybdenum (μg)	All	Food sources	50 ± 50	40 ± 40	55 ± 50	60 ± 60	50 ± 40	50–100
		Adequate intake (%)	30.0%	16.2%	37.5%	35.1%	33.3%	
	Nonusers	Food sources	50 ± 50	40 ± 40	55 ± 50	60 ± 60	60 ± 50	
		Adequate intake (%)	30.0%	13.9%	38.7%	34.3%	38.9%	
	DS users [+]		7.7% (N = 10)	2.7% (N = 1) [c]	3.1% (N = 1) [e]	5.4% (N = 2) [f]	25.0% (N = 6)	
		Food sources	40 ± 20	50	30	40 ± 40	30 ± 20	
		Adequate intake (%)	30.0%	100%	0%	50.0%	16.7%	
		Food sources + DS	60 ± 30	70	40	80 ± 70	60 ± 30	
		Adequate intake (%)	50.0%	100%	0%	50.0%	50.0%	
[2] Sodium (mg)		Food sources	2400 ± 1100	2650 ± 1000	2400 ± 1200	2200 ± 1100	2300 ± 1000	1500
[2] Chloride (mg)		Food sources	3800 ± 1600	4200 ± 1600	3900 ± 1700	3400 ± 1600	3400 ± 1500	2300

LCHF—low-carbohydrate high-fat; DS—dietary supplement; RV—Reference Values for Slovene population. [+] $p < 0.05$, Kruskal-Wallis H test of DS use prevalence between dietary groups; [c,e,f]—$p < 0.05$, Mann-Whitney test between: [c]—omnivorous and LCHF group; [e]—vegan and LCHF group; [f]—vegetarian and LCHF group. [1]—[24]. [2]—Micronutrients used for improving taste in form of salt.

3.4. Micronutrient Content in Multimicronutrient Dietary Supplements (MMN DS)

MMN DSs were the fourth most popular DS in our sample, as 35 (26.9%) participants took them. A total of 30 different MMN DSs were used. The content of MMN DSs was analyzed. Three MMN DSs were taken by more than one participant (Figure 2A, numbers 3, 13 and 25). One participant concomitantly took two different MMN DSs.

The most abundant components of MMN DSs were B group vitamins. MMN DSs differed in composition in terms of the vitamins and minerals they contained and in their amounts. For example, the content of riboflavin in different MMN DSs differed from 4% to 2564% of the daily RV (Figure 2A). Many participants who took MMN DSs (26; 74.3% of MMN DS users), also took other DSs at the same time.

Intake adequacy of some micronutrients with food alone was low, such as vitamin D, vitamin B_{12}, calcium, and molybdenum (colored in blue, Figure 2B). Intake adequacy was increased with MMN DSs (Figure 2C), seen as a switch from blue to yellow (100% RV) mostly for B group vitamins. Intake adequacy was further improved with all added DSs (Figure 2D), seen especially in vitamin D supplementation. On the other hand, high-dose supplementation of some micronutrients was also present (red color), vitamin B_{12} was the most commonly supplemented micronutrient in high doses, even to above 3000% of the RV.

3.5. Tolerable Upper Intake Level

Exceeding the tolerable upper intake level (UL) was rare in our participants; 6.9% of participants exceeded the UL for niacin intake with food alone and 15.4% with included DSs. There were also individual examples of exceeding the UL with some other micronutrients, namely selenium, zinc, folate, iron, copper, pyridoxine, vitamin A, calcium, vitamin D, and vitamin C, as shown in Table 11. Vitamin E has a UL of 300 mg and molybdenum has a UL of 600 μg [25], but no participant had exceeded these levels.

Table 11. Prevalence of participants exceeding the tolerable upper intake level (UL) with food alone and with included dietary supplement intake.

Variable	Food Alone (%)	Food + DS (%)	UL
Niacin	6.9	15.4	35 mg [1]
Selenium	3.1	3.1	255 μg [2]
Zinc	1.5	6.2	25 mg [1]
Folate	1.5	3.8	1000 μg [1]
Iron	1.5	3.1	45 mg [1]
Copper	1.5	1.5	5 mg [1]
Pyridoxine	0.8	3.1	12 mg [3]
Vitamin A	0.8	0.8	3000 μg [1]
Calcium	0.8	0.8	2500 mg [4]
Vitamin D	0	1.5	100 μg [5]
Vitamin C	0	0.8	2000 mg [1]

DS—dietary supplement; [1] [25], [2] [26], [3] [27], [4] [28], [5] [29].

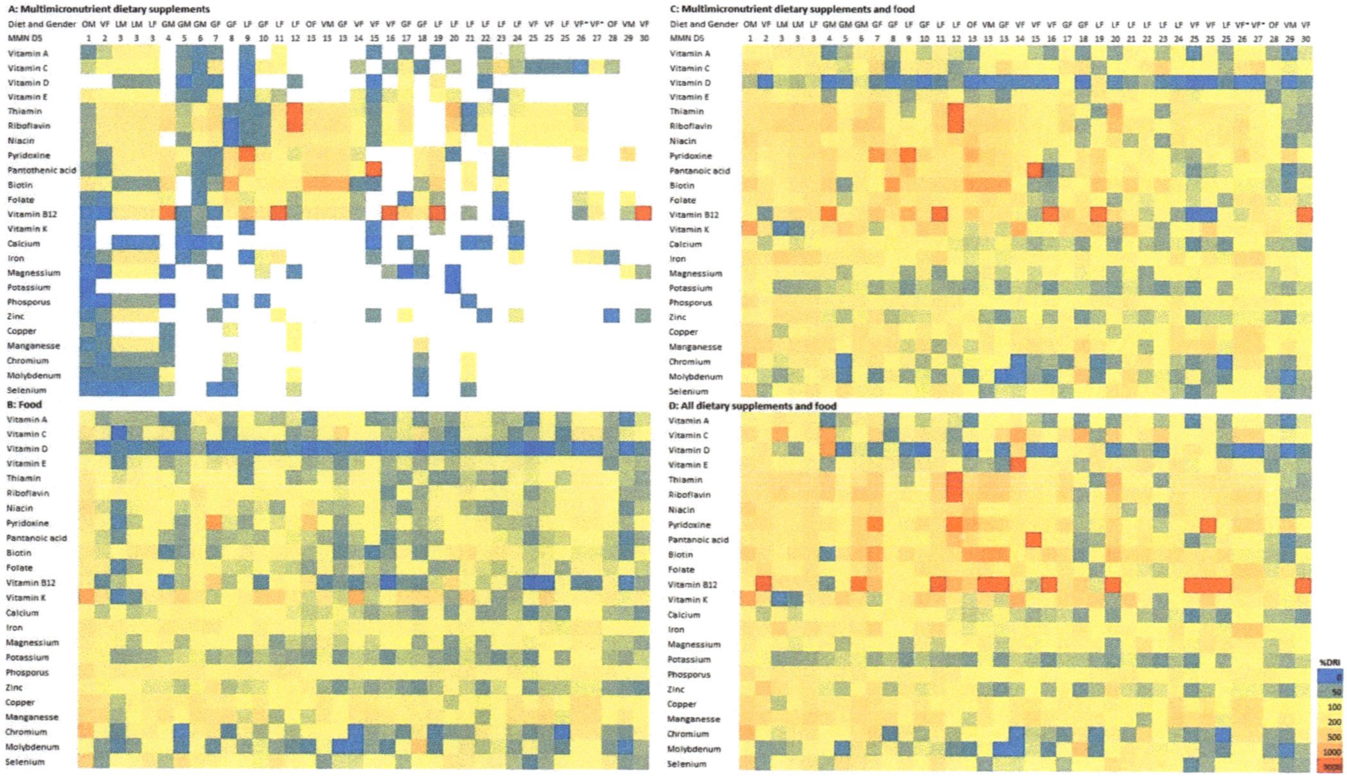

Figure 2. (**A**) Micronutrient content of multimicronutrient dietary supplements taken by our participants. (**B**) Micronutrient intake adequacy with food alone. (**C**) Micronutrient intake adequacy with food and multimicronutrient dietary supplements intake. (**D**) Micronutrient intake adequacy with food, multimicronutrient, and other dietary supplements intake. Diet and gender: O—omnivore; V—vegan, G—vegetarian; L—low-carbohydrate high-fat diet; M—male; F—female; MMN DS—number of multimicronutrient dietary supplements; %DRI—intake in % of daily recommended intake. * Multimicronutrient dietary supplement used by the same participant.

4. Discussion

Micronutrient intake adequacy was analyzed in healthy adult participants with habitual omnivorous, vegan, vegetarian, and LCHF dietary patterns with normal BMI and high interest in healthy nutrition. We observed the lowest prevalence of adequate micronutrient intake with food alone for vitamin D, iodine, potassium, molybdenum, pantothenic acid, and calcium, regardless of the nutritional pattern. A low prevalence of adequate vitamin B_{12} intake was present in vegans and vegetarians and it was also relatively low in omnivores. Many participants did not reach the recommended intake for numerous micronutrients, despite adequate mean intake in the group. We observed the highest prevalence of DS use among vegans followed by those practicing LCHF, which indicates awareness of possible diet shortages, although not all insufficiencies were tackled specifically. Participants in the LCHF group took the highest number of DSs at the same time, 21% of the LCHF group took three DSs and 12% of the group took four or more DSs.

There were no significant differences in micronutrient intake with food alone between DS users and nonusers, except for calcium in the vegetarian group, which is in line with some previously reported data [19], despite some reports of higher nutrient adequacy with food alone in DS users [30]. Despite no significant difference in mean intake, a higher prevalence of adequate intake with food alone was seen in vegetarian DS users for vitamin E. We did not find any differences between DS users and nonusers in age, education, physical activity, smoking, or self-reported health, which is contrary to other studies [18,19,31], but this is probably due to our sample, which included healthy participants with normal BMI and an interest in nutrition.

4.1. Frequently Used DS

Vitamin B_{12} was the most popular DS, especially in the vegan group, where 78% of participants took it, which is comparable to a study from Germany [32]. Dietary intake of vitamin B_{12} was low in our vegan group and therefore supplementation was necessary. The vegetarian group had a lower prevalence of vitamin B_{12} supplementation (30%), despite the low prevalence of adequate intake of vitamin B_{12} with food alone in their group (16%), which is in line with previous findings that vegetarians are less likely to take DSs with vitamin B_{12} than vegans [7]. The highest proportion of participants with adequate vitamin B_{12} intake with food alone was in the LCHF group, followed by the omnivorous group (83% and 43%, respectively). A recent study on a Slovenian representative sample showed that 32% of the adult population did not meet the recommended vitamin B_{12} intake, but the prevalence of serum vitamin B_{12} deficiency was present was only 1.2% in the adult population [33]. Despite a high prevalence of adequate vitamin B_{12} intake with diet alone in the LCHF group, more than 40% of the participants from the group took DSs containing vitamin B_{12}, the majority as part of MMN DS. We observed that many participants who a took vitamin B_{12}-only supplement, with the highest proportion in the vegan group, took high doses, such as 1200 µg, 1000 µg, 500 µg, and 400 µg daily, which were doses recommended by the DS manufacturers. Such recommendations by the manufacturers exceed the maximum level for the addition of vitamin B_{12} to foods including food supplements published by official institutions; the German Federal Institute for Risk Assessment recommends the maximum level of daily recommended dose of vitamin B_{12} per DS to be 25 µg [34,35]. Some participants combined a vitamin B_{12} DS with MMN DSs that also contained vitamin B_{12} and reached daily doses as high as 5000 µg daily. The tolerable upper intake level (UL) for vitamin B_{12} is not set [36], but nevertheless there is some evidence of adverse side effects of chronic high-dose vitamin B_{12} supplementation, especially with combined high pyridoxine intake [37]. High vitamin B_{12} intake in combination with high pyridoxine intake was observed in four participants, of which one had an intake of both micronutrients above 3000% of the RV. It is known that vitamin B_{12} is better absorbed when it is regularly included in food than from a one-time high dose [38], but this does not justify the high daily dosage observed. The efficiency of absorption of vitamin B_{12} decreases with supplement dose, from 56% of a 1 µg dose to 1.3% of a 1000 µg dose [38]. Additionally, a 350 μg dosage per week distributed among 50 μg doses per day was comparable in terms of effectiveness to a single 2000 μg dose per week in restoring normal cobalamine plasma levels in vegetarians and vegans with mild deficiency [39]. This points towards such high doses of vitamin B_{12} in healthy vegetarians and vegans being needless. Moreover, a study of a Canadian representative sample showed that doses up to 10–25 μg for adults efficiently decrease the prevalence of vitamin B_{12} deficiency, whereas higher doses did not contribute further [40].

The second most popular DS was vitamin D. A total of 38% of participants took it, which is similar to a study from Germany [32], but a lot less compared to a Finnish report on vegan and omnivorous groups [41]. The highest prevalence of use of this DS was found in the vegan and LCHF groups (44% and 42%, respectively), followed by the vegetarian group and the omnivorous group (35% and 19%, respectively). The vegan group had the lowest and the LCHF group had the highest vitamin D intake with food alone, which is in line with previous reports [7,8,11], but regardless of these differences, the intakes were too low in all groups. Vitamin D can be biosynthesized internally in skin with sun exposure, but at our latitudes (above 35° north) the incident angle of the sun is too small in wintertime for the biosynthesis of vitamin D in the skin to occur [11]. In a Slovenian representative sample, a high prevalence of vitamin D deficiency was shown in the winter months and this was lower but still high in the summer months, which points to the need of vitamin D supplementation, at least in the winter months [11]. It is important to note that we do not have data regarding sun exposure of the participants that participated in the study during summer, and thus we cannot know if suitable levels were reached through photoreaction in skin. None of our participants reached adequate vitamin D intake with food alone. Only 43% of participants who participated to the study in the winter months took a DS with vitamin D and nearly one-quarter of them did not reach the recommended intake of 20 μg per day [24], despite the DS use. Only two omnivorous participants (11%) took a DS with vitamin D in winter and only one of them reached the RV. Our results point to an insufficient awareness in the population of the need of vitamin D supplementation in the winter months and a lack of knowledge regarding the suitable dose. The majority of MMN DSs reported by our participants had low doses of vitamin D (Figure 2A). In European regulation for food labeling, the RV for vitamin D is still set at 5 μg per day [42], so the relatively low doses of vitamin D in DSs appear high when expressed in %RV. Furthermore, the dose of vitamin D in DSs is often reported in international units while in the reference values for the Slovene population, the dose is expressed in μg [24]. Although the RV contains a conversion factor in the footnote, the information might not be easy to obtain and/or understand by the public. Despite relatively low vitamin D DS use in comparison to recommended supplementation DS use increased the prevalence of adequate vitamin D intake from 0 to 68% in DS users.

DSs with vitamin C were also commonly used among our participants, more than a fourth of participants took them. Not all the participants that used vitamin C DSs would need supplementation (60% of users had adequate vitamin C intake), but vitamin C supplementation increased vitamin C intake adequacy in vitamin DS users to 91%. The highest prevalence of vitamin C DS use was in the LCHF group, followed by the vegan group. The vegetarian and omnivorous groups had the lowest prevalence of vitamin C DS use, despite the fact that the omnivorous group also had the lowest prevalence of adequate vitamin C intake with food alone, which amounted to only 37% among non-users in the omnivorous group. Vitamin C is present in a wide range of food; hence, vitamin C deficiency should be rare. However, forty percent of participants did not reach the vitamin C RV with food alone. Insufficient intake of vitamin C was present in all groups, including vegans, where intakes were the highest and which were also reported to have the highest intakes of vitamin C by the literature [7]. Low intake of fruit and vegetables is generally observed in the Slovenian population [43]; additionally, high carbohydrate fruits and vegetables are intentionally excluded in the LCHF diet, and this is a risk factor for insufficient vitamin C intake with food. A recent representative study of the USA population showed a 22% decline in vitamin C intake across a 20-year period, mostly due to lower intake of fruit juices, while relatively low intakes of vegetables persisted [44]. As fruit juice contributes substantially to energy intake, its use was low in our sample and the preferable beverages were water and herbal tea.

Single-mineral DS use was rarely reported by our participants, except for DSs with magnesium. Insufficient magnesium intake with food alone was observed in 40% of participants. The lowest magnesium intake was in the LCHF group where only 40% of participants reached the RV with food alone, which is consistent with previous studies [8]. However, LCHF was also the group with the highest prevalence of magnesium DS use (50%). Magnesium supplementation in this group increased magnesium intake adequacy, but only in participants who took a magnesium DS and not a MMN DS, since the doses in the latter were too low (Figure 2C). Vegans, followed by vegetarians, had higher magnesium intake adequacy with food alone (81% and 65%, respectively), which is in line with previous outcomes [7].

Iron intake with food alone was the highest in the vegan group, where 97% of participants reached the RV, followed by the omnivorous, LCHF, and vegetarian group (92%, 88% and 84%, respectively); however, the iron intake was not corrected for lower bioavailability from plant sources. The observed higher iron intakes of vegans, but not vegetarians, are in line with previous studies [7]. Reports also show that even though bioavailability of iron is higher from animal products, such as meat and meat products, and vegan diet contains more inhibitors of absorption, participants on the vegetarian or vegan diet had normal iron status due to high iron intake [45]. In contrast, iron intake in our vegetarian group was more comparable with the omnivorous and LCHF group, than with the vegan group (Tables 2–10). Higher iron intake in vegans might show better awareness of low iron bioavailability in their diet, which is also shown in the case of vitamin B_{12} supplementation and points to the need of raising awareness in the vegetarian group.

4.2. Inadequate Intake with Food and Low or No Supplementation

Intake adequacy for some micronutrients was low, and many of them were rarely supplemented, and even when they were, the DS had insufficient doses.

Folate intake with food sources alone was insufficient in more than 40% of our participants. The Slovenian representative sample reports an even higher prevalence of folate insufficiency, with 58% [43]. The vegan group had the highest folate intake, with 81% of participants reaching RV, followed by vegetarians, omnivores, and those practicing LCHF. Contrary to Swedish reports [8], our LCHF participants had low folate intakes with food alone, with 58% of participants not reaching the RV. Only 22% of participants used folate DS. Importantly, everyone who took DSs with folate reached the RV, regardless of the type of DS: single-vitamin DS or MMN DS with folate. This shows that in case folate DSs were used, they would be properly chosen and dosed; however, almost half of participants who needed folate supplementation did not take it.

Pantothenic acid intake was low in our participants; only 31% reached the RV and low supplementation was also seen. The highest intake of pantothenic acid with food alone was observed in the LCHF group with half of participants with adequate intake. Interestingly, the LCHF group also most commonly used DSs with pantothenic acid. In total, 20% of all participants supplemented pantothenic acid, the majority of them as part of a MMN DS. Almost all participants (92%) who took a DS with pantothenic acid reached the RV. With this in mind, foods high in pantothenic acid and/or suitable DSs should be promoted more.

DSs with potassium are rare in Slovenia and so is potassium DS use; only three (2.3%) participants supplemented potassium, two of them as part of a MMN DS. Less than a quarter of participants reached the RV for potassium with food alone and no one who took potassium DSs increased potassium intake enough to reach the RV. The latest data showed that potassium intake is low in Europe [46]. Potassium DSs in Slovenia are rare and have low doses in comparison to the Slovene recommended intake, the highest dose we found was 375 mg, which is only 19% of the recommended daily intake, despite reports that potassium supplementation up to 3 g per day showed no adverse effects [25].

The prevalence of calcium supplementation with DS was low in our sample (10%), despite low calcium intake with food alone in all dietary groups; only 24% of participants reached the RV. The highest prevalence of adequate calcium intake was in the omnivorous group, 43% met RV, followed by LCHF, vegetarian, and vegan (25%, 24%, and 13%, respectively). Low calcium intake was previously reported among vegetarians and was even lower among vegans [7], but in our study we also observed low calcium intake in the LCHF and omnivorous group, which is in contrast to previous studies reporting significantly lower calcium intake in vegans compared with vegetarians and omnivores [7,41]. It is concerning that among calcium DS users, 31% of participants did not reach the RV despite calcium supplementation. Low calcium supplementation points to a low awareness of low calcium intake in all dietary groups, because calcium DSs are widely available in different doses: 60%, 80%, and 100% of the RV.

Molybdenum intake in our participants was relatively low, only 30% of participants reached the RV. Molybdenum was also rarely supplemented, only 8% of participants supplemented it, all with a MMN DS. MMN DSs with molybdenum had low doses and only 50% of participants who supplemented molybdenum reached the RV.

Only ten participants of our study reached the iodine RV, only two of them without a DS. Iodine is systematically supplemented in Slovenia through salt iodization; therefore, iodine is rarely present in DSs. Iodine sufficiency is periodically assessed in a representative sample of the population, for which sufficient iodine status is reported due to highly excessive salt intake [47]. Our participants had lower salt intake than reported for the general population in Slovenia [48]. Low iodine intake was reported before along with low urinary excretion of iodine in vegans but also in the vegetarian and omnivorous group [32,41]. Iodine intakes in our participants could be even lower than assessed, as non-iodized salt is on the market and some laic nutritional information sources preferred by people on special dietary patterns, especially vegetarians and vegans, promote it as more natural and healthy [49]. Eleven participants supplemented iodine as part of a MMN DS.

4.3. Multimicronutrient Dietary Supplements (MMN DS)

MMN DSs were very commonly used, more than a quarter of participants took them, as was also reported before in [50,51]. The LCHF group had the highest prevalence of MMN DS use among groups (54%), followed by the vegan and vegetarian groups (28% and 27%, respectively) and the lowest prevalence of MMN DS use was in the omnivorous group (8%). Three MMN DSs were used by more than one participant: the first MMN DS included both vitamins and minerals, the second MMN DS included only vitamins from group B, and the third MMN DS was composed of vitamin C, thiamin, riboflavin, and niacin (Figure 2A).

MMN DSs had a wide range of included vitamins and minerals and a wide range of dosages. Of the micronutrients that we identified to have the lowest prevalence of adequate intake with food, vitamin D was found in only ten MMN DSs used by our participants, only two of which contained an adequate daily amount of vitamin D. It was previously reported that vitamin D is often present in a low dose in MMN DSs, nevertheless the incidence of deficiency in vitamin D was also decreased with MMN DS use [51]. Calcium was found in ten MMN DSs and the highest amount of calcium in a MMN DS was 20% of the RV. Low calcium intake adequacy and also low calcium intake with a MMN DS was reported previously [50,51], which indicates the need to use a calcium-only DS to reach sufficient intakes. Furthermore, potassium was only present in two MMN DSs with amounts of only 1 and 2% of the RV, which was also indicated by other authors [51]. We observed that some micronutrients were supplemented only in the form of MMN DSs, these were potassium, calcium, chromium, molybdenum, iodine, and vitamins from group B, except vitamin B_{12}.

Some micronutrients are often present in MMN DSs and also in an adequate amount, such as vitamins from group B and vitamin E. MMN DSs often improved adequacy of micronutrient intake of vitamins and minerals. In our study, this was mostly seen for group B vitamins. B group vitamins were also those that most commonly exceeded the UL. DS use increased the prevalence of exceeded UL for niacin, folate, and pyridoxine, which is in line with previous reports [19,52]. On the other hand, MMN DSs were often missing vitamins and minerals that were shown to have low adequacy in many dietary groups, such as vitamin D, potassium, calcium, and iodine.

4.4. Adequacy of Supplementation

DS use was common, but often did not answer the needs of an individual or dietary pattern. Some micronutrients were correctly chosen and supplemented, such as vitamin B_{12} and vitamin D. The use of DSs with vitamin B_{12} and vitamin D increased the prevalence of adequate intake of those vitamins, even if doses were often misaligned with the need or the RV. Vitamin D was insufficiently (with too low a dose) supplemented in 32% of vitamin D DS users through the whole year and also in 23% in the winter months. On the other hand, vitamin B_{12} was often supplemented in extra high doses, which is not recommended, despite the absence of a UL for vitamin B_{12}. Furthermore, some micronutrients were supplemented despite adequate intake with food. For example, among vitamin K DS users, 87% of them had adequate intake with food alone. Use of MMN DSs with B group vitamins was frequent among the LCHF group, despite high intakes of riboflavin, biotin, and vitamin B_{12} with food alone. Riboflavin and biotin intakes were also adequate with food alone in omnivorous DS users. Iron intake with food alone was adequate in all iron DS users, except in DS users from the vegetarian group. On the contrary, we saw low supplementation of micronutrients that were not sufficiently provided with food, such as potassium and iodine. Low adequate intake with food alone and low supplementation were also observed for calcium in vegans, vegetarians, and the LCHF group, and for vitamin A and vitamin E in the omnivorous and vegetarian groups.

DS users were more likely to exceed the UL for niacin, zinc, folate, iron, pyridoxine, and vitamins D and C than nonusers. Exceeding the UL for niacin with DS use was previously reported [19], but the same study also reported an exceeded UL for folate, vitamin A, and iron with DS use, which in our study was present in very few cases. Exceeded UL in DS users for zinc was also previously reported [30]. Overall, exceeding the UL in our participants was lower than previously reported [51,52].

Our sample was carefully chosen to be able to compare groups, because previous vegan and vegetarian samples were associated with better lifestyle choices and this made those two groups hard to compare with others, especially a representative sample of omnivores. In the present study, we invited participants with an interest in nutrition, and our groups were matched for BMI, physical activity, fat, and fat-free mass, as well as smoking status. Furthermore, we also did not find any differences between DS users and nonusers in education level, income, gender, age, and diet quality, which also made the two groups easy to compare.

The present study pointed to many micronutrient intake shortages compared to reference values in different dietary patterns, but further research on the serum levels of micronutrients is needed. Dietary characteristics of different dietary patterns might influence bioavailability of micronutrients. Magnesium bioavailability, for example, is lower with high phytic acid intake, as often seen in the vegan group [53]. Iron bioavailability is higher from animal sources in the form of heme-iron, but it is also dependent on other dietary factors such as intake of vitamin C [54]. Additionally, some micronutrients in doses lower than the RV do not cause clinical effects; for example, molybdenum was researched for its positive effects on treating anemia and arthritis, but healthy adults are unlikely to develop clinical deficiencies [55].

5. Conclusions

We can conclude that DS use can increase the prevalence of micronutrient intake adequacy if DSs are chosen properly, which was not always the case. Vitamin B_{12} and vitamin D were supplemented to fill nutritional gaps, but the doses were not always appropriate. The fact that several nutrients, such as vitamin K, riboflavin, biotin, and iron were supplemented needlessly, whereas other nutrients, such as potassium, calcium, and iodine were not supplemented, even if intakes with food alone were insufficient, indicates a need for more accurate public education. While it is obvious that participants following diets that omit whole food groups are well aware of certain shortages, such as vitamin B_{12} and iron in the vegan group, and, to a degree, vitamin C and calcium in the LCHF group, the other risks of inadequate intakes are not well known. Increased awareness of possible diet shortages and how to fill them is needed among people without dietary supervision, where it should be acknowledged that several dietary components, typical for the investigated dietary patterns, may influence the micronutrient bioavailability.

Regardless of diet, inadequate micronutrient intake is common among participants who hold the opinion that their diet is balanced and beneficial to health. This raises the need for food counseling and help with selecting proper DSs with a suitable dose. Also, certain adjustments of MMN DSs' composition, such as decreased doses of B group vitamins and increased potassium and vitamin D doses, could be considered.

Author Contributions: Conceptualization, N.M. and Z.J.P.; methodology, N.B.J., K.Š.N., S.K., A.P., Z.J.P. and N.M.; software, N.B.J. and K.Š.N.; validation, N.B.J.; formal analysis, N.B.J.; investigation, N.B.J., K.Š.N., S.K., A.P., Z.J.P. and N.M.; resources, Z.J.P. and N.M.; data curation, N.B.J.; writing—original draft preparation, N.B.J.; writing—review and editing, N.M. and S.K.; visualization, N.B.J. and N.M.; supervision, N.M.; project administration, N.M. and Z.J.P. All authors have read and agreed to the published version of the manuscript.

Funding: The study was supported by the Slovenian Research and Innovation Agency (Programmes P5-0443, P1-0386 and I0-0035).

Institutional Review Board Statement: The study was conducted according to the guidelines of Declaration of Helsinki and approved by the Slovenian National Medical Ethics Committee (No. 0120-557/2017/4, on 10 November 2017) and was registered on ClinicalTrials.gov (Identifier: NCT04347213).

Informed Consent Statement: Informed consent was obtained from all participants involved in the study.

Data Availability Statement: The raw data supporting the conclusions of this article will be made available by the authors on request.

Acknowledgments: Authors thank the participants for participating in the study.

Conflicts of Interest: The authors declare no conflict of interest.

References

1. Medawar, E.; Huhn, S.; Villringer, A.; Veronica Witte, A. The Effects of Plant-Based Diets on the Body and the Brain: A Systematic Review. *Transl. Psychiatry* **2019**, *9*, 226. [CrossRef] [PubMed]
2. Bogataj Jontez, N.; Kenig, S.; Šik Novak, K.; Petelin, A.; Jenko Pražnikar, Z.; Mohorko, N. Habitual Low Carbohydrate High Fat Diet Compared with Omnivorous, Vegan, and Vegetarian Diets. *Front. Nutr.* **2023**, *10*, 1106153. [CrossRef] [PubMed]
3. Huskisson, E.; Maggini, S.; Ruf, M. The Role of Vitamins and Minerals in Energy Metabolism and Well-Being. *J. Int. Med. Res.* **2007**, *35*, 277–289. [CrossRef]
4. Kim, M.; Basharat, A.; Santosh, R.; Mehdi, S.F.; Razvi, Z.; Yoo, S.K.; Lowell, B.; Kumar, A.; Brima, W.; Danoff, A.; et al. Reuniting Overnutrition and Undernutrition, Macronutrients, and Micronutrients. *Diabetes Metab. Res. Rev.* **2019**, *35*, e3072. [CrossRef] [PubMed]
5. Govers, C.; Calder, P.C.; Savelkoul, H.F.J.; Albers, R.; van Neerven, R.J.J. Ingestion, Immunity, and Infection: Nutrition and Viral Respiratory Tract Infections. *Front. Immunol.* **2022**, *13*, 841532. [CrossRef] [PubMed]
6. Tulchinsky, T.H. Micronutrient Deficiency Conditions: Global Health Issues. *Public Health Rev.* **2010**, *32*, 243–255. [CrossRef]
7. Schüpbach, R.; Wegmüller, R.; Berguerand, C.; Bui, M.; Herter-Aeberli, I. Micronutrient Status and Intake in Omnivores, Vegetarians and Vegans in Switzerland. *Eur. J. Nutr.* **2017**, *56*, 283–293. [CrossRef] [PubMed]

8. Hagström, H.; Hagfors, L.N.; Tellström, A.; Hedelin, R.; Lindmark, K. Low Carbohydrate High Fat-Diet in Real Life Assessed by Diet History Interviews. *Nutr. J.* **2023**, *22*, 14. [CrossRef]
9. Gallego-Narbón, A.; Zapatera, B.; Barrios, L.; Vaquero, M.P. Vitamin B12 and Folate Status in Spanish Lacto-Ovo Vegetarians and Vegans. *J. Nutr. Sci.* **2019**, *8*, e7. [CrossRef]
10. Hansen, T.H.; Madsen, M.T.B.; Jørgensen, N.R.; Cohen, A.S.; Hansen, T.; Vestergaard, H.; Pedersen, O.; Allin, K.H. Bone Turnover, Calcium Homeostasis, and Vitamin D Status in Danish Vegans. *Eur. J. Clin. Nutr.* **2018**, *72*, 1046–1054. [CrossRef]
11. Hribar, M.; Hristov, H.; Gregorič, M.; Blaznik, U.; Zaletel, K.; Oblak, A.; Osredkar, J.; Kušar, A.; Žmitek, K.; Rogelj, I.; et al. Nutrihealth Study: Seasonal Variation in Vitamin D Status Among the Slovenian Adult and Elderly Population. *Nutrients* **2020**, *12*, 1838. [CrossRef]
12. Pravst, I.; Lavriša, Ž.; Hribar, M.; Hristov, H.; Kvarantan, N.; Seljak, B.K.; Gregorič, M.; Blaznik, U.; Gregorič, N.; Zaletel, K.; et al. Dietary Intake of Folate and Assessment of the Folate Deficiency Prevalence in Slovenia Using Serum Biomarkers. *Nutrients* **2021**, *13*, 3860. [CrossRef] [PubMed]
13. Churuangsuk, C.; Griffiths, D.; Lean, M.E.J.; Combet, E. Impacts of Carbohydrate-Restricted Diets on Micronutrient Intakes and Status: A Systematic Review. *Obes. Rev. Off. J. Int. Assoc. Study Obes.* **2019**, *20*, 1132–1147. [CrossRef] [PubMed]
14. Kenig, S.; Petelin, A.; Poklar Vatovec, T.; Mohorko, N.; Jenko-Pražnikar, Z. Assessment of Micronutrients in a 12-Wk Ketogenic Diet in Obese Adults. *Nutrition* **2019**, *67–68*, 110522. [CrossRef] [PubMed]
15. Food Supplements | EFSA. Available online: https://www.efsa.europa.eu/en/topics/topic/food-supplements (accessed on 27 February 2023).
16. Mishra, S.; Stierman, B.; Gahche, J.J.; Potischman, N. Dietary Supplement Use Among Adults: United States, 2017–2018. NCHS Data Brief 2021; pp. 1–8. Available online: https://www.cdc.gov/nchs/data/databriefs/db399-H.pdf (accessed on 28 October 2022).
17. Burnett, A.J.; Livingstone, K.M.; Woods, J.L.; McNaughton, S.A. Dietary Supplement Use among Australian Adults: Findings from the 2011–2012 National Nutrition and Physical Activity Survey. *Nutrients* **2017**, *9*, 1248. [CrossRef] [PubMed]
18. Iłowiecka, K.; Maślej, M.; Czajka, M.; Pawłowski, A.; Więckowski, P.; Styk, T.; Gołkiewicz, M.; Kuzdraliński, A.; Koch, W. Lifestyle, Eating Habits, and Health Behaviors among Dietary Supplement Users in Three European Countries. *Front. Public Health* **2022**, *10*, 892233. [CrossRef] [PubMed]
19. Dickinson, A.; MacKay, D. Health Habits and Other Characteristics of Dietary Supplement Users: A Review. *Nutr. J.* **2014**, *13*, 14. [CrossRef] [PubMed]
20. Bizjak, M.; Jenko-Pražnikar, Z.; Koroušić Seljak, B. Development and Validation of an Electronic FFQ to Assess Food Intake in the Slovene Population. *Public Health Nutr.* **2014**, *17*, 1729–1737. [CrossRef] [PubMed]
21. Korošec, M.; Golob, T.; Bertoncelj, J.; Stibilj, V.; Seljak, B. The Slovenian Food Composition Database. *Food Chem.* **2013**, *140*, 495–499. [CrossRef]
22. Souci, S.W.; Fachmann, W.; Kraut, H. *Food Composition and Nutrition Tables*; Medpharm: Guildford, UK, 2000.
23. Hayowitz, D.B.; Ahuja, J.K.C.; Wu, X.; Somanchi, M.; Nickle, M.; Nguyen, Q.A.; Roseland, J.M.; Williams, J.R.; Patterson, K.Y.; Pehrsson, P.R. *USDA National Nutrient Database for Standard Reference, Legacy Release 2019*; USDA: Washington, DC, USA, 2019.
24. NIJZ Referenčne Vrednosti Za Energijski Vnos Ter Vnos Hranil. Available online: https://www.nijz.si/sl/referencne-vrednosti-za-energijski-vnos-ter-vnos-hranil (accessed on 21 June 2020).
25. European Food Safety Authority, Scientific Committee on Food. Tolerable Upper Intake Levels for Vitamins and Minerals. 2006. Available online: https://www.efsa.europa.eu/sites/default/files/assets/ndatolerableuil.pdf (accessed on 21 September 2023).
26. EFSA Panel on Nutrition, Novel Foods and Food Allergens (NDA); Turck, D.; Bohn, T.; Castenmiller, J.; de Henauw, S.; Hirsch-Ernst, K.-I.; Knutsen, H.K.; Maciuk, A.; Mangelsdorf, I.; McArdle, H.J.; et al. Scientific Opinion on the Tolerable Upper Intake Level for Selenium. *EFSA J.* **2023**, *21*, e07704. [CrossRef]
27. EFSA Panel on Nutrition, Novel Foods and Food Allergens (NDA); Turck, D.; Bohn, T.; Castenmiller, J.; de Henauw, S.; Hirsch-Ernst, K.-I.; Knutsen, H.K.; Maciuk, A.; Mangelsdorf, I.; McArdle, H.J.; et al. Scientific Opinion on the Tolerable Upper Intake Level for Vitamin B6. *EFSA J.* **2023**, *21*, e08006. [CrossRef] [PubMed]
28. EFSA Panel on Dietetic Products, Nutrition and Allergies (NDA). Scientific Opinion on the Tolerable Upper Intake Level of Calcium. *EFSA J.* **2012**, *10*, 2814. [CrossRef]
29. EFSA Panel on Nutrition, Novel Foods and FoodAllergens (NDA); Turck, D.; Bohn, T.; Castenmiller, J.; de Henauw, S.; Hirsch-Ernst, K.-I.; Knutsen, H.K.; Maciuk, A.; Mangelsdorf, I.; McArdle, H.J.; et al. Scientific Opinion on the Tolerable Upper Intake Level for Vitamin D, Including the Derivation of a Conversion Factor for Calcidiol Monohydrate. *EFSA J.* **2023**, *21*, e08145. [CrossRef] [PubMed]
30. Murphy, S.P.; White, K.K.; Park, S.-Y.; Sharma, S. Multivitamin-Multimineral Supplements' Effect on Total Nutrient Intake. *Am. J. Clin. Nutr.* **2007**, *85*, 280S–284S. [CrossRef] [PubMed]
31. Sicinska, E.; Madej, D.; Szmidt, M.K.; Januszko, O.; Kaluza, J. Dietary Supplement Use in Relation to Socio-Demographic and Lifestyle Factors, Including Adherence to Mediterranean-Style Diet in University Students. *Nutrients* **2022**, *14*, 2745. [CrossRef] [PubMed]

32. Weikert, C.; Trefflich, I.; Menzel, J.; Obeid, R.; Longree, A.; Dierkes, J.; Meyer, K.; Herter-Aeberli, I.; Mai, K.; Stangl, G.I.; et al. Vitamin and Mineral Status in a Vegan Diet. *Dtsch. Ärztebl. Int.* **2020**, *117*, 575–582. [CrossRef]
33. Lavriša, Ž.; Hristov, H.; Hribar, M.; Žmitek, K.; Kušar, A.; Koroušić Seljak, B.; Gregorič, M.; Blaznik, U.; Gregorič, N.; Zaletel, K.; et al. Dietary Intake and Status of Vitamin B12 in Slovenian Population. *Nutrients* **2022**, *14*, 334. [CrossRef] [PubMed]
34. Bundesinstitut Für Risikobewertung. Updated Recommended Maximum Levels for the Addition of Vitamins and Minerals to Food Supplements and Conventional Foods: BfR Opinion No 009/2021 of 15 March 2021. *BfR-Stellungnahmen* **2021**, *2021*, 9. [CrossRef]
35. Bundesinstitut Für Risikobewertung. Maximum Levels for the Addition of Vitamin B12 to Foods Including Food Supplements. 2021. Available online: https://www.bfr.bund.de/cm/349/maximum-levels-for-the-addition-of-vitamin-b12-to-foods-including-food-supplements.pdf (accessed on 14 February 2024).
36. EFSA Panel on Dietetic Products, Nutrition, and Allergies (NDA). Scientific Opinion on Dietary Reference Values for Cobalamin (Vitamin B12). *EFSA J.* **2015**, *13*, 4150. [CrossRef]
37. Meyer, H.E.; Willett, W.C.; Fung, T.T.; Holvik, K.; Feskanich, D. Association of High Intakes of Vitamins B6 and B12 From Food and Supplements with Risk of Hip Fracture Among Postmenopausal Women in the Nurses' Health Study. *JAMA Netw. Open* **2019**, *2*, e193591. [CrossRef]
38. Carmel, R. How I Treat Cobalamin (Vitamin B12) Deficiency. *Blood* **2008**, *112*, 2214–2221. [CrossRef] [PubMed]
39. Del Bo', C.; Riso, P.; Gardana, C.; Brusamolino, A.; Battezzati, A.; Ciappellano, S. Effect of Two Different Sublingual Dosages of Vitamin B12 on Cobalamin Nutritional Status in Vegans and Vegetarians with a Marginal Deficiency: A Randomized Controlled Trial. *Clin. Nutr.* **2019**, *38*, 575–583. [CrossRef] [PubMed]
40. MacFarlane, A.J.; Shi, Y.; Greene-Finestone, L.S. High-Dose Compared with Low-Dose Vitamin B-12 Supplement Use Is Not Associated with Higher Vitamin B-12 Status in Children, Adolescents, and Older Adults. *J. Nutr.* **2014**, *144*, 915–920. [CrossRef] [PubMed]
41. Elorinne, A.-L.; Alfthan, G.; Erlund, I.; Kivimäki, H.; Paju, A.; Salminen, I.; Turpeinen, U.; Voutilainen, S.; Laakso, J. Food and Nutrient Intake and Nutritional Status of Finnish Vegans and Non-Vegetarians. *PLoS ONE* **2016**, *11*, e0148235. [CrossRef] [PubMed]
42. Regulation (EU) No 1169/2011 of the European Parliament and of the Council of 25 October 2011 on the Provision of Food Information to Consumers, Amending Regulations (EC) No 1924/2006 and (EC) No 1925/2006 of the European Parliament and of the Council, and Repealing Commission Directive 87/250/EEC, Council Directive 90/496/EEC, Commission Directive 1999/10/EC, Directive 2000/13/EC of the European Parliament and of the Council, Commission Directives 2002/67/EC and 2008/5/EC and Commission Regulation (EC) No 608/2004 (Text with EEA Relevance)Text with EEA Relevance. Available online: https://eur-lex.europa.eu/legal-content/EN/TXT/PDF/?uri=CELEX:32011R1169&from=EN (accessed on 14 February 2024).
43. Gregorič, M.; Hristov, H.; Blaznik, U.; Koroušić Seljak, B.; Delfar, N.; Pravst, I. Dietary Intakes of Slovenian Adults and Elderly: Design and Results of the National Dietary Study SI.Menu 2017/18. *Nutrients* **2022**, *14*, 3618. [CrossRef] [PubMed]
44. Brauchla, M.; Dekker, M.J.; Rehm, C.D. Trends in Vitamin C Consumption in the United States: 1999–2018. *Nutrients* **2021**, *13*, 420. [CrossRef]
45. Henjum, S.; Groufh-Jacobsen, S.; Stea, T.H.; Tonheim, L.E.; Almendingen, K. Iron Status of Vegans, Vegetarians and Pescatarians in Norway. *Biomolecules* **2021**, *11*, 454. [CrossRef]
46. McLean, R.M.; Wang, N.X. Potassium. *Adv. Food Nutr. Res.* **2021**, *96*, 89–121. [CrossRef] [PubMed]
47. Stimec, M.; Kobe, H.; Smole, K.; Kotnik, P.; Sirca-Campa, A.; Zupancic, M.; Battelino, T.; Krzisnik, C.; Fidler Mis, N. Adequate Iodine Intake of Slovenian Adolescents Is Primarily Attributed to Excessive Salt Intake. *Nutr. Res.* **2009**, *29*, 888–896. [CrossRef]
48. Ribič, C.H.; Zakotnik, J.M.; Vertnik, L.; Vegnuti, M.; Cappuccio, F.P. Salt Intake of the Slovene Population Assessed by 24 h Urinary Sodium Excretion. *Public Health Nutr.* **2010**, *13*, 1803–1809. [CrossRef]
49. Žmitek, K.; Pravst, I. Iodisation of Salt in Slovenia: Increased Availability of Non-Iodised Salt in the Food Supply. *Nutrients* **2016**, *8*, 434. [CrossRef] [PubMed]
50. Shakur, Y.A.; Tarasuk, V.; Corey, P.; O'Connor, D.L. A Comparison of Micronutrient Inadequacy and Risk of High Micronutrient Intakes among Vitamin and Mineral Supplement Users and Nonusers in Canada. *J. Nutr.* **2012**, *142*, 534–540. [CrossRef] [PubMed]
51. Wallace, T.C.; Frankenfeld, C.L.; Frei, B.; Shah, A.V.; Yu, C.-R.; van Klinken, B.J.-W.; Adeleke, M. Multivitamin/Multimineral Supplement Use Is Associated with Increased Micronutrient Intakes and Biomarkers and Decreased Prevalence of Inadequacies and Deficiencies in Middle-Aged and Older Adults in the United States. *J. Nutr. Gerontol. Geriatr.* **2019**, *38*, 307–328. [CrossRef] [PubMed]
52. Biesalski, H.K. Nutrition Meets the Microbiome: Micronutrients and the Microbiota. *Ann. N. Y. Acad. Sci.* **2016**, *1372*, 53–64. [CrossRef] [PubMed]
53. Barbagallo, M.; Veronese, N.; Dominguez, L.J. Magnesium in Aging, Health and Diseases. *Nutrients* **2021**, *13*, 463. [CrossRef] [PubMed]

54. Perera, D.N.; Palliyaguruge, C.L.; Eapasinghe, D.D.; Liyanage, D.M.; Seneviratne, R.A.C.H.; Demini, S.M.D.; Jayasinghe, J.A.S.M.; Faizan, M.; Rajagopalan, U.; Galhena, B.P.; et al. Factors Affecting Iron Absorption and the Role of Fortification in Enhancing Iron Levels. *Nutr. Bull.* **2023**, *48*, 442–457. [CrossRef]
55. Grech, B.J. Mechanistic Insights into the Treatment of Iron-Deficiency Anemia and Arthritis in Humans with Dietary Molybdenum. *Eur. J. Clin. Nutr.* **2021**, *75*, 1170–1175. [CrossRef]

nutrients

MDPI

Article

Dietary Intake among Lebanese Adults: Findings from the Updated LEBANese natiONal Food Consumption Survey (LEBANON-FCS)

Maha Hoteit [1,2,*], Maroun Khattar [2], Dana Malli [2], Esraa Antar [2], Zahraa Al Hassani [2], Maher Abdallah [2], Dalia Hachem [2], Elham Al Manasfi [3], Abdulrahman Chahine [3], Nikolaos Tzenios [4,*] and the Adults-LEBANON-FCS Group †

1 Food Sciences Unit, National Council for Scientific Research-Lebanon (CNRS-L), Beirut P.O. Box 11-8281, Lebanon
2 Faculty of Public Health, Section 1, Lebanese University, Beirut P.O. Box 6573, Lebanon; dana.malli@st.ul.edu.lb (D.M.); e.antar@st.ul.edu.lb (E.A.); zahraa.al-hassani@st.ul.edu.lb (Z.A.H.)
3 Arab Group for Scientific Research, Beirut 1103, Lebanon
4 Faculty of Public Health, Charisma University, London EC1V 7QE, UK
* Correspondence: maha.hoteit@cnrs.edu.lb (M.H.); nicolas@trccolleges.com (N.T.)
† The members of the Adults-LEBANON-FCS Group listed in Appendix A are considered as co-authors.

Abstract: Background: The rates of obesity, undernutrition, and other non-communicable diseases are on the rise among Lebanese adults. Therefore, it is crucial to evaluate the food consumption habits of this population to understand diet quality, analyze consumption trends, and compare them to healthy diets known to reduce risks of non-communicable diseases. Aim: To evaluate the food consumption patterns, energy intake, as well as macro- and micro-nutrient intake among a nationally representative sample of Lebanese adults aged 18–64 years old. Methods: A cross-sectional study was carried out from May to September 2022 involving 444 participants from all eight Lebanese governorates. Sociodemographic and medical information was gathered through a questionnaire, food consumption was evaluated using a validated FFQ and 24 h recall, and anthropometric measurements were recorded. Results: There was a notable lack of adherence to three healthy diets (Mediterranean, EAT-Lancet, USDA) among Lebanese adults. Their dietary pattern is characterized by high energy, added sugars, sodium, and saturated fat intake while being low in healthy fats, vitamin A, D, and E. Adult women are falling short of meeting their daily calcium, vitamin D, iron, and vitamin B12 requirements, putting them at increased risk of anemia, osteoporosis, and other health issues. Grains and cereals were the most consumed food groups, and most participants were found to be overweight or obese. Conclusions: In conclusion, the results highlight the need for public health policies and interventions aimed at encouraging Lebanese adults to make healthier food choices and transition towards diets like the Mediterranean, EAT-Lancet, or USDA diet. These diets have been shown to promote overall health and wellbeing.

Keywords: adult; food consumption; food groups; macronutrients; micronutrients; healthy diets

1. Introduction

In an era marked by rapid globalization, urbanization, demographic and epidemiological transitions, and economic volatility, the dynamics of nutrition transition and food insecurity have become critical focal points for policymakers, researchers, and public health practitioners worldwide. The intricate interplay between nutrition transition—the shift in dietary patterns towards higher consumption of high-caloric food and a decrease in consumption of healthy foods [1]—and food insecurity—the inadequate access to sufficient, safe, and nutritious food—is emblematic of multifaceted challenges facing contemporary societies. This transition is often accompanied by a rise in sedentary lifestyles, reduced physical activity, and changing patterns of food preparation and consumption, heralding a new era of dietary diversity but also posing significant challenges to public health and nutrition. The current pattern of nutrition transition (consumption of high-caloric food and sedentary lifestyle) is characterized by the rising of nutrition-related non-communicable diseases (NR-NCDs) that seems to be accelerating in the lower- and middle-income transitional countries [2], which now carry more than 75% of the global non-communicable disease (NCD) burden [3]. This is the case in Lebanon, where Lebanese adults aged 18 years and older dietary patterns have shifted, and where the prevalences of obesity and undernourishment are increasing significantly. For instance, the prevalences of obesity (in 2016) and undernourishment (in 2020) increased and reached about 32% and 9.5%, respectively [4,5]. This is mainly due to the limited progress towards achieving the diet-related NCD targets, mainly obesity targets [6], although several diets were established and contributed to limit the development of NCDs, such as the Mediterranean, the EAT-Lancet and USDA diets, and dietary guidelines. This dietary shift is the result of changes the country has faced, and is still facing, since the past decade, such as increased urbanization, economic development, modernization in lifestyle, the COVID-19 pandemic, the massive blast that hit the Beirut port on 4 August 2020, and, most recently, the Ukraine–Russia war. The recent events have heightened the risk of food insecurity in the Lebanese population, affecting their nutritional behaviors and status [7–9]. This increased the risk of undernutrition, micronutrient deficiencies, and overweight/obesity in this population because of insufficient or imbalanced macro- and micro-nutrient intakes [10], which in turn can increase the risk of diet-related health conditions such as diabetes, hypertension, hyperlipidemia, and metabolic syndrome, among other conditions [11–14].

Given the significance of adopting healthy food choices to reduce the risk of non-communicable diseases, and with the rising rates of obesity, undernutrition, and other non-communicable diseases among Lebanese adults, it is essential to examine the dietary habits of this population. In addition, the current available data on adults' food consumption in the country reflect the consumption of this population up to the year 2009, which, although important, is now outdated due to the changes that have occurred in the country since then and have affected food consumption. This highlights the importance of having new reliable data that reflect the recent trends of consumption in this population. Thus, this examination aims to understand the quality of Lebanese adults' diets, analyze consumption trends, and compare them to proven healthy diets that can mitigate the risks of non-communicable diseases. By doing so, actionable steps can be taken to improve the dietary patterns of the population and eventually improve their overall health and wellbeing.

2. Methods

2.1. Study Design and Eligibility Criteria

This was a cross-sectional study that was conducted over a period of 5 months between May and September 2022 on a nationally representative sample of Lebanese adults. To be eligible, a participant had to be Lebanese and aged between 18 and 64 years old.

2.2. Sampling Method and Recruitment Process

For the sample to be nationally representative, a minimum number of 400 participants was required. The sample size was calculated based on the population estimates from 2018 to 2019 using the following formula:

$$n = [p\ (1 - p)] \times [(Z_{\alpha/2})^2/(e)^2]$$

where 'n' refers to the sample size; '$Z_{\alpha/2}$' refers to the standard error's reliability coefficient at a 5% level of significance and is equal to 1.96; 'p' denotes the probability of adults (18–64 y) who were not capable of taking precautions regarding the diseases (50%); and 'e' represents the standard error's tolerated level (5%), as stated by Hosmer and Lemeshow [15]. Overall, 449 participants (184 males and 265 females) from the 8 Lebanese governorates were included. The sampling technique was a combination of stratified cluster sampling, with the stratified groups being the two genders and the clusters being the Lebanese governorates. The process of recruiting participants involved various channels, including volunteers, charitable organizations, first-aid and medical centers, so a broad range of participants could be reached. Participants recruited in this stage were then encouraged to invite other individuals within their outreach to participate. This allowed us to reach participants that were difficult to reach physically due to budget constraints and timing. The individuals willing to participate were informed about the study nature and then assessed for eligibility. Eligible participants provided an electronic written consent indicating their willingness to participate in the study. One individual per Lebanese household was allowed to participate in the study so that a wide representation of households could be guaranteed. Overall, the study involved 444 participants, as 5 participants were excluded after checking for missing data, errors, and outliers. Participant distribution across the 8 governorates is shown in Figure 1.

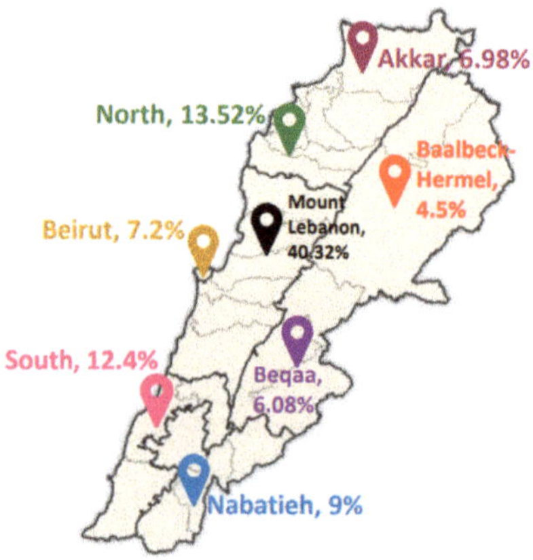

Figure 1. Participant distribution across the Lebanese governorates (Map template adapted from https://en.m.wikipedia.org/wiki/File:Lebanon_districts.png, accessed on 1 May 2024).

2.3. Data Collection

2.3.1. Phase 1: Administration of Sociodemographic Questionnaire

During the initial data collection phase, a pre-tested questionnaire was utilized in interviews with participants. This questionnaire covered demographic and socioeconomic details along with the medical background of the participants. For example, participants were queried about their age, gender, weight, height, place of residence, marital status, living space, household size, number of rooms in their residence, educational level, occupation, and any existing chronic illnesses. Questions pertaining to household size and number of rooms were included to compute the crowding index (CI), which serves as an indicator of a household's socioeconomic standing [16].

2.3.2. Phase 2: Food Frequency Questionnaire

Following the completion of the sociodemographic questionnaire, trained dietitians conducted 30-min interviews with participants to administer a 157-item semi-quantitative food frequency questionnaire (FFQ), which had been validated previously among the adult Lebanese population [17]. To assist the participants in remembering how much food they had consumed and in estimating portion sizes as precisely as possible, instructions and visual aids were given to them. The interviewers recorded how many servings and how often the stated portions (daily, weekly, or monthly) for each food item were consumed. Trained dietitians administered the FFQ. Furthermore, two 24 h recalls were conducted—one on a typical weekday and another on a weekend day. The FFQ captured the frequency of consuming various foods over the past year, with interviewees noting servings, grams, and consumption frequency (daily, weekly, or monthly). The consumption of each specific food and beverage was comprehensively recorded through the two 24 h recalls. Visual aids and instructions were provided to aid participants in accurately recalling food intake and estimating portion sizes.

2.3.3. Phase 3: Anthropometric Measurements

During this stage, anthropometric measurements (weight and height) of the participants were taken at a designated center or facility within their respective governorates. Standardized protocols and calibrated equipment, including a digital scale for weight and a stadiometer for height, were employed to ensure precise measurements. To enhance accuracy, each participant's height and weight were measured thrice, and the Body Mass Index (BMI) was calculated by averaging the three recorded readings.

2.4. Data Management and Data Analysis

Excel 2016 was used to code and organize the data. The CI was calculated by dividing the total number of people living in the home (apart from infants) by the total number of rooms (apart from bathrooms and kitchens) [16]. The food items were divided into food groups according to the classifications of the following three distinct diets: the 'Mediterranean Diet' [18], the 'EAT-Lancet Diet' [19,20], and the 'USDA Diet' [21]. The food group intake (g/day) was then calculated and compared to the recommendations of each of these three diets. To calculate the food group consumption (g/day), the following method was used: The daily consumption of each food item was determined using the FFQ data. To calculate the daily frequency (serving/day), a serving that was reported as being consumed on a weekly or monthly basis was divided by 7 or 30, respectively. Then, the quantity of each food item consumed (g/day) was calculated by multiplying the daily frequencies that resulted by the corresponding serving sizes of the individual food items (g/serving). After that, the individual foods were divided into categories according to the three diets. The total intake (g/day) for a food group was then determined by adding the quantities consumed of each food item belonging to the corresponding group.

After calculating the amounts of food consumed in grams per day, extraction of energy, macro- and micro-nutrients and the fiber content of the food consumed was undertaken using 'Nutritionist Pro' (version 5.1.0, 2014, First Data Bank, Nutritionist Pro, Axxya Systems, San Bruno, CA, USA), which is a software that permits the nutritional analysis of individual foods, menu items, and recipe ingredients [22]. The extracted nutritional value of food consumed was then compared to the age-specific Dietary Reference Intakes (DRIs), which were created by the 'Food and Nutrition Board, Institute of Medicine, National Academies' (NIH) and include the 'Acceptable Macronutrient Distribution Range' (AMDR), the 'Adequate Intake' (AI) and the 'Recommended Dietary Allowance' (RDAs) [23], 'Dietary Cholesterol and Cardiovascular Risk: A Science Advisory From the American Heart Association' [24], 'Development of a Lebanese food exchange system based on frequently consumed Eastern Mediterranean traditional dishes and Arabic sweets' [25], and 'Nutritional value of the Middle Eastern diet: analysis of total sugar, salt, and iron in Lebanese traditional dishes' [26]. Energy requirements were extracted from the 'Dietary Guidelines for Americans 2020–2025' [21].

2.5. Statistical Analysis

The sample was classified based on genders into 4 age categories in accordance with the 'Food and Nutrition Board, Institute of Medicine, National Academies' (NIH) [23] as follows: 18 years; 19–30 years; 31–50 years; and 51–64 years.

The Statistical Package for the Social Sciences (SPSS; Version 25.0, IBM Corp: Armonk, NY, USA) was used to analyze the data at a 95% confidence interval. Frequencies (N) and percentages (%) were calculated for categorical variables, while means and standard deviations (SD) were calculated for the continuous variables.

2.6. Ethical Considerations

The protocol for this study underwent review and approval by the Ethical Committee at Al Zahraa University Medical Center (#57/2022) and was carried out in compliance with the ethical principles set forth in the Declaration of Helsinki. Prior to participation, participants provided informed consent and were informed that their involvement was voluntary, with the option to withdraw at any point.

3. Results

3.1. Population Characteristics

The demographic and socioeconomic characteristics of the study population are shown in Table 1, and the study population's health characteristics are shown in Table 2. Most participants were females (58.8%), and the mean age ± SD (years) was 34.1 ± 12.7. Most of the participants were residing in Mount Lebanon (40.32%), and most households were found to be crowded (62.84%), which reflects a lower socioeconomic status in these households compared to the non-crowded ones. Almost one-third of the participants (33.8%) had a normal BMI, while the majority (61.9%) were found to be overweight or obese. In addition, 25% of the participants reported having one or more chronic diseases, with anemia (32.4%) being the most prevalent disease, followed by hypertension (30.6%). Regarding the type of disease, more women were shown to be affected by the majority of diseases, except for kidney disease (similar between genders) and liver disease (more men are affected).

Table 1. Demographic and socioeconomic characteristics of the study population, overall and by gender.

KERRYPNX		Overall (n = 444)	Male (n = 183)	Female (n = 261)	p-Value
		n (%)	n (%)	n (%)	
Age Category	18 Years	20 (4.5%)	5 (25%)	15 (75%)	0.167
	19–30 Years	187 (42.1%)	78 (41.7%)	109 (58.3%)	
	31–50 Years	174 (39.2%)	79 (45.4%)	95 (54.6%)	
	51–64 Years	63 (14.2%)	21 (33.3%)	42 (66.7%)	
Residency (Governorate)	Akkar	31 (6.98%)	11 (35.5%)	20 (64.5%)	0.006 *
	Mount Lebanon	179 (40.32%)	73 (40.8%)	106 (59.2%)	
	Beqaa	27 (6.08%)	5 (18.5%)	22 (81.5%)	
	North Lebanon	60 (13.52%)	33 (55%)	27 (45%)	
	Baalbek-Hermel	20 (4.5%)	10 (50%)	10 (50%)	
	South Lebanon	55 (12.4%)	30 (54.5%)	25 (45.5%)	
	Beirut	32 (7.2%)	10 (31.2%)	22 (68.8%)	
	Nabatiyeh	40 (9%)	11 (27.5%)	29 (72.5%)	
Marital Status	Single	202 (45.5%)	81 (40.1%)	121 (59.9%)	0.139
	Married	223 (50.23%)	97 (43.5%)	126 (56.5%)	
	Widowed	7 (1.57%)	0 (0.0%)	7 (100%)	
	Divorced	12 (2.7%)	5 (41.7%)	7 (58.3%)	
Crowding index	No crowding	165 (37.16%)	79 (47.9%)	86 (52.1%)	0.028 *
	Crowding	279 (62.84%)	104 (37.3%)	175 (62.7%)	
Number of children	0	217 (48.87%)	87 (40.1%)	130 (59.9%)	0.124
	1–3	159 (35.81%)	74 (46.5%)	85 (53.5%)	
	>3	68 (15.32%)	22 (32.4%)	46 (67.6%)	
Education level	Illiterate	3 (0.68%)	1 (33.3%)	2 (66.7%)	0.961
	School	175 (39.41%)	72 (41.1%)	103 (58.9%)	
	University	266 (59.91%)	110 (41.4%)	156 (58.6%)	
Current Occupation	Unemployed	218 (49.1%)	40 (18.3%)	178 (81.7%)	0.000 *
	Employed	226 (50.9%)	143 (63.3%)	83 (36.7%)	

Table 1. *Cont.*

KERRYPNX		Overall (*n* = 444)	Male (*n* = 183)	Female (*n* = 261)	*p*-Value
		n (%)	*n* (%)	*n* (%)	
Monthly salary changes after economic crisis	No Impact	129 (29%)	63 (48.8%)	66 (51.2%)	0.000 *
	Decline in Salary	123 (27.7%)	51 (41.5%)	72 (58.5%)	
	Increase in Salary	70 (15.8%)	42 (60%)	28 (40%)	
	Already have no Salary	122 (27.5%)	27 (22.1%)	95 (77.9%)	
Household Monthly Income	None	39 (8.78%)	17 (43.6%)	22 (56.4%)	0.000 *
	Less than 1.5 million LBP	58 (13.1%)	15 (25.9%)	43 (74.1%)	
	>=1.5 million LBP	211 (47.5%)	79 (37.4%)	132 (62.6%)	
	<=300 USD	92 (20.72%)	41 (44.6%)	51 (55.4%)	
	More than 300 USD	44 (9.9%)	31 (70.5%)	13 (29.5%)	

* *p*-value < 0.05 is significant.

Table 2. Health characteristics of the study population, overall and by gender.

Variable		Overall (*n* = 444)		Male (*n* = 183)		Female (*n* = 261)		
		Mean	SD	Mean	SD	Mean	SD	*p*-Value
Weight (kg)		73.8	17.1	81.8	16.6	68.3	15.1	<0.001 *
Height (cm)		165.3	9.4	173.5	7	159.5	5.9	<0.001 *
Body mass index (kg/m^2)		27	5.8	27.2	5.3	26.9	6.1	0.626
		n	%	*n*	%	*n*	%	
BMI classification	Underweight	19	4.3	4	21.1	15	78.9	0.084
	Normal	150	33.8	57	38	93	62	
	Overweight and Obese	275	61.9	122	44.4	153	55.6	
Disease status	No disease	333	75	150	45	183	55	0.005 *
	Having disease	111	25	33	29.7	78	70.3	
Disease type	Cardiovascular disease	14	12.6	5	15.2	9	11.5	0.004 *
	Diabetes	3	2.7	1	3	2	2.6	
	Hypertension	34	30.6	16	48.5	18	23.1	
	Kidney disease	4	3.6	2	6.1	2	2.6	
	Liver disease	1	0.9	1	3	0	0	
	Osteoporosis	14	12.6	1	3	13	16.7	
	Asthma/Respiratory diseases	12	10.8	2	6.1	10	12.8	
	Anemia	36	32.4	5	15.2	31	39.7	
	Others [a]	32	28.8	6	18.2	26	33.3	

* *p*-value < 0.05 is significant. [a] Includes other self-reported diseases: (1) Allergies (seasonal, food, dust, skin); (2) vertebral column problems; (3) sarcoidosis; (4) migraine; (5) thyroid disease; (6) gastrointestinal problems; (7) psychological conditions; (8) neurological conditions; (9) hypovitaminosis D; (10) hypocalcemia; (11) iron deficiency; (12) urinary tract infection; (13) hypercholesterolemia; (14) Raynaud's syndrome; (15) varicose veins; (16) autoimmune diseases; (17) cancer; (18) thrombosis; (19) polycystic ovarian syndrome.

Significant differences between genders existed when it comes to residency (*p*-value = 0.006), crowding index (*p*-value = 0.028), occupation (*p*-value = 0.000), household income (*p*-value = 0.000), salary change (*p*-value = 0.000), the presence of chronic diseases (*p*-value = 0.005) and the disease type (*p*-value = 0.004).

3.2. *Food Groups Consumption and Comparison to Different Diets' Recommendations*

3.2.1. Food Groups Consumption

Mean intake of the different food groups by age and by gender are shown in Tables 3 and 4, respectively. The description of food items included in each food group is shown in Table S1. In the overall study population, intake of bread/cereals/grains was the highest (317.18 g/d), followed by fruits (254.33 g/d) then vegetables (206.49 g/d). Among age categories, the mean intake of bread/cereals/grains was the highest compared to other food groups in all age categories except for participants in the 51–64 age group, in which the mean intake of fruits was the highest compared to other food groups (330 g/d). Significant differences in consumption existed among age categories when it comes to the consumption of processed meat (*p*-value = 0.000), poultry (*p*-value = 0.003), fresh fruit juices (*p*-value = 0.001), sweets (*p*-value = 0.000), and added fats/oils (*p*-value = 0.002). Regarding consumption based on gender, our results showed that, on average, male participants had a higher consumption compared to women from all the food groups except for vegetables, with significant differences in consumption existing when it comes to consuming nuts/seeds (*p*-value = 0.04), dairy products (*p*-value = 0.011), red meat (*p*-value = 0.000), processed meat (*p*-value = 0.000), poultry (*p*-value = 0.000), fish (*p*-value = 0.000), eggs (*p*-value = 0.000), drinking water (*p*-value = 0.000), non-alcoholic beverages (*p*-value = 0.000), and alcoholic beverages (*p*-value = 0.01).

Table 3. Food groups consumption by Lebanese adults, by age category.

	Dietary Intake (g/day)				
	Overall (*n* = 444)				
Food Groups	**18 Years (*n* = 20)**	**19–30 Years (*n* = 187)**	**31–50 Years (*n* = 174)**	**51–64 Years (*n* = 63)**	***p*-Value**
Bread, Cereals and Grains	312 ± 89.78	329.88 ± 146.19	312.94 ± 132.31	292.61 ± 115.57	0.268
Legumes	73.03 ± 56.1	61.98 ± 59.97	67.95 ± 50.1	76.34 ± 50.01	0.297
Nuts and Seeds	2.56 ± 2.73	6.24 ± 16.52	3.84 ± 8.26	5.3 ± 9.37	0.246
Starchy Vegetables	43.5 ± 21.96	54.52 ± 49.02	48.21 ± 36.26	46.98 ± 48.94	0.391
Vegetables	177.86 ± 107.46	211.38 ± 118.85	194.73 ± 118.31	233.55 ± 112.69	0.087
Dairy Products	162.16 ± 128.4	201.19 ± 184.49	168.14 ± 150.94	187.19 ± 146.2	0.26
Meat and Meat Products, Poultry, Fish, Eggs					
Red Meat	39.35 ± 27.06	48.38 ± 52.85	36.73 ± 50.72	33.83 ± 26.19	0.069
Processed Meat	2.14 ± 2.46	4.71 ± 7.04	2.03 ± 3.17	1.66 ± 3.19	0.000 *
Poultry	30.96 ± 15.32	42.16 ± 41.42	30.62 ± 49.31	21.58 ± 20.28	0.003 *
Fish	7.97 ± 6.82	13.72 ± 26.05	10.08 ± 17.93	9.22 ± 13.45	0.244
Eggs	20.62 ± 19.47	26.58 ± 35.65	20.07 ± 34.12	15.84 ± 17.7	0.087
Fruits, Total					
Fruits	272.63 ± 229.84	231.99 ± 251.28	248.79 ± 293.12	330.09 ± 356.76	0.124
Fresh Juices (100% fruit juices) [a]	52.39 ± 59.71	52.8 ± 95.58	29.84 ± 60.07	12.78 ± 24.97	0.001 *
Sweets and Added Sugars					
Sweets	178.53 ± 399.44	81.32 ± 93.52	44.77 ± 54.66	38.92 ± 52.19	0.000 *
Added Sugars, Jams, Honey, Molasses	23.75 ± 26.72	18.3 ± 22.36	18.9 ± 21.3	19.69 ± 22.66	0.761
Added Fats and Oils	14.15 ± 11.77	9.47 ± 9.44	11.89 ± 12.84	15.68 ± 13.13	0.002 *
Non-Alcoholic Beverages [a]	104.6 ± 184.74	82.89 ± 127.27	60.99 ± 113.91	50.13 ± 87.95	0.093
Alcoholic Beverages [a]	0 ± 0	0.41 ± 5.05	1.04 ± 7.79	0.19 ± 1.51	0.649

Values are Mean ± Standard deviation. * *p*-value < 0.05 is significant. [a] Beverages presented in mL/day.

Table 4. Food groups consumption by Lebanese adults, overall and by gender.

Food Groups	Dietary Intake (g/day)			
	Overall (*n* = 444)	**Male (*n* = 183)**	**Female (*n* = 261)**	***p*-Value**
Bread, Cereals and Grains	317.18 ± 134.85	390.58 ± 139.96	265.71 ± 104.04	0.000
Legumes	66.85 ± 54.77	68.24 ± 62.25	65.89 ± 48.96	0.657
Nuts and Seeds	5 ± 12.46	6.45 ± 13.08	3.99 ± 11.93	0.04 *
Starchy Vegetables	50.48 ± 43.48	54.34 ± 42.38	47.78 ± 44.13	0.118
Vegetables	206.49 ± 117.79	197.76 ± 115.39	212.61 ± 119.29	0.191
Dairy Products	184.5 ± 164.72	208.33 ± 186.13	167.78 ± 145.94	0.011 *

Table 4. *Cont.*

Food Groups	Dietary Intake (g/day)			
	Overall (n = 444)	Male (n = 183)	Female (n = 261)	p-Value
Meat and Meat Products, Poultry, Fish, Eggs				
Red Meat	41.34 ± 48.39	54.45 ± 59.22	32.15 ± 36.47	0.000 *
Processed Meat	3.11 ± 5.32	4.35 ± 6.79	2.24 ± 3.76	0.000 *
Poultry	34.21 ± 42.34	46.55 ± 53.88	25.56 ± 28.98	0.000 *
Fish	11.39 ± 21.02	16.86 ± 28.22	7.56 ± 12.63	0.000 *
Eggs	22.23 ± 32.6	32.36 ± 44.33	15.13 ± 17.76	0.000 *
Fruits, Total				
Fruits	254.33 ± 284.95	275.91 ± 286.66	239.19 ± 283.32	0.182
Fresh Juices (100% fruit juices) [a]	38 ± 75.5	40.58 ± 80.49	36.36 ± 71.94	0.563
Sweets and Added Sugars				
Sweets	65.36 ± 114.08	77.73 ± 159.17	56.69 ± 65.24	0.056
Added Sugars, Jams, Honey, Molasses	18.97 ± 22.15	20.47 ± 23.76	17.93 ± 20.94	0.235
Added Fats and Oils	11.51 ± 11.68	12.21 ± 13.75	11.02 ± 9.98	0.289
Herbs and Spices	47.87 ± 44.1	50.1 ± 46.08	46.31 ± 42.67	0.373
Hot Beverages [a]	546.83 ± 427.36	543.56 ± 454.43	549.12 ± 408.19	0.893
Drinking Water [a]	1440.48 ± 843.19	1819.37 ± 866.39	1236.91 ± 747.44	0.000 *
Non-alcoholic beverages [a]	70.63 ± 120.94	97.04 ± 160.6	52.12 ± 77.66	0.000 *
Alcoholic beverages [a]	0.6 ± 5.9	1.47 ± 9.14	0 ± 0	0.01 *

Values are Mean ± Standard deviation. * p-value < 0.05 is significant. [a] Beverages presented in mL/day.

3.2.2. Comparison of Food Groups Consumed to the Mediterranean, the EAT-Lancet, and the USDA Diet Recommendations

Pyramids showing comparisons of the current consumption to the Mediterranean, EAT-Lancet, and USDA diet recommendations are shown in Figure 2. In general, the dietary pattern of Lebanese adults showed low adherence to the recommendations of the three healthy diets.

For instance, the current consumption showed low adherence to the Mediterranean recommendations, especially the consumption of 'sweets', 'red meat', 'white meat', and 'legumes', for which consumption exceeded the recommended daily intake by 1106.4%, 516.8%, 427.5%, and 267.4%, respectively. Our results also showed that the consumption of 'dairy products', 'fruits', 'vegetables', 'olive oil', 'olives/nuts/seeds', and 'grains/cereals' was lower than the amounts recommended by the Mediterranean diet. As for the EAT-Lancet recommendations, the consumption of 'added sugar', 'beef, lamb, pork', 'grains', 'chicken and other poultry', and 'fruits' exceeded the recommended daily intake by 499.9%, 295%, 132%, 118%, and 146.16%, respectively. In addition, most of the consumed grains (92% of the amount consumed) are refined grains, which is far from this diet's recommendation, as it recommends consuming 232 g/d of whole grains (compared to only 24 g/d in our study) and very low amounts (or nothing) of refined grains, in contrast to 274 g/d in our study. Our results also showed that the consumption of 'vegetables', 'dairy products', 'fish', 'nuts', and 'unsaturated oils' was lower than the amounts recommended by the EAT-Lancet diet. Regarding the USDA diet recommendations, the current consumption of 'vegetables', 'fruits' and 'meat and poultry' exceeded the recommendations by 174.37%, 146.17% and 104.57%, respectively. Additionally, a lower consumption of 'grains', 'dairy products', 'fish', 'oils', and 'nuts, seeds, soy products' was observed compared to the recommendations.

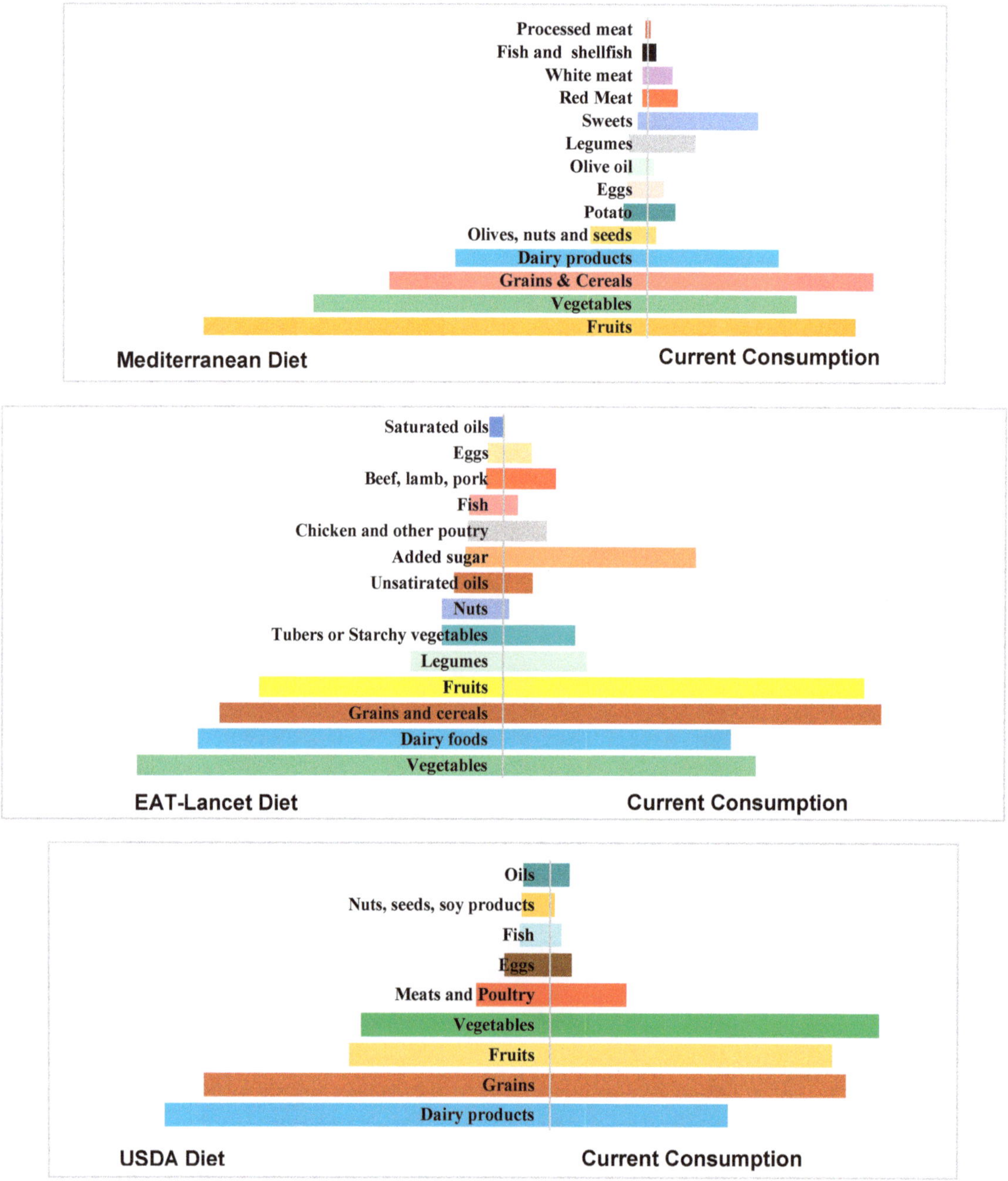

Figure 2. Comparison of the current food consumption to three different diets.

3.3. Energy Content of Food Consumed

The energy content of the food consumed by the study participants is shown in Table 5. The mean estimated energy requirement (EER) for a participant in our study was 2237.47 kcal/day, and a participant consumed on average 2237.49 kcal/day, which represents 100% of the mean EER. Our findings showed that, on average, participants of both genders and in all age categories exceeded their EER, except females in the '31–50 years' age group, of which almost all consumed their EER (97%). Males and females in the '18 years' age group had the highest consumption among male and female participants. Significant differences in the energy content of food consumed existed between genders (p-value = 0.000) and among age categories (p-value = 0.019).

Table 5. Energy content of food consumed by Lebanese adults and the corresponding percentage contribution to the estimated energy requirement per age and per gender.

	Consumption				
	Age Group (n = 444)				p-Value *
Estimated Energy Intake	**18 Years (n = 20)**	**19–30 Years (n = 187)**	**31–50 Years (n = 174)**	**51–64 Years (n = 63)**	**0.019**
	Mean ± SD				
Energy Content of Food Consumed (Kcal)	M: 3032 ± 959 F: 2156 ± 760.78	M: 2830.6 ± 1397.8 F: 2153.9 ± 1437	M: 2490.5 ± 1184.69 F: 1751.5 ± 806.7	M: 2566.5 ± 662.8 F: 1746.1 ± 675.47	0.000
EER (kcal/d)	M: 2200 F: 1800	M: 2400 F: 2000	M: 2200 F: 1800	M: 2000 F: 1600	
% EER [a]	M: 137.8% F: 119.78%	M: 117.92% F: 107.69%	M: 113.18% F: 97.3%	M: 128.3% F: 109.12%	

[a] %EER = Energy Content/EER × 100. * p-value < 0.05 is significant. Abbreviations: d day, EER Estimated Energy Requirement, F female, kcal kilocalories, M male, n number of participants, SD Standard Deviation.

3.4. Macronutrient Content of Food Consumed

The macronutrient content of food consumed by the study population is shown in Table 6. Our findings showed that the consumption of carbohydrates and fat exceeded the AMDR in participants from all age categories and genders, except the fat for the females in the 31–50 years group (97.4%). As for proteins, the AMDR was not reached in any of the age groups and genders, ranging from 65.3% for the female participants aged 31–50 years to 93.6% for the male participants aged 51–64 years. The consumption of monounsaturated fatty acids (MUFAs) did not exceed 60% of the RDA for all age categories and genders, except for males in the 51–64 years group (75.29%). In addition, participants from all age categories and genders exceeded the recommended daily limit of saturated fats, except for females in the 31–50 years group, who almost reached the recommended level (99.6%). Plus, the saturated fat content of food consumed exceeded 10% of the energy intake for males in the 19–30 years group and almost exceeded this limit for the other groups (>8% for all age groups and genders).

3.5. Micronutrient Content of Food Consumed

The micronutrient content of food consumed by the study population is shown in Table 7. Our results showed that participants in all age groups and genders had a low consumption of fat soluble vitamins (A, D, E), especially vitamin D, for which content in the consumed food was not 20% of the RDA. As for vitamin K, the RDA was exceeded for participants in all age groups and genders. Concerning water soluble vitamins, participants in all age groups and genders had a high consumption for all the vitamins except for biotin and B12. In general, the consumption of biotin did not exceed 85% of the RDA in all age groups and genders, and B12 consumption did not exceed 75% of the RDA in females belonging to the 51–64 years age group. In addition, our results revealed that females of reproductive age (belonging to the age groups 18, 19–30, 31–50) did not reach their daily requirements of iron, while females in all age categories had a low consumption of calcium, not exceeding 80% of the RDA in all the age categories. Moreover, our findings showed that the food consumed by Lebanese adults was high in sodium, with levels exceeding 150% of the RDA for all age groups and genders.

Table 6. Macronutrient content of food consumed by Lebanese adults and the percent contribution to daily value, per age and per gender.

Age Group	**18 Years (n = 20)**						**19–30 Years (n = 187)**					
Gender	**Male (n = 5)**			**Female (n = 15)**			**Male (n = 78)**			**Female (n = 109)**		
Nutrient	**DRI (RDA/ AMDR)**	**Mean ± SD**	**% DV**	**DRI (RDA/ AMDR)**	**Mean ± SD**	**% DV**	**DRI (RDA/ AMDR)**	**Mean ± SD**	**% DV**	**DRI (RDA/ AMDR)**	**Mean ± SD**	**% DV**
Macronutrients												
Total Fat (g/d)	**73**	95.18 ± 38.39	130.38%	**60**	75.78 ± 32.47	126.3%	**80**	96.53 ± 54.75	120.66%	**66.7**	75.75 ± 64.89	113.57%
Cholesterol (mg/d) [a]	<300	344.83 ± 171.76	114.94%	<300	204.28 ± 92.56	68.1%	< 300	368.24 ± 274.83	122.75%	<300	237.72 ± 166.55	79.24%
Saturated fat (g/d) [b]	22	32 ± 13.92	145.45%	18	22.96 ± 10.93	127.56%	24	31.74 ± 20.38	132.25%	20	22.81 ± 13.18	114.05%
Monounsaturated fat (g/d) [b]	48.4	29.03 ± 14.54	59.98%	39.6	23.78 ± 10.33	60.05%	52.8	30.41 ± 17.32	57.59%	44	23.51 ± 17.62	53.43%
Polyunsaturated fat (g/d) [b]	24.2	17.69 ± 6.63	73%	19.8	17.93 ± 9.06	90.56%	26.4	18.86 ± 11.27	71.44%	22	14.3 ± 9.16	65%%
Linoleic acid (g/d)	16	15.05 ± 7.04	94%	11	16.46 ± 8.69	149.63%	17	16.35 ± 10.35	96.18%	12	12.69 ± 8.52	105.75%
Alpha linolenic acid (g/d)	1.6	1.03 ± 0.27	64.37%	1.1	0.92 ± 0.35	83.63%	1.6	1.26 ± 0.77	78.75%	1.1	0.95 ± 0.54	86.36%
Trans Fat (g/d) [b]	2.42	0.36 ± 0.23	14.87%	1.98	0.36 ± 0.45	18.18%	2.64	0.38 ± 0.35	14.39%	2.2	0.28 ± 0.28	12.73%
Carbohydrate (g/d)	**275**	455.8 ± 169.3	165.74%	**225**	310.5 ± 119.99	138%	**300**	390.1 ± 195	130%	**250**	300.3 ± 180.64	120.12%
Total sugar (g/d) [c]	161.7	192.56 ± 154.85	119.08%	132.3	114 ± 76.54	86.17%	176.4	120.5 ± 90.41	68.3%	147	100.52 ± 73.3	68.38%
Protein (g/d)	**110**	97.82 ± 37.66	88.9%	**90**	68.1 ± 17.93	75.67%	**120**	106.55 ± 58.81	88.79%	**100**	76.32 ± 47.28	76.32%
Dietary fiber (g/d)	38	25.25 ± 11.09	66.45%	26	24.17 ± 9.67	92.96%	38	27.44 ± 15.47	72.21%	25	33.79 ± 105.35	135.16%
As percentage of EI												
Total Fat (%)	**25–30%**	27.89%	Within range	**25–30%**	31%	More than required	**20–35%**	30.42%	Within range	**20–35%**	31.15%	Within range
Saturated fat (%) [b]	<10%	9.37%	Did not exceed	<10%	9.4%	Did not exceed	<10%	10%	Exceeded	<10%	9.38%	Did not exceed
Carbohydrate (%)	**45–65%**	59.37%	Within range	**45–65%**	56.6%	Within range	**45–65%**	54.65%	Within range	**45–65%**	54.9%	Within range
Total sugar (%) [c]	<30%	25%	Did not exceed	<30%	20.76%	Did not exceed	<30%	16.88%	Did not exceed	<30%	18.37%	Did not exceed
Protein (%)	**10–30%**	12.74%	Within range	**10–30%**	12.4%	Within range	**10–35%**	14.93%	Within range	**10–35%**	13.95%	Within range

Table 6. *Cont.*

Age Group	31–50 years (n = 174)						51–64 Years (n = 63)					
Gender	Male (n = 79)			Female (n = 95)			Male (n = 21)			Female (n = 42)		
Nutrient	DRI (RDA/ AMDR)	Mean ± SD	% DV	DRI (RDA/ AMDR)	Mean ± SD	% DV	DRI (RDA/ AMDR)	Mean ± SD	% DV	DRI (RDA/ AMDR)	Mean ± SD	% DV
Macronutrients												
Total Fat (g/d)	**73**	80.34 ± 46.37	110.05%	**60**	58.44 ± 36.74	97.4%	**66.7**	91.15 ± 42.85	136.66%	**53**	56.94 ± 25.82	107.44%
Cholesterol (mg/d) [a]	<300	262.29 ± 222.5	60.76%	<300	179.9 ± 141.7	59.97%	<300	293.25 ± 116.63	97.75%	<300	139.82 ± 66.55	46.61%
Saturated fat (g/d) [b]	22	23.67 ± 14.28	107.59%	18	17.93 ± 15.24	99.61%	20	26.58 ± 12.41	132.9%	16	16.14 ± 7.77	100.88%
Monounsaturated fat (g/d) [b]	48.4	26.48 ± 18.85	54.71%	39.6	17.74 ± 11.84	44.8%	44	33.13 ± 19.22	75.29%	35.2	18.47 ± 9.56	52.47%
Polyunsaturated fat (g/d) [b]	24.2	17.08 ± 11.61	70.58%	19.8	12.76 ± 7.83	64.44%	22	18.91 ± 10.16	85.95%	17.6	13.15 ± 7.48	74.71%
Linoleic acid (g/d)	17	15.22 ± 10.56	89.53%	12	11.47 ± 7.18	95.58%	14	16.32 ± 9.06	116.57%	11	11.69 ± 6.79	106.27%
Alpha linolenic acid (g/d)	1.6	1.1 ± 1.01	68.75%	1.1	0.81 ± 0.58	73.64%	1.6	1.32 ± 0.95	82.5%	1.1	0.75 ± 0.37	68.18%
Trans Fat (g/d) [b]	2.42	0.32 ± 0.43	13.22%	1.98	0.19 ± 0.15	9.59%	2.2	0.24 ± 0.2	10.91%	1.76	0.18 ± 0.13	10.23%
Carbohydrate (g/d)	**275**	353.93 ± 170	128.7%	**225**	254.5 ± 107.9	113.11%	**250**	351.58 ± 71.5	140.63%	**200**	261.24 ± 110.53	130.62%
Total sugar (g/d) [c]	161.7	98.27 ± 67.59	60.77%	132.3	81.26 ± 60.63	61.42%	147	99.4 ± 42.86	67.62%	117.6	86.97 ± 61.44	73.95%
Protein (g/d)	**110**	94.36 ± 59.89	85.78%	**90**	58.77 ± 27.56	65.3%	**100**	93.61 ± 31.44	93.6%	**80**	56.47 ± 19.51	70.59%
Dietary fiber (g/d)	38	29.54 ± 27.66	77.74%	25	21.31 ± 9.36	85.24%	30	29.22 ± 9.93	97.4%	21	25.24 ± 10.82	120.19%
As percentage of EI												
Total Fat (%)	**20–35%**	29%	Within range	**20–35%**	29.56%	Within range	**20–35%**	31.5%	Within range	**20–35%**	28.74%	Within range
Saturated fat (%) [b]	<10%	8.47%	Did not exceed	<10%	9.07%	Did not exceed	<10%	9.2%	Did not exceed	<10%	8.14%	Did not exceed
Carbohydrate (%)	**45–65%**	56%	Within range	**45–65%**	57.22%	Within range	**45–65%**	54.1%	Within range	**45–65%**	58.6%	Within range
Total sugar (%) [c]	<30%	15.62%	Did not exceed	<30%	18.27%	Did not exceed	<30%	15.28%	Did not exceed	<30%	19.51%	Did not exceed
Protein (%)	**10–35%**	15%	Within range	**10–35%**	13.21%	Within range	**10–35%**	14.4%	Within range	**10–35%**	12.66%	Within range

Abbreviations: AMDR Acceptable Macronutrient Distribution Range, d day, DRI Dietary Reference Intake, DV Daily Value, g grams, n number of participants, RDA Recommended Dietary Allowance, SD Standard Deviation. Values in bold are AMDR (50% carbohydrates, 20% proteins, 30% fat) based on the estimated energy requirement of each age group. [a] [24–26], [b,c] Values were extracted based on a 2000 kcal-diet then adjusted to each age group's estimated energy requirements.

Table 7. Micronutrient content of food consumed by Lebanese adults and the percent contribution to daily value per age and gender.

Age Group	18 Years						19–30 Years					
Gender	Male			Female			Male			Female		
Nutrient	DRI (RDA/AI)	Mean ± SD	%DV	DRI (RDA/AI)	Mean±SD	%DV	DRI (RDA/AI)	Mean±SD	%DV	DRI (RDA/AI)	Mean ± SD	%DV
Antioxidants												
Vitamin C (mg/d)	75	129.8 ± 75.82	173%	65	116.31 ± 87.1	178.94%	90	130.6 ± 116.18	145.11%	75	122.1 ± 155.26	162.67%
B Vitamins												
Thiamin (mg/d)	1.2	1.38 ± 0.43	115%	1	1.08 ± 0.3	108%	1.2	1.57 ± 0.79	130.83%	1.1	1.11 ± 0.51	100.91%
Riboflavin (mg/d)	1.3	1.64 ± 0.57	126.15%	1	1.19 ± 0.4	119%	1.3	1.85 ± 1.14	142.31%	1.1	1.35 ± 0.85	122.73%
Niacin (mg/d)	16	22.44 ± 5.78	140.25%	14	16.8 ± 5.17	120%	16	29.1 ± 20.93	181.87%	14	17.95 ± 9.27	128.2%
Vitamin B-6 (mg/d)	1.3	1.79 ± 0.67	137.69%	1.2	1.78 ± 1.03	148.33%	1.3	2.84 ± 3.41	218.46%	1.3	1.62 ± 0.92	124.61%
Folate (µg dietary folate equivalent/d)	400	432.81 ± 191.86	108.2%	400	355.6 ± 107.4	88.91%	400	448.53 ± 247.1	121.13%	400	364.85 ± 177.65	91.21%
Vitamin B-12 (µg/d)	2.4	3 ± 1.3	125%	2.4	2.39 ± 1.09	99.58%	2.4	4.41 ± 3.96	183.75%	2.4	2.75 ± 1.99	114.58%
Biotin (µg/d) *	25	20.97 ± 9.15	83.88%	25	15.28 ± 9.14	61.12%	30	23.41 ± 17.5	78%	30	18.53 ± 20.69	61.77%
Pantothenic Acid (mg/d) *	5	5.1 ± 1.55	102%	5	4.53 ± 1.55	90.6%	5	6.43 ± 4.42	128.6%	5	4.6 ± 2.48	92%
Bone-Related Nutrients												
Calcium (mg/d) *	1300	1023.4 ± 334.54	78.72%	1300	701.25 ± 233	53.94%	1000	1086.1± 567.55	108.6%	1000	761.17 ± 321.66	76.11%
Phosphorus (mg/d)	1250	1325 ± 496.28	106%	1250	903.8 ± 254.2	72.3%	700	1366.8 ± 811.48	195.26%	700	990.24 ± 510.5	141.46%
Magnesium (mg/d)	410	394 ± 58.6	96.1%	360	291.6 ± 82.83	81%	400	421.49 ± 225.55	105.37%	310	319.21 ± 147.85	102.97%
Vitamin D (IU/d) *	600	84 ± 53.6	14%	600	46.8 ± 34.8	7.8%	600	100 ± 109.6	16.67%	600	67.6 ± 58.4	9.73%
Other Micronutrients												
Vitamin A (µg retinol activity equivalent/d)	900	448.9 ± 219.86	49.88%	700	435 ± 260.46	62.14%	900	595.88 ± 548.11	66.21%	700	511.1 ± 1295.87	73%
Vitamin E of alpha-Tocopherol Equivalents (mg/d)	15	8.32 ± 4.77	55.47%	15	9.36 ± 5.3	62.4%	15	8.58 ± 5.45	57.2%	15	7.37 ± 5.57	49.13%
Vitamin K (µg/d) *	75	123 ± 54.23	164%	75	100.9 ± 50.49	134.53%	120	124.38 ± 84.03	103.65%	90	103.76 ± 71.03	115.29%
Iron (mg/d)	11	18.81 ± 6.92	171%	15	13.45 ± 4.21	89.67%	8	18.21 ± 8.93	227.62%	18	14.84 ± 18.99	82.44%
Zinc (mg/d)	11	9.97 ± 3.36	90.64%	9	8.4 ± 3.1	93.33%	11	11.87 ± 7.4	107.91%	8	8.81 ± 5.02	110.25%
Sodium (g/d) *	1.5	3.99 ± 1.19	266%	1.5	2.88 ± 0.95	192%	1.5	4.04 ± 1.92	269.33%	1.5	3.37 ± 4.93	224.67%
Potassium (g/d) *	3.4	2.86 ± 0.86	84.11%	3.4	2.5 ± 0.99	73.53%	3.4	3.1 ± 1.72	91.17%	3.4	2.63 ± 1.28	77.35%
Copper (mcg/d)	890	1730 ± 650	194.38%	890	1410 ± 340	158.43%	900	2000 ± 1300	222.22%	900	1700 ± 2480	188.89%
Manganese (mg/d) *	2.2	4.17 ± 1.92	189.54%	1.6	3.21 ± 0.9	200.6%	2.3	4.32 ± 2.68	187.83%	1.8	3.57 ± 2.15	198.33%
Selenium (µg/d)	55	61.49 ± 24.52	111.8%	55	42.9 ± 16.59	78%	55	79.64 ± 58.51	144.8%	55	53.48 ± 34.49	97.24%
Fluoride (mg/d) *	3	1.82 ± 1.34	60.67%	3	0.86 ± 0.67	28.67%	4	1.33 ± 1.457	33.25%	3	1.76 ± 2.15	58.67%
Chromium (mcg/d) *	35	30 ± 20	85.71%	24	20 ± 20	83.33%	35	30 ± 30	85.71%	25	20 ± 40	80%
Molybdenum (µg/d)	43	17.43 ± 8.68	40.53%	43	18.88 ± 13.75	43.91%	45	21.36 ± 18.44	47.47%	45	17.83 ± 15.35	39.62%

Table 7. *Cont.*

Age Group	31–50 years						51–64 years					
Gender	Male			Female			Male			Female		
Nutrient	DRI (RDA/AI)	Mean ± SD	%DV	DRI (RDA/AI)	Mean ± SD	%DV	DRI (RDA/AI)	Mean ± SD	%DV	DRI (RDA/AI)	Mean ± SD	%DV
Antioxidants												
Vitamin C (mg/d)	90	110.63 ± 98.1	192.22%	75	86.56 ± 79.39	115.41%	90	123.49 ± 63.46	137.21%	75	110.68 ± 110.75	147.57%
B Vitamins												
Thiamin (mg/d)	1.2	1.42 ± 0.68	118.33%	1.1	0.96 ± 0.4	87.27%	1.2	1.5 ± 0.4	125%	1.1	0.98 ± 0.38	89.1%
Riboflavin (mg/d)	1.3	1.68± 0.86	129.23%	1.1	1.2 ± 0.76	109.1%	1.3	1.81 ± 0.5	139%	1.1	1.17 ± 0.47	106.36%
Niacin (mg/d)	16	25.8 ± 15.59	161.25%	14	15.68 ± 9.41	112%	16	25.43 ± 10.39	158.94%	14	16.29 ± 7.3	116.35%
Vitamin B-6 (mg/d)	1.3	1.8 ± 1.38	138.46%	1.3	1.26 ± 0.85	96.92%	1.7	2.01 ± 1.27	118.23%	1.5	1.32 ± 0.72	88%
Folate (μg dietary folate equivalent/d)	400	471.12 ± 555.79	117.78%	400	330.59 ± 148.51	82.65%	400	429.98 ± 112.59	107.49%	400	359.66 ± 155.74	89.91%
Vitamin B-12 (μg/d)	2.4	3.21 ± 2.42	133.75%	2.4	2.12 ± 1.71	88.33%	2.4	3.66 ± 2.12	152.5%	2.4	1.78 ± 1.02	74.17%
Biotin (μg/d) *	30	19.85 ± 17.08	66.17%	30	13.34 ± 10.34	44.47%	30	23.64 ± 11.99	78.8%	30	13.67 ± 10.29	45.57%
Pantothenic Acid (mg/d) *	5	5.14 ± 2.69	102.8%	5	3.83 ± 2.25	76.6%	5	5.43 ± 1.52	108.6%	5	3.6 ± 1.53	72%
Bone-Related Nutrients												
Calcium (mg/d) *	1000	962.51 ± 420.83	96.25%	1000	701.82 ± 359.83	70.18%	1000	1110.3 ± 379.9	111%	1200	659 ± 234.1	54.92%
Phosphorus (mg/d)	700	1200.3 ± 760.1	171.47%	700	813.97 ± 406.04	116.28%	700	1234.3 ± 432.1	176.33%	700	771.55 ± 286.14	110.22%
Magnesium (mg/d)	420	450 ± 265.6	107.14%	320	318.34 ± 156.1	99.48%	420	477.81 ± 123.6	113.76%	320	341.52 ± 140	106.72%
Vitamin D (IU/d) *	600	71.2 ± 71.6	11.87%	600	50 ± 60	8.33%	600	80 ± 58	13.33%	600	39.2 ± 34.8	6.53%
Other Micronutrients												
Vitamin A (μg retinol activity equivalent/d)	900	484.83 ± 432.1	53.87%	700	357 ± 317.8	51%	900	613.12 ± 349.17	68.12%	700	320 ± 207.6	45.71%
Vitamin E of alpha-Tocopherol Equivalents (mg/d)	15	8.9± 6.1	59.33%	15	6.41 ± 4.46	42.73%	15	10.26 ± 5.42	68.4%	15	7.23 ± 4.66	48.2%
Vitamin K (μg/d) *	120	124.81 ± 106.97	104%	90	91.69 ± 62.7	101.88%	120	206.59 ± 206.23	172.16%	90	100.35 ± 53.89	111.5%
Iron (mg/d)	8	17.36 ± 11.76	217%	18	11.54 ± 4.74	64.11%	8	17.43 ± 4.96	217.87%	8	12.66 ± 5.22	158.25%
Zinc (mg/d)	11	10.82 ± 7.33	98.36%	8	7.31 ± 3.7	91.37%	11	11.05 ± 3.86	100.45%	8	7.05 ± 2.55	88.12%
Sodium (g/d) *	1.5	3.62 ± 1.69	241.33%	1.5	2.5 ± 0.99	166.67%	1.3	3.7 ± 0.91	284.61%	1.3	2.49 ± 0.81	191.5%
Potassium (g/d) *	3.4	3.03 ± 1.87	89.12%	3.4	2.26 ± 1.16	66.47%	3.4	3.25 ± 0.88	95.59%	3.4	2.46 ± 1.22	72.35%
Copper (mcg/d)	900	2010 ± 1400	223.33%	900	1370 ± 560	152.22%	900	1990 ± 580	221.11%	900	1380 ± 540	153.33%
Manganese (mg/d) *	2.3	4.66 ± 3.95	202.61%	1.8	3.17 ± 1.47	176.11%	2.3	4.86 ± 1.58	211.3%	1.8	3.52 ± 1.68	195.56%
Selenium (μg/d)	55	65.1 ± 54.57	118.36%	55	36.46 ± 24.1	66.3%	55	64.29 ± 34.2	116.89%	55	33.18 ± 16.23	60.33%
Fluoride (mg/d) *	4	2.04 ± 2.73	51%	3	4.02 ± 8.99	134%	4	3.05 ± 2.57	76.25%	3	2.97 ± 3.1	99%
Chromium (mcg/d) *	35	30 ± 30	85.71%	25	10 ± 10	40%	30	30 ± 20	100%	20	10 ± 10	50%
Molybdenum (μg/d)	45	19.62 ± 17.31	43.6%	45	16.88 ± 14.88	37.51%	45	29.48 ± 18.23	65.51%	45	17.72 ± 15.14	39.38%

Abbreviations: AI Adequate Intake, d day, DRI Dietary Reference Intake, DV Daily Value, g grams, n number of participants, RDA Recommended Dietary Allowance, SD Standard Deviation. * Values are AIs.

4. Discussion

This is the most updated study undertaken in Lebanon to assess the dietary consumption patterns of adults and report the energy, macro- and micro-nutrients of this consumption. Our results showed a low adherence to the following three different healthy diets: the Mediterranean, the EAT-Lancet, and the USDA diet. In addition, participants, especially women, failed to meet the RDA for many essential vitamins and minerals, notably vitamin D, calcium, and iron. Also, it was shown that Lebanese adults follow dietary patterns that are high in sodium, added sugars, and saturated fats, and low in potassium and MUFAs. Plus, the consumption of refined grains, red meat, and poultry exceeded the recommended amounts when compared to each of the three diets. A low consumption of seafood and nuts was observed which did not reach the recommendations when compared to each of the three diets. Our findings aligned with the results of a previous national study, which showed that Lebanese adults have low adherence to the Mediterranean diet [27]. Similarly in Italy [28], a study showed that Italian adult participants had a medium adherence to the Mediterranean diet, highlighting the need for public health policies to improve dietary habits. As for the EAT-Lancet diet, our findings align with a study conducted in Brazil [29] involving adults aged 20 years and above that showed a low adherence to the recommendations of this diet. The low adherence to the healthy and sustainable diets in our study population might be due to the shift in dietary patterns, as shown in a national study published in 2019 regarding the consumption patterns between the years 1997 and 2008/2009, which showed that the adult Lebanese population is shifting towards the Westernized dietary patterns and departing from the traditional Lebanese dietary pattern [30]. This low adherence to the healthy diets, particularly the Mediterranean diet, highlights the importance of shifting towards a healthier dietary pattern in this population, which can be achieved in many ways. For instance, Lebanese adults' consumption of fruits, vegetables, nuts and seeds, and whole grains is lower than the recommended levels. In contrast, the consumption of red and processed meat, and sweets and added sugars exceeds the limits by far. Thus, reducing the consumption of sweets and red and processed meats and shifting to consuming more nuts, seeds, fruits, and vegetables can improve this population's adherence to the Mediterranean and other healthy diets. In addition, Lebanese adults can replace red, processed and white meats with seafood, which will increase the consumption of the latter, as it was shown that consumption of fish and seafood, which contain healthy fats, is below the recommendations. These few changes can eventually improve the nutritional status of Lebanese adults, as fruits, vegetables and nuts/seeds/fish are rich in essential vitamins, minerals and healthy fats that are cardio-protective.

Our results showed that the food consumed by Lebanese adults is high in energy, with participants in all age groups and genders (except females in the 31–50 years group) exceeding their EER. This is reflected by most participants (61.9%) being overweight or obese. The following findings reveal that Lebanese adults are at a high risk of developing NR-NCDs, especially as the high-energy diet of this population is also very high in sodium and saturated fats and low in healthy fats (due to the low consumption of fish, nuts, and seeds). For instance, a systematic analysis conducted in 2017 showed that diets high in sodium are the leading cause of global deaths attributable to diet, while diets low in nuts and seeds were the fourth cause of global death attributable to diet, with the most deaths occurring from cardiovascular disease, followed by diabetes [31]. This is compounded by a low vitamin D intake for participants in all ages and genders and low iron and calcium intakes in female participants, which puts female Lebanese adults at a high risk of anemia and osteoporosis. For instance, women aged 50 years and above have a four times higher prevalence of osteoporosis and a two times higher prevalence of osteopenia in comparison to men [32], and low calcium intake is considered a modifiable risk factor for osteoporosis [33]. In addition, the amount of females of reproductive age (18–49 years) requiring higher amounts of iron and not meeting their requirements from food intake, as revealed in our study, is alarming, especially as 65.6% of the female participants in our study failed to meet their requirements. Concerning vitamin D deficiency, similar findings were found in Libya [34], Egypt [35], Iran [36], Qatar [37], and Saudi Arabia [38], where a high deficiency of vitamin D was prevalent within the populations. As for vitamins E, A, and K, our findings revealed that participants had a low intake of vitamins A and E and a high intake of vitamin K, which is consistent with a study performed in Jordan that showed that vitamin A and E daily dietary intakes were below the RDAs [39]. Furthermore, in Greece, a low nutrient intake of vitamin E was found in all age groups [40], while in Kuwait, around 80% of the population was shown to consume less than the RDAs of vitamins A and E [41]. Some studies showed different results when it comes to the consumption of vitamins A and E. A study conducted in Egypt revealed that the intakes of both vitamins A and E were within or above recommendations [35]. Similarly, in Pakistan, vitamin A intake seemed quite high at the national level [42]. The low consumption of vitamin A and E in our study might be due to the reduction in intake of animal products, fruit/vegetables for vitamin A and vegetable oils/nuts for vitamin E. As for vitamin B12, despite the mean intake being 2.9 μg/day, which is higher than the RDA (2.4 μg/day), and despite the mean intake for most age categories exceeding this RDA, more than half of the participants (52.5%) failed to meet this RDA, indicating a low intake in the adult population. Notably, in our study, younger adults (<30 years) were found to significantly consume more sweets and non-alcoholic beverages than older adults. This can be explained by younger generations being more willing to try new and trendy meals compared to older adults, who stick to old traditions [43].

When it comes to consumption patterns between the two genders, disparities may indeed exist. This could be attributed to various factors, such as cultural norms, access to resources, household dynamics, and societal roles. For instance, based on the 'Food and Agriculture Organization of the United Nations' (FAO), denying women's rights is one of the leading causes of food and nutrition insecurity, making women more vulnerable to chronic nutrition and food insecurity [44]. Our findings align with studies that tackled gender disparities in food consumption. A study conducted in Bangladesh [45] showed that men had higher food intakes compared to females, as well as higher portion sizes. In addition, in Lebanon, a study showed that males had significantly higher energy intakes than females [46].

Compared to the findings of the nationally representative survey [30] that addressed the adult dietary consumption in the years 2008/2009 (see Table 8), our results showed a shift in the consumption of most of the food groups. For instance, an increased consumption of bread/cereals/grains (228 g/d vs. 317 g/d), legumes (40.87 g/d vs. 66.85 g/d), vegetables (190.93 g/d vs. 206.49 g/d), dairy products (88.21 g/d vs. 184.5 g/d), fruits (111.59 g/d vs. 254.33 g/d), fresh juices (8.53 mL/d vs. 38 mL/d), eggs (7.3 g/d vs. 22.23 g/d), chips and salty crackers (2.79 g/d vs. 8.35 g/d), hot beverages (217.75 mL vs. 546.83 mL/d), sweets (32.74 g/d vs. 65.36 g/d), and added sugars (7.3 g/d vs. 18.97 g/d) was observed. The consumption of red meat, processed meat, poultry, and fish underwent a slight change, while a significant decrease occurred in the consumption of nuts/seeds (9.44 g/d vs. 5 g/d), sugar sweetened beverages (165.76 mL/d vs. 75.86 mL/d), and alcoholic beverages (12.7 mL/d vs. 0.6 mL/d). This dietary shift in consumption occurred in both genders, with the consumption of a food group either increasing or decreasing simultaneously in both genders, except for vegetables consumption. In short, the increased consumption of fruits and vegetables and the decreased consumption of alcoholic beverages between the years 2009 and 2022 are considered positive shifts. However, this positive shift is faced by a negative shift characterized by decreased consumption of healthy fats, especially nuts and seeds, and a significant increase in the consumption of sweets, added sugars, sugar sweetened beverages, chips and salty crackers, and bread/cereals/grains, which include many refined items such as pasta, rice, and breakfast cereals. In addition, although the consumption of meat, poultry, and fish remained stable, the consumption of red meat remained higher than the limit set by the healthy diets, while the consumption of fish remained particularly low. This high consumption of red meat is alarming, since red meat is classified as a Group 2A carcinogen, meaning that it is "probably carcinogenic to humans", with a 17% increase in the risk of developing cancer with every 100 g consumed per day [47]. Plus, excess red meat consumption is associated with higher risk of developing cardiovascular disease, type 2 diabetes and other NR-NCDs [47]. Moreover, the high consumption of sweets, especially in the younger adults' generation, accompanied by an increased consumption of refined carbohydrates predispose Lebanese adults to increased adiposity levels and eventually overweight and obesity [48]. For instance, sweets and refined carbohydrates are energy-dense and low in proteins, fiber and essential macro- and micro-nutrients, and their high consumption is associated with increased risk of developing cardiometabolic diseases and dental caries, among other issues [48,49]. In short, our findings showed that Lebanese adults, especially women, are at high risk of developing NR-NCDs and hidden hunger.

Table 8. Comparison of the current adult food-group consumption to the consumption of the year 2009.

Food Groups	Mean Dietary Intake (g/d)					
	Males (n = 1319)		Females (n = 1643)		Overall (n = 2962)	
	2009	2022	2009	2022	2009	2022
Bread	148.27	183.01	79.3	146.73	109.18	161.68
Cereals and cereal based products	145.88	207.56	96.49	118.98	119.08	155.5
Legumes	53.99	68.24	30.8	65.89	40.87	66.85
Nuts and Seeds	10.97	6.45	8.35	3.99	9.44	5
Starchy Vegetables	42.78	46.01	29.56	39.42	35.34	42.13
Vegetables	209.87	197.76	176.3	212.61	190.93	206.49
Dairy Products	95.94	208.33	82.16	167.78	88.21	184.5
Meat and Meat Products, Poultry, Fish, Eggs						
Red Meat	58.01	54.45	29.96	32.15	42.26	41.34
Processed Meat	5.99	4.35	3.27	2.24	4.49	3.11
Poultry	38.68	46.55	21.02	25.56	29.07	34.21
Fish	18.09	16.86	8.44	7.56	12.78	11.39
Eggs	10.75	32.36	4.76	15.13	7.3	22.23
Fruits, Total						
Fruits	115.96	275.91	108.29	239.19	111.59	254.33
Fresh Juices (100% fruit juices) *	9.48	40.58	7.7	36.36	8.53	38
Chips and Salty Crackers	2.98	8.33	2.73	8.36	2.79	8.35
Sweets and Added Sugars						
Sweets	33.54	77.73	32.16	56.69	32.74	65.36
Added Sugars, Jams, Honey, Molasses	8.56	20.47	5.99	17.93	7.08	18.97
Added Fats and Oils	21.12	12.21	10.39	11.02	15.1	11.51
Hot Beverages *	198.7	543.56	237.51	549.12	217.75	546.83
Sugar Sweetened Beverages *	171.44	96.18	156.85	62.49	165.76	75.86
Alcoholic Beverages *	23.84	1.47	4.02	0	12.7	0.6

* Values in mL/day.

5. Strengths and Limitations

This study has the major strength of being the most updated regarding assessing the dietary patterns of Lebanese adults and the corresponding nutritional value of these patterns following the economic crisis, providing valuable insights into the significance of this crucial matter. In addition, the study was performed on a nationally representative sample covering all the Lebanese governorates, which allows for the generalization of the results to the Lebanese adult population. However, this study has some limitations. The data collected in the study relied on self-reported data. This type of data is subject to inaccuracies due to recall bias, which might lead to inaccuracies in estimating portion sizes and under- and/or over-reporting of food consumption.

6. Conclusions

Our findings highlight unhealthy food consumption patterns in the Lebanese adult population characterized by high sodium, added sugars, and saturated fat intake, as well as low intakes of healthy fats, essential vitamins, and minerals, with the consumption of sweets and added sugars doubling compared to the year 2009. In a country where 91% of all deaths are attributed to NCDs [50], and where the prevalence of NR-NCDs is rising, these results are alarming, as the current dietary pattern has put the Lebanese adult population at high risk of developing NR-NCDs, NR-NCD complications, and hidden hunger. The findings of our study thus call for public health policies and interventions that allow for the adoption of healthy food choices and the shift towards healthier diets, such as the Mediterranean, the EAT-Lancet, or the USDA diet, which are proven to be healthy diets. This might require changes across the food system to focus on promoting healthier diets and ensuring their affordability, availability, accessibility, and acceptability for all [51].

Supplementary Materials: The following supporting information can be downloaded at: https://www.mdpi.com/article/10.3390/nu16111784/s1, Table S1: Food items included in each food group.

Author Contributions: Conceptualization, M.H. and N.T.; methodology, M.K., D.M., E.A., Z.A.H., D.H. and M.A.; validation, M.H. and N.T.; formal analysis, M.K., D.M., E.A., Z.A.H., D.H. and M.A.; investigation, M.K., D.M., E.A., Z.A.H., D.H., E.A.M. and A.C.; data curation, M.K., D.M. and E.A.; writing—original draft preparation, M.H. and MK.; writing—review and editing, all the authors. All authors have read and agreed to the published version of the manuscript.

Funding: This research received no external funding.

Institutional Review Board Statement: The study was conducted in accordance with the Declaration of Helsinki and was approved by the Ethics Committee of Al Zahraa University Medical Center (Approval Code: #57/2022; Approval Date: 5 October 2022).

Informed Consent Statement: Informed consent was obtained from all subjects involved in the study. In addition, written informed consent has been obtained from the patient(s) to publish this paper.

Data Availability Statement: The original contributions presented in the study are included in the article, further inquiries can be directed to the corresponding author.

Acknowledgments: We extend our gratitude to the team at the Achrafieh Biomedical Center Laboratory for their valuable contributions to data collection. Additionally, we appreciate the support received from individuals and organizations who assisted in participant recruitment and graciously hosted us at their centers for data collection, with special thanks to Hala Mohsen.

Conflicts of Interest: The authors declare that the research was conducted in the absence of any commercial or financial relationships that could be construed as a potential conflict of interest.

Appendix A

Adults-LEBANON-FCS group: Zahraa Fadlallah, Razan Khadra (Faculty of Public Health, Lebanese University); Mohamad Chahine, Omasyarifa Binti Jamal Poh (Kursk State University, Russia).

References

1. Popkin, B.M. Nutrition Transition and the Global Diabetes Epidemic. *Curr. Diab. Rep.* **2015**, *15*, 64. [CrossRef] [PubMed]
2. Popkin, B.M. The nutrition transition: An overview of world patterns of change. *Nutr. Rev.* **2004**, *62*, S140–S143. [CrossRef] [PubMed]
3. Noncommunicable Diseases: Mortality. Available online: https://www.who.int/data/gho/data/themes/topics/topic-details/GHO/ncd-mortality (accessed on 24 April 2024).
4. FAOSTAT. Available online: https://www.fao.org/faostat/en/#country/121 (accessed on 24 April 2024).
5. Food Systems Profile—Lebanon. Available online: https://openknowledge.fao.org/items/c6cb0242-28e1-4ac4-8a51-361bb945a998 (accessed on 24 February 2024).

6. Global Nutrition Report | Country Nutrition Profiles—Global Nutrition Report. Available online: https://globalnutritionreport.org/resources/nutrition-profiles/ (accessed on 24 April 2024).
7. UN-Habitat Lebanon-Urban Issues. Available online: https://unhabitat.org/lebanon (accessed on 15 April 2019).
8. Available online: https://www.ers.usda.gov/webdocs/publications/102076/err-298.pdf (accessed on 14 May 2024).
9. Hamzeh, R.A. Assessing Nutritional Status and Purchasing Ability Amongst Adults in Mount Lebanon during the Economic Crisis 2022. Available online: https://papers.ssrn.com/sol3/papers.cfm?abstract_id=4373846 (accessed on 24 April 2024).
10. The State of Food Security and Nutrition in the World. Available online: https://www.fao.org/publications/home/fao-flagship-publications/the-state-of-food-security-and-nutrition-in-the-world/2022/en (accessed on 24 February 2024).
11. Seligman, H.K.; Schillinger, D. Hunger and socioeconomic disparities in chronic disease. *N. Engl. J. Med.* **2010**, *363*, 6–9. [CrossRef] [PubMed]
12. Seligman, H.K.; Laraia, B.A.; Kushel, M.B. Food Insecurity Is Associated with Chronic Disease among Low-Income NHANES Participants. *J. Nutr.* **2010**, *140*, 304–310. [CrossRef] [PubMed]
13. Parker, E.; Widome, R.; Nettleton, J.; Pereira, M. Food security and metabolic syndrome in U.S. adults and adolescents: Findings from the National Health and Nutrition Examination Survey, 1999–2006. *Ann. Epidemiol.* **2010**, *20*, 364–370. [CrossRef] [PubMed]
14. Hoteit, M.; Khadra, R.; Fadlallah, Z.; Mourad, Y.; Chahine, M.; Skaiki, F.; Al Manasfi, E.; Chahine, A.; Poh, O.B.J.; Tzenios, N. Prevalence and Time Trends of Low Serum B12 Levels and Inadequate B12 Dietary Intake in Lebanese Adults amidst the Food Insecurity Situation: Findings from a Nationally Representative Cross-Sectional Study. *Nutrients* **2024**, *16*, 226. [CrossRef] [PubMed]
15. Lwanga, S.K.; Lemeshow, S.; World Health Organization. Sample Size Determination in Health Studies: A Practical Manual. Available online: https://iris.who.int/handle/10665/40062 (accessed on 25 February 2024).
16. WHO Housing and Health Guidelines. Available online: https://www.who.int/publications-detail-redirect/9789241550376 (accessed on 25 February 2024).
17. Aoun, C.; Bou Daher, R.; El Osta, N.; Papazian, T.; Khabbaz, L. Reproducibility and relative validity of a food frequency questionnaire to assess dietary intake of adults living in a Mediterranean country. *PLoS ONE* **2019**, *14*, e0218541. [CrossRef] [PubMed]
18. Bach-Faig, A.; Berry, E.M.; Lairon, D.; Reguant, J.; Trichopoulou, A.; Dernini, S.; Medina, F.X.; Battino, M.; Belahsen, R.; Miranda, G.; et al. Mediterranean diet pyramid today. Science and cultural updates. *Public Health Nutr.* **2011**, *14*, 2274–2284. [CrossRef] [PubMed]
19. Available online: https://eatforum.org/content/uploads/2019/07/EAT-Lancet_Commission_Summary_Report.pdf (accessed on 14 May 2024).
20. The Eat-Lancet Commission on Food, Planet, Health—Eat Knowledge. 2024. Available online: https://eatforum.org/eat-lancet-commission/ (accessed on 14 May 2024).
21. Dietary Guidelines for Americans, 2020–2025 and Online Materials | Dietary Guidelines for Americans. Available online: https://www.dietaryguidelines.gov/resources/2020-2025-dietary-guidelines-online-materials (accessed on 25 February 2024).
22. Diet Analysis, Food Label, Menu Creation Software. 2022. Available online: https://nutritionistpro.com/ (accessed on 11 March 2024).
23. Available online: https://www.nationalacademies.org/fnb/food-and-nutrition-board (accessed on 9 February 2024).
24. Carson, J.A.S.; Lichtenstein, A.H.; Anderson, C.A.; Appel, L.J.; Kris-Etherton, P.M.; Meyer, K.A.; Petersen, K.; Polonsky, T.; Van Horn, L.; on behalf of the American Heart Association Nutrition Committee of the Council on Lifestyle; et al. Dietary Cholesterol and Cardiovascular Risk: A Science Advisory from the American Heart Association. *Circulation* **2020**, *141*, E39–E53. [CrossRef]
25. Hoteit, M.; Zoghbi, E.; Rady, A.; Shankiti, I.; Al-Jawaldeh, A. Development of a Lebanese food exchange system based on frequently consumed Eastern Mediterranean traditional dishes and Arabic sweets. *F1000Research* **2021**, *10*, 12. [CrossRef]
26. Hoteit, M.; Zoghbi, E.; Al Iskandarani, M.; Rady, A.; Shankiti, I.; Matta, J.; Al-Jawaldeh, A. Nutritional value of the Middle Eastern diet: Analysis of total sugar, salt, and iron in Lebanese traditional dishes. *F1000Research* **2020**, *9*, 1254. [CrossRef] [PubMed]
27. Naja, F.; Itani, L.; Hamade, R.; Chamieh, M.C.; Hwalla, N. Mediterranean Diet and Its Environmental Footprints Amid Nutrition Transition: The Case of Lebanon. *Sustainability* **2019**, *11*, 6690. [CrossRef]
28. Cardamone, E.; Iacoponi, F.; Di Benedetto, R.; Lorenzoni, G.; Di Nucci, A.; Zobec, F.; Gregori, D.; Silano, M. Adherence to Mediterranean Diet and its main determinants in a sample of Italian adults: Results from the ARIANNA cross-sectional survey. *Front. Nutr.* **2024**, *11*, 1346455. [CrossRef] [PubMed]
29. Neta, R.S.d.O.; Lima, S.C.V.C.; de Medeiros, M.F.A.; Neta, A.d.C.P.d.A.; Jacob, M.C.M.; Marchioni, D.M.L.; Lyra, C.d.O.; Oliveira, A.G.R.d.C. Adherence to the EAT-Lancet Dietary Recommendations for a Healthy and Sustainable Diet—The Case of the Brazuca Natal Study. *Sustainability* **2023**, *15*, 16526. [CrossRef]
30. Nasreddine, L.; Ayoub, J.J.; Hachem, F.; Tabbara, J.; Sibai, A.M.; Hwalla, N.; Naja, F. Differences in Dietary Intakes among Lebanese Adults over a Decade: Results from Two National Surveys 1997–2008/2009. *Nutrients* **2019**, *11*, 1738. [CrossRef] [PubMed]
31. GBD 2017 Diet Collaborators. Health effects of dietary risks in 195 countries, 1990–2017: A systematic analysis for the global burden of disease study 2017. *Lancet* **2019**, *393*, 1958–1972. [CrossRef] [PubMed]
32. Alswat, K. Gender disparities in osteoporosis. *J. Clin. Med. Res.* **2017**, *9*, 382–387. [CrossRef]
33. Keen, M. *Osteoporosis in Females*; StatPearls: St. Petersburg, FL, USA, 2023.

34. Faid, F.; Nikolic, M.; Milesevic, J.; Zekovic, M.; Kadvan, A.; Gurinovic, M.; Glibetic, M. Assessment of vitamin D intake among Libyan women—Adaptation and validation of specific food frequency questionnaire. *Libyan J. Med.* **2018**, *13*, 1502028. [CrossRef] [PubMed]
35. Brouzes, C.M.C.; Darcel, N.; Tomé, D.; Dao, M.C.; Bourdet-Sicard, R.; Holmes, B.A.; Lluch, A. Urban Egyptian Women Aged 19–30 Years Display Nutrition Transition-Like Dietary Patterns, with High Energy and Sodium Intakes, and Insufficient Iron, Vitamin D, and Folate Intakes. *Curr. Dev. Nutr.* **2020**, *4*, nzz143. [CrossRef]
36. Ziaee, A.; Javadi, A.; Javadi, M.; Zohal, M.; Afaghi, A. Nutritional Status Assessment of Minodar Residence in Qazvin City, Iran: Vitamin D Deficiency in Sunshine Country, a Public Health Issue. *Glob. J. Health Sci.* **2012**, *5*, 174–179. [CrossRef]
37. Mahdy, S.; Al-Emadi, S.A.; Khanjar, I.A.; Hammoudeh, M.M.; Sarakbi, H.A.; Siam, A.M.; Abdelrahman, M.O. Vitamin D status in health care professionals in Qatar. *Saudi Med. J.* **2010**, *31*, 74–77. [PubMed]
38. Hussain, A.N.; Alkhenizan, A.H.; El Shaker, M.; Raef, H.; Gabr, A. Increasing trends and significance of hypovitaminosis D: A population-based study in the Kingdom of Saudi Arabia. *Arch. Osteoporos.* **2014**, *9*, 190. [CrossRef] [PubMed]
39. El-Qudah, J.; Al-Widyan, O.; Alboqai, O.; Suleiman, A.; Quasem, J.M. Fat Soluble Vitamins (A, E and K) Intake among a Sample of Jordanian University Students. 2008. Available online: https://www.academia.edu/117248418/Fat_Soluble_Vitamins_A_E_and_K_Intake_Among_a_Sample_of_Jordanian_University_Students (accessed on 14 May 2024).
40. Manios, Y.; Moschonis, G.; Mavrogianni, C.; Bos, R.; Singh-Povel, C. Micronutrient Intakes among Children and Adults in Greece: The Role of Age, Sex and Socio-Economic Status. *Nutrients* **2014**, *6*, 4073–4092. [CrossRef] [PubMed]
41. Zaghloul, S.; Al-Hooti, S.N.; Al-Hamad, N.; Al-Zenki, S.; Alomirah, H.; Alayan, I.; Al-Attar, H.; Al-Othman, A.; Al-Shami, E.; Al-Somaie, M.; et al. Evidence for nutrition transition in Kuwait: Over-consumption of macronutrients and obesity. *Public Health Nutr.* **2012**, *16*, 596–607. [CrossRef] [PubMed]
42. Analysis of Food and Nutrition Security in Pakistan: A Contribution to Zero Hunger Policies. Available online: https://www.researchgate.net/publication/353275981_Analysis_of_Food_and_Nutrition_eSecurity_in_Pakistan_A_Contribution_to_Zero_Hunger_Policies (accessed on 14 May 2024).
43. Hu, E.A.; Toledo, E.; Diez-Espino, J.; Estruch, R.; Corella, D.; Salas-Salvado, J.; Vinyoles, E.; Gomez-Gracia, E.; Aros, F.; Fiol, M.; et al. Lifestyles and Risk Factors Associated with Adherence to the Mediterranean Diet: A Baseline Assessment of the PREDIMED Trial. *PLoS ONE* **2013**, *8*, e60166. [CrossRef] [PubMed]
44. Available online: https://www.fao.org/fileadmin/templates/cfs/Docs1920/Gender/GEWE_Scoping_Paper-FINAL040ct.pdf (accessed on 28 May 2024).
45. Sudo, N.; Sekiyama, M.; Watanabe, C.; Bokul, A.T.M.M.H.; Ohtsuka, R. Gender differences in food and energy intake among adult villagers in northwestern Bangladesh: A food frequency questionnaire survey. *Int. J. Food Sci. Nutr.* **2004**, *55*, 499–509. [CrossRef] [PubMed]
46. Nasreddine, L.; Chamieh, M.C.; Ayoub, J.; Hwalla, N.; Sibai, A.-M.; Naja, F. Sex disparities in dietary intake across the lifespan: The case of Lebanon. *Nutr. J.* **2020**, *19*, 24. [CrossRef]
47. World Health Organization. 2023. Available online: https://iris.who.int/bitstream/handle/10665/370775/9789240074828-eng.pdf?sequence=1 (accessed on 20 May 2024).
48. Prada, M.; Saraiva, M.; Garrido, M.V.; Sério, A.; Teixeira, A.; Lopes, D.; Silva, D.A.; Rodrigues, D.L. Perceived Associations between Excessive Sugar Intake and Health Conditions. *Nutrients* **2022**, *14*, 640. [CrossRef] [PubMed]
49. Henney, A.E.; Gillespie, C.S.; Alam, U.; Hydes, T.J.; Boyland, E.; Cuthbertson, D.J. Ultra-processed food and non-communicable diseases in the United Kingdom: A narrative review and thematic synthesis of literature. *Obes. Rev.* **2024**, *25*, e13682. [CrossRef]
50. Zablith, N.; Diaconu, K.; Naja, F.; El Koussa, M.; Loffreda, G.; Bou-Orm, I.; Saleh, S. Dynamics of non-communicable disease prevention, diagnosis and control in Lebanon, a fragile setting. *Confl. Health* **2021**, *15*, 4. [CrossRef]
51. NERC/22/5—Transforming Agrifood Systems to Promote Healthy Diets for All. Available online: https://openknowledge.fao.org/items/4970790c-8086-4315-8944-43351fa44932 (accessed on 28 May 2024).

nutrients

Article

A Pilot Study on Dietary Choices at Universities: Vending Machines, Canteens, and Lunch from Home

Leandro Oliveira [1,2,*], Mona N. BinMowyna [3], Ibrahim Alasqah [4,5], Renata Puppin Zandonadi [6], Edite Teixeira-Lemos [7], Cláudia Chaves [8], Hmidan A. Alturki [9], Najla A. Albaridi [10], Fatmah Fahad Alribdi [11] and António Raposo [1,*]

1 CBIOS (Research Center for Biosciences and Health Technologies), Universidade Lusófona de Humanidades e Tecnologias, Campo Grande 376, 1749-024 Lisboa, Portugal
2 Polytechnic Institute of Coimbra, Coimbra Health School, Rua 5 de Outubro–S. Martinho do Bispo, Apartado 7006, 3046-854 Coimbra, Portugal
3 College of Education, Shaqra University, Shaqra 11911, Saudi Arabia; m.mwena@su.edu.sa
4 Department of Community, Psychiatric and Mental Health Nursing, College of Nursing, Qassim University, Buraydah 51452, Saudi Arabia; i.alasqah@qu.edu.sa
5 School of Health, University of New England, Armidale, NSW 2351, Australia
6 Department of Nutrition, School of Health Sciences, University of Brasilia (UnB), Campus Darcy Ribeiro, Asa Norte, Brasilia 70910-900, Brazil; renatapz@unb.br
7 CERNAS Research Centre, Polytechnic University of Viseu, 3504-510 Viseu, Portugal; etlemos3@gmail.com
8 ESSV, Centre for Studies in Education and Innovation (CI&DEI), Polytechnic University of Viseu, 3504-510 Viseu, Portugal; claudiachaves21@gmail.com or cchaves@essv.ipv.pt
9 King Abdulaziz City for Science & Technology, Wellness and Preventive Medicine Institute—Health Sector, Riyadh 11442, Saudi Arabia; halturki@kacst.edu.sa
10 Department of Health Science, College of Health and Rehabilitation, Princess Nourah bint Abdulrahman University, P.O. Box 84428, Riyadh 11671, Saudi Arabia; naalbaridi@pnu.edu.sa
11 Director of Model of Care, Qassim Health Cluster, Buraydah 52367, Saudi Arabia; falribdi@moh.gov.sa
* Correspondence: leandroliveira.nut@gmail.com (L.O.); antonio.raposo@ulusofona.pt (A.R.)

Abstract: Commercial environments and food acquisition methods significantly shape dietary practices and impact health. This study assesses dietary choices among Portuguese university students regarding vending machines, canteens, and lunches from home. It also evaluates their use of the university canteen and their tendency to bring lunch from home. This pilot cross-sectional study used a self-administered electronic questionnaire, made available in early 2023. Participants were recruited through snowball sampling. The study included 137 students from Portuguese higher education institutions, mainly women (74.5%), pursuing degrees or integrated Master's degrees (83.2%), primarily in health-related fields (55.5%). The median age was 21 years (20 to 23.5 years). About 70.0% regularly consumed food from vending machines, while approximately 60.0% brought lunch from home, avoiding the canteen. Factors such as convenience (48.5%), price (47.5%), product availability (40.6%), and taste (39.6%) mainly influenced vending machine choices. Monthly, chocolates, water, coffee, cookies, treats, and soft drinks were the most commonly acquired items, with coffee being the most frequent daily purchase. These findings provide insights for creating policies and initiatives to promote healthier and more accessible food options for students and strategies to encourage positive eating behaviors.

Keywords: vending machines; canteen; lunch; nutrition; university; students

1. Introduction

The university food environment is characterized by the availability of foods, preparations, and beverages (FPB); their physical and financial accessibility; the promotion of FPB; and the presence of nutritional information and advertising on campus, as well as in the surrounding areas [1]. It is known that this environment influences the eating habits of those who frequent it, potentially facilitating or hindering healthy choices [2,3]. Meals consumed at the university constitute an important part of the diet for students, teachers, and staff, highlighting the relevance of this environment in promoting healthy eating habits [1,2].

In addition to the university food environment, other factors influence the dietary choices of higher education students [2]. Studies indicate that the primary determinants of food choices among university students include lack of time, convenience, cost, taste, health status, social and physical environment, concerns about weight control [4–6], and even food sustainability [7,8].

One significant aspect of the university food environment is the increasing prominence of vending machines, which provide food and beverages across various settings, including higher education institutions. The presence of vending machines on university campuses offers numerous advantages for students. Firstly, they offer convenience and accessibility [9], allowing students to obtain food and drinks quickly between classes or during short breaks. Furthermore, vending machines provide diverse options, ranging from quick snacks to complete meals, catering to students' preferences and dietary restrictions [10,11].

However, acquiring food and beverages in vending machines also has challenges. Often, the options available from these machines are commonly highly processed foods, rich in sugars, saturated fats, and sodium, which can lead to an unbalanced diet and contribute to the increase in the consumption of unhealthy foods, as evidenced in national studies conducted in Portugal [10,12–14] and internationally [9,11,15,16]. In addition, the lack of detailed nutritional information on product packaging and the absence of clear guidelines on healthy eating choices can make it difficult for students to make informed decisions [17].

University students are not exempt from the global health challenge of overweight and obesity, with a considerable proportion of this group being affected [18–21]. In a study encompassing 22 nations across various regions of the world with diverse economic and social conditions, statistics revealed that approximately 22% of university students are affected by overweight or obesity [22]. In Portugal, the prevalence of excess weight among higher education students reaches nearly 25% [23]. Furthermore, a report on the health and well-being behaviors of polytechnic higher education students indicates that 77.70% of students consider their diet to be reasonably healthy, while 12.90% admit to having an unhealthy diet. Conversely, 8.30% perceive their diet as very wholesome, with only 1.10% of students reporting an unhealthy diet [24]. Just as a conducive teaching environment is essential for academic success, a balanced and healthy diet is vital for students' cognitive function, energy levels, and overall well-being. However, studies show that the regular consumption of vending machine food is associated with a greater risk of developing a variety of chronic diseases, including obesity, diabetes, cardiovascular diseases, and hypertension [25,26].

Alternatives to vending machines include canteens and bringing meals from home. Several factors influence both the choice of the canteen for meals and the overall satisfaction with the canteen's services. Some of these factors include the quality of meals and beverages, encompassing the quality of ingredients used and the taste of the food [27,28]; the quality of service, which includes team performance, service efficiency, and the service environment [27,28]; and the waiting time for service [29], among others. Just as a conducive teaching environment is essential, having a balanced and healthy diet is equally important. Canteens should provide healthy menu options without restricting choices and should adhere to current nutritional trends [28]. However, this assertion fails to capture the complexity of the current situation, as it neglects the intricate nutritional requirements of students. These needs hint at a larger issue of nutritional imbalance, which demands deeper exploration. For example, this exploration would entail scrutinizing specific dietary deficiencies or excesses contributing to this imbalance, alongside investigating underlying factors such as socioeconomic influences, cultural norms, and the accessibility of nutritious food options [28,30,31].

Bringing lunch from home to the university is another aspect to consider in the university food environment. Healthy food consumption through packed lunches depends on various factors, including culinary skills. A systematic review of observational studies revealed that cooking at home was associated with healthier food consumption [32]. Furthermore, cross-sectional research involving university students found that more frequent cooking was correlated with an increased consumption of fruits and vegetables [33]. However, studies have indicated a lack of cooking skills and infrequent meal preparation among university students, particularly males [32,34,35]. Additionally, the decision to consume packed lunches can be influenced by various factors, such as meeting specific nutritional requirements, satisfying food preferences, overcoming time constraints for on-campus meals, identifying suitable places for university dining, and managing individual food budgets [36].

Given these challenges (e.g., the prevalence of unhealthy options in vending machines and nutritional imbalances), it is essential to implement strategies that promote healthy food choices in the university environment. For this, information about the acquisition of food and beverages in vending machines, the use of the university canteen, and the habit of taking lunch from home is necessary, especially because there is a lack of studies in Portugal in this regard. Thus, dietary choices considering vending machines, canteens, and lunch from home of a sample of Portuguese university students were investigated.

Therefore, this study is expected to provide some insights, including specific dietary interventions, aimed at enhancing the dietary habits of university students.

2. Materials and Methods

2.1. Study Design and Participants

This is a cross-sectional study in which a self-administered electronic questionnaire (Supplementary Material) was available during the first semester of 2023. The target population comprised a convenience sample of public and private Portuguese university students invited to participate in the online survey. The snowball sampling method was used to ensure a wide distribution and recruitment of participants. A web URL link was obtained for the inquiry and distributed through invitations sent by the university's internal email system and social networking platforms. All participants completed an electronic informed consent form before participating and had the right to give up at any time during the research. The university students who consented to participate in the survey, completed the questionnaire, and submitted their answers were included in the study. All information was collected anonymously, without indicating personal data, and participants did not receive any reward. This study followed the ethical code for web-based research [37] and the recommendations of the Declaration of Helsinki [38]. The study protocol was approved by the Ethics Commission of the School of Health Sciences and Technologies of the Lusophone University (P02-23).

2.2. Survey Questionnaire

The questionnaire was structured into the following three main sections: sociodemographic characterization, eating habits, and acquisition of food and drinks in vending machines. This questionnaire was initially prepared and applied in Portuguese and was subsequently translated into English to facilitate its publication in international settings. This translation process involved ensuring the accuracy and clarity of the questions and responses to maintain the integrity of the data collected. The sociodemographic characterization section comprised inquiries regarding gender, age, nationality, academic level, field of study, weight, and height. The section on eating habits focused on bringing food to the university and lunch in the canteen. Thus, participants were asked if they used to take lunch from home to lunch at the university (yes or no), and if so, they were asked what the main reason was (open response). Moreover, they were asked if they used to have lunch at the university canteen (yes or no); if negative, they were asked what the main reason was (open response). Finally, participants were asked if they used to consume food or beverages purchased from vending machines. The participants who answered "no" ended the questionnaire at that point.

Regarding the section on the acquisition of food and beverages from vending machines, participants who reported purchasing food and drinks from vending machines were asked about the top three factors influencing the items they buy. These factors, adapted from a previous study [33], included: I do not know; habit or routine; the taste of food; food price; control your weight; food availability; presentation or packaging; someone else decides most of the foods that I eat; vegetarian food or other special habits; content in additives, dyes, and preservatives; my cultural, religious, or ethnic roots; ease or convenience of preparation; try to make a healthy diet; and quality or freshness of food.

Subsequently, participants were asked about their purchasing frequency of various foods and beverages that are accessible from vending machines. The products available in vending machines on the campus's periphery were assessed and categorized into the following distinct food groups: 1. Coffee; 2. Other hot drinks with coffee; 3. Hot chocolate or other beverages with chocolate; 4. Bottled water; 5. Sparkling water; 6. Soft drinks (Coca-Cola, Sumol, Iced Tea); 7. Energy Drinks; 8. Sandwiches; 9. Cakes and pastry products; 10. Cookies; 11. Cereal bars; 12. Potato chips; 13. Solid yogurt; 14. Liquid yogurt; 15. Fresh fruit; 16. Chocolates, 17. Sweets (gums; candies); and 18. Other Snacks. Respondents were presented with a nine-point scale for indicating the frequency of acquiring these food items and beverages, encompassing the following options: "Never", "Once a month", "2 to 3 times a month", "Once a week", "2–3 times a week", "4–6 times a week", "Daily", "2 to 3 times a day", and "More than three times a day". The questionnaire was inserted into the Google Forms platform and was distributed to university students.

2.3. Data Analysis

To authenticate participant responses and minimize the potential for contamination from non-human sources, data validation techniques were implemented. These methods involved identifying and eliminating any responses that appeared suspicious or inconsistent. This scrutiny included analyzing response patterns, such as unusually rapid completion times or repetitive answers, which could suggest non-human activity. Additionally, participant information was cross-referenced with demographic data to confirm the coherence of responses and ensure alignment with the characteristics of our target population.

Open-ended responses were analyzed using content analysis to extract valuable insights beyond quantitative data. This involved systematically coding and categorizing the responses to identify recurring themes and patterns. Each response was carefully reviewed to ensure comprehensive data coverage, allowing us to gain deeper insights into the participants' choices. It is important to note that in some responses, more than one reason was identified. Additionally, the 94 different reasons were derived from the question of why they take food from home to university, while the 76 reasons referred to the question about reasons for not usually having lunch in the canteen. This process involved thoroughly reviewing all responses to identify common themes and group them according to their relevance for the analysis. Excel 365 software (for windows) was used for data management and content analysis. Two independent coders were involved in the analysis and they coded the data separately to enhance reliability. Any discrepancies or disagreements between the coders were resolved through discussion and consensus. In cases where consensus could not be reached, a third coder was consulted to adjudicate the discrepancies.

The respondents' weight and height information were used to calculate their BMI (Body Mass Index) using the Quetlet formula, as follows: BMI = weight (kg)/height $(m)^2$. The cohort was established according to the World Health Organization's criteria, which categorizes BMI as underweight (<18.5 kg/m^2), normal weight (18.5–24.9 kg/m^2), overweight (25.0–29.9 kg/m^2), or obese ($\geq$30.0).

The statistical analysis was conducted using the Statistical Package for the Social Sciences (SPSS), version 26.0, for Windows. Categorical variables were summarized in counts and percentages. The Kolmogorov–Smirnov test was employed to assess variable distributions. The chi-square test or Fisher's exact test was used to determine the variables' independence, while the Mann–Whitney test was used to compare medians in independent samples. Regarding the inquiry about the frequency of acquiring food and beverages from vending machines, specific response categories were grouped due to the dispersion of responses and the low frequency of specific scale options. This consolidation was performed as follows: "Once a month" and "2 to 3 times a month" responses were combined into a single category named "Monthly"; "Once a week", "2–3 times a week", and "4–6 times a week" responses were grouped into a category labeled "Weekly"; and "2 to 3 times a day" and "more than three times a day" responses were unified into the "Daily" category. This approach of consolidating responses aimed to simplify and enhance the coherence of the analysis concerning the frequency of acquiring food and beverages from vending machines. Results were considered significant at a p-value < 0.05.

3. Results

This study included 137 individuals attending Portuguese higher education institutions. Most were women (74.5%) and participated in a degree or integrated Master's degree (83.2%) in the health area (55.5%). The participants' median age was 21 (20; 23.5) years. About 70% consume food from vending machines, 60% typically bring lunch from home to the university, and 40% eat lunch in the institution's canteen (Table 1).

Table 1. Demographic and behavioral characteristics of the university students (n = 137).

Studied Parameters	Median (P25; P75)
Age	21 (20.0; 23.5)
	n (%)
Gender	
Men	35 (25.5)
Woman	102 (74.5)
Education	
Bachelor's or Licentiate/Integrated Master's Degree	114 (83.2)
Master's degree	18 (13.1)
Doctorate	2 (1.5)
Postgraduate Course *	3 (2.2)
Area of the Course	
Health	76 (55.5)
Other areas	61 (44.5)
Body mass index classification	
Underweight	6 (4.4)
Normal weight	99 (72.3)
Overweight	32 (23.4)
Do you usually take lunch from home to university?	
Yes	82 (59.9)
No	55 (40.1)
Do you usually have lunch in the university canteen?	
Yes	59 (43.1)
No	78 (56.9)
Do you usually consume food or beverages from vending machines?	
Yes	101 (73.7)
No	36 (26.3)

* Courses undertaken after completing a Bachelor's degree, without the conferral of an academic degree. For example, this includes courses with a duration of one academic year or less. P25: 25th percentile; P75: 75th percentile.

The relationships between the questions "Do you usually take lunch from home to university?", "Do you usually have lunch in the university canteen?", and "Do you usually consume food or beverages from vending machines?" were examined in relation to other sociodemographic characteristics, namely gender, age, level of education, field of study, and nutritional status (normal weight versus overweight). However, these data were not presented in the tables. From this analysis, it was observed that participants enrolled in health-related courses tended to take lunch from home to university ($\chi^2 = 11.1$; $p = 0.01$) and usually did not have lunch in the university canteen ($\chi^2 = 9.2$; $p = 0.02$), unlike their counterparts (n = 55; 72.4% and n = 52; 72.4% versus n = 27; 44.3% and n = 26; 42.6%, respectively). No relationships were found between the other aforementioned variables.

The questions "Do you usually take lunch from home to university?", "Do you usually have lunch in the university canteen?", and "Do you usually consume food or beverages from vending machines?" were also examined for their interrelationships. It was observed that, as expected, participants who brought lunch from home did not usually have lunch in the university canteen ($\chi^2 = 22.0$; $p < 0.01$), unlike their counterparts (n = 60; 73.2% versus n = 18; 32.7%, respectively). There was no relationship found between the questions "Do you usually take lunch from home to university?" or "Do you usually have lunch in the university canteen?" and "Do you usually consume food or beverages from vending machines?".

In total, 74 participants answered the question of why they take food from home to university; content analysis allowed us to extract 94 reasons, based on the following: 56.4% economic reasons (saving money, having expensive lunch in the canteen, etc.); 18.1% health-related reasons; 12.8% personal tastes; 8.5% logistics/time reasons; and 4.3% reasons related to the lack of quality of canteen meals. A total of 66 participants provided reasons for not usually having lunch in the canteen. The content analysis allowed us to extract 76 reasons, based on the following: 43.4% economic reasons (price, being expensive to have lunch in the canteen, etc.); 27.6% logistics/time reasons (including taking the home meal); 13.2% personal tastes; 10.5% health-related reasons; and 5.3% reasons related to the lack of quality of canteen meals—Table 2.

Table 2. Emergent factors from responses to open-ended questions.

Emergent Factors	Definition/Description	Number of Mentions	%
Do you usually bring lunch from home to eat at the university? If YES, what is the main reason? (n = 74)			
Logistics/time reasons	I do not have a cafeteria and I save more time; because it is more practical; lack of time.	8	8.5
Economic Reasons	Having expensive lunch in the canteen; more economical; lower price; savings; be cheaper; not spending money; spend less money.	53	56.4
Health-related reasons	Lack of healthy options; specific diet; diet; I can bring healthier options	17	18.1
Personal taste	I like home food more; I prefer my food to the canteen; I usually do not like eating outside the home.	12	12.8
Quality	Quality; food quality; variety.	4	4.3
Do you usually have lunch at the university canteen? If NO, what is the main reason? (n = 66)			
Logistics/time reasons	Have lunch at home; I take food when necessary; schedule allows for lunch at home; be practical/convenient.	21	27.6
Economic Reasons	Price; being expensive to have lunch in the canteen; too expensive; to save.	33	43.4
Health-related reasons	Lack of healthy options; go on a diet.	8	10.5
Personal taste	Prefiro a minha comida (I prefer my food); food not well prepared; porque normalmente não gosto da comida (because I usually don't like the food)	10	13.2
Quality	Quality; food quality.	4	5.3

The factors that have the most significant influence on dietary choices made by university students when buying from vending machines are presented in Table 3. In general, the main factors that affect the food choice and drinks in vending machines are convenience (48.5%), price (47.5%), and product availability (40.6%), as well as the taste of food (39.6%). Male participants, those who attend healthcare courses, and those who often have lunch in the canteen reported that convenience is more influential than their counterparts. In addition, students who have lunch in the canteen considered that the content of additives, dyes, and preservatives is more critical than those who do not have lunch in the canteen. Younger participants (median age: 21; P25: 19; P75: 24) indicated that price influences food choices at vending machines more than older participants (median age: 22; P25: 20; P75 24)—$p = 0.045$. No relationship was found between the factors influencing the food choice on vending machines and whether participants brought lunch food at the university, or with nutritional status (average weight versus overweight), or with level of education (Bachelor's or Licentiate/Integrated Master's Degree versus other courses).

Regarding acquiring food and beverages in vending machines (Table 4), more than 90% never acquired sparkling water, energy drinks, solid yogurts, liquid yogurts, and fresh fruit. At the monthly level, the most frequently acquired foods were chocolates (47.5%), water (44.6%), coffee (34.7%), cookies (35.6%), treats (30.7%), and soft drinks (24.8). At the weekly level, the most frequently acquired foods were coffee (25.7%), bottled water (19.8%), other hot beverages with coffee (9.9%), and chocolates (9.9%). At the daily level, the most acquired food was coffee (15.8%). Next, an analysis was conducted to examine the relationship between the acquisition of food and beverages from vending machines and variables such as gender, study area, canteen lunching habits, and the practice of bringing lunch from home. Male participants were observed to have a higher frequency of acquiring coffee, water, energy drinks, potato chips, and solid yogurt from vending machines than their women counterparts. Moreover, students who regularly had lunch in the canteen displayed a greater frequency of acquiring sandwiches and hot chocolate or other chocolate beverages from vending machines compared to students who did not use the cafeteria for their meals. Health students had a lower frequency of cereal bar acquisition in vending machines than students from other areas. On the other hand, they had a higher frequency of water acquisition in vending machines than students from different areas. No differences were found in the acquisition of food and beverages in vending machines among students who had the habit of bringing lunch from home to university and those who did not have this habit.

Table 3. Most significant factors influencing food choices made by university students when purchasing food and beverages from vending machines (n = 101).

	Total		Gender			Course			Do You Usually Have Lunch in the University Canteen?		
	No	Yes	Men	Woman	p	Health	Others	p	Yes	No	p
I do not know	98 (97.0)	3 (3.0)	0 (0.0)	3 (3.8)	1.000 [a]	1 (1.9)	2 (4.2)	0.603 [a]	2 (4.3)	1 (1.9)	0.596 [a]
Habit or routine	66 (65.3)	35 (34.7)	10 (43.5)	25 (32.1)	0.312 [b]	20 (37.7)	15 (31.3)	0.494 [b]	13 (27.7)	22 (40.7)	0.168 [b]
The taste of food	61 (60.4)	40 (39.6)	11 (47.8)	29 (37.2)	0.359 [b]	19 (35.8)	21 (43.8)	0.417 [b]	17 (36.2)	23 (42.6)	0.510 [b]
Food price	53 (52.5)	48 (47.5)	8 (34.8)	40 (51.3)	0.164 [b]	26 (49.1)	22 (45.8)	0.746 [b]	23 (48.9)	25 (46.3)	0.791 [b]
Control your weight	92 (91.1)	9 (8.9)	1 (4.3)	8 (10.3)	0.680 [a]	4 (7.5)	5 (10.4)	0.733 [a]	4 (8.5)	5 (9.3)	1.000 [a]
Food availability	60 (59.4)	41 (40.6)	10 (43.5)	31 (39.7)	0.749 [b]	17 (32.1)	24 (50.0)	0.067 [b]	19 (40.4)	22 (40.7)	0.974 [b]
Presentation or packaging	97 (96.0)	4 (4.0)	1 (4.3)	3 (3.8)	1.000 [a]	2 (3.8)	2 (4.2)	1.000 [a]	2 (4.3)	2 (3.7)	1.000 [a]
Someone else decides most of the foods that I eat	101 (100.0)	0 (0.0)	0 (0.0)	0 (0.0)	...	0 (0.0)	(0.0)	...	0 (0.0)	0 (0.0)	...
Vegetarian food or other particular habits	94 (93.1)	7 (6.9)	0 (0.0)	7 (9.0)	0.346 [a]	3 (5.7)	4 (8.3)	0.706 [a]	5 (10.6)	2 (3.7)	0.246 [a]
Content in additives, dyes, and preservatives	97 (96.0)	4 (4.0)	1 (4.3)	3 (3.8)	1.000 [a]	1 (1.9)	3 (6.3)	0.344 [a]	4 (8.5)	0 (0.0)	0.044 [a]*
My cultural, religious, and ethnic roots	101 (100.0)	0 (0.0)	0 (0.0)	0 (0.0)	...	0 (0.0)	0 (0.0)	...	0 (0.0)	0 (0.0)	...
Ease of convenience of preparation	52 (51.5)	49 (48.5)	16 (69.6)	33 (42.3)	0.022 [b]*	31 (58.5)	18 (37.5)	0.035 [b]*	17 (36.2)	32 (59.3)	0.021 [b]*
Try to make a healthy diet	81 (80.2)	20 (19.8)	4 (17.4)	16 (20.5)	1.000 [a]	11 (20.8)	9 (18.8)	0.801 [b]	7 (14.9)	13 (24.1)	0.248 [b]
Quality or freshness of food	90 (89.1)	11 (10.9)	2 (8.7)	9 (11.5)	1.000 [a]	4 (7.5)	7 (14.6)	0.257 [b]	8 (17.0)	3 (5.6)	0.065 [b]

* $p < 0.05$; Gender, course, and "Do you usually have lunch in the university canteen?": [a] Fisher's or [b] chi-square test based on the expected frequencies in each cell. Note: The data for gender, course, and food/beverage acquisition in vending machines are only presented for participants who answered "Yes" in the total column.

Table 4. Acquisition of food and beverages in vending machines (n = 101).

		n	Never	Monthly	Weekly	Daily	*p*
1. Coffee	Men	23	2 (8.7)	8 (34.8)	7 (30.4)	6 (26.1)	0.031
	Woman	78	22 (28.2)	27 (34.6)	19 (24.4)	10 (12.8)	
	Total	101	24 (23.8)	35 (34.7)	26 (25.7)	16 (15.8)	...
2. Other hot drinks with coffee	Total	101	57 (56.4)	31 (30.7)	10 (9.9)	3 (3.0)	...
3. Hot chocolate or other drinks with chocolate	Lunch in the canteen	47	25 (53.2)	14 (29.8)	7 (14.9)	1 (2.1)	0.007 *
	Do not have lunch in the canteen	54	42 (77.8)	9 (16.7)	3 (5.6)	0 (0.0)	
	Total	101	67 (66.3)	23 (22.8)	10 (9.9)	1 (1.0)	...
4. Bottled water	Health	76	36 (47.4)	26 (34.2)	13 (17.1)	1 (1.3)	0.048 *
	Other	61	21 (34.4)	26 (42.6)	8 (13.1)	6 (9.8)	
	Total	101	30 (29.7)	45 (44.6)	20 (19.8)	6 (5.9)	...
5. Sparkling water	Men	23	19 (82.6)	3 (13.0)	1 (4.3)	0 (0.0)	0.024 *
	Woman	78	75 (96.2)	3 (3.8)	0 (0.0)	0 (0.0)	
	Total	101	94 (93.1)	6 (5.9)	1 (1.0)	0 (0.0)	...
6. Soft drinks (Coca-Cola, Sumol, Iced Tea)	Total	101	74 (73.3)	25 (24.8)	2 (2.0)	0 (0.0)	...
7. Energy Drinks	Men	23	18 (78.3)	1 (4.3)	4 (17.4)	0 (0.0)	<0.001 *
	Woman	78	78 (100.0)	0 (0.0)	0 (0.0)	0 (0.0)	
	Total	101	96 (95.0)	1 (1.0)	4 (4.0)	0 (0.0)	...
8. Sandwiches	Lunch in the canteen	47	32 (68.1)	11 (23.4)	4 (8.5)	0 (0.0)	0.036 *
	Do not have lunch in the canteen	54	46 (85.2)	7 (13.0)	1 (1.9)	0 (0.0)	
	Total	101	78 (77.2)	18 (17.8)	5 (5.0)	0 (0.0)	...
9. Cakes and pastry products	Total	101	75 (74.3)	21 (20.8)	5 (5.0)	0 (0.0)	...
10. Cookies	Total	101	61 (60.4)	36 (35.6)	4 (4.0)	0 (0.0)	...
11. Cereal bars	Health	76	69 (90.8)	7 (9.2)	0 (0.0)	0 (0.0)	0.040 *
	Another course	61	48 (78.7)	10 (16.4)	3 (4.9)	0 (0.0)	
	Total	101	83 (82.2)	15 (14.9)	3 (3.0)	0 (0.0)	...
12. Potato chips	Men	23	16 (69.6)	5 (21.7)	2 (8.7)	0 (0.0)	
	Woman	78	69 (88.5)	9 (11.5)	0 (0.0)	0 (0.0)	0.023 *
	Total	101	85 (84.2)	14 (13.9)	2 (2.0)	0 (0.0)	
13. Solid yogurt	Men	23	20 (87.0)	1 (4.3)	1 (4.3)	1 (4.3)	
	Woman	78	76 (97.4)	2 (2.6)	0 (0.0)	0 (0.0)	0.039 *
	Total	101	96 (95.0)	3 (3.0)	1 (1.0)	1 (1.0)	
14. Liquid yogurt	Total	101	94 (93.1)	5 (5.0)	2 (2.0)	0 (0.0)	...
15. Fresh fruit	Total	101	94 (93.1)	6 (5.9)	0 (0.0)	1 (1.0)	...
16. Chocolates	Total	101	42 (41.6)	48 (47.5)	10 (9.9)	1 (1.0)	...
17. Sweets (gums; candies)	Total	101	65 (64.4)	31 (30.7)	4 (4.0)	1 (1.0)	...
18. Other Snacks	Total	101	78 (77.2)	19 (18.8)	4 (4.0)	0 (0.0)	...

* $p < 0.05$; Men/Woman, Lunch in the canteen/Do not have lunch in the canteen, and Health/Other course: Mann–Whitney test. Only detailed data are presented for the results where significant differences exist.

4. Discussion

The present study aimed to assess the purchasing behaviors of food and beverages from vending machines among higher education students in Portugal, alongside examining their utilization of university canteens and their propensity to bring lunch from home. The study revealed that a significant proportion of participants (73.7%) bring their own lunch to the university, while over half do not utilize the university canteen. These findings are consistent with a prior study conducted in 2018 among 620 Spanish and Portuguese university students, which indicated that 83.9% of respondents used vending machines [39].

Since the economic crisis of 2013, there has been an increasing trend toward consumer rationalization and a heightened focus on managing household budgets. Consequently, approximately 31% of Portuguese consumers have reduced their frequency of dining out at restaurants. This shift has led to a rise in home-cooked meals and the prevalence of packed lunches. A study conducted in 2020 during the COVID-19 pandemic found that nearly half of the participants opted for packed lunches for meals consumed outside the home [40]. Regarding the utilization of university canteens, findings from a study conducted in Indonesia indicate that over half of university students who dine away from home prefer to have their meals in the canteen [30]. Conversely, another study conducted at Polish universities found that only 35.5% of students and staff members regularly use the cafeterias daily or at least once a week [28]. Unlike some other countries, Portugal observes a customary lunch hour [28]. However, this allocated time may not be adequate for lunch in the canteen due to logistical and time constraints. For instance, the closure of university canteens and their distance from academic buildings contribute to time spent commuting and waiting in line for meals [41]. Furthermore, the cost of a full meal in private canteens significantly exceeds that of public institution canteens (EUR 2.80) [41], potentially influencing the decision to bring lunch from home. It is noteworthy that students identified logistical, time-related, and economic factors as reasons for abstaining from using the canteen and opting to bring lunch from home. Food and beverage vending machines are prevalent, particularly on a weekly basis, akin to findings in the Caruso, Klein, and Kaye [42] study. Convenience, price, product availability, and taste emerged as primary factors influencing these choices, consistent with previous research [9,27,42,43]. Moreover, the analysis of specific demographic groups revealed notable nuances. Male participants and those enrolled in health courses have shown a greater tendency to consider convenience as an influential factor than their colleagues. This may suggest that these groups may be more oriented towards practicality and efficiency in choosing foods on sales machines. However, it is essential to mention that students from health courses should be aware of opting for healthier choices than other university students due to their knowledge about food and health.

The finding suggests that students who utilize the canteen exhibit a heightened awareness of additives, dyes, and preservatives, indicating a greater consciousness regarding the nutritional quality of food. This implies that the canteen could potentially play a significant role in promoting healthier food choices among this group of students [31]. However, no correlation was identified between the factors influencing food choices from vending machines and the practice of bringing lunch from home. This indicates that the motivations driving these two behaviors may differ and that additional factors may be influential in determining such behaviors. Finally, the absence of correlation between food choice factors and participants' nutritional status (normal weight versus overweight) emphasizes the complexity of food decisions, the influence of multiple contextual factors, and food's simple energy value.

It was observed that a significant portion, more than 90%, never acquired items such as sparkling water, energy drinks, solid yogurts, liquid yogurts, and fresh fruits from the vending machines. However, when considering the monthly frequency, foods such as chocolates, bottled water, coffee, cookies, sweets, and soft drinks were purchased more regularly. In the weekly context, the most common acquisitions included coffee, bottled water, and other hot beverages, along with chocolates. Daily analysis revealed that coffee stood out as the most frequently acquired item. These results are consistent with other studies reporting that the most consumed foods in the university's food environment (including vending machines) are hot drinks (coffee, hot chocolate, etc.), bottled water, and sandwiches or hamburgers, while the least consumed are healthier options like fatty fruits and fresh fruits [3,44]. This suggests a preference for convenience and quick energy boosts over healthier choices among university students.

In a study that evaluated the quality of snacks and beverages sold in vending machines, most food items sold had a high energy density and none satisfied low sugar or high fiber content criteria [45,46]. The researchers pointed out that the shortage of time, high food prices, limited availability of healthy options, and lack of motivation were the most frequently mentioned barriers by students, as obstacles to healthy eating [46,47].

The study of the relationships between the acquisition of food and beverages from vending machines and variables such as gender, area of study, the habit of having lunch in the canteen, and bringing lunch from home has brought to light some differences. The results indicated that male students had a higher frequency of acquiring certain items, such as coffee, water, energy drinks, potato chips, and solid yogurts, than female students. According to Hasan et al. [9], male students consume more soda and energy drinks than female students. Yet, another study reveals that male students consumed significantly more energy from sugary drinks than female students [48]. The findings underscore the need to consider these differences when designing strategies to promote healthier eating habits on campus. By understanding different student groups' specific preferences and behaviors, universities can better tailor their interventions to encourage more balanced and nutritious dietary choices. Furthermore, the frequency of purchasing products such as sandwiches and hot chocolate or other chocolate beverages from the vending machines was higher among students who had lunch in the canteen than those who did not. According to the work of Czarniecka-Skubina et al. [28], students who used the canteen often choose to buy soups (39.2%) and sandwiches (28%), i.e., meals that can be consumed relatively rapidly. Thus, the hypothesis can be that students resort to vending machines to complement the meals consumed in the canteen. In addition, health students have demonstrated specific consumer standards, with a lower frequency of cereal bar acquisition and a higher frequency of water acquisition in machines than students from other areas. These findings can be associated with variations in the demographic and economic profile [49], in addition to personal factors, such as cooking skills, level of information and perspectives, as well as social influences, such as the role of friends and norms in the purchase decision, among others [50]. These insights underscore the importance of considering diverse student needs and behaviors when designing interventions to promote healthier eating habits within the university environment.

These results provide a comprehensive overview of vending machines' food and beverage consumption habits, highlighting purchase preferences at different time intervals and the influence of demographic and behavioral variables. Additionally, they can help understand participants' eating standards and inform health promotion strategies and healthier eating habits.

Strengths, Limitations, and Implications

This pilot study has several strengths. Its findings offer insights into acquiring food and beverages from vending machines, presenting intervention opportunities for institutions offering products in these machines. Additionally, the study provides the questionnaire used, enabling other researchers to replicate it and establish points of comparison with future studies. Considering changes to the food options offered in vending machines is crucial to improving consumer choices and promote healthier eating habits. Providing nutritious food options in vending machines is especially relevant, given that many participants indicated that they consume less healthy foods on a regular basis. Moreover, investing in food education to guide consumers in making healthier decisions, along with enhancing university meal spaces such as canteens to offer nutritious meals, as well as lunch spaces for students who bring lunch from home, would be important steps.

While our study provides insights, it is important to recognize several limitations. Given the utilization of an online questionnaire, several measures were implemented to ensure the authenticity of participant responses. Data validation techniques were employed to identify and remove any suspicious or inconsistent responses, including scrutinizing response patterns for signs of non-human activity. Additionally, participant information was cross-referenced with demographic data to verify response consistency and alignment with our target population's characteristics. These measures aimed to uphold the integrity and reliability of our data, minimizing the risk of contamination from non-human responses. However, it is acknowledged that no method is entirely foolproof, and there may still be potential limitations associated with web-based survey platforms. Future research could explore additional strategies or technologies to further enhance data validity and mitigate the influence of non-human responses.

Another limitation of this study is that using a self-report questionnaire may introduce the possibility of inaccurate information due to respondent bias or error. Additionally, relying on a convenience sample limits the generalizability of our findings to other contexts within Portugal.

One additional limitation stems from our decision to restrict open-ended questions solely to students who indicated "no" to using canteens and vending machines. While this approach aimed to focus on understanding the specific factors influencing students' decisions not to use these facilities, it may have overlooked valuable insights from students who responded affirmatively. Including perspectives from both groups could have provided a more comprehensive understanding of the factors influencing food choices among university students.

Another constraint is the absence of a comprehensive analysis of potential confounding factors, such as students' socioeconomic status. It is known that socioeconomic status can play a crucial role in dietary choices, influencing both access to certain foods and dietary preferences. The lack of consideration of these factors may have impacted the conclusions' accuracy.

Regarding the statistical analyses, categorical variables were summarized in counts and percentages, and the Kolmogorov–Smirnov test was used to assess variable distributions. The chi-square test or Fisher's exact test was utilized to determine the independence of variables, while the Mann–Whitney test was employed to compare medians in independent samples. While these methods are appropriate for basic statistical analysis, they come with limitations. For instance, the Kolmogorov–Smirnov test is sensitive to sample size and may not perform well with small samples. Similarly, the chi-square and Fisher's exact tests, while useful for categorical data, do not account for potential confounding variables. The Mann–Whitney test is non-parametric and does not provide insights into the effects of multiple variables simultaneously. Additionally, the consolidation of response categories into "Monthly", "Weekly", and "Daily" was necessary due to the dispersion and low frequency of specific options. This simplification aimed to enhance the coherence of our analysis, but may have resulted in a loss of detailed information regarding the frequency of acquiring food and beverages from vending machines.

To address these limitations and improve the robustness of our analysis in future studies, more sophisticated statistical methods will be incorporated. Mixed-effects models will allow data with multiple levels of variability, such as individual and group differences, to be handled, providing a more nuanced understanding of the factors influencing vending machine usage. Structural equation modeling can help explore complex relationships between variables, including mediating and moderating effects, offering deeper insights into the determinants of food and beverage choices. By employing these advanced techniques, the aim is to overcome the constraints of the current methodology and enable the accounting for of confounding factors and interactions between variables, ultimately leading to more accurate and reliable results.

Recognizing and addressing these factors in future studies is essential to ensure the validity and generalizability of the results. The inclusion of measures to control for participants' socioeconomic status, such as family income questionnaires or parental education levels, could provide a more comprehensive and accurate understanding of the associations between dietary habits and other relevant factors. Thus, it is important to emphasize that the inadequate consideration of these factors may have limited the comprehensive interpretation of the results of this study. In future research, expanding our data collection to include qualitative insights from all respondents, irrespective of their utilization of canteens and vending machines, can significantly enhance our comprehension of students' food choices and underlying motivations. This inclusive approach would enable a more nuanced exploration of the multifaceted factors influencing food-related decisions within university settings.

Furthermore, by delving into potential interventions, such as incorporating healthier alternatives in vending machines or implementing nutritional education programs, we can make substantial strides in promoting healthier eating habits among students. These interventions hold promise in fostering a supportive environment for making nutritious and balanced food choices, even amidst the demanding schedules of university life.

By embracing these measures, higher education institutions can play a pivotal role in advocating for and facilitating healthy eating practices among students. Ensuring access to wholesome food options and imparting nutritional knowledge not only bolsters student well-being and academic performance but also instills lifelong healthy eating habits. This proactive approach underscores the commitment of universities to the holistic development and flourishing of their student communities.

5. Conclusions

This pilot study offers valuable insights into the eating habits of a subset of university students in Portugal. A significant portion of higher education students in Portugal bring lunch from home to the university rather than using the canteen. Food and beverage vending machines are extensively used by university students, mainly driven by convenience, price, product availability, and flavor preferences. Economic reasons and health concerns are key factors that influence the dietary choices of this sample of students, namely concerning lunch in the canteen and taking home lunch. The most often purchased foods were chocolates, bottled water, coffee, cookies, sweets, and sodas. In addition, the frequency of vending machines varies according to gender, area of study, and canteen use. Male students tend to purchase certain items more frequently than female students, and health students exhibit distinct consumer preferences, emphasizing the influence of demographic and behavioral factors on food choices. These results could potentially provide insights for future large-scale studies aimed at informing policies and programs promoting healthy and accessible food choices for students. Additionally, gaining insight into consumer preferences could pave the way for developing effective strategies to foster healthy eating behaviors among Portuguese university students. Forthcoming investigations could delve into specific areas such as the impact of vending machine placement on food choices or the effectiveness of educational interventions in promoting healthier eating habits.

Supplementary Materials: The following supporting information can be downloaded at: https://www.mdpi.com/article/10.3390/nu16111722/s1, Questionnaire applied to participants.

Author Contributions: Conceptualization, L.O.; methodology, L.O.; software, L.O.; validation, L.O. and A.R.; formal analysis, L.O., R.P.Z. and A.R.; investigation, L.O. and A.R.; resources, L.O.; data curation, L.O., R.P.Z. and A.R.; writing—original draft preparation, L.O.; writing—review and editing, L.O., M.N.B., I.A., R.P.Z., E.T.-L., C.C., H.A.A., N.A.A., F.F.A. and A.R.; visualization, L.O. and A.R.; project administration, L.O. and A.R.; funding acquisition, M.N.B., I.A., E.T.-L., C.C., H.A.A., N.A.A., F.F.A. and A.R. All authors have read and agreed to the published version of the manuscript.

Funding: This research was funded by the Fundação para a Ciência e a Tecnologia (FCT) through the CBIOS projects https://doi.org/10.54499/UIDB/04567/2020, accessed on 15 March 2024 and https://doi.org/10.54499/UIDP/04567/2020, accessed on 15 March 2024. This work was also funded by National Funds through the FCT—Foundation for Science and Technology, I.P., within the scope of the projects Ref. UIDB/05507/2020 and DOI identifier https://doi.org/10.54499/UIDB/05507/2020, accessed on 15 March 2024, as well as Ref. UIDB/00681/2020 and DOI identifier https://doi.org/10.54499/UIDB/00681/2020, accessed on 15 March 2024.

Institutional Review Board Statement: This study followed the ethical code for web-based research and the recommendations of the Declaration of Helsinki. The study protocol was approved by the

Ethics Commission of the School of Health Sciences and Technologies of the Lusophone University (P02-23) 5 June 2023.

Informed Consent Statement: Informed consent was obtained from all subjects involved in the study.

Data Availability Statement: Data are contained within the article.

Acknowledgments: We are grateful to all participants who kindly participated in this study. Furthermore, we would like to thank the Centre for Studies in Education and Innovation (CI&DEI), Centre for Natural Resources, Environment and Society (CERNAS), and the Institute Polytechnic of Viseu for their support. Author N.A.A. would like to thank Princess Nourah bint Abdulrahman University Researchers supporting project number (PNURSP2024R130), Princess Nourah bint Abdulrahman University, Riyadh, Saudi Arabia.

Conflicts of Interest: The authors declare no conflicts of interest.

References

1. Dahl, A.A.; Fandetti, S.M.; Ademu, L.O.; Harris, R.; Racine, E.F. Assessing the Healthfulness of University Food Environments: A Systematic Review of Methods and Tools. *Nutrients* **2024**, *16*, 1426. [CrossRef] [PubMed]
2. Li, X.; Braakhuis, A.; Li, Z.; Roy, R. How Does the University Food Environment Impact Student Dietary Behaviors? A Systematic Review. *Front. Nutr.* **2022**, *9*, 840818. [CrossRef] [PubMed]
3. Martinez-Perez, N.; Telleria-Aramburu, N.; Insúa, P.; Hernández, I.; Telletxea, S.; Ansotegui, L.; Rebato, E.; Basabe, N.; de Pancorbo, M.M.; Rocandio, A.; et al. On-campus food purchase behaviors, choice determinants, and opinions on food availability in a Spanish university community. *Nutrition* **2022**, *103–104*, 111789. [CrossRef] [PubMed]
4. Sousa, B.; Pacheco, C.A.; Pereira, C.; Batalha, M.; Santos, T.; de Carvalho, R.V. Factors influencing healthy food choices of university students: Fatores que influenciam a escolha de comida saudável nos estudantes universitários. *Biomed. Biopharm. Res. J.* **2020**, *17*, 2–11. [CrossRef]
5. Oliveira, L.; Raposo, A. Factors That Most Influence the Choice for Fast Food in a Sample of Higher Education Students in Portugal. *Nutrients* **2024**, *16*, 1007. [CrossRef] [PubMed]
6. Skalkos, D.; Kalyva, Z.C.; Kosma, I.S. The Impact of the COVID-19 Pandemic on College Students' Food Choice Motives in Greece. *Sustainability* **2023**, *15*, 9865. [CrossRef]
7. Mastora, A.; Chatzitheodoridis, F.; Skalkos, D. Perceptions from Member-Consumers of a University Community for Sustainable and Healthy Eating: Evidence from Greece. *Sustainability* **2024**, *16*, 2213. [CrossRef]
8. Sánchez, L.A.; Roa-Díaz, Z.M.; Gamba, M.; Grisotto, G.; Londoño, A.M.M.; Mantilla-Uribe, B.P.; Méndez, A.Y.R.; Ballesteros, M.; Kopp-Heim, D.; Minder, B.; et al. What Influences the Sustainable Food Consumption Behaviours of University Students? A Systematic Review. *Int. J. Public Health* **2021**, *66*, 1604149. [CrossRef] [PubMed]
9. Hasan, H.; Faris, M.A.-I.E.; Mohamad, M.N.; Al Dhaheri, A.S.; Hashim, M.; Stojanovska, L.; Al Daour, R.; Rashid, M.; El-Farra, L.; Alsuwaidi, A.; et al. Consumption, Attitudes, and Trends of Vending Machine Foods at a University Campus: A Cross-Sectional Study. *Foods* **2021**, *10*, 2122. [CrossRef]
10. Dias, I.C.; Tavares, R.; Franchini, B.; Rodrigues, S. Máquinas de venda automática de alimentos/bebidas da Universidade do Porto: Caracterização da oferta alimentar. *Acta Port. Nutr.* **2021**, *24*, 46–49. [CrossRef]
11. Martinez-Perez, N.; Arroyo-Izaga, M. Availability, Nutritional Profile and Processing Level of Food Products Sold in Vending Machines in a Spanish Public University. *Int. J. Environ. Res. Public Health* **2021**, *18*, 684. [CrossRef] [PubMed]
12. Alegre, A.; Magalhães, S.; Lemos, C.; Brito, M.; JReis Lima, M.; Teixeira de Lemos, E. Máquinas de Venda Automática de Alimentos Promotoras de Diabesidade no Ensino Superior Politécnico. *Rev. Port. Diabetes* **2014**, *9*, 166–172.
13. Luís, A. Avaliação da Oferta Alimentar das Máquinas de Venda Automática de Alimentos e Bebidas das Instituições do Ensino Superior em Portugal. Master's Thesis, Universidade do Porto, Porto, Portugal, 2019.
14. Ferreira, A.; Castro, D.; Valada, E.; Costa, P.; Samorinha, C.; Precioso, J. Caracterização da oferta alimentar dos bufetes e máquinas de venda automática de alimentos da universidade do Minho. *Aliment. Hum.* **2009**, *15*, 80–85.
15. Park, H.; Papadaki, A. Nutritional value of foods sold in vending machines in a UK University: Formative, cross-sectional research to inform an environmental intervention. *Appetite* **2016**, *96*, 517–525. [CrossRef] [PubMed]
16. Raposo, A.; Carrascosa Iruzubieta, C.; Pérez, E.; Tavares, A.; Sanjuán, E.; Saavedra, P.; Millán, R. Vending machine foods: Evaluation of nutritional composition. *Ital. J. Food Sci.* **2016**, *28*, 448–463. [CrossRef]
17. Prowse, R.J.; Tomlin, D.L.; Naylor, P.J.; Raine, K.D. Exploring Nutrition Labelling of Food and Beverages in Vending Machines in Canadian Recreational Sport Settings. *Can. J. Diet. Pract. Res.* **2019**, *80*, 55–62. [CrossRef]
18. de Faria, H.C.; Garcez, A.; da Costa, J.S.D.; Ramos, M.; Paniz, V.M.V. Overweight and obesity among Brazilian healthcare university students: Prevalence and associated factors. *Arq. Bras. Endocrinol. Metabol.* **2023**, *67*, 416–426. [CrossRef] [PubMed]
19. Zamsad, M.; Banik, S.; Ghosh, L. Prevalence of overweight, obesity and abdominal obesity in Bangladeshi university students: A cross-sectional study. *Diabetes Metab. Syndr. Clin. Res. Rev.* **2018**, *13*, 480–483. [CrossRef] [PubMed]
20. Al Banna, H.; Brazendale, K.; Hasan, M.; Khan, S.I.; Sayeed, A.; Kundu, S. Factors associated with overweight and obesity among Bangladeshi university students: A case-control study. *J. Am. Coll. Health* **2022**, *70*, 2327–2333. [CrossRef] [PubMed]

21. Du, T.; Zhu, E.; Jiao, S. Poor Physical Performance is Associated with Obesity Among University Students in China. *Med. Sci. Monit. Basic Res.* **2017**, *23*, 173–178. [CrossRef]
22. Peltzer, K.; Pengpid, S.; Samuels, T.A.; Özcan, N.K.; Mantilla, C.; Rahamefy, O.H.; Wong, M.L.; Gasparishvili, A. Prevalence of overweight/obesity and its associated factors among university students from 22 countries. *Int. J. Environ. Res. Public Health* **2014**, *11*, 7425–7441. [CrossRef]
23. Ferreira, M.M.S.V.; Santos, J.M.; Sampaio, F.; Moreira, M.T.; Nogueira, A.; Guerra, M.; Brito, I. Estilos de vida dos estudantes do ensino superior: Contributos para a promoção da saúde. *Rev. Enferm. Ref.* **2023**, *6*, 1–10. [CrossRef]
24. Bento, M.C.; Barroso, T.; Ferreira, T.; Henriques, C.; Pimentel, H.; Ramos, L.; Rosa, A.; Vinagre, M.G. Comportamentos de Saúde e Bem-Estar dos Estudantes do Ensino Superior Politécnico—Um Diagnóstico a Partir da Perspetiva dos Estudantes. 2021. Available online: https://ccisp.pt/wp-content/uploads/2021/06/Relatorio-Saude.pdf (accessed on 20 March 2024).
25. Rousham, E.K.; Goudet, S.; Markey, O.; Griffiths, P.; Boxer, B.; Carroll, C.; Petherick, E.S.; Pradeilles, R. Unhealthy Food and Beverage Consumption in Children and Risk of Overweight and Obesity: A Systematic Review and Meta-Analysis. *Adv. Nutr. Int. Rev. J.* **2022**, *13*, 1669–1696. [CrossRef]
26. Elizabeth, L.; Machado, P.; Zinöcker, M.; Baker, P.; Lawrence, M. Ultra-Processed Foods and Health Outcomes: A Narrative Review. *Nutrients* **2020**, *12*, 1955. [CrossRef]
27. Garg, A.; Kumar, J. Exploring customer satisfaction with university cafeteria food services. An empirical study of Temptation Restaurant at Taylor's University, Malaysia. *Eur. J. Tour. Hosp. Recreat.* **2017**, *8*, 96–106. [CrossRef]
28. Czarniecka-Skubina, E.; Górska-Warsewicz, H.; Laskowski, W.; Jeznach, M. Consumer Choices and Service Quality in the University Canteens in Warsaw, Poland. *Int. J. Environ. Res. Public Health* **2019**, *16*, 3699. [CrossRef]
29. Min, H.; Min, H. Benchmarking the service quality of fast-food restaurant franchises in the USA. *Benchmarking Int. J.* **2011**, *18*, 282–300. [CrossRef]
30. Sakai, Y.; Rahayu, Y.Y.S.; Araki, T. Nutritional Value of Canteen Menus and Dietary Habits and Intakes of University Students in Indonesia. *Nutrients* **2022**, *14*, 1911. [CrossRef]
31. Fernández Torres, Á.; Moreno-Rojas, R.; Cámara Martos, F. Nutritional content of foods offered and consumed in a Spanish university canteen. *Nutr. Hosp.* **2014**, *31*, 1302–1308. [CrossRef]
32. Mills, S.; White, M.; Brown, H.; Wrieden, W.; Kwasnicka, D.; Halligan, J.; Robalino, S.; Adams, J. Health and social determinants and outcomes of home cooking: A systematic review of observational studies. *Appetite* **2017**, *111*, 116–134. [CrossRef]
33. Hanson, A.J.; Kattelmann, K.K.; McCormack, L.A.; Zhou, W.; Brown, O.N.; Horacek, T.M.; Shelnutt, K.P.; Kidd, T.; Opoku-Acheampong, A.; Franzen-Castle, L.D.; et al. Cooking and Meal Planning as Predictors of Fruit and Vegetable Intake and BMI in First-Year College Students. *Int. J. Environ. Res. Public Health* **2019**, *16*, 2462. [CrossRef] [PubMed]
34. Soldavini, J.; Berner, M. Characteristics associated with cooking frequency among college students. *Int. J. Gastron. Food Sci.* **2021**, *23*, 100303. [CrossRef]
35. Wilson, C.K.; Matthews, J.I.; Seabrook, J.A.; Dworatzek, P.D. Self-reported food skills of university students. *Appetite* **2017**, *108*, 270–276. [CrossRef] [PubMed]
36. Gavioli, F. Motivações e Fatores Envolvidos no Preparo e Consumo de Marmitas por Estudantes de uma Universidade Pública de Florianópolis/SC. Master's Thesis, Universidade Pública de Florianópolis/SC, Florianópolis, Brazil, 2021.
37. Holmes, S. Methodological and ethical considerations in designing an Internet study of quality of life: A discussion paper. *Int. J. Nurs. Stud.* **2009**, *46*, 394–405. [CrossRef]
38. World Medical Association. World Medical Association Declaration of Helsinki: Ethical principles for medical research involving human subjects. *JAMA* **2013**, *310*, 2191–2194. [CrossRef]
39. Raposo, A.; Pérez, E.; Sanjuán, E.; Saavedra, P.; Millán, R.; Carrascosa Iruzubieta, C. Vending machines and university students' consumption trends. *J. Food Nutr. Res.* **2018**, *57*, 295–306.
40. Alves, A. Tendências Alimentares no Setor do Food Service em Portugal. Master's Thesis, Universidade do Porto, Porto, Portugal, 2021.
41. Fernandes, V. Cantinas Universitárias: A Evolução Necessária para Alimentar o Conhecimento. P3. 2023. Available online: https://www.publico.pt/2023/08/09/p3/cronica/cantinas-universitarias-evolucao-necessaria-alimentar-conhecimento-2058029 (accessed on 20 March 2024).
42. Caruso, M.L.; Klein, E.G.; Kaye, G. Campus-Based Snack Food Vending Consumption. *J. Nutr. Educ. Behav.* **2014**, *46*, 401–405. [CrossRef]
43. Brown, M.V.; Flint, M.; Fuqua, J. The effects of a nutrition education intervention on vending machine sales on a university campus. *J. Am. Coll. Health* **2014**, *62*, 512–516. [CrossRef] [PubMed]
44. Roy, R.; Soo, D.; Conroy, D.; Wall, C.R.; Swinburn, B. Exploring University Food Environment and On-Campus Food Purchasing Behaviors, Preferences, and Opinions. *J. Nutr. Educ. Behav.* **2019**, *51*, 865–875. [CrossRef]
45. Faris, M.E.; Hasan, H.; Ismail, L.C.; Jahrami, H.; Rajab, D.; Almashgouni, A.A.; Alshehhi, A.; Aljabry, A.; Aljarwan, M.; Alnaqbi, M.; et al. Assessment of nutritional quality of snacks and beverages sold in university vending machines: A qualitative assessment. *Br. Food J.* **2021**, *123*, 2449–2460. [CrossRef]
46. Ashton, L.M.; Hutchesson, M.J.; Rollo, M.E.; Morgan, P.J.; Collins, C.E. Motivators and Barriers to Engaging in Healthy Eating and Physical Activity. *Am. J. Men's Health* **2016**, *11*, 330–343. [CrossRef]

47. Allom, V.; Mullan, B. Maintaining healthy eating behaviour: Experiences and perceptions of young adults. *Nutr. Food Sci.* **2014**, *44*, 156–167. [CrossRef]
48. Bawadi, H.; Khataybeh, T.; Obeidat, B.; Kerkadi, A.; Tayyem, R.; Banks, A.D.; Subih, H. Sugar-Sweetened Beverages Contribute Significantly to College Students' Daily Caloric Intake in Jordan: Soft Drinks Are Not the Major Contributor. *Nutrients* **2019**, *11*, 1058. [CrossRef] [PubMed]
49. Wills, W.; Danesi, G.; Kapetanaki, A.B.; Hamilton, L. Socio-Economic Factors, the Food Environment and Lunchtime Food Purchasing by Young People at Secondary School. *Int. J. Environ. Res. Public Health* **2019**, *16*, 1605. [CrossRef]
50. Kabir, A.; Miah, S.; Islam, A. Factors influencing eating behavior and dietary intake among resident students in a public university in Bangladesh: A qualitative study. *PLoS ONE* **2018**, *13*, e0198801. [CrossRef] [PubMed]

nutrients

MDPI

Article

Determinants of Weight Status and Body, Health and Life Satisfaction in Young Adults

Julia Suwalska [1,*], Sylwia Łukasik [2], Maciej Cymerys [3], Aleksandra Suwalska [4] and Paweł Bogdański [1]

1 Department of Treatment of Obesity, Metabolic Disorders and Clinical Dietetics, Poznan University of Medical Sciences, 60-569 Poznan, Poland
2 Institute of Human Biology and Evolution, Faculty of Biology, Adam Mickiewicz University in Poznan, 61-614 Poznan, Poland
3 Department of Internal Medicine, Poznan University of Medical Sciences, 60-786 Poznan, Poland
4 Department of Mental Health, Chair of Psychiatry, Poznan University of Medical Sciences, 60-572 Poznan, Poland
* Correspondence: jsuwalska@ump.edu.pl

Abstract: Health behaviors include behavioral patterns and habits that relate to health maintenance, restoration and improvement. They do not only affect the physical condition; they are also associated with life satisfaction. In our study, we focused on young adulthood, a specific lifespan period for establishing long-term health behavior patterns. The aim of the present study was to investigate depressive symptoms, lifestyle and eating behaviors and delineate their associations with overweight/obesity and body, health and life satisfaction in young adults in Poland. We enrolled 800 students (81.4% females and 18.6% males). Diet, physical activity, depressive symptoms, eating behaviors and body, health and life satisfaction were assessed. Multivariate logistic regression models were employed. Almost half of the participants in our study had at least mild symptoms of depression. Symptoms of depression significantly reduced the odds of satisfaction with body, health and life, whereas physical activity increased them. Overweight/obesity significantly reduced the odds of body and health satisfaction. In women, a history of depression and emotional eating increased the odds of being overweight/obese. The results of our study may contribute to the development of educational programs and intervention strategies for young adults.

Keywords: emotional eating; obesity; young adults; depression; physical activity; life satisfaction

1. Introduction

A quarter of a century ago, the World Health Organization (WHO) described a healthy lifestyle as a way of living that lowers the risk of being seriously ill or dying early [1]. According to this definition, a healthy lifestyle means engaging in regular physical activity, refraining from smoking, limiting alcohol consumption, and eating healthily to prevent being overweight. These behaviors contribute to better physical health and foster mental well-being [1,2]. A healthy lifestyle is further defined as a combination of lifestyle components associated with lower mortality and better health outcomes [3]. Health behaviors include behavioral patterns and habits that relate to health maintenance, health restoration and health improvement [4,5].

Most studies on lifestyle investigate smoking, diet, physical activity and overweight or obesity, and some also take alcohol use into account [3]. It has been found that smoking, physical inactivity, an unhealthy diet, obesity and other lifestyle behaviors are associated with the development of diseases such as cancer, heart disease, stroke and diabetes [6]. Individuals with four or more healthy behaviors have a 66% reduced risk of all-cause mortality [7] compared to those with an unhealthy lifestyle.

Health behaviors do not only affect the physical condition; they are also associated with subjective well-being (SWB) [8]. SWB comprises life satisfaction and the balance between positive and negative affect [9]. Life satisfaction reflects the extent to which various aspects of an individual's life are considered satisfying or fulfilling. It can be evaluated globally or divided into various domains, including, among others, satisfaction with self, health, work, family and leisure [10]. College students rate life satisfaction as very important [11]. In youth, body satisfaction may protect against excessive weight gain and eating disorders [12,13].

It is particularly important to investigate health behaviors in young adults (18–25 years of age) [14]. This is a period in life when young people experience dynamic and complex changes and set themselves on the path to adulthood, change their living arrangements, end their education, start working and change their primary relationships [15–17]. This is the time of transition from parental supervision to individual responsibility [13], from adolescent/dependent roles to adult/independent roles [17]. These life transitions may affect health behaviors [18]. During the shift from adolescence into young adulthood, a decline in physical activity and dietary habits is observed [15,19,20]. Young adulthood is often associated with poor lifestyle behaviors [21]. Unhealthy behaviors tend to continue into middle and late adulthood, predisposing individuals to preventable chronic conditions such as cardiovascular and respiratory diseases and diabetes [22].

An analysis of data from over 24,000 adults aged 18–24 years from the Behavioral Risk Factor Surveillance System (BRFSS) showed that almost half of them had at least one chronic condition. The most prevalent conditions were obesity (25.5%) and depression (21.3%) [23]. An increase in weight in young people may be attributed to a poor diet, excessive alcohol intake and low levels of physical activity [24]. Compared to other age groups, young adults are more likely to manage stress by engaging in unhealthy and weight-promoting behaviors, such as excessive eating and drinking alcohol [25]. Young adulthood represents a critical period for weight control, as the rate of weight gain is greatest at this time of life [25].

Young adults are also exposed to a high risk of developing mental health problems, as the onset of 75% of lifetime mental disorders occurs before the age of 25 [26]. The beginning of higher education coincides with the age of onset of problem behaviors (e.g., alcohol abuse and internet addiction) and mental health problems (e.g., depression and anxiety) [27]. One in five university students experiences mental health concerns, a five-fold increase over the past decade [28]. Mental disorders like depression and anxiety may negatively affect global and domain-specific life satisfaction [29,30].

The aim of this study was to investigate depressive symptoms, lifestyle and eating behaviors and delineate their associations with overweight/obesity and body, health and life satisfaction in young adults in Poland.

2. Materials and Methods

2.1. Study Procedure and Participants

The study was approved by the Ethical Committee of the Poznan University of Medical Sciences on 6 September 2018 by Resolution No. 857/18. The study was designed as a cross-sectional study and conducted among undergraduate health sciences students at the Poznan University of Medical Sciences, Poland. Data were collected between October 2019 and March 2022. Questionnaires were distributed by researchers to 985 students in their 1st-3rd year of physiotherapy, midwifery, nursing, public health, emergency medicine, occupational therapy, cosmetology, or dietetics during study courses. Eight hundred and five questionnaires were returned (response rate 81.7%), and five forms were excluded due to missing data (sex, age, weight). All participants enrolled voluntarily and provided written informed consent. The final study sample (800 students) included 81.4% females and 18.6% males, with a mean age of 20.4 ± 1.7 (range 18–25 years).

2.2. Measures

Sociodemographic characteristics (gender, age, sex, financial situation, self-reported health data, etc.) were collected. Smoking status was assessed with a question from the

European Health and Behavior Study (EHBS) [31]. Participants were classified as current smokers or non-smokers.

BMI (body mass index) was calculated as body mass (kg) divided by height squared (m^2) from the students' self-reported height and weight. According to the World Health Organization, participants were classified as underweight (BMI < 18.5 kg/m^2), healthy weight (BMI 18.5 to 24.9 kg/m^2), overweight (BMI 25.0 to 29.9 kg/m^2), and obese (BMI 30.0 kg/m^2 or higher) [32]. For the purpose of statistical analysis, the categories of overweight and obese were merged into one category.

Symptoms of depression were assessed with the Beck Depression Inventory (BDI) [33], a 21-item multiple-choice questionnaire. For every question, the severity of the symptom is assessed on a scale of 0 to 3, and the score is the sum of the points. The cut-off scores were as follows: 0–9, normal range; 10–18, mild-to-moderate depression; 19–29, moderate-to-severe depression; and 30–63, severe depression [34].

The Food Frequency Questionnaire (FFQ) [35] was used to collect information on the frequency of consumption of 62 product groups. Consumption frequency for each food item was indicated by choosing one of six answers: never or very rarely, once a month or less, several times a month, several times a week, daily, or a few times a day. Subsequently, the answers were converted into daily frequency and aggregated into twenty-five food categories [36]. Alcohol consumption was assessed by a question from FFQ [35] following the same conversion procedure.

The International Physical Activity Questionnaire (IPAQ) [37] was used to evaluate the level of physical activity. The short form of IPAQ asks about three specific types of activity (walking, moderate-intensity activities, and vigorous-intensity activities) undertaken in the last 7 days. Based on the results, participants were divided into three levels of physical activity (low, moderate or high). In the analyses, moderate/high activities were compared to low physical activity as a reference category.

To assess eating behaviors, a Polish validated version of the Three Factor Eating Questionnaire (TFEQ-18) was used [38,39]. This questionnaire measures three aspects of eating behaviors: restrained eating (6 items, conscious restriction of food intake in order to control body weight or to promote weight loss), uncontrolled eating (9 items, tendency to eat more than usual due to a loss of control over intake), and emotional eating (3 items, inability to resist emotional cues) [38]. Seventeen items were answered on a 4-point scale and one on an 8-point scale. The results were summated into scale scores for cognitive restraint, uncontrolled eating, and emotional eating and transformed to a 0–100 scale [40].

Body satisfaction was assessed using the question "How satisfied are you with your body appearance?", health satisfaction using the question "How satisfied are you with your health?" and life satisfaction using the question "How satisfied are you with your life, overall?" For each item, there were five Likert response categories: (1) very dissatisfied, (2) dissatisfied, (3) neither dissatisfied nor satisfied, (4) satisfied and (5) very satisfied [41,42]. Answers were dichotomized into 'not satisfied' (1–3) and 'satisfied' (4–5).

2.3. Statistical Analysis

Data were analyzed using the Statistica 13 package (Statsoft, Kraków, Poland). Continuous data are presented as mean and standard deviation (SD), whereas categorical variables are expressed as frequencies and percentages. A *T*-test for continuous variables and a chi-squared test for categorical variables (with Yates's correction when the class size did not exceed 10 items) were used. The level of significance was set at $p < 0.05$.

To address the research purposes, logistic regression models were employed. All of the analyses were also conducted separately for women and men.

First, a univariate logistic regression was conducted to assess the potential association between dependent variables, i.e., overweight/obesity, body satisfaction, health satisfaction and life satisfaction, and independent variables. The independent variables tested for their association with overweight/obesity included sociodemographic factors (sex, financial status, smoking), medical history (history of depression, hypothyroidism), eating behaviors (emotional eating, cognitive restraint, uncontrolled eating), symptoms of depression (no/yes), physical activity (low/moderate/high) and consumption of food products measured by FFQ. The independent variables tested for their association with body satisfaction, health satisfaction and life satisfaction included sociodemographic factors (sex, financial status, smoking), medical history (history of depression, hypothyroidism), eating behaviors (emotional eating, cognitive restraint, uncontrolled eating), symptoms of depression (no/yes), physical activity (low/moderate/high) and overweight/obesity.

Then, hypotheses of how different independent variables (factors) may act together to affect the dependent variables (overweight/obesity, body satisfaction, health satisfaction and life satisfaction) and the nature (positive or negative) and significance of the relationship were tested. For this purpose, variables identified as statistically significant in the univariate analysis ($p < 0.05$) were entered into the multivariate analysis.

3. Results

3.1. Characteristics of the Studied Group

The main characteristics of the participants are summarized in Table 1.

The studied group consisted of 800 students: 651 (81.4%) female and 149 (18.6%) male; mean age 20.4 ± 1.7. The participants were students in their 1st–3rd year of physiotherapy (336; 42.0%), midwifery (278; 34.8%), nursing (108; 13.5%), public health (21; 2.6%), emergency medicine (34; 4.3%), occupational therapy (17; 1.5%), cosmetology (4; 0.5%), or dietetics (2; 0.3%). In the study group, 9.3% of the participants were underweight, 71.8% had a normal weight, 14.3% were overweight and 4.8% were obese. Hypothyroidism was reported by 68 subjects (8.5%) and a history of depression by 52 (6.5%). One hundred and fifty-seven participants (19.6%) reported smoking tobacco. Of the 800, 63.3% of the participants reported body satisfaction, 57.3% reported health satisfaction and 76.2% reported life satisfaction. In terms of physical activity, 20.5% of the participants had a low level, 46.1% had a moderate level, and 33.4% had a high level (IPAQ). Almost half of the respondents (49.6%) showed symptoms of depression.

Table 1. Characteristics of the participants.

Characteristic	N (%)
Weight status	
Underweight	74 (9.3)
Normal range	574 (71.8)
Overweight	114 (14.3)
Obese	38 (4.8)
Symptoms of depression	
Normal range	401 (50.4)
Mild to moderate	255 (32.1)
Moderate to severe	104 (13.1)
Severe	35 (4.4)
History of depression	
Yes	52 (6.5)
No	748 (93.5)
Hypothyroidism	
Yes	68 (8.5)
No	732 (91.5)
Smoking	
Yes	157 (19.6)
No	643 (80.4)

Table 1. *Cont.*

Characteristic	N (%)
Level of physical activity	
Low	164 (20.5)
Moderate	369 (46.1)
High	267 (33.4)
Body satisfaction	
Yes	498 (63.3)
No	289 (36.7)
Health satisfaction	
Yes	454 (57.3)
No	338 (42.7)
Life satisfaction	
Yes	607 (76.2)
No	190 (23.8)

3.2. Comparison between Men and Women

The results are presented in Table 2.

Table 2. Participants' body mass index, symptoms of depression, eating behaviors, diet, hypothyroidism, physical activity and body, health and life satisfaction broken down by gender.

	Men		Women		*p*
	Mean	SD	Mean	SD	
Body mass index	23.7	3.5	22.1	3.7	<0.001
Beck depression inventory	7.6	7.3	11.9	8.8	<0.001
Three-Factor Eating Questionnaire					
Cognitive restraint	39.5	18.6	44.2	20.3	0.010
Uncontrolled eating	36.1	18.9	33.5	18.0	n.s.
Emotional eating	28.0	25.6	39.7	27.3	<0.001
Food Frequency Questionnaire (aggregated)					
Sugar, sweets and snacks	1.4	1.1	1.6	1.2	n.s.
Milk, fermented milk drinks and curd cheese	1.2	0.9	1.1	0.8	n.s.
Sweetened milk products	0.4	0.5	0.3	0.4	0.008
Cheese	0.6	0.5	0.6	0.4	n.s.
Eggs and egg dishes	0.5	0.4	0.4	0.4	0.005
Breakfast cereals	0.2	0.3	0.2	0.3	n.s.
Whole-grain products	0.8	0.6	0.8	0.7	n.s.
Refined-grain products	1.0	0.6	0.8	0.5	<0.001
Butter and cream	0.8	0.6	0.6	0.6	0.023
Other animal fats	0.0	0.1	0.0	0.1	n.s.
Vegetable oils	0.5	0.4	0.5	0.4	n.s.
Other fats	0.4	0.5	0.2	0.4	0.003
Fruits	0.7	0.6	0.8	0.5	n.s.
Dried fruit, fruit preserves and fruit condiments	0.3	0.4	0.2	0.4	n.s.
Vegetables	0.9	0.5	0.9	0.6	n.s.
Dry and processed pulses	0.2	0.4	0.2	0.3	n.s.
Potatoes	0.5	0.4	0.4	0.3	0.004
Nuts and seeds	0.4	0.5	0.4	0.6	n.s.
Processed meats	0.9	0.8	0.5	0.6	<0.001
Red meat and venison	0.3	0.3	0.1	0.2	<0.001
White meat	0.4	0.3	0.3	0.3	<0.001

Table 2. *Cont.*

	Men		Women		*p*
	Mean	**SD**	**Mean**	**SD**	
Fish	0.2	0.3	0.1	0.2	n.s.
Juices	0.5	0.6	0.4	0.5	0.004
Sweetened beverages and energy drinks	0.4	0.6	0.2	0.4	<0.001
Alcohol	0.4	0.4	0.2	0.3	<0.001
	N	%	*N*	%	*p*
Hypothyroidism					
Yes	3	2.0	65	10.0	0.003 [Y]
No	146	98.0	586	90.0	
International Physical Activity Questionnaire					
Low activity	18	12.1	146	22.4	0.005
Moderate/high activity	131	87.9	505	77.6	
Smoking					
Yes	38	25.5	119	18.3	0.045
No	111	74.5	532	81.7	
Body satisfaction					
Yes	110	74.8	388	60.6	0.001
No	37	25.2	252	39.4	
Health satisfaction					
Yes	104	70.7	350	54.3	<0.001
No	43	29.3	295	45.7	
Life satisfaction					
Yes	125	84.5	482	74.3	0.009
No	23	15.5	167	25.7	

SD—standard deviation; n.s.—not significant; [Y] Yates' correction.

Women significantly more often reported hypothyroidism than men. Men significantly more often showed moderate/high physical activity levels according to the IPAQ category and significantly more often reported that they smoked tobacco. They also reported a higher consumption of refined grains, butter, other fats, potatoes, processed meat, red and white meat, alcohol, sweetened beverages and juices. Women had a significantly higher severity of depressive symptoms. Furthermore, symptoms of depression were more frequently observed in women than in men (53.2% vs. 33.8%, $p < 0.05$). Women were significantly less likely to be satisfied with their body, health and life. Cognitive restraint and emotional eating were significantly more pronounced in women.

3.3. Overweight/Obesity

In the multivariate analysis (Table 3), male gender, cognitive restraint, emotional eating and the consumption of red meat and sweetened beverages were identified as statistically significant risk factors in predicting overweight/obesity, whereas the consumption of refined grains reduced the risk. In women, the odds of being overweight/obese were increased by hypothyroidism, a history of depression, emotional eating, and red meat consumption. After adjusting for other factors in the model, only cognitive restraint significantly increased the odds of overweight/obesity in men.

Table 3. Multivariate logistic regression to predict overweight/obesity (separate models for all subjects, women, and men).

Variable	OR	95%CI	*p*
		All participants	
Male gender	2.17	1.32–3.57	0.002
History of depression	1.95	0.98–3.87	n.s.
Cognitive restraint	1.01	1.00–1.02	0.019
Uncontrolled eating	0.99	0.98–1.01	n.s.
Emotional eating	1.02	1.01–1.03	<0.001
Refined grains	0.58	0.40–0.85	0.005
Red meat	3.15	1.40–7.08	0.005
Sweetened beverages	1.54	1.02–2.32	0.041
Alcohol	1.32	0.79–2.19	n.s.
		Women	
Hypothyroidism	2.22	1.17–4.22	0.015
History of depression	2.24	1.07–4.67	0.032
Emotional eating	1.02	1.01–1.03	<0.001
Red meat	5.43	1.78–16.56	0.003
		Men	
Cognitive restraint	1.03	1.01–1.05	0.011
Cereals	0.21	0.04–1.06	n.s.
Refined grains	0.73	0.35–1.52	n.s.
Oil	0.33	0.09–1.18	n.s.
Vegetables	0.45	0.18–1.09	n.s.

OR—odds ratio; CI—confidence interval; n.s.—not significant.

3.4. Body Satisfaction

Table 4 shows the results of a multivariate logistic regression analysis predicting body satisfaction. The odds of body satisfaction were significantly reduced by overweight/obesity, symptoms of depression, cognitive restraint and uncontrolled eating, whereas moderate/high physical activity significantly increased the odds. The model for women included the same significant factors. In men, only overweight/obesity and symptoms of depression remained significant after adjustment for other factors.

Table 4. Multivariate logistic regression to predict body satisfaction (separate models for all subjects, women, and men).

Variable	OR	95%CI	*p*
	All Participants		
Male gender	1.56	0.94–2.58	n.s.
History of depression	0.63	0.31–1.27	n.s.
Overweight/obesity	0.33	0.21–0.51	<0.001
Symptoms of depression	0.16	0.11–0.23	<0.001
Cognitive restraint	0.98	0.97–0.99	<0.001
Uncontrolled eating	0.99	0.98–1.00	0.041
Emotional eating	1.00	0.99–1.01	n.s.
Moderate/high physical activity	2.08	1.36–3.19	0.001
	Women		
History of depression	0.62	0.29–1.33	n.s.
Overweight/obesity	0.38	0.23–0.63	<0.001

Table 4. *Cont.*

Variable	OR	95%CI	p
Symptoms of depression	0.18	0.12–0.26	<0.001
Cognitive restraint	0.98	0.97–0.99	<0.001
Uncontrolled eating	0.99	0.97–1.00	0.024
Emotional eating	1.00	0.99–1.01	n.s.
Moderate/high physical activity	2.09	1.33–3.28	0.001
	Men		
Overweight/obesity	0.14	0.05–0.39	<0.001
Symptoms of depression	0.08	0.03–0.23	<0.001
Emotional eating	1.00	0.98–1.02	n.s.
Moderate/high physical activity	1.82	0.51–6.47	n.s.

OR—odds ratio; CI—confidence interval; n.s.—not significant.

3.5. Health Satisfaction

Table 5 presents the multivariate logistic regression model for predicting health satisfaction. Hypothyroidism, history of depression, overweight/obesity, symptoms of depression measured by BDI and emotional eating reduced the odds of health satisfaction, whereas moderate/high physical activity significantly increased the odds. In women, the same factors had a significant impact. Symptoms of depression and uncontrolled eating significantly reduced the odds of health satisfaction in men.

Table 5. Multivariate logistic regression to predict health satisfaction (separate models for all subjects, women, and men).

Variable	OR	95%CI	p
	All participants		
Male gender	1.35	0.86–2.12	n.s.
Average financial status [a]	1.52	0.86–2.69	n.s.
High financial status [a]	1.88	0.92–3.83	n.s.
Hypothyroidism	0.23	0.13–0.44	<0.001
History of depression	0.19	0.08–0.44	<0.001
Overweight/obesity	0.60	0.40–0.91	0.016
Symptoms of depression	0.39	0.28–0.54	<0.001
Uncontrolled eating	1.00	0.99–1.01	n.s.
Emotional eating	0.99	0.98–1.00	0.004
Moderate/high physical activity	1.58	1.07–2.35	0.022
	Women		
Average financial status [a]	1.43	0.74–2.77	n.s.
High financial status [a]	1.95	0.84–4.50	n.s.
Hypothyroidism	0.20	0.10–0.39	<0.001
History of depression	0.18	0.07–0.44	<0.001
Overweight/obesity	0.59	0.36–0.96	0.034
Symptoms of depression	0.39	0.27–0.56	<0.001
Uncontrolled eating	1.00	0.99–1.02	n.s.
Emotional eating	0.99	0.98–0.99	0.001
Moderate/high physical activity	1.65	1.08–2.52	0.022
	Men		
Symptoms of depression	0.35	0.16–0.77	0.008
Uncontrolled eating	0.98	0.96–1.00	0.041

OR—odds ratio; CI—confidence interval; n.s.—not significant; [a] compared to low financial status.

3.6. Life Satisfaction

In the multivariate analysis (Table 6), the odds of life satisfaction were reduced by smoking and symptoms of depression. An average or high financial status compared to a low financial status and moderate/high physical activity compared to low physical activity increased the odds of life satisfaction. In women, the odds were reduced by symptoms of depression and increased by an average or high financial status and moderate/high physical activity. In men, the odds were significantly reduced by depressive symptoms.

Table 6. Multivariate logistic regression to predict life satisfaction (separate models for all subjects, women, and men).

Variable	OR	95%CI	p
	All participants		
Male gender	1.17	0.67–2.04	n.s.
Average financial status [a]	2.49	1.39–4.45	0.002
High financial status [a]	8.67	3.43–21.95	<0.001
History of depression	0.55	0.28–1.08	n.s.
Smoking	0.60	0.38–0.94	0.027
Symptoms of depression	0.19	0.12–0.30	<0.001
Uncontrolled eating	0.99	0.98–1.01	n.s.
Emotional eating	1.00	0.99–1.00	n.s.
Moderate/high physical activity	1.70	1.11–2.61	0.015
	Women		
Average financial status [a]	2.95	1.53–5.67	0.001
High financial status [a]	10.04	3.45–29.24	<0.001
History of depression	0.57	0.27–1.18	n.s.
Smoking	0.61	0.37–1.01	n.s.
Overweight/obesity	0.73	0.43–1.23	n.s.
Symptoms of depression	0.20	0.12–0.32	<0.001
Uncontrolled eating	0.99	0.98–1.01	n.s.
Emotional eating	1.00	0.99–1.01	n.s.
Moderate/high physical activity	1.66	1.05–2.63	0.030
	Men		
Symptoms of depression	0.16	0.06–0.43	<0.001

OR—odds ratio; CI—confidence interval; n.s.—not significant; [a] compared to low financial status.

4. Discussion

In our study, we focused on young adulthood, a specific lifespan period during which many people experience weight gain. This is also the time to establish long-term health behavior patterns [15]. As overweight and obesity are associated with many negative health consequences, including increased risk of cardiovascular diseases and cancer [43], it is important to redirect resources towards the targeted primary prevention of weight gain in early adulthood [44]. To do this, it is important to analyze risk factors such as emotional eating, poor diet or depressive symptoms, which are potential targets for intervention.

Our study also analyzed factors influencing body, health and life satisfaction in young adults. It is believed that focusing on the health and well-being of young adults is especially important as it may help them to successfully embrace adult roles as healthy citizens, workers and parents [16].

Only approximately 57% of the subjects in our study were satisfied or very satisfied with their health (men significantly more often than women: 70.7% vs. 54.3%). According to the American College Health Association (ACHA), in 2019, over eighty percent of college students described their health as 'good', 'very good' or 'excellent' [45]. Among Italian students, having good or very good health has been declared by 77% [46], and in the United Kingdom, 47.5% have perceived their own health as 'very good' or 'excellent' [47]. Higher health satisfaction among men is in line with other studies [46,48]. Three-quarters of the subjects in our study were satisfied with their life, this being significantly more frequent in men. The results of previous studies on gender differences as regards to life satisfaction are inconsistent and vary across countries [42,49]. Body satisfaction was observed in 63.3% of our study participants, significantly more often in men. Compared with men, women have shown lower body satisfaction in a study by Godoy-Izquierdo et al. [50].

Both an average and high financial status increase the odds of life satisfaction (2.5 times and 8.7 times, respectively). In a study by Prémusz et al. [51], financial status was the strongest predictor of life satisfaction among women, whereas in a study by He et al., women in households with a lower wealth status reported poorer subjective health, life satisfaction and happiness [52]. Similar results were obtained in a Spanish study [48].

In our study, smoking decreased the odds of life satisfaction. The results of a longitudinal study by Lappan et al. revealed that smoking predicted poorer life satisfaction, less optimism, positive affect and less purpose in life [53]. In a study by Grant et al. [42], life satisfaction was positively associated with non-smoking among students from 21 countries. The literature rarely considers decreasing life satisfaction as a negative consequence of smoking [53]. However, the relationship might be bidirectional—smoking contributes to low life satisfaction and life dissatisfaction leads to smoking [42].

4.1. Physical Activity

In our study, as many as 79.5% of the participants reported a moderate/high level of physical activity. In a study by Pengpid and Peltzer [41], 42.2% of the participants reported a low level of activity, 36.5% a moderate level of activity, and 21.2% a high level of physical activity. The higher level of physical activity in our study may be due to the fact that it was conducted among students of health sciences, including 42.0% of physiotherapy students who are generally engaged in sports and are more health-oriented. Regular physical activity is proven to help prevent and manage noncommunicable diseases (NCDs), such as heart disease, stroke, diabetes and obesity. It can improve mental health, quality of life and well-being [54].

We found a significantly higher level of physical activity among men, which is in line with previous studies [55–57]. Possible causes of these gender discrepancies include cultural standards and values, traditional roles and the lack of social and community support for women's participation in physical activity [58]. More opportunities for safe and accessible leisure-time activity need to be provided to women in order to increase their overall levels of activity [55].

In our study group, moderate/high physical activity significantly increased the odds of body, health and life satisfaction. The results of the aforementioned study by Pengpid et al. [41] revealed that moderate/high physical activity increases the odds of higher life satisfaction, greater happiness and better perceived health, whereas longer sedentary behavior decreases them. In previous studies among students, physical activity has been associated with happiness and better perceived health [47,59]. A large European study conducted among women of reproductive age has shown that regular physical activity results in better life satisfaction [51]. Leisure-time physical exercise has also been associated with better life satisfaction in a large population of students [42]. Physical activity can and should be integrated into the settings in which people live, work and play [54]. Quality physical education and supportive environments can contribute to long-lasting healthy, active lifestyles [54]. Universities can encourage physical activity among students by offering extra physical education classes and exercise facilities and promoting walking and cycling as means of transportation and active recreation.

4.2. Overweight/Obesity

Overweight/obesity was observed in almost 20% of the study's participants. Overweight/obesity significantly reduced the odds of body satisfaction (3.0 times) and health satisfaction (1.7 times). In a study by Godoy-Izquierdo et al. among Spanish adults, a higher BMI was associated with lower body satisfaction among men and women. Similar results were presented by Streeter et al. for a group of young adults in Canada [60]. Among Portuguese and Brazilian students, a higher BMI has been associated with greater dissatisfaction with general body appearance in men and body shape in women [61]. In a systematic review by Weinberger et al. [62], individuals with obesity reported higher levels of body dissatisfaction than normal-weight individuals. In a systematic review by Puhl and Heuer, obesity was shown to increase the risk of depression, low self-esteem and poor body image and was associated with stigmatizing attitudes [63].

In our study, a poorer quality of diet in men (a higher consumption of refined grains, butter and other fats, meat, sweetened beverages and alcohol) was observed. Data from other studies indicate that, compared to men, women are more likely to report eating fruits, vegetables, cereals, milk, dairy and whole-grain products and avoiding red meat, eggs, alcohol and high-sucrose foods [64–67].

We noted that the consumption of red meat and sweetened beverages increased the risk of overweight/obesity, and the intake of refined grains decreased it. Whereas the role of red meat and sweetened beverages as risk factors for weight gain is well established [68,69], our results concerning refined grains are somewhat counterintuitive since refined grain intake is widely assumed to be associated with adverse health outcomes. However, the results of 11 meta-analyses of prospective cohort studies demonstrated that refined grain intake has not been associated with all-cause mortality, type 2 diabetes, cardiovascular disease, coronary heart disease, stroke, hypertension or cancer [70]. Furthermore, white bread is included in a common Polish breakfast, and a link between skipping breakfast and overweight/obesity has been reported previously [71].

4.3. Depression

Almost half of the participants in our study had at least mild symptoms of depression, and 6.5% reported a history of depression. Depressive symptoms were significantly more common in women than in men. The 2019 data from the American College Health Association showed that within the previous 12 months, 20.0% of students (11.7% of men and 22.5% of women) had been diagnosed with or treated by a professional for depression [45], and 45.1% of the participants reported feeling so depressed that it was difficult to function [45]. According to Lipson et al. [72], there was a 134.6% increase in symptoms of depression among U.S. students between 2013 and 2021 (from 17.4% to 40.8%). Depressive disorders are the leading cause of years lost due to disability (YLDs) for females aged 15–24 years and affect more females than males in all young people's age groups [73].

In our study, symptoms of depression significantly reduced the odds of satisfaction with body (6.3 times), health (2.6 times) and life (5.3 times). Moreover, a history of depression significantly reduced the odds of health satisfaction. In a longitudinal study, Fergusson et al. [74] showed a bidirectional association between mental health problems (including major depression) and life satisfaction.

In this group of women, a history of depression increased the odds of developing obesity by 2.2 times. In a longitudinal study by Konttinen et al., depression predicted higher BMI and waist circumference gain over 7 years [75]. In a systematic review and meta-analysis of longitudinal studies by Luppino et al. [76], baseline depression (symptoms and disorder) increased the odds of developing obesity. Therefore, patients with obesity should be screened for depression, and patients diagnosed with depression should have their body mass monitored [77].

4.4. Hypothyroidism

In our study, hypothyroidism was significantly associated with overweight/obesity. The common symptoms of hypothyroidism in adults, such as fatigue, mood impairment, weight gain, constipation and menstrual disturbance [78], are not specific and can be confused with those of obesity [79]. A higher prevalence of overt and subclinical hypothyroidism in obesity has been shown [80], but some studies suggest that changes in thyroid hormones could be the consequence, rather than the cause, of weight gain [81]. The European Society of Endocrinology Clinical Practice Guideline recommends an assessment of thyroid function in people with obesity [79].

4.5. Eating Behaviors

We confirmed the results of previous studies showing that emotional and restrained eating are more common in women [40,82,83]. Our results showed that higher levels of emotional eating increased the odds of overweight/obesity in women. This is in line with the results of a 5-year study by van Strien et al. [84], which showed that emotional eating predicted future body weight gain in women but not in men. Also, in a study by Anglé, higher scores of cognitive restraint and emotional eating were associated with a higher BMI [85].

In a study on a Swedish population, cognitive restraint was associated with a higher body weight in adolescents, whereas this was the case for uncontrolled eating and emotional eating in adult women [86]. High levels of emotional eating were associated with overweight in a study by Lluch et al. [83]. An association between emotional eating and BMI has also been reported in young people [87,88].

In our study, cognitive restraint was significantly associated with overweight/obesity in men. An association between cognitive restraint and overweight/obesity has been reported previously [83,89]. It should be noted, however, that in view of the fact that it is a cross-sectional study, it is possible that the dependence is the other way around: a higher body weight makes people eat in a more restrained way in order to control their weight [85]. In a French longitudinal study, restrained eating was not associated with an increase in adiposity over time, but a higher initial BMI was associated with a greater increase in cognitive restraint scores in participants [90].

In women, a higher level of emotional eating reduced the odds of health satisfaction, whereas cognitive restraint reduced the odds of body satisfaction. A higher level of uncontrolled eating reduced body satisfaction in women and health satisfaction in men. In a study by Jáuregui-Lobera et al. [89], cognitive restraint was associated with the perception of being overweight.

These results are of significance since they show that poor eating behaviors can lead to overweight and obesity and can reduce body, health and life satisfaction. This is why eating behaviors should be considered in the development of lifestyle interventions [91], for example, by teaching emotion regulation skills [92].

4.6. Limitations

Several limitations should be acknowledged. First, the results were obtained using self-reported questionnaires and self-reported height and weight data. The diagnosis of hypothyroidism was self-reported and was not confirmed by laboratory tests. Second, the sample is gender-imbalanced, with male respondents being in the minority, which is due to the high proportion of female students in health-related studies. This limitation was addressed by performing a separate analysis of the data for women and for men. Third, body, health and life satisfaction measurements were performed using a single-item measure, which is not as reliable or valid as multi-item measures but is widely used in research surveys and has been reviewed as acceptably valid [10,93]. Fourth, this study was conducted with health science students, who are more aware of the importance of health behaviors, including physical activity and diet; therefore, caution is needed when extrapolating the results to broader populations.

Although this study identified significant predictors of weight status, body, health and life satisfaction in a large sample of university students, the findings should be interpreted with caution due to the cross-sectional design. Longitudinal research is required in the future to verify the findings of the current study.

5. Conclusions

Our study provides valuable insights into the impact of lifestyle, symptoms of depression and eating behaviors on the weight status and body, health and life satisfaction of young adults, laying the groundwork for future research and interventions in this population.

The health behaviors developed in this period can persist into later life. Young adulthood is a key period for promoting healthy behaviors such as a healthy diet and a good level of physical activity, which, as shown herein, have a positive impact on body, health and life satisfaction. The lifestyle assessment of young adults should not focus on a single behavior; the co-occurrence and interaction of multiple health behaviors should be taken into consideration. It is also important to pay more attention to emotional eating and its negative consequences.

The importance of the high prevalence of depressive symptoms among young adults should also be highlighted. These symptoms were associated with reduced body, health and life satisfaction, while a history of depression significantly increased the risk of overweight/obesity in women. Screening for depression in young adults is necessary. Collaboration between specialists in obesity medicine, dietetics, psychology and psychiatry is needed for the treatment of people with obesity and depression.

Young adulthood is considered a critical life stage for interventions designed to improve health behaviors. We hope that the results of our study may contribute to the development of educational programs and intervention strategies.

Author Contributions: Conceptualization, J.S.; methodology, J.S. and P.B.; formal analysis, J.S. and A.S.; investigation, J.S. and S.Ł.; resources, J.S.; data curation, J.S.; writing—original draft preparation, J.S.; writing—review and editing, J.S., A.S., M.C. and P.B.; visualization, J.S. and S.Ł; supervision, A.S., M.C. and P.B.; project administration, J.S.; funding acquisition, J.S. All authors have read and agreed to the published version of the manuscript.

Funding: This research was funded by the Ministry of Science and Higher Education—DiamondGrant (grant number: 0185/DIA/2018/47).

Institutional Review Board Statement: This study was conducted according to the guidelines of the Declaration of Helsinki and approved by the Bioethics Committee of the Poznan University of Medical Sciences (protocol code 857/18; date of approval: 6 September 2018).

Informed Consent Statement: Informed consent was obtained from all subjects involved in the study.

Data Availability Statement: The data presented in this study are available upon request from the corresponding author.

Conflicts of Interest: The authors declare no conflicts of interest. The funders had no role in the design of the study; in the collection, analyses, or interpretation of the data; in the writing of the manuscript; or in the decision to publish the results.

References

1. World Health Organization. *Healthy Living: What Is a Healthy Lifestyle?* WHO Regional Office for Europe: Copenhagen, Denmark, 1999; pp. 1–24.
2. Velten, J.; Bieda, A.; Scholten, S.; Wannemüller, A.; Margraf, J. Lifestyle choices and mental health: A longitudinal survey with German and Chinese students. *BMC Public Health* **2018**, *18*, 632. [CrossRef] [PubMed]
3. Adams, M.L.; Katz, D.L.; Shenson, D. A healthy lifestyle composite measure: Significance and potential uses. *Prev. Med.* **2016**, *84*, 41–47. [CrossRef] [PubMed]
4. Gochman, D.S. *Handbook of Health Behavior Research II: Provider Determinants*; Springer Science & Business Media: Berlin/Heidelberg, Germany, 2013.
5. Conner, M.; Norman, P. Health behaviour: Current issues and challenges. *Psychol. Health* **2017**, *32*, 895–906. [CrossRef] [PubMed]
6. Lopez, A.D.; Mathers, C.D.; Ezzati, M.; Jamison, D.T.; Murray, C.J. Global and regional burden of disease and risk factors, 2001: Systematic analysis of population health data. *Lancet* **2006**, *367*, 1747–1757. [CrossRef] [PubMed]
7. Loef, M.; Walach, H. The combined effects of healthy lifestyle behaviors on all cause mortality: A systematic review and meta-analysis. *Prev. Med.* **2012**, *55*, 163–170. [CrossRef]
8. Stenlund, S.; Koivumaa-Honkanen, H.; Sillanmäki, L.; Lagström, H.; Rautava, P.; Suominen, S. Changed health behavior improves subjective well-being and vice versa in a follow-up of 9 years. *Health Qual. Life Outcomes* **2022**, *20*, 66. [CrossRef] [PubMed]
9. Keyes, C.L.; Shmotkin, D.; Ryff, C.D. Optimizing well-being: The empirical encounter of two traditions. *J. Pers. Soc. Psychol.* **2002**, *82*, 1007. [CrossRef] [PubMed]
10. Diener, E.; Suh, E.M.; Lucas, R.E.; Smith, H.L. Subjective well-being: Three decades of progress. *Psychol. Bull.* **1999**, *125*, 276–302. [CrossRef]

11. Larsen, R.J.; Eid, M. Ed Diener and the science of subjective well-being. In *The Science of Subjective Well-Being*; Eid, M., Larsen, R.J., Eds.; Guilford Publications: New York, NY, USA, 2008; pp. 1–13.
12. Loth, K.A.; Watts, A.W.; van den Berg, P.; Neumark-Sztainer, D. Does Body Satisfaction Help or Harm Overweight Teens? A 10-Year Longitudinal Study of the Relationship between Body Satisfaction and Body Mass Index. *J. Adolesc. Health* **2015**, *57*, 559–561. [CrossRef]
13. Sonneville, K.R.; Calzo, J.P.; Horton, N.J.; Haines, J.; Austin, S.B.; Field, A.E. Body satisfaction, weight gain and binge eating among overweight adolescent girls. *Int. J. Obes.* **2012**, *36*, 944–949. [CrossRef]
14. SAHM. Young Adult Health and Well-Being: A Position Statement of the Society for Adolescent Health and Medicine. *J. Adolesc. Health* **2017**, *60*, 758–759. [CrossRef] [PubMed]
15. Nelson, M.C.; Story, M.; Larson, N.I.; Neumark-Sztainer, D.; Lytle, L.A. Emerging adulthood and college-aged youth: An overlooked age for weight-related behavior change. *Obesity* **2008**, *16*, 2205–2211. [CrossRef] [PubMed]
16. Bonnie, R.J.; Stroud, C. *Investing in the Health and Well-Being of Young Adults*; National Academies Press: Washington, DC, USA, 2015.
17. Wood, D.; Crapnell, T.; Lau, L.; Bennett, A.; Lotstein, D.; Ferris, M.; Kuo, A. Emerging Adulthood as a Critical Stage in the Life Course. In *Handbook of Life Course Health Development*; Halfon, N., Forrest, C.B., Lerner, R.M., Faustman, E.M., Eds.; Springer International Publishing: Cham, Switzerland, 2018; pp. 123–143.
18. Burns, R.D. Public Health Implications of the Dose-Response Association between Physical Activity and Cardiometabolic Health in Young Adults. *J. Adolesc. Health* **2020**, *67*, 155–156. [CrossRef] [PubMed]
19. Caspersen, C.J.; Pereira, M.A.; Curran, K.M. Changes in physical activity patterns in the United States, by sex and cross-sectional age. *Med. Sci. Sports Exerc.* **2000**, *32*, 1601–1609. [CrossRef] [PubMed]
20. Deforche, B.; Van Dyck, D.; Deliens, T.; De Bourdeaudhuij, I. Changes in weight, physical activity, sedentary behaviour and dietary intake during the transition to higher education: A prospective study. *Int. J. Behav. Nutr. Phys. Act.* **2015**, *12*, 16. [CrossRef] [PubMed]
21. Sharkey, T.; Whatnall, M.C.; Hutchesson, M.J.; Haslam, R.L.; Bezzina, A.; Collins, C.E.; Ashton, L.M. Effectiveness of gender-targeted versus gender-neutral interventions aimed at improving dietary intake, physical activity and/or overweight/obesity in young adults (aged 17–35 years): A systematic review and meta-analysis. *Nutr. J.* **2020**, *19*, 78. [CrossRef] [PubMed]
22. Lau, J.S.; Adams, S.H.; Irwin, C.E.; Ozer, E.M. Receipt of Preventive Health Services in Young Adults. *J. Adolesc. Health* **2013**, *52*, 42–49. [CrossRef] [PubMed]
23. Watson, K.B.; Carlson, S.A.; Loustalot, F.; Town, M.; Eke, P.I.; Thomas, C.W.; Greenlund, K.J. Chronic Conditions among Adults Aged 18–34 Years—United States, 2019. *MMWR Morb. Mortal. Wkly. Rep.* **2022**, *71*, 964–970. [CrossRef] [PubMed]
24. Quick, V.M.; Byrd-Bredbenner, C. Disordered eating, socio-cultural media influencers, body image, and psychological factors among a racially/ethnically diverse population of college women. *Eat. Behav.* **2014**, *15*, 37–41. [CrossRef]
25. Lanoye, A.; Brown, K.L.; LaRose, J.G. The Transition into Young Adulthood: A Critical Period for Weight Control. *Curr. Diab. Rep.* **2017**, *17*, 114. [CrossRef]
26. Kessler, R.C.; Amminger, G.P.; Aguilar-Gaxiola, S.; Alonso, J.; Lee, S.; Ustun, T.B. Age of onset of mental disorders: A review of recent literature. *Curr. Opin. Psychiatry* **2007**, *20*, 359. [CrossRef] [PubMed]
27. Wynaden, D.; Wichmann, H.; Murray, S. A synopsis of the mental health concerns of university students: Results of a text-based online survey from one Australian university. *HERD* **2013**, *32*, 846–860. [CrossRef]
28. Thorley, C. *Not by Degrees: Improving Student Mental Health in the UK's Universities*; IPPR: London, UK, 2017.
29. Henning, E.R.; Turk, C.L.; Mennin, D.S.; Fresco, D.M.; Heimberg, R.G. Impairment and quality of life in individuals with generalized anxiety disorder. *Depress. Anxiety* **2007**, *24*, 342–349. [CrossRef]
30. Daig, I.; Herschbach, P.; Lehmann, A.; Knoll, N.; Decker, O. Gender and age differences in domain-specific life satisfaction and the impact of depressive and anxiety symptoms: A general population survey from Germany. *Qual. Life Res.* **2009**, *18*, 669–678. [CrossRef] [PubMed]
31. Steptoe, A.; Wardle, J.; Cui, W.; Bellisle, F.; Zotti, A.M.; Baranyai, R.; Sanderman, R. Trends in smoking, diet, physical exercise, and attitudes toward health in European university students from 13 countries, 1990–2000. *Prev. Med.* **2002**, *35*, 97–104. [CrossRef] [PubMed]
32. CDC. Centres for Disease Control and Prevention. In *About Adult BMI*. Available online: https://www.cdc.gov/healthyweight/ssessing/bmi/adult_bmi/index.html (accessed on 17 December 2023).
33. Beck, A.T. An Inventory for Measuring Depression. *Arch. Gen. Psychiatry* **1961**, *4*, 561. [CrossRef]
34. Beck, A.T.; Steer, R.A.; Carbin, M.G. Psychometric properties of the Beck Depression Inventory: Twenty-five years of evaluation. *Clin. Psychol. Rev.* **1988**, *8*, 77–100. [CrossRef]
35. Lidia Wądołowska Website. Available online: www.uwm.edu.pl/edu/lidiawadolowska (accessed on 15 December 2023).
36. Niedzwiedzka, E.; Wadolowska, L.; Kowalkowska, J. Reproducibility of A Non-Quantitative Food Frequency Questionnaire (62-Item FFQ-6) and PCA-Driven Dietary Pattern Identification in 13–21-Year-Old Females. *Nutrients* **2019**, *11*, 2183. [CrossRef] [PubMed]
37. Biernat, E.; Stupnicki, R.; Lebiedziński, B.; Janczewska, L. Assessment of physical activity by applying IPAQ questionnaire. *Phys. Educ. Sport* **2008**, *52*, 46–52. [CrossRef]

38. Karlsson, J.; Persson, L.O.; Sjöström, L.; Sullivan, M. Psychometric properties and factor structure of the Three-Factor Eating Questionnaire (TFEQ) in obese men and women. Results from the Swedish Obese Subjects (SOS) study. *Int. J. Obes. Relat. Metab. Disord.* **2000**, *24*, 1715–1725. [CrossRef]
39. Brytek-Matera, A.; Rogoza, R.; Czepczor-Bernat, K. The Three-Factor Eating Questionnaire-R18 Polish version: Factor structure analysis among normal weight and obese adult women. *Arch. Psychiatry Psychother.* **2017**, *19*, 81–90. [CrossRef]
40. de Lauzon, B.; Romon, M.; Deschamps, V.; Lafay, L.; Borys, J.M.; Karlsson, J.; Ducimetière, P.; Charles, M.A. The Three-Factor Eating Questionnaire-R18 is able to distinguish among different eating patterns in a general population. *J. Nutr.* **2004**, *134*, 2372–2380. [CrossRef] [PubMed]
41. Pengpid, S.; Peltzer, K. Sedentary Behaviour, Physical Activity and Life Satisfaction, Happiness and Perceived Health Status in University Students from 24 Countries. *Int. J. Environ. Res. Public Health* **2019**, *16*, 2084. [CrossRef] [PubMed]
42. Grant, N.; Wardle, J.; Steptoe, A. The relationship between life satisfaction and health behavior: A cross-cultural analysis of young adults. *Int. J. Behav. Med.* **2009**, *16*, 259–268. [CrossRef] [PubMed]
43. Afshin, A.; Forouzanfar, M.H.; Reitsma, M.B.; Sur, P.; Estep, K.; Lee, A.; Marczak, L. Health Effects of Overweight and Obesity in 195 Countries over 25 Years. *N. Engl. J. Med.* **2017**, *377*, 13–27. [CrossRef] [PubMed]
44. Katsoulis, M.; Lai, A.G.; Diaz-Ordaz, K.; Gomes, M.; Pasea, L.; Banerjee, A.; Denaxas, S.; Tsilidis, K.; Lagiou, P.; Misirli, G.; et al. Identifying adults at high-risk for change in weight and BMI in England: A longitudinal, large-scale, population-based cohort study using electronic health records. *Lancet Diabetes Endocrinol.* **2021**, *9*, 681–694. [CrossRef]
45. American College Health Association (ACHA); National College Health Assessment II (NCHA II). *Reference Group Executive Summary Spring 2019*; American College Health Association (ACHA): Silver Spring, MD, USA, 2020.
46. de Waure, C.; Soffiani, V.; Virdis, A.; Poscia, A.; Di Pietro, M.L. Italian university students' self-perceived health and satisfaction of life. *Ann. Ist. Super Sanita* **2015**, *51*, 121–125. [CrossRef]
47. El Ansari, W.; Stock, C.; Phillips, C.; Mabhala, A.; Stoate, M.; Adetunji, H.; Deeny, P.; John, J.; Davies, S.; Parke, S.; et al. Does the association between depressive symptomatology and physical activity depend on body image perception? A survey of students from seven universities in the UK. *Int. J. Environ. Res. Public Health* **2011**, *8*, 281–299. [CrossRef] [PubMed]
48. Cabiedes-Miragaya, L.; Diaz-Mendez, C.; García-Espejo, I. Well-Being and the Lifestyle Habits of the Spanish Population: The Association between Subjective Well-Being and Eating Habits. *Int. J. Environ. Res. Public Health* **2021**, *18*, 1553. [CrossRef]
49. Zweig, J.S. Are women happier than men? Evidence from the Gallup World Poll. *J. Happiness Stud.* **2015**, *16*, 515–541. [CrossRef]
50. Godoy-Izquierdo, D.; González-Hernández, J.; Rodríguez-Tadeo, A.; Lara, R.; Ogallar, A.; Navarrón, E.; Ramírez, M.J.; López-Mora, C.; Arbinaga, F. Body Satisfaction, Weight Stigma, Positivity, and Happiness among Spanish Adults with Overweight and Obesity. *Int. J. Environ. Res. Public Health* **2020**, *17*, 4186. [CrossRef]
51. Prémusz, V.; Makai, A.; Ács, P.; Derkács, E.; Laczkó, T. Association of Outdoor Physical Activity and Sports with Life Satisfaction among Women of Reproductive Age According to a European Representative Sample—A Longitudinal Analysis. *Eur. J. Investig. Health Psychol. Educ.* **2023**, *13*, 1859–1879. [CrossRef] [PubMed]
52. He, Z.; Cheng, Z.; Bishwajit, G.; Zou, D. Wealth Inequality as a Predictor of Subjective Health, Happiness and Life Satisfaction among Nepalese Women. *Int. J. Environ. Res. Public Health* **2018**, *15*, 2836. [CrossRef] [PubMed]
53. Lappan, S.; Thorne, C.B.; Long, D.; Hendricks, P.S. Longitudinal and Reciprocal Relationships between Psychological Well-Being and Smoking. *Nicotine Tob. Res.* **2020**, *22*, 18–23. [CrossRef] [PubMed]
54. World Health Organization. *Global Action Plan on Physical Activity 2018–2030: More Active People for a Healthier World*; World Health Organization: Geneva, Switzerland, 2018.
55. Guthold, R.; Stevens, G.A.; Riley, L.M.; Bull, F.C. Worldwide trends in insufficient physical activity from 2001 to 2016: A pooled analysis of 358 population-based surveys with 1.9 million participants. *Lancet Glob. Health* **2018**, *6*, e1077–e1086. [CrossRef] [PubMed]
56. Althoff, T.; Sosič, R.; Hicks, J.L.; King, A.C.; Delp, S.L.; Leskovec, J. Large-scale physical activity data reveal worldwide activity inequality. *Nature* **2017**, *547*, 336–339. [CrossRef] [PubMed]
57. Mielke, G.I.; da Silva, I.C.M.; Kolbe-Alexander, T.L.; Brown, W.J. Shifting the Physical Inactivity Curve Worldwide by Closing the Gender Gap. *Sports Med.* **2018**, *48*, 481–489. [CrossRef] [PubMed]
58. World Health Organization, Regional Office for the Eastern Mediterranean. *Promoting Physical Activity in the Eastern Mediterranean Region through a Life-Course Approach*; World Health Organization: Geneva, Switzerland, 2014.
59. Murphy, M.H.; Carlin, A.; Woods, C.; Nevill, A.; MacDonncha, C.; Ferguson, K.; Murphy, N. Active Students Are Healthier and Happier Than Their Inactive Peers: The Results of a Large Representative Cross-Sectional Study of University Students in Ireland. *J. Phys. Act. Health* **2018**, *15*, 737–746. [CrossRef]
60. Streeter, V.M.; Milhausen, R.R.; Buchholz, A.C. Body Image, Body Mass Index, and Body Composition: In Young Adults. *Can. J. Diet. Pract. Res.* **2012**, *73*, 78–83. [CrossRef]
61. Silva, W.R.D.; Campos, J.; Marôco, J. Impact of inherent aspects of body image, eating behavior and perceived health competence on quality of life of university students. *PLoS ONE* **2018**, *13*, e0199480. [CrossRef]
62. Weinberger, N.A.; Kersting, A.; Riedel-Heller, S.G.; Luck-Sikorski, C. Body Dissatisfaction in Individuals with Obesity Compared to Normal-Weight Individuals: A Systematic Review and Meta-Analysis. *Obes. Facts* **2016**, *9*, 424–441. [CrossRef] [PubMed]
63. Puhl, R.M.; Heuer, C.A. The stigma of obesity: A review and update. *Obesity* **2009**, *17*, 941–964. [CrossRef] [PubMed]

64. Kiefer, I.; Rathmanner, T.; Kunze, M. Eating and dieting differences in men and women. *J. Men's Health Gend.* **2005**, *2*, 194–201. [CrossRef]
65. Wardle, J.; Haase, A.M.; Steptoe, A.; Nillapun, M.; Jonwutiwes, K.; Bellisle, F. Gender differences in food choice: The contribution of health beliefs and dieting. *Ann. Behav. Med.* **2004**, *27*, 107–116. [CrossRef]
66. Wicki, M.; Kuntsche, E.; Gmel, G. Drinking at European universities? A review of students' alcohol use. *Addict. Behav.* **2010**, *35*, 913–924. [CrossRef] [PubMed]
67. Kriaučionienė, V.; Grincaitė, M.; Raskilienė, A.; Petkevičienė, J. Changes in Nutrition, Physical Activity, and Body Weight among Lithuanian Students during and after the COVID-19 Pandemic. *Nutrients* **2023**, *15*, 4091. [CrossRef]
68. Malik, V.S.; Hu, F.B. The role of sugar-sweetened beverages in the global epidemics of obesity and chronic diseases. *Nat. Rev. Endocrinol.* **2022**, *18*, 205–218. [CrossRef]
69. Rouhani, M.H.; Salehi-Abargouei, A.; Surkan, P.J.; Azadbakht, L. Is there a relationship between red or processed meat intake and obesity? A systematic review and meta-analysis of observational studies. *Obes. Rev.* **2014**, *15*, 740–748. [CrossRef]
70. Gaesser, G.A. Perspective: Refined Grains and Health: Genuine Risk, or Guilt by Association? *Adv. Nutr.* **2019**, *10*, 361–371. [CrossRef]
71. Ma, X.; Chen, Q.; Pu, Y.; Guo, M.; Jiang, Z.; Huang, W.; Long, Y.; Xu, Y. Skipping breakfast is associated with overweight and obesity: A systematic review and meta-analysis. *Obes. Res. Clin. Pract.* **2020**, *14*, 1–8. [CrossRef]
72. Lipson, S.K.; Zhou, S.; Abelson, S.; Heinze, J.; Jirsa, M.; Morigney, J.; Patterson, A.; Singh, M.; Eisenberg, D. Trends in college student mental health and help-seeking by race/ethnicity: Findings from the national healthy minds study, 2013–2021. *J. Affect. Disord.* **2022**, *306*, 138–147. [CrossRef] [PubMed]
73. Mokdad, A.H.; Forouzanfar, M.H.; Daoud, F.; Mokdad, A.A.; El Bcheraoui, C.; Moradi-Lakeh, M.; Kyu, H.H.; Barber, R.M.; Wagner, J.; Cercy, K.; et al. Global burden of diseases, injuries, and risk factors for young people's health during 1990-2013: A systematic analysis for the Global Burden of Disease Study 2013. *Lancet* **2016**, *387*, 2383–2401. [CrossRef] [PubMed]
74. Fergusson, D.M.; McLeod, G.; Horwood, L.J.; Swain, N.R.; Chapple, S.; Poulton, R. Life satisfaction and mental health problems (18 to 35 years). *Psychol. Med.* **2015**, *45*, 2427–2436. [CrossRef] [PubMed]
75. Konttinen, H.; Van Strien, T.; Männistö, S.; Jousilahti, P.; Haukkala, A. Depression, emotional eating and long-term weight changes: A population-based prospective study. *Int. J. Behav. Nutr. Phys. Act.* **2019**, *16*, 1–11. [CrossRef] [PubMed]
76. Luppino, F.S.; Wit, L.M.; Bouvy, P.F. Overweight, obesity, and depression: A systematic review and meta-analysis of longitudinal studies. *Arch. Gen. Psychiatry* **2010**, *67*, 220–229. [CrossRef] [PubMed]
77. Olszanecka-Glinianowicz, M.; Mazur, A.; Chudek, J.; Kos-Kudła, B.; Markuszewski, L.; Dudek, D.; Major, P.; Małczak, P.; Tarnowski, W.; Jaworski, P.; et al. Obesity in Adults: Position Statement of Polish Association for the Study on Obesity, Polish Association of Endocrinology, Polish Association of Cardiodiabetology, Polish Psychiatric Association, Section of Metabolic and Bariatric Surgery of the Association of Polish Surgeons, and the College of Family Physicians in Poland. *Nutrients* **2023**, *15*, 1641. [CrossRef]
78. Chaker, L.; Bianco, A.C.; Jonklaas, J.; Peeters, R.P. Hypothyroidism. *Lancet* **2017**, *390*, 1550–1562. [CrossRef] [PubMed]
79. Pasquali, R.; Casanueva, F.; Haluzik, M.; van Hulsteijn, L.; Ledoux, S.; Monteiro, M.P.; Salvador, J.; Santini, F.; Toplak, H.; Dekkers, O.M. European Society of Endocrinology Clinical Practice Guideline: Endocrine work-up in obesity. *Eur. J. Endocrinol.* **2020**, *182*, G1–G32. [CrossRef] [PubMed]
80. Michalaki, M.A.; Vagenakis, A.G.; Leonardou, A.S.; Argentou, M.N.; Habeos, I.G.; Makri, M.G.; Psyrogiannis, A.I.; Kalfarentzos, F.E.; Kyriazopoulou, V.E. Thyroid function in humans with morbid obesity. *Thyroid* **2006**, *16*, 73–78. [CrossRef]
81. Soriguer, F.; Valdes, S.; Morcillo, S.; Esteva, I.; Almaraz, M.C.; de Adana, M.S.R.; Tapia, M.J.; Dominguez, M.; Gutierrez-Repiso, C.; Rubio-Martin, E.; et al. Thyroid hormone levels predict the change in body weight: A prospective study. *Eur. J. Clin. Investig.* **2011**, *41*, 1202–1209. [CrossRef]
82. Henning, C.; Schroeder, S.; Steins-Loeber, S.; Wolstein, J. Gender and Emotional Representation Matter: Own Illness Beliefs and Their Relationship to Obesity. *Front. Nutr.* **2022**, *9*, 799831. [CrossRef] [PubMed]
83. Lluch, A.; Herbeth, B.; Méjean, L.; Siest, G. Dietary intakes, eating style and overweight in the Stanislas Family Study. *Int. J. Obes. Relat. Metab. Disord.* **2000**, *24*, 1493–1499. [CrossRef] [PubMed]
84. van Strien, T.; Konttinen, H.; Homberg, J.; Engels, R.; Winkens, L. Emotional eating as a mediator between depression and weight gain. *Appetite* **2016**, *100*, 216–224. [CrossRef] [PubMed]
85. Anglé, S.; Engblom, J.; Eriksson, T.; Kautiainen, S.; Saha, M.T.; Lindfors, P.; Lehtinen, M.; Rimpelä, A. Three factor eating questionnaire-R18 as a measure of cognitive restraint, uncontrolled eating and emotional eating in a sample of young Finnish females. *Int. J. Behav. Nutr. Phys. Act.* **2009**, *6*, 41. [CrossRef] [PubMed]
86. Elfhag, K.; Linné, Y. Gender differences in associations of eating pathology between mothers and their adolescent offspring. *Obes. Res.* **2005**, *13*, 1070–1076. [CrossRef] [PubMed]
87. Guerrini-Usubini, A.; Cattivelli, R.; Scarpa, A.; Musetti, A.; Varallo, G.; Franceschini, C.; Castelnuovo, G. The interplay between emotion dysregulation, psychological distress, emotional eating, and weight status: A path model. *Int. J. Clin. Health Psychol.* **2023**, *23*, 100338. [CrossRef] [PubMed]
88. Lazarevich, I.; Irigoyen Camacho, M.E.; Velázquez-Alva, M.D.C.; Zepeda Zepeda, M. Relationship among obesity, depression, and emotional eating in young adults. *Appetite* **2016**, *107*, 639–644. [CrossRef] [PubMed]

89. Jáuregui-Lobera, I.; García-Cruz, P.; Carbonero-Carreño, R.; Magallares, A.; Ruiz-Prieto, I. Psychometric properties of Spanish version of the Three-Factor Eating Questionnaire-R18 (Tfeq-Sp) and its relationship with some eating- and body image-related variables. *Nutrients* **2014**, *6*, 5619–5635. [CrossRef] [PubMed]
90. de Lauzon-Guillain, B.; Basdevant, A.; Romon, M.; Karlsson, J.; Borys, J.M.; Charles, M.A. Is restrained eating a risk factor for weight gain in a general population? *Am. J. Clin. Nutr.* **2006**, *83*, 132–138. [CrossRef]
91. Suwalska, J.; Kolasińska, K.; Łojko, D.; Bogdański, P. Eating Behaviors, Depressive Symptoms and Lifestyle in University Students in Poland. *Nutrients* **2022**, *14*, 1106. [CrossRef]
92. Konttinen, H. Emotional eating and obesity in adults: The role of depression, sleep and genes. *Proc. Nutr. Soc.* **2020**, *79*, 283–289. [CrossRef] [PubMed]
93. Headey, B.; Muffels, R.; Wagner, G.G. Choices Which Change Life Satisfaction: Similar Results for Australia, Britain and Germany. *Soc. Indic. Res.* **2013**, *112*, 725–748. [CrossRef]

nutrients

MDPI

Communication

The Paradox of Alcohol and Food Affordability: Minimal Impact of Leading Beer and Cachaça Brands on Brazilian Household Income Amid Hazardous Drinking Patterns

Ian C. C. Nóbrega [1,*], Rhennan V. L. Marques [1], Matheus A. Ferreira [1] and Dirk W. Lachenmeier [2,*]

1 Department of Food Engineering, Universidade Federal da Paraíba (UFPB), João Pessoa 58051-900, Paraíba, Brazil; rhennan.victor@gmail.com (R.V.L.M.); mas22702@gmail.com (M.A.F.)

2 Chemisches und Veterinäruntersuchungsamt (CVUA) Karlsruhe, Weissenburger Strasse 3, 76187 Karlsruhe, Germany

* Correspondence: ian.nobrega@academico.ufpb.br (I.C.C.N.); lachenmeier@web.de (D.W.L.)

Abstract: Alcohol consumption, associated with various cancers, mental disorders, and aggressive behavior, leads to three million deaths globally each year. In Brazil, the alcohol per capita consumption among drinkers aged 15 and over is 41.7 g of pure alcohol/day (~1 L beer/day), which falls into the risky consumption category and exceeds the global average by almost 30%. An effective way to mitigate alcohol-related harm is to increase its retail price. This study assesses the costs of consuming leading brands of beer and sugarcane spirit cachaça (Brazil's most popular alcoholic beverages) against the expenditure on staple foods. Data on food and alcoholic beverage prices were collected in João Pessoa, Brazil, for 2020 and 2021. The cost per gram of pure alcohol and food were considered to establish consumption patterns of 16.8 g/day (moderate), 41.7 g/day, and 83.4 g/day (heavy), distributed in three scenarios involving the beverages alone or combined (64% beer and 36% cachaça), and a balanced 2000 kcal/day staple diet. The study finds that all heavy consumption scenarios cost less or significantly less (cachaça alone) than a 2000 kcal/day staple diet, highlighting an urgent need for fiscal policies, such as a minimum unit pricing for alcohol, to address public health concerns.

Keywords: alcohol consumption; household income; beer; dietary expenditure; Brazil; minimum unit pricing; alcohol pricing; risky drinking patterns

1. Introduction

Globally, alcohol consumption presents a significant public health challenge, with nearly half of the population aged 15 and over having never consumed alcohol, and approximately 43% identified as current drinkers. The World Health Organization (WHO) reported an average annual per capita consumption of 6.4 L of pure alcohol worldwide in 2016, a figure that significantly increases to 15.1 L when considering only those who drink [1]. A substantial portion of this consumption, up to 25.5% globally, involves unrecorded alcohol, which poses additional risks due to a lack of quality control and potential for higher alcohol content [1,2]. The WHO aims to reduce alcohol consumption by 10% by 2025, emphasizing the need for tailored national policies to address this issue.

In Brazil, alcohol consumption rates exceed the global average, with the drinking population consuming an average of 19.3 L of pure alcohol per year. This consumption pattern is predominantly driven by beer (62%), followed by spirits (34%), and wine (3%), reflecting a preference that aligns with the broader Region of the Americas [1]. The First National Survey on Alcohol Consumption Patterns in the Brazilian Population reveals that over half of Brazilians aged 18 and older consume alcohol, with significant disparities between genders and drinking frequency. The south of Brazil shows higher rates of regular drinking, contrasting with the northeast, where half of the population abstains [3].

The impact of alcohol consumption extends beyond individual health, contributing to significant morbidity and mortality worldwide [4]. In 2016, alcohol-related harm resulted in approximately three million deaths globally, surpassing deaths caused by diseases such as tuberculosis, HIV/AIDS, and diabetes. The health consequences of alcohol consumption include toxic effects on organs, alcohol dependence, and the immediate psychoactive effects of intoxication. In Brazil, alcohol consumption was responsible for a considerable number of deaths from liver cirrhosis, traffic accidents, and cancer in 2016, highlighting the urgent need for effective interventions to mitigate these harms [1].

Alcohol policies may encompass a broad spectrum of regulations that address the relationship between alcohol consumption and its implications for safety, health, and social welfare [5]. These policies extend from the production processes over the pricing strategies and availability of alcoholic beverages to bans or comprehensive restrictions on alcohol advertising.

In the context of Brazil, the enactment and implementation of alcohol policies have encountered considerable delays and exhibit substantial shortcomings. Despite the introduction of the first restrictions on hazardous substances in the Republican Code of 1890, it was not until the early 21st century that Brazil formulated and enacted concrete alcohol policies. An important moment in this trajectory was in 2005, during Brazil's hosting of the 1st Pan-American Conference on Public Policies on Alcohol, supported by the Pan-American Health Organization. This conference catalyzed the development of intercontinental policies aimed at mitigating the adverse effects associated with alcohol consumption. It advocated for the nations in the Americas to devise strategies and programs dedicated to curtailing and preventing the harms of excessive alcohol use [6].

Following this critical juncture, the Brazilian government, in 2007, issued Decree No. 6.117 [7], sanctioning the National Alcohol Policy. This decree delineates a comprehensive strategy aimed at diminishing the misuse of alcohol and its correlation with violence and crime, alongside introducing other related measures. It embodies a concerted effort to mitigate health and life risks associated with alcohol use.

Internationally, various strategies have been deployed by governments to manage alcohol-related issues, with the regulation of pricing and taxation on alcoholic beverages being the predominant approach [8]. In this vein, Scotland's implementation of the Minimum Unit Pricing (MUP) in 2018 stands as a significant exemplar. The MUP policy, predicated on setting a minimum price per unit of alcohol (10 mL or 8 g of pure alcohol) for retail sales, encompasses a holistic suite of policy measures and legislative initiatives aimed at reducing alcohol consumption across the population and thereby diminishing the consequent health and social detriments [9].

An investigation conducted by O'Donnel et al. [10] into the immediate repercussions of the MUP policy unveiled that the initiative successfully achieved its objectives. Notably, the most significant reductions in consumption were observed among high-alcohol-content beverages, which experienced a relative price increase compared to lower-alcohol-content alternatives. This outcome underscores the efficacy of MUP in steering consumption patterns towards safer levels, highlighting the potential of targeted policy interventions in addressing public health concerns related to alcohol consumption.

In summary, the most promising strategies for reducing alcohol-related death and damage include increasing the retail price of alcoholic beverages. Implementing such a policy in Brazil necessitates a comprehensive understanding of alcohol pricing and its impact on the nation's average per capita income. This study aims to evaluate the effects of home consumption scenarios of beer and cachaça, the country's two most popular alcoholic drinks, on national per capita household income. The assessment will reference the per capita expenditure on a staple balanced diet of 2000 kcal/day, providing critical insights into the economic implications of alcohol consumption patterns within Brazil.

2. Materials and Methods

2.1. Defining Levels of Alcohol Consumption

To accurately assess the impact of alcohol consumption on health outcomes, it is essential to delineate specific levels of consumption that reflect realistic quantities of alcohol intake. Following the classification system proposed by Rumgay et al. [11], alcohol consumption was categorized into three distinct levels: moderate consumption (<20 g pure ethanol/day), risky consumption (20 to 60 g/day), and heavy consumption (>60 g/day). These categorizations facilitate a nuanced analysis of alcohol's effects across different consumption patterns.

For the purpose of this study, precise levels within these categories were established to align with the specific context of alcohol consumption in Brazil. Moderate consumption was set at 16.8 g/day, mirroring the per capita consumption of the Brazilian population over the age of 15 in 2016, as reported by the WHO [1]. Risky consumption was defined at 41.7 g/day, corresponding to the per capita consumption among Brazilian men and women over 15 who consume alcohol. Heavy consumption was determined at 83.4 g/day, a figure derived by doubling the per capita consumption indicative of risky consumption (Table 1). The selection of these specific levels was informed by the WHO's guidelines, which acknowledge that no level of alcohol consumption is entirely devoid of health risks [12]. The chosen levels for moderate and risky drinking were based on Brazil's alcohol per capita consumption (APC) for 2016, adjusted from liters of pure alcohol per year to grams of pure alcohol per day using a standardized formula. The heavy drinking threshold was similarly calculated, emphasizing the study's alignment with recognized standards and the relevance of these levels to Brazil's drinking patterns in 2016 [1].

Table 1. Categories of alcohol per capita consumption (APC) by range (in grams of pure alcohol per day) [1], APC levels considered in the study, and their relevance to Brazil.

Categories (Range) [2]	Considered Level of APC	Relevance of the APC to Brazil [5]
Moderate drinking (<20 g per day)	16.8 g per day [3]	General population (15+) consumption, 2016
Risky drinking (20–60 g per day)	41.7 g per day [3]	Drinkers only (15+) consumption, 2016
Heavy drinking (>60 g per day)	83.4 g per day [4]	-

[1] Although categories of the APC by range are accepted as references for assessing consumption patterns of populations and individuals, current WHO guidelines state that there is no safe level of alcohol consumption that does not affect human health [12]. [2] Categories, by range of grams of pure alcohol consumption per day, according to Rumgay et al. [11]. [3] The levels for moderate and risky drinking (in g of pure alcohol per day) were chosen because they coincide with the APC (15+, both sexes) in Brazil in 2016 [1], namely 7.8 L of pure alcohol per year (general population) and 19.3 L of pure alcohol per year (drinkers-only population); the APC in 2016 was converted from liters of pure alcohol/year to g of pure alcohol/day using the following formula: (APC in liters of pure alcohol per year × 1000 × 0.79)/366 days. [4] The APC considered for heavy drinking was obtained multiplying the APC for risky consumption by 2. [5] Relevance of chosen levels considering WHO GISAH data from Brazil in 2016 [1].

2.2. Selection of Beverage Brands

The study considered the distribution of alcohol consumption by beverage type, based on publicly available WHO data from 2016 [1], with beer and cachaça identified as the primary alcoholic beverages consumed in Brazil. This distribution informed the selection of low-price leading national beer and cachaça brands for surveying in 2020 and 2021, based on data from the Brazilian Association of Supermarkets (ABRAS) [13].

The top-selling beer and cachaça brands in 2019, as identified by ABRAS [13], were selected for inclusion in the study. This selection aimed to reflect the most widely consumed and accessible brands in Brazil, facilitating a realistic assessment of alcohol purchase and consumption patterns. The number of beer and cachaça samples corresponded to the availability of selected brands in visited supermarkets/grocery stores, ensuring a representative collection of data on popular alcoholic beverages. Regular prices for the selected beer and cachaça brands were collected from local supermarkets or grocery stores, excluding promotional or limited-time discount offers to maintain consistency in price analysis.

The average price per gram of pure alcohol was determined by dividing the average product price (in Brazilian reals, BRL) by the mass of ethanol in the beverage, using the density of ethanol (0.79 g/mL) as a conversion factor. This calculation provides a basis for comparing the cost-effectiveness of different alcoholic beverages in relation to their alcohol content, offering insights into consumption preferences based on price and alcohol content.

2.3. *Choice of Alcoholic Beverages and Definition of Consumption Scenarios*

To accurately assess the expenditure on alcohol at the defined daily consumption levels, the selection of alcoholic beverages for price investigation in the retail market was guided by prevalent consumption patterns in Brazil. Utilizing the WHO's 2018 distribution data on per capita alcohol consumption in Brazil for individuals over 15 years old, the following beverage types were identified: beer (61.8%), spirits (34.3%), wine (3.4%), and other alcoholic beverages (0.5%) (Table 2). Given the lack of specificity in the WHO (2018) report regarding the types of spirits consumed, further refinement was necessary for this study.

Table 2. Scenarios of alcohol per capita consumption (15+, both sexes) in Brazil for moderate (16.8 g pure alcohol per day), risky (41.7 g pure alcohol per day), and heavy (83.4 g pure alcohol per day) drinking, considering the consumption of beer only, cachaça only, or a combination of the two beverages (64% beer + 36% cachaça).

Type of Alcoholic Beverage	Category of Alcohol Consumption	Consumption in g of Pure Alcohol/Day [1]	Consumption in mL of Beverage/Week [2]
Beer only	Moderate	16.8	3167.2
	Risky	41.7	7861.6
	Heavy	83.4	15,723.1
Cachaça only	Moderate	16.8	376.9
	Risky	41.7	935.4
	Heavy	83.4	1870.9
Combination of beverages (64% + 36%) [3]	Moderate	10.8 + 6.0	2036.1 + 134.6
	Risky	26.7 + 15.0	5033.7 + 336.5
	Heavy	53.4 + 30.0	10,067.3 + 673.0

[1] Values were obtained according to Table 1. [2] The corresponding volume (mL) of the beverages (beer or cachaça) was calculated as follows: [(consumption in g of pure alcohol per day)/0.79] × (1/alcohol content of each beverage in % vol) × 7. The alcohol contents of beer and cachaça used were 4.7% and 39.5%, respectively, because they correspond to the average alcohol contents displayed on labels of beers and cachaças selected for the present study. The density of alcohol is 0.79 g/mL. [3] Recorded alcohol per capita consumption (15+; in liters of pure alcohol) values by type of alcoholic beverage in 2016 according to WHO GISAH [1] were the following: 61.8% beer, 34.3% spirits, 3.4% wine, and 0.5% other beverages. Distribution in the spirits category is not provided by WHO GISAH [1], but according to a large Brazilian survey [3], cachaça is by far the most consumed spirit in Brazil. The rationale behind the combined consumption of beer and cachaça considered, first, cachaça as the only spirit consumed in the WHO GISAH spirit category; then, the consumptions of wine and other beverages (3.9%) were distributed equally to beer (61.8%) and spirits (34.3%), resulting in the 64% beer + 36% cachaça scenario.

The research by Laranjeira et al. [3], which examines alcohol consumption patterns within the Brazilian population, indicated cachaça as the predominant spirit, accounting for approximately 42% of spirit consumption. Vodka followed with an 18% consumption rate. Based on these insights, and to streamline the research process, this study focused exclusively on the price analysis of selected brands of cachaça and beer. This decision reflects both the prominence of these beverages in the Brazilian market and their relevance to the study's objectives of determining alcohol expenditure at specified consumption levels.

The choice to limit the study to these two types of beverages is aimed at ensuring both the manageability of the research process and the relevance of the findings to the broader context of alcohol consumption in Brazil. This approach facilitates a focused examination of spending behaviors associated with the most popular alcoholic beverages, thereby enabling the derivation of insights that are both meaningful and actionable within the context of Brazilian alcohol consumption trends.

2.4. Choosing Food and Defining a Daily Diet

The selection of food staples and the definition of a 2000 kcal/day diet for this study were planned to reflect the dietary habits prevalent in Brazil as a whole; for this purpose, aspects of Brazilian dietary patterns and healthy meal options, as described by the dietary guidelines for the Brazilian population [14], were considered (Table 3). This entailed surveying local supermarkets/grocery stores to identify the reference weight (kg) or volume (mL) for the sale of essential food items, alongside determining their corresponding values for edible conversion factors (ECFs), cooking conversion factors (CCFs), and total conversion factor (TCF). Additionally, the energy content (kcal per 100 g or 100 mL) and selected nutrient content (g or mg per 100 g or 100 mL) of these foods in their usual form of consumption were assessed based on the Brazilian Food Composition Table [15].

Table 3. Levels and recommendations of selected dietary components for adults (both sexes) used as references in the preparation of a balanced/adequate diet from surveyed food staples.

Component	Level/Recommendation	Source
Energy	2000 kcal/day	Health Regulatory Agency, Brazil [16]
Carbohydrates (sugars and starches)	45–65% energy	Institute of Medicine, USA [17]
Free sugars	<10% energy	Institute of Medicine [17] and WHO [18]
Protein	10–35% energy	Institute of Medicine, USA [17]
Total fat	<30% energy	WHO [18]
Saturated fat	<10% energy	WHO [18]
Trans fat	<1% energy	WHO [18]
Sodium	<2000 mg/day	WHO [18]
Fruits and vegetables [1]	≥400 g/day	WHO [18]
Fiber	≥25 g/day	Health Regulatory Agency, Brazil [16]
Natural or minimally processed foods	Basis of diet	Dietary Guidelines, Brazil [14]
Processed foods	Limit	Dietary Guidelines, Brazil [14]
Ultra-processed foods	Avoid	Dietary Guidelines, Brazil [14]

[1] Excluding potatoes and starchy roots, according to World Health Organization [18].

The basic food staples surveyed included whole/fresh banana, rice, beans, tomato, beef chuck, and other staples integral to the Brazilian diet. The average weights for these items were sourced from various studies and reports, such as Almeida et al. [19] for pineapple and CEAGESP [20] for lettuce (see also the details in Appendix A, Table A1).

The usual form of food consumption was aligned with known dietary habits in Brazil, incorporating preparation methods that are commonplace in Brazilian cuisine, such as steaming for corn couscous and sautéing for white rice. Serving sizes for each food item, such as soybean oil, fluid milk, raw banana, and cooked rice, were determined based on estimations from authoritative sources like ANVISA and the Ministry of Health [16,21].

ECFs, CCFs, and TCF for the surveyed food commodities were calculated to convert the weight or volume of food as sold into its edible form post-preparation. For instance, the TCF calculation for raw beef chuck eye steak involved dividing the CCF by the ECF, providing a quantifiable measure of the food in its final form of consumption. The calorie and nutrient content of each food item, including trace levels, were sourced from TBCA [15], ensuring the accurate representation of their nutritional value in the typical Brazilian diet. Levels and recommendations for selected dietary components for adults were referenced from various health guidelines, including the Agência Nacional de Vigilância Sanitária (ANVISA) and the World Health Organization (WHO) [16,18]. These references guided the formulation of a balanced and adequate diet from the surveyed food staples, adhering to the latest dietary guidelines and nutrient requirements.

2.5. Place and Period of Price Collection for Alcoholic Beverages and Foodstuffs

The data collection for the prices of alcoholic beverages and foodstuffs was conducted in João Pessoa, the capital city of the northeastern state of Paraíba, Brazil. This region, with a population of approximately 800,000, served as the focal area for this study. The period designated for price collection spanned two phases: between August and September of both 2020 and 2021, allowing for an assessment of price variations over time within the context of the COVID-19 pandemic.

To ensure a comprehensive and representative dataset, the selection process for supermarkets and grocery stores was comprehensively planned. Initial research was conducted through internet searches, supplemented by site visits, to identify potential establishments for data collection. These establishments were located within a circular geographic area with a radius of 15 km, centered around the Universidade Federal da Paraíba (UFPB), encompassing an area of approximately 700 km^2. This strategy was aimed at capturing a wide range of retail environments within the city, from large supermarkets to smaller grocery stores, to accurately reflect the retail landscape of João Pessoa.

Given the unique challenges posed by the COVID-19 pandemic, specific health and safety measures were rigorously observed during all visits to supermarkets and grocery stores. Researchers equipped themselves with N-95 disposable respirators to mitigate the risk of virus transmission. In adherence to guidelines issued by health authorities, additional precautions included maintaining increased space and practicing distancing from other individuals during site visits. These measures ensured the safety of both the researchers and the public, allowing for the successful collection of price data amidst the pandemic.

2.6. Determining the Final Price of Meals

To accurately assess the economic implications of dietary choices, the final price of meals, incorporating both branded and non-branded food items, was calculated. For non-branded food items such as oranges, onions, and raw/chilled beef chuck, the regular price recorded was the one available at each visited supermarket or grocery store. This approach captures the typical market price for staple food items that do not vary significantly by brand. For branded food items like soybean oil, rice, and ground coffee, where multiple brands were often available, the lowest regular price was consistently selected. This decision was made to reflect cost-effective purchasing habits, excluding "best buys" or temporary discount offers to maintain price consistency across data collection periods.

The number of food staple samples correlates directly with the number of supermarkets and grocery stores visited where the specific item was available, ensuring a broad and representative dataset for price analysis. To derive the average price of food per reference weight or volume as sold, the calculated cost per gram or milliliter of the converted food is adjusted by the TCF and the reference sale weight or volume.

This structured methodology for calculating meal prices allows for a comprehensive analysis of dietary economics, factoring in the variations in food preparation and consumption practices. It provides a detailed basis for evaluating the cost implications of dietary choices within the context of Brazilian households.

2.7. Assessing the Impact of Alcohol and Food Consumption on National Per Capita Household Income

The economic burden of alcohol and food consumption on Brazilian households was analyzed by comparing these expenditures to the national per capita household income. Such an analysis reveals the percentage of income that households dedicate to alcohol and food, offering insights into the economic pressures they face.

National per capita household income data were sourced from the Brazilian Institute of Geography and Statistics (IBGE), Ministry of Economy. According to the IBGE, the nominal monthly per capita household income of the resident population in Brazil was BRL 1380.00 in 2020 and slightly decreased to BRL 1367.00 in 2021 [22,23]. These figures provide a basis for evaluating the relative economic impact of alcohol and food expenditures on household budgets. The expenditure on alcohol and food was calculated using price data collected from supermarkets and grocery stores in João Pessoa, as specified above.

The total expenditure on alcohol and food for an average household was then calculated. This amount was divided by the national per capita household income to determine the expenditure ratio. This ratio, expressed as a percentage, illustrates the share of household income consumed by these expenditures.

3. Results

3.1. Average Price of Pure Alcohol from Leading Brands of Beer and Cachaça

Selected leading national brands of beer and sugarcane spirit cachaça surveyed in local (João Pessoa, Brazil) supermarkets/grocery stores in 2020 and 2021, and corresponding average prices (per product and per gram of pure alcohol), are shown in Table 4.

Table 4. Selected low-price leading national brands of alcoholic beverages (beer and cachaça) [1] surveyed in local (João Pessoa, Brazil) supermarkets/grocery stores in August–September/2020 and August–September/2021, number of samples, average price (Brazilian reals, BRL) of the alcoholic beverage and average price of corresponding g of pure alcohol.

Alcoholic Beverages [1] and Alcohol Content (Labels), as Sold in Local Supermarkets	Number of Samples [2]		Average Price (BRL) of Branded Product [3] ± Std. Deviation		Average Price (BRL) of g Pure Alcohol [4]	
	2020	2021	2020	2021	2020	2021
Beer, can, 350 mL						
Brand B1 (5.0% vol.)	14	24	1.95 ± 0.15	2.09 ± 0.17	0.11	0.15
Brand B2 (4.7% vol.)	13	26	1.97 ± 0.22	2.35 ± 0.19	0.13	0.18
Brand B3 (4.5% vol.)	10	19	2.06 ± 0.16	2.25 ± 0.23	0.12	0.18
Average price (B1–B3 brands)			1.99	2.23	0.12	0.17
Cachaça, can, 350 mL						
Brand C1 (39% vol.)	9	17	3.84 ± 0.49	4.39 ± 0.58	0.03	0.04
Brand C2 (40% vol.)	15	14	4.28 ± 0.56	4.49 ± 0.48	0.03	0.04
Average price (C1 and C2 brands)			4.06	4.44	0.03	0.04

[1] To define low-price leading national beer and cachaça brands to be surveyed in 2020 and 2021, data from the Brazilian Association of Supermarkets regarding leading (best-selling) brands in the year 2019 were used [13]. The 5 best-selling beer brands (brand name/manufacturer) in 2019, all manufactured in Brazil, were Skol pilsen/AMBEV, Brahma chopp/AMBEV, Budweiser/AMBEV, Heineken/Heineken Brasil, and Itaipava Pilsen/Grupo Petrópolis. The 5 best-selling cachaça brands (brand name/manufacturer) in 2019, all manufactured in Brazil, were Pirassununga 51/Müller, Velho Barreiro/Tatuzinho, Ypióca/Diageo, Pitú/Engarrafamento Pitú, and Salinas/Lactalis. Due to greater availability in local supermarkets and/or relatively lower regular prices (among the top 5 best-selling brands), 3 brands of beer (named in this study as B1, B2, and B3; all "American Lager" in beer style) and 2 brands of cachaça (named in this study as C1 and C2; all colorless/"white" sweetened column still type cachaças) were chosen to be surveyed. [2] The number of samples of beer and cachaça corresponds to the number of visited supermarkets/grocery stores where the specific brands of beer and cachaça (in aluminum cans of 350 mL) were available. [3] Regular price of product collected in local supermarkets or grocery stores ("best buys" or limited-time discount offers were not considered). [4] Average price per g of pure alcohol was calculated by dividing the average price (BRL) of the product by the mass of ethanol in the beverage (volume of alcoholic beverage × alcohol content in % vol. × 0.79); 0.79 g/mL is the density of ethanol.

Price variations of the branded beverages in different supermarkets/grocery stores surveyed in 2020 and 2021 were within expectations. The coefficient of variation (CV, standard deviation divided by the average and multiplied by 100) of all brands ranged from 7.7% (brand B1 in 2020) to 13.2% (brand C1 in 2021), with an overall CV of 10.2%.

From 2020 to 2021, the average price of the beer and cachaça brands rose by 11.9% and 9.6%, respectively, and these increases are aligned with the official annual inflation rate of 10.6% in 2021 (in 2020, the inflation was 4.52%) [24,25].

On average, the price per gram of pure alcohol from cachaça is approximately four times cheaper than that from beer, both in 2020 and 2021 (Table 4). This difference in price may be related to the fact that beer produced in Brazil depends heavily on imported raw materials (especially malt and hops), which are more subjected to price variations in the international market, a fact that does not apply to cachaça (Brazil is the world's largest producer of sugarcane). Despite the peculiarities in production costs between beer and cachaça, such an impressive discrepancy in price per gram of pure alcohol was unexpected.

As the significant difference in average price of pure alcohol from brands of cachaça (BRL 0.03 and BRL 0.04) and beer (BRL 0.12 and BRL 0.17) could have been the result of specific market disruptions during the COVID-19 pandemic in 2020 and 2021, in February 2024, while this article was being written, a representative supermarket chain in João Pessoa, Paraíba, Brazil, was visited to check how different the prices were from the 2021 survey. Brands B1, B2, B3, C1, and C2 were available in the visited supermarket, all in the same type of packaging material/volume (aluminum cans of 350 mL). After more than two years since the last survey, both the B1 (5.0% vol.) and B2 (4.7% vol.) beer brands were being sold at BRL 3.19 while the price of B3 (4.5% vol.) was BRL 2.87. Regarding the cachaça brands, prices of both C1 (39% vol.) and C2 (40% vol.) were BRL 4.99. Assuming this single price collection in 2024 represents the current average prices in the Brazilian market, it appears that while prices of the leading beer brands rose sharply since 2021, with an average increase of 38.6%, the price of cachaça rose 12.4%. After applying the same conversion procedure indicated in Table 4, prices per gram of pure alcohol in February 2024 were 0.23 (B1), 0.25 (B2), 0.23 (B3), 0.05 (C1), and 0.04 (C2); in this respect, the average gram of pure alcohol from cachaça (BRL 0.045) would be five times cheaper than that from beer (BRL 0.24) in 2024.

It should be highlighted that the leading brands of cachaça surveyed in 2020 and 2021, which are known to be low-price, were not the cheapest brand available in some supermarkets. For example, a 38% vol. recorded brand of cachaça that was being sold at BRL 2.69 in a PET bottle contained 480 mL, which converts into BRL 0.02 per gram of pure alcohol. Furthermore, in the 2020 and 2021 survey, some brands of vodka, the second most consumed spirit in Brazil [3], which is usually produced from sugarcane [26], have prices that are similar to the leading brands of cachaça.

3.2. *Average Price Per Gram of Converted Food Staples*

Table 5 presents a summary of average prices (BRL) per gram of 24 converted food staples (i.e., food without inedible/unwanted parts and then cooked, if applicable) collected from supermarkets and grocery stores in 2020 and 2021. For detailed information on food characteristics/composition, forms of consumption, forms of preparations, standard serving size, edible conversion factor, cooking conversion factor, etc., see Appendix A Table A1.

Food price variations in different supermarkets/grocery stores surveyed in 2020 and 2021 were greater than values observed for the leading brands of beer and cachaça (9.6% to 11.9%). Price variations in food, given as a coefficient of variation (CV), ranged from 3.9% (mozzarella-type cheese in 2020) to 58.3% (raw tomato cv Italiano in 2021), with a 16.7% average CV of all surveyed foods. Compared to the three brands of beer and two brands of cachaça, the greater variation in food prices in different outlets may simply reflect a more complex nature associated with the production and logistics of 24 different types of foods.

Regarding variations in average prices of the 24 food staples from 2020 to 2021, the majority (21) experienced increases while prices fell for only 2 of them (raw garlic, −20.8%; salt, −31.2%). In one case, beans cv Carioca, the average price remained the same in 2021. Foods that experienced increases in prices ranged from 2.3% (UHT whole fluid milk) to 70.8% (raw butterhead lettuce), with an overall increase in food of 30.9%. As the official inflation rate in Brazil was reported as 10.06% in 2021 [24], price increases in most surveyed food staples were well above the annual inflation rate and, again, they may have been compounded by market disruptions due to the COVID-19 pandemic.

A quick price update in February 2024 in a representative supermarket in João Pessoa, Paraíba, Brazil, was conducted to check how different the prices of 10 selected food staples were from the 2021 survey. Similar to the 2020 and 2021 surveys, the lowest price available for each item was collected. After applying the conversion factors when necessary, prices per gram or mL of the 10 selected food items in February 2024 were the following (price increase relative to the 2021 survey in brackets): banana, BRL 7.4/g (+32.1%); papaya, BRL 9.8/g (+84.9%); tomato, BRL 6.7/g (+85.8%); lettuce, BRL 17.6/g (+114.1%); milk, BRL

5.3/mL (+17.6%); rice, BRL 3.2/g (+59.0%); beans, BRL 2.7/g (+6.4%); sugar, BRL 4.2/g (+12.3%); chicken, BRL 64.6/g (+12.3%); and beef, BRL 49.3/g (+8.3%).

Table 5. Selected low-price [1] food staples available in local (João Pessoa, PB, Brazil) supermarkets/grocery stores in August–September/2020 (2020) and August–September/2021 (2021), number of samples, and average price per g or mL of converted food.

Food Staples [2], as Sold in Local Supermarkets/Grocery Stores	Number of Samples [3]		Form of Consumption/ Use of Edible Portion [2]	Average Price (BRL) of Converted Food [4] per g or mL ± SD (×10³)	
	2020	2021		2020	2021
Orange cv. Pera, raw/natural	12	26	Squeezed	4.1 ± 0.5	4.9 ± 1.3
Banana cv. Pacovã, raw/natural	12	29	Sliced	3.5 ± 0.8	5.6 ± 1.4
Papaya cv. Formosa, raw/natural	12	28	Sliced	3.5 ± 0.8	5.3 ± 1.6
Pineapple cv. Pérola, raw/natural	17	23	Sliced	5.1 ± 1.0	5.4 ± 1.3
White onion, raw/natural	13	28	As ingredient	3.1 ± 0.6	4.2 ± 1.0
Carrot, raw/natural	13	28	Grated	3.8 ± 0.5	4.7 ± 0.9
Garlic, raw/natural	19	26	As ingredient	30.7 ± 5.4	24.3 ± 3.9
Tomato cv. Italiano, raw/natural	12	26	Sliced	2.9 ± 0.3	3.6 ± 2.1
Green butterhead lettuce, raw/natural	11	26	Sliced	4.8 ± 1.5	8.2 ± 2.7
Flaked cornmeal, pre-cooked/dry, branded	13	30	Steamed	1.5 ± 0.1	1.7 ± 0.2
White/polished rice, dry/raw, branded	22	30	Cooked	1.9 ± 0.2	2.0 ± 0.3
Beans cv. Carioca, dry/raw, branded	16	29	Cooked	2.5 ± 0.2	2.5 ± 0.4
Spaghetti-type wheat pasta, dry/raw, branded	23	29	Cooked	1.4 ± 0.1	1.8 ± 0.3
Granulated cane sugar, white, branded	20	26	As sweetener	2.5 ± 0.1	3.7 ± 0.3
Table salt, refined, branded	13	26	As ingredient	1.6 ± 0.2	1.1 ± 0.3
Soybean oil, refined, branded	12	30	As ingredient	6.2 ± 1.9	9.6 ± 0.6
Mozzarella-type cheese, cow's, branded	9	38	Sliced	36.2 ± 1.4	37.2 ± 6.0
Butter, unsalted, branded	8	14	As spread	50.3 ± 6.3	51.9 ± 5.8
Long-life/UHT whole fluid milk, cow's, branded	20	29	As such	4.4 ± 0.3	4.5 ± 0.4
Chicken breast, bone-in, skin-on, frozen/raw, branded	13	27	Cooked	34.8 ± 3.8	57.5 ± 8.8
Beef chuck eye steak, chilled/raw	13	19	Cooked	32.3 ± 4.4	45.5 ± 2.0
Chicken egg, large size, raw, branded	13	17	Cooked	9.0 ± 0.9	14.1 ± 1.7
Brazilian wheat bread roll (*pão francês*), baked	13	20	As such	9.7 ± 2.3	11.3 ± 2.9
Ground coffee, branded	21	30	Brewed, 8%	1.4 ± 0.1	1.7 ± 0.2

[1] For non-branded food items (e.g., orange, onion, raw/chilled beef chuck, etc.), the collected regular price was the one available in each visited supermarket/grocery store; for branded food items (e.g., soybean oil, rice, and ground coffee), where more than one brand was frequently available in each supermarket, the collected regular price was always the lowest; "best buys" or limited-time discount offers were not considered. [2] For detailed information on food characteristics/composition, forms of consumption, forms of preparations, standard serving size, edible conversion factor, cooking conversion factor, etc., see Appendix A Table A1. [3] The number of samples of food staples corresponds to the number of visited supermarkets/grocery stores where the item was found. [4] To obtain the average price per g or mL of a given converted food (i.e., food without inedible/unwanted parts and then cooked, if applicable), first the reference weight (in grams) or volume (in mL) of food for sale in supermarkets/grocery stores (see Appendix A Table A1) is transformed into weight or volume of edible/cleaned/cooked food (this is conducted by multiplying the reference weight or volume of food for sale by the total conversion factor, TCF; see Appendix A Table A1 for values). Then, the average price (in Brazilian reals, BRL) of the food per reference weight (in g) or volume (in mL), as collected in supermarkets/grocery stores (not shown), is divided by the weight (g) or volume (mL) of the converted food (e.g., 1000 g of raw beef chuck eye steak, with TCF = 0.5882, converts into 588.2 g of cooked beef prepared/shallow fried with onion, garlic, vegetable oil, and salt; visible fat trimmed before cooking). To obtain the average price of food per reference weight (g) or volume (mL), as sold in supermarkets/grocery stores, multiply the average cost (in BRL) of converted food per g or mL (see table above) by the TCF and by the reference weight (g) or volume (mL) for sale (e.g., the average cost per g of edible/cooked beef chuck eye steak in August–September/2020 is BRL 0.0323; thus, BRL 0.0323/g × 0.5882 × 1000 g = BRL 19.00 per kg or 1000 g of raw/chilled beef chuck eye steak).

Assuming the single price collection in 2024 represents the current average prices in the Brazilian market, it appears that food prices have been rising at different paces since 2021. In some cases, prices rose sharply for some foods, such as lettuce, papaya, tomato, and rice (between 59 and 114%); in other cases, such as beef, chicken, sugar, and beans, a more discrete price increase (between 6 and 13%) was observed.

3.3. Daily Expenditures on Alcohol and Food Consumption

Tables 6 and 7 present daily expenditures on alcohol and food consumption, respectively, both in 2020 and 2021. Table 6 shows spending in nine specific consumption scenarios involving different types of drinks (beer and/or cachaça) and the level of consumption (moderate, risky, and heavy). Table 7, on the other hand, presents the expenditure on a low-price balanced staple diet of 2000 kcal that includes 24 different types of food. The daily expenditures on alcohol and food were obtained by multiplying the daily per capita consumption of pure alcohol (in grams) and converted food (in grams or mL) by the average price of each item, which have already been specified in Sections 3.1 and 3.2 (Tables 4 and 5).

Table 6. Daily expenditure (BRL) in 9 scenarios of alcohol per capita consumption in Brazil for moderate (16.8 g pure alcohol/day), risky (41.7 g/g/day), and heavy (83.4 g/day) drinking, considering the consumption of beer only, cachaça only, or a combination of the two beverages (64% beer + 36% cachaça).

Type of Alcoholic Beverage [1]	Consumption in g of Pure Alcohol/Day [2]	Consumption in mL of Beverage per Day [3]	Daily Expenditure (BRL) [4]	
			2020	2021
Beer only	16.8 41.7 83.4	452.5 1123.1 2246.2	2.52 6.26 12.51	2.86 7.09 14.18
Cachaça only	16.8 41.7 83.4	53.8 133.6 267.3	0.67 1.67 3.34	0.67 1.67 3.34
Combination (64% beer + 36% cachaça)	10.8 + 6.0 26.7 + 15.0 53.4 + 30.0	290.9 + 19.2 719.1 + 48.1 1438.2 + 96.1	1.86 4.61 9.21	2.08 5.14 10.28

[1] Alcoholic beverages (beer and cachaça) were all low-price leading national brands surveyed in local (João Pessoa, Brazil) supermarkets/grocery stores in August–September/2020 and August–September/2021 (see Table 4 for more details). [2] Values (g of pure alcohol/day) for moderate, risky, and heavy drinking were obtained as described in Table 1. [3] The corresponding volume (mL) of the beverages (beer or cachaça) was calculated as follows: [(consumption in g of pure alcohol per day)/0.79] × (1/alcohol content of each beverage in %vol). The alcohol contents of beer and cachaça used were 4.7% and 39.5%, respectively, because they correspond to the average alcohol contents displayed on labels of beers and cachaças selected for the present study. The density of alcohol is 0.79 g/mL. Values were calculated as described in Table 2. [4] See Table 4 for average prices of beers, cachaças, and of g of pure alcohol of corresponding beverage.

With respect to price variations that occurred from 2020 to 2021, expenses rose when the consumed beverages were beer alone and beer + cachaça by approximately 13% and 12%, respectively; however, there was no change when the beverage consumed was cachaça only. Compared to alcohol consumption, there was a much higher increase in food (staple diet of 2000 kcal/day) spending in 2021, around 25%. In brief, spending on alcohol consumption either did not rise or rose much less sharply than spending on food in 2021. Based on the recent single survey on the prices of alcoholic beverages (beer and cachaça) and selected foods (see Sections 3.1 and 3.2), it is assumed that the higher rate of increase in food spending (in relation to alcohol) remains or even increased in 2024.

All expenses related to the nine alcohol consumption scenarios in 2020 and 2021 (Table 6), which varied from BRL 0.67/day (moderate consumption of cachaça, equivalent to 0.4 L/week) up to BRL 13.34/day (heavy beer consumption, equivalent to 15.7 L/week), cost less than the expenditure on a staple balanced diet of 2000 kcal (BRL 14.73/day). It should be noted that all scenarios of heavy alcohol consumption are cheaper than the staple diet; in this sense, it is concerning that the scenario involving heavy daily consumption of cachaça (equivalent to 1.9 L/week) has an average cost of only one-fifth (or 20%) of the amount spent on the staple diet.

Although the beers and cachaças surveyed are considered leading brands, therefore "popular alcoholic beverages" in Brazil, when looking at cachaça and beer drunk separately, the cost of drinking the same amount of alcohol from cachaça is approximately four times lower than that from beer. As mentioned previously, a possible explanation for this discrepancy is the fact that the main raw material for manufacturing cachaça—sugar cane—is very abundant and cheap in Brazil (compared to raw materials used in breweries, especially imported malt and hops).

Table 7. Daily expenditure (BRL) on a balanced [1] staple diet of 2000 kcal, consisting of 5 meals, and corresponding consumed quantities (g or mL) of each food item and their calories (kcal).

Converted [2] Low-Price Food Staples [3]	Consumption [4]	kcal [5]	Expenditure (BRL) [6]	
			2020	2021
Breakfast (517.2 kcal): various				
Papaya cv Formosa, raw/natural, sliced	60 g	28.2	0.21	0.32
Salted/steamed flaked cornmeal ("Brazilian corn couscous")	220 g	246.4	0.33	0.37
Salted/shallow fried (soybean oil) chicken egg	48 g	111.8	0.43	0.68
Unsalted butter, spread on "corn couscous"	10 g	77.6	0.50	0.52
Black coffee (via infusion brewing at 8%)	165 mL	13.2	0.23	0.28
White granulated sugar (added to coffee)	10 g	40.0	0.02	0.04
Morning snack (134.0 kcal): milk banana smoothie				
Long-life/UHT whole fluid milk	100 mL	65.0	0.44	0.45
Banana cv. Pacovã, raw/natural, sliced (blended with milk)	60 g	69.0	0.21	0.33
Lunch (594.5 kcal)				
Cooked/boiled beans cv Carioca (prepared with onion, garlic, water, soybean oil, and salt; served with 50% beans and 50% broth)	100 g	79.0	0.25	0.25
Cooked/boiled white rice (prepared with onion, garlic, water, and soybean oil)	250 g	347.5	0.48	0.49
Green butterhead lettuce, raw/natural, sliced	50 g	6.5	0.24	0.41
Carrot, raw/natural, grated	50 g	15.5	0.19	0.23
Cooked/shallow fried beef chuck eye steak (prepared with onion, garlic, soybean oil, and salt; served drained)	50 g	106.0	1.61	2.27
Orange juice, raw/natural, squeezed/strained	120 mL	40.0	0.49	0.59
Afternoon snack (306.0 kcal): cheese sandwich				
Brazilian wheat bread roll (pão francês)	70 g	210.0	0.68	0.79
Mozzarella-type cheese, cow's, sliced	30 g	96.0	1.08	1.12
Dinner (448.3 kcal): various				
Cooked/boiled spaghetti-type wheat pasta, unsalted, drained	250 g	315.0	0.35	0.45
Cooked/shallow fried chicken breast (prepared with soybean oil and salt; served drained, boned, and skinned)	50 g	93.0	1.74	2.88
Tomato cv. Italiano, raw/natural, sliced	85 g	15.3	0.24	0.30
Pineapple cv. Pérola, raw/natural, sliced	50 g	25.0	0.26	0.27
Approximate quantities of converted food ingredients [7] and cooking gas used in all culinary preparations.				
Soybean oil, refined	65 mL	- [9]	0.40	0.62
White onion, raw	120 g	- [9]	0.37	0.50
Garlic, raw	57 g	- [9]	1.75	1.39

Table 7. *Cont.*

Converted [2] Low-Price Food Staples [3]	Consumption [4]	kcal [5]	Expenditure (BRL) [6]	
			2020	2021
Table salt, refined	5 g	- [9]	0.01	0.01
Cooking gas (liquefied petroleum gas, LPG) [8]	0.11 kg	-	0.60	0.80
	Total [10]	2000.0	13.11	16.36

[1] The above diet is considered balanced because its daily energy and nutrient profile [Energy, 2000 kcal; carbohydrates (starches and sugars), 296.02 g (59.2% energy); estimated free sugars, 48.76 g (9.8% energy); protein, 82.10 g (16.4% energy); total fat, 48.32 g (21.7% energy); saturated fat, 18.71 g (8.4% energy); sodium, 1852.91 mg; fruits and vegetables, 475.0 g; fiber, 26.05 g]—calculated from the energy and nutrient content values in Appendix A Tables A1 and A2—is in line with levels/recommendations of dietary components presented in Table 3; estimates of free sugars intake were based on the quantities of selected sugar-containing food in the diet and their corresponding free sugar contents (%), namely fruits—papaya, 8%; banana, 15%; orange, 9%; pineapple, 9% [27]; vegetables—carrot, 6%; tomato, 2% [28]; whole milk, 5% [29]; granulated sugar, 99.6% [15]. [2] Converted food is the edible food (i.e., without inedible parts) that has been prepared (cooked, if applicable) in a specific way and that is ready to be consumed or used; the food preparation and consumption in this study considered known dietary habits in Brazil and information from the Brazilian Food Composition Table [15]. [3] For detailed information on food characteristics/composition, forms of consumption, forms of preparations, standard serving size, edible conversion factor, etc., see Appendix A Table A1. [4] Quantities (g or mL) of converted food consumed in each meal (for information on standard serving size of each food item, see Appendix A Table A1). [5] Energy (kcal) in the converted food, as shown in Appendix A Table A1. [6] The average expenditure on food items, as collected in August–September 2020 (2020) and August–September 2021 (2021), was calculated by multiplying the consumed quantities by the corresponding average price of converted food presented in Table 5. [7] The quantity of ingredients used in all culinary preparations was estimated by multiplying the standard serving size of each ingredient (13 mL, soybean oil; 40 g, onion; 19 g, garlic; 1 g, salt; see Appendix A Table A1) by the number of preparations in which they were used, namely 5 (soybean oil), 3 (onion), 3 (garlic), and 5 (salt). [8] The following formula was used to calculate the daily per capita expenditure (BRL) on LPG in 2020 and 2021, respectively: (0.11 kg/13 kg) × BRL 71.42 and (0.11 kg/13 kg) × BRL 94.30; where 0.11 kg is the estimated daily LPG demand per capita in Brazilian households and 13 kg is the most common size of LPG bottle used in Brazilian households [30]; BRL 71.42 and BRL 94.30 are the average prices of a 13 kg LPG bottle in the city of João Pessoa, as collected in 19 and 23 LPG retail outlets by the city of João Pessoa Consumer Protection Agency (Procon-JP) in August 2020 and August 2021, respectively [31,32]. [9] Individual energy (kcal) and nutrition values of food ingredients used in culinary preparations (soybean oil, onion, garlic, and salt) are not considered for calculations in the diet because they are already included in the energy and nutrient content of the converted food. [10] "Total" refers to total energy (kcal) in the diet (sum of calories of each consumed converted food item) and total expenditure (BRL) on the diet (sum of average cost of each consumed item) in 2020 and 2021.

Although a scenario of moderate consumption was tested (Table 6), it is worth noticing that the latest epidemiological evidence indicates that there is no safe amount of alcohol that can be consumed (to the point of excluding risks associated with alcohol completely), as alcohol is toxic to the human body at any level; therefore, the level of alcohol consumption that minimizes health loss is zero [33]. However, moderate levels of alcohol consumption have been defined, such as less than 20 g of pure alcohol per day [11].

3.4. *Impact of Daily Expenditures in Alcohol and Food Consumption on National Per Capita Household Income*

The question that arises is to what extent food and alcohol spending scenarios impact on the finances of the average Brazilian. In other words, how much of the national income does food and alcohol consumption represent? It is currently understood that alcohol consumption, in any of the presented scenarios, represents a smaller portion of a Brazilian's income compared to a 2000 kcal staple diet.

The first aspect to consider is that food spending is necessary for survival and, therefore, mandatory. Let us consider, then, that the expenditure on the balanced staple diet of 2000 kcal would already be at the minimum possible cost (average of BRL 14.73/day) and, therefore, with no more room for reductions. In this case, one can ask the following: would there be, in theory, room in the household income to allow for the inclusion of the alcohol consumption scenarios, in particular the risky and heavy scenarios, without compromising other mandatory expenses (housing, transport, health, clothing, etc.)?

According to the Brazilian Institute of Geography and Statistics—IBGE—the monthly national household income per capita in Brazil in 2020 and 2021 was BRL 1380.00 and BRL 1367.00, respectively. Per capita household income is calculated as the ratio between the total household income and the total number of residents [22,23]. Considering the 2020–2021 income average and dividing the value by 30, the daily household income in those years was BRL 45.78.

Figure 1 shows the impact (%) of daily alcohol and food consumption on the daily national per capita household income. They were obtained by dividing average daily expenditure values (2020 and 2021) on food and alcohol (Tables 6 and 7) by BRL 45.78 and multiplying by 100.

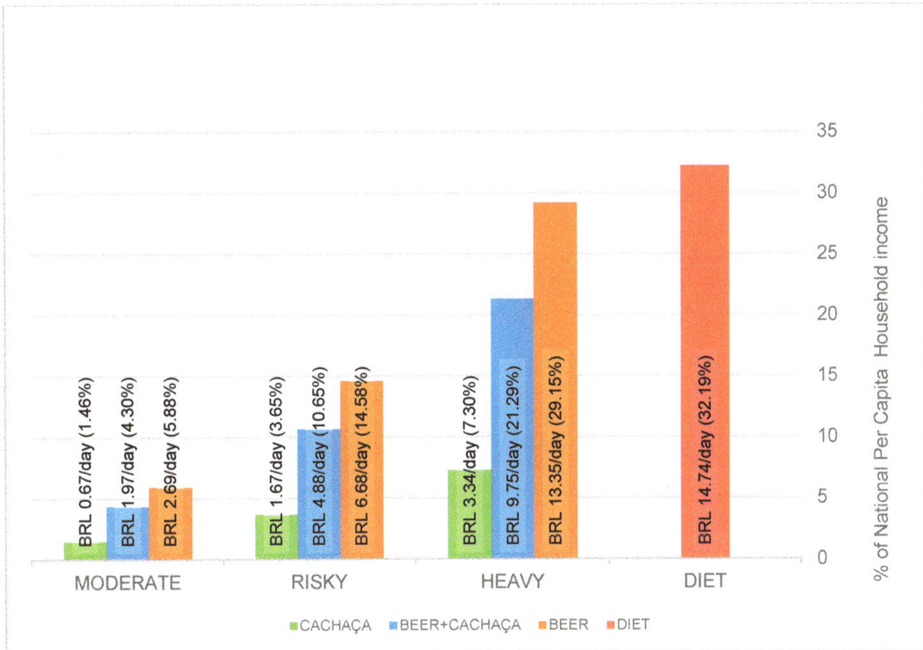

Figure 1. Impact (%) of alcohol and food expenditures on national per capita household income, average 2020 and 2021.

The balanced diet of 2000 kcal/day (BRL 14.7 3/day, average over 2020 and 2021) represents a significant portion of household income, 32%, the biggest impact of all the scenarios analyzed (Figure 1). The variations in the impact of daily expenditures on national per capita household income between 2020 and 2021, calculated as a coefficient of variation (CV), ranged from 0.0% (all cachaça scenarios) to 11.0% (diet), with an overall value of 4.6%.

Taking into account the moderate scenario (16.8 g of pure alcohol per day) only, the consumption of cachaça alone, cachaça + beer, or beer alone has very little impact on household income, namely 1.5%, 4.3%, and 5.9%, respectively. If the consumption moves to a risky (41.7 g/day) scenario, which corresponds to the per capita consumption among Brazilian men and women over 15 who consume alcohol, impacts on the domestic income are 3.6% (cachaça alone), 10.6% (beer + cachaça), and 14.6% (beer alone) (Figure 1).

Finally, in a scenario of heavy alcohol consumption (83.4 g/day), impacts on household income are 7.3% (cachaça alone), 21.3% (beer + cachaça), and 29.1% (beer alone), all below the expenditure on a 2000 kcal staple diet. Although the volumes of beverage consumption in the heavy scenario are all very high, it is the cachaça scenario and its impact on household income that draws the attention most: consumption of a large amount of cachaça (equivalent to 1.9 L per week) has minimal impact, 7.3%, on the household income (Figure 1). From the financial point of view, the result suggests that it is entirely possible for average Brazilians to engage in a heavy alcohol consumption pattern, especially from drinking leading brands of cachaça, without compromising other mandatory household expenses. Engaging in a risky scenario of drinking is thus even more economically viable.

4. Discussion

The health and economic burdens associated with alcohol consumption disproportionately affect various socioeconomic groups, with the most economically disadvantaged and less educated groups experiencing more significant health impacts and financial strain. This strain includes compromises in family income and the ability to afford essential dietary needs [1]. The World Health Organization advocates for increasing the retail price of alcohol as an effective measure to mitigate the harm caused by its consumption [34]. This approach has proven successful in reducing alcohol-related harm, morbidity, and mortality when properly implemented [1]. However, the application of such a policy in Brazil necessitates a thorough understanding of alcohol's relative pricing and its impact on household income. To date, there has been limited research in this area.

The study by Abramson et al. [35] stands out as a pioneering effort to explore this issue within Brazil. Their research involved a comparison of the prices of popular alcoholic beverages (such as cachaça, beer, and table wine) with basic food groups (cheese, milk, rice, vegetables, and meat), based on data collected from 32 retail supermarkets across eight municipalities in Paraíba. Their findings highlighted a discrepancy in pricing, with alcoholic beverages, particularly popular brands of cachaça and beer, being significantly cheaper than basic food items. This disparity suggests that interventions aimed at addressing alcohol dependence must consider the economic accessibility of alcohol relative to essential dietary foods. While Abramson et al. [35] offered crucial insights, they did not account for the typical expenditure on alcohol consumption (e.g., grams of pure alcohol per day) or compare it against the expenditure on a reference diet (e.g., 2000 kcal/day). Despite this limitation, their conclusion that consuming popular alcoholic beverages is more affordable than adhering to dietary staples remains a critical observation, underscoring the need for policy interventions that consider both the economic and health impacts of alcohol consumption within Brazil.

In relation to the per capita household income in 2020 and 2021, both approximately BRL 46.00 per day [22,23], the daily household expenditure on a 2000 kcal diet in 2020 (BRL 13.11) and 2021 (BRL 16.36) represents 28% and 36%, respectively. It is assumed that this increase is related to the official inflation measured in Brazil in those years, which jumped from 4.52% in 2020 to 10.06% in 2021 [24,25].

In addition to eating, the population must also direct their income to meet all other basic needs, such as transport, health, clothing, and housing. Therefore, committing between 28% and 36% of income to food alone is concerning. This monthly commitment percentage of 28–36% on a diet of 2000 kcal/day is in line with the latest Family Budget Survey (POF) 2017–2018 by IBGE, according to which families with up to two minimum wages a month in Brazil (in 2018, BRL 63.60/day) spent 22% on food [36].

This research approach faces some limitations that must be acknowledged. The study's focus on beer and cachaça, while providing valuable insights into these popular beverages, may overlook the diversity of alcohol consumption patterns across different segments of the Brazilian population. This could limit the generalizability of the findings to the broader context of alcohol use in Brazil. Furthermore, the reliance on retail prices from supermarkets in Greater João Pessoa may not accurately reflect price variations and consumption patterns in other regions, particularly in rural areas or among different socioeconomic groups, as well as the phenomenon of unrecorded alcohol, which might be prevalent specifically for sugarcane spirits. This geographic limitation suggests the need for further research encompassing a broader array of locations and demographic profiles to capture the full spectrum of alcohol's economic impact on Brazilian households.

Another limitation stems from the study's methodological focus on economic impacts, which may not fully account for the complex social and cultural factors influencing alcohol consumption in Brazil [37]. While economic measures like Minimum Unit Pricing have the potential to mitigate harmful drinking patterns, their effectiveness can be influenced by cultural attitudes toward alcohol, social drinking norms, and the availability of informal alcohol markets. For instance, in Brazil, social gatherings and celebrations often center around alcohol, potentially reinforcing and normalizing high consumption rates. Moreover, the stigma associated with seeking help for alcohol dependency varies culturally, which can affect the effectiveness of public health interventions. Moreover, dietary habits may be intrinsically linked to alcohol consumption. In many cultures, including Brazil, alcohol is often consumed in conjunction with meals, and the types of food available or preferred can affect the amount and type of alcohol consumed. For instance, the prevalence of heavy fat- and carbohydrate-rich foods may traditionally correlate with the preference for spirits like cachaça. Understanding these dietary patterns can provide insights into the contextual factors that drive alcohol consumption. Moreover, dietary habits can also reflect broader socioeconomic conditions that influence drinking behaviors, such as income levels and access to food diversity. Addressing these multifaceted drivers of alcohol use requires a comprehensive approach that combines economic interventions with social and cultural strategies.

This article contributes to a deeper understanding of alcohol consumption's economic impacts on Brazilian households. By focusing on beer and cachaça, the most popular alcoholic beverages in Brazil, the study provides targeted insights into consumption patterns that have significant implications for public health and economic well-being. This specificity allows for a nuanced analysis of how these beverages contribute to household expenditures and potentially displace essential dietary needs. Additionally, using the per capita expenditure on a balanced diet as a reference point offers a tangible measure of the trade-offs households may face between alcohol consumption and nutritional requirements, highlighting the broader societal impacts of alcohol affordability.

5. Conclusions

This study highlights a significant public health and economic concern due to the affordability of alcoholic beverages relative to essential dietary needs in Brazil. Notably, alcoholic drinks such as cachaça are often more affordable than staple foods, which may facilitate hazardous drinking patterns within average Brazilian households. This finding indicates that a reevaluation of alcohol pricing policies, including the consideration of Minimum Unit Pricing (MUP), could be beneficial. However, the actual effectiveness of such measures requires careful consideration and further empirical validation. Combining educational campaigns with strategic pricing could also offer a more comprehensive approach to mitigating alcohol-related harm. Developing effective policy responses will necessitate a multifaceted strategy that encompasses regulatory, educational, and economic measures, tailored to the complex interplay between alcohol affordability, consumption, and public health. It is essential for future research to explore the long-term impacts of these policies on alcohol consumption patterns, health outcomes, and the economic burden on households to ensure that policies are both effective and equitable.

Author Contributions: Conceptualization, I.C.C.N.; methodology, I.C.C.N.; formal analysis, R.V.L.M. and M.A.F.; investigation, R.V.L.M. and M.A.F.; resources, I.C.C.N.; data curation, R.V.L.M. and M.A.F.; writing—original draft preparation, I.C.C.N. and D.W.L.; writing—review and editing, R.V.L.M. and M.A.F.; visualization, R.V.L.M.; supervision, I.C.C.N.; project administration, I.C.C.N. All authors have read and agreed to the published version of the manuscript.

Funding: This research received no external funding. Institutional funding within the research project 23074.041057/2018-38 UFPB is acknowledged.

Institutional Review Board Statement: Not applicable.

Informed Consent Statement: Not applicable.

Data Availability Statement: The raw data supporting the conclusions of this article will be made available by the authors on request.

Acknowledgments: Yuri Ishihara (UFPB), Aline Dantas (UFPB), Celiane Silva (UFRPE), and Éder Souza Leão (UFRPE) are thanked for their assistance and/or helpful advice. In the development of this manuscript, ChatGPT, an AI language model developed by OpenAI (San Francisco, CA, USA) was utilized. An individualized version of ChatGPT was employed, which was customized to provide targeted assistance in academic research and writing. This adaptation involved fine-tuning the model to focus on alcohol research, particularly in the context of the article's topics. The model was provided with access to all references in full text. Notably, the GPT-4 version of the model was used. GPT-4 was used to translate Portuguese language drafts into clear, concise, and scientifically coherent English narratives. It also played a role in shortening the abstract. Finally, it was applied as a tool in referencing by converting the various reference sources into BibTeX format for further processing with Zotero v. 6.0.36.

Conflicts of Interest: The authors declare no conflicts of interest.

Appendix A

Table A1. Food staples surveyed in this study, their reference weight (kg) or volume (mL) for sale in local (João Pessoa, PB, Brazil) supermarkets/grocery stores, and corresponding values of edible conversion factors (ECFs), cooking conversion factors (CCFs), total conversion factor (TCF), energy (kcal per 100 g or 100 mL of food in its usual form of consumption or use), and content of selected nutrients (g or mg per 100 g or 100 mL of edible food in its usual form of consumption or use).

Surveyed Food Staples	Reference Weight or Volume for Sale [1]	Form of Consumption/ Use of Edible Portion [5]	Standard Portion/ Serving Size [12]	ECF; CCF [20]	TCF [25]	Contents of Energy (kcal), Available Carbohydrates (Carb; g), Dietary Fiber (Fiber; g), Protein (g), Total Fat (Tot. Fat; g), Saturated Fat (Sat. Fat; g), and Sodium (mg) per 100 g (Solid Food) or 100 mL (Liquid Food) of Converted Food (Edible Portion of Food in Its Usual Form of Consumption of Use) [26]						
						Energy	Carb.	Fiber	Protein	Tot. Fat	Sat. Fat	Sodium
Orange cv. Pera, raw/natural	1000 g	Squeezed	200 mL [13]	2.13 [21]; 1.0	0.4695	33	7.58	tr [27]	0.74	0.07	0.00	tr [27]
Banana cv. Pacovã, raw/natural	1000 g	Sliced	86 g [14]	1.51 [21]; 1.0	0.6623	115	25.3	2.80	1.69	0.11	0.03	0.88
Papaya cv. Formosa, raw/natural	1000 g	Sliced	160 g [14]	1.63 [21]; 1.0	0.6135	47	9.74	1.81	0.82	0.12	0.04	3.26
Pineapple cv. Pérola, raw/natural	1350 g [2]	Sliced	130 g [14]	1.89 [21]; 1.0	0.5291	50	10.5	1.12	0.68	0.33	0.02	2.84
White onion, raw/natural	1000 g	As ingredient	40 g [15]	1.73 [21]; 1.0	0.5780	41	7.16	2.04	1.76	0.13	0.05	0.62
Carrot, raw/natural	1000 g	Grated	38 g [16]	1.17 [21]; 1.0	0.8547	31	4.56	2.98	1.12	0.21	0.03	11.1
Garlic, raw/natural	1000 g	As ingredient	19 g [17]	1.08 [21]; 1.0	0.9259	121	22.6	3.19	5.70	0.20	0.04	5.43
Tomato cv. Italiano, raw/natural	1000 g	Sliced	80 g [16]	1.25 [21]; 1.0	0.8000	18	2.22	1.60	1.04	0.17	0.02	3.13
Green butterhead lettuce, raw/natural	275 g [3]	Sliced	32 g [18]	1.21 [21]; 1.0	0.8264	13	0.10	2.33	1.69	0.12	0.00	4.23
Flaked cornmeal, pre-cooked/dry, branded	500 g	Steamed [6]	100 g [17]	1.0; 2.0 [22]	2.0000	112	23.2	2.05	2.16	0.68	0.20	247
White/polished rice, dry/raw, branded	1000 g	Cooked [7]	125 g [14]	1.0; 2.5 [21]	2.5000	139	28.0	1.28	2.41	1.59	0.33	1.60
Beans cv. Carioca, dry/raw, branded	1000 g	Cooked [8]	50 g [14]	1.0; 3.0 [21]	3.0000	79	7.77	6.84	4.69	1.72	0.28	190
Granulated cane sugar, white, branded	1000 g	As sweetener	5 g [13]	1.0; 1.0	1.0000	400	99.6	0.00	0.32	tr [27]	0.00	tr [27]
Table salt, refined, branded	1000 g	As ingredient	1 g [19]	1.0; 1.0	1.0000	0	0.00	0,00	0.00	0.00	0.00	39943
Soybean oil, refined, branded	900 mL	As ingredient	13 mL [13]	1.0; 1.0	1.0000	828	0.00	0.00	0.00	92.0	14.00	0.00
"Mozzarella-type" cheese, cow's, branded	1000 g	Sliced	30 g [13]	1.0; 1.0	1.0000	320	1.97	0.00	23.8	24.1	13.60	506
Butter, unsalted, branded	200 g	As spread	10 g [13]	1.0; 1.0	1.0000	776	0.00	0.00	0.40	86.0	51.5	3.85

Table A1. *Cont.*

Surveyed Food Staples	Reference Weight or Volume for Sale [1]	Form of Consumption/ Use of Edible Portion [5]	Standard Portion/ Serving Size [12]	ECF; CCF [20]	TCF [25]	Contents of Energy (kcal), Available Carbohydrates (Carb; g), Dietary Fiber (Fiber; g), Protein (g), Total Fat (Tot. Fat; g), Saturated Fat (Sat. Fat; g), and Sodium (mg) per 100 g (Solid Food) or 100 mL (Liquid Food) of Converted Food (Edible Portion of Food in Its Usual Form of Consumption of Use) [26]						
						Energy	Carb.	Fiber	Protein	Tot. Fat	Sat. Fat	Sodium
Long-life/UHT whole fluid milk, cow's, branded	1000 mL	As such	200 mL [13]	1.0; 1.0	1.0000	65	7.16	0.00	2.35	3.04	1.40	63.8
Chicken breast, bone-in, frozen/raw, branded	1000 g	Cooked [9]	100 g [14]	2.38 [21]; 0.7 [21]	0.2941	186	0.00	0.00	29.7	7.94	1.79	233
Beef chuck eye steak, chilled/raw	1000 g	Cooked [10]	100 g [16]	1.19 [21]; 0.7 [21]	0.5882	212	1.16	0.12	26.0	11.4	5.39	233
Chicken egg, large size, raw, branded	57 g [4]	Cooked [9]	45 g [16]	1.12 [21]; 0.9 [23]	0.8036	233	1.19	0.00	15.5	18.5	4.10	353
Brazilian wheat bread roll, baked	1000 g	As such	50 g [16]	1.0; 1.0	1.0000	300	59.0	2.61	9.83	2.12	0.68	681
Ground coffee, branded	250 g	Brewed, 8% [11]	165 mL [17]	1.0; 12.5 [24]	12.5000	8	1.34	0.00	0.54	0.06	0.01	0.82
Spaghetti-type wheat pasta, dry/raw, branded	500 g	Cooked [6]	105 g [14]	1.0; 3.0 [21]	3.0000	126	26.1	0.91	3.56	0.57	0.16	1.92

[1] Reference weights (g) or volumes (mL) of surveyed food staples were obtained from local supermarkets/grocery stores. [2] Whole/fresh pineapple was sold by unit (not by weight); to facilitate some calculations, the average weight of a pineapple unit (1350 g) was obtained from [19]. [3] Butterhead lettuce was sold by unit/head; to facilitate some calculations, the average weight of a lettuce head (275 g; "especial" type) was obtained from CEAGESP [20]. [4] Surveyed eggs were packed in a 15 units' case; to facilitate some calculations, the average weight of an egg unit (57 g, "large" type) was obtained from [38]. [5] Form of consumption or use of edible food portion in this study considered known dietary habits in Brazil and data from the Brazilian Food Composition Table [15]. [6] Soaked in water, salted then steamed for the preparation of so-called *Brazilian corn couscous*. [7] Boiled in unsalted water; in the case of white rice, previously sautéed (fried quickly) in vegetable oil with onion and garlic. [8] Boiled in water and then sautéed in vegetable oil with onion, garlic, and salt; served with 50% beans and 50% broth. [9] Chicken breast (bone-in/skin-on) and chicken egg prepared/shallow fried with vegetable oil and salt (both served drained; chicken breast served without bone and skin). [10] Prepared/shallow fried with onion, garlic, vegetable oil, and salt; visible fat trimmed before cooking. [11] Coffee drink prepared through infusion brewing at 8% (8 g roasted coffee/100 mL water) was obtained from TBCA [15]. [12] Serving size of edible food in the form of consumption/use described in column 2. [13] Serving size obtained from ANVISA/Ministry of Health [16]. [14] Serving size obtained from Ministry of Health [21]. [15] Serving size of onion (40 g) as ingredient (equals ~4 tablespoons of chopped onion) was estimated for this study. [16] Serving size of Brazilian wheat bread roll, known in Brazil as *pão francês*, was obtained from Philippi [39]. [17] Serving size was obtained from TBCTA [15]. [18] Lettuce serving size of 32 g (equals ~4 medium/large leaves) was estimated for this study. [19] Serving size of table salt (1 g) was obtained from pack labels/nutrition facts. [20] Edible conversion factors (ECFs) and cooking conversion factors (CCFs) of food commodities or branded food surveyed in this study. [21] ECF and CCF obtained from Ornellas [40]. [22] A CCF estimation of 2.0 (10 g of pre-cooked flaked cornmeal yields 20 g of soaked/steamed "corn couscous") was based on the preparation method/yield displayed on pack labelling (one part of pre-cooked flaked cornmeal is soaked with one part of water followed by quick steaming). [23] Estimated for this study. [24] CCF of 12.5 estimated from an infusion brewing at 8% [15]. [25] Total conversion factor (TCF) of surveyed foods, as sold in supermarkets/grocery stores (see column 1), to edible food in its usual form of consumption (see column 2) was calculated dividing the cooking conversion factor (CCF) by the edible conversion factor (ECF), by multiplying the weight or volume of surveyed food by the TCF results in a given amount of food in its final form of consumption (e.g., 1000 g of raw beef chuck eye steak, with TCF = 0.5882, converts into 588.2 g of cooked beef prepared/shallow fried with onion, garlic, vegetable oil, and salt; visible fat trimmed before cooking). [26] Calories and nutrient contents were obtained from TBCA [15]. [27] Present in trace levels, according to TBCA [15].

Table A2. Energy and nutrient contents of converted foods in each meal (from Appendix A Tables 7 and A1).

Meal	Energy and Nutrients Conversion
Breakfast	60 g papaya (energy, 28.2 kcal; carbohydrates/starches and sugars; fiber, 1.09 g; protein, 0.49 g; total fat, 0.07 g; saturated fat, 0.02 g; sodium, 1.96 mg) + 220 g salted/steamed flaked cornmeal (energy, 246.4 kcal; carbohydrates/starches and sugars, 51.04 g; fiber, 4.51 g; protein, 4.75 g; total fat, 1.5 g; saturated fat, 0.44 g; sodium, 543.4 mg) + 48 g salted/shallow fried (soybean oil) chicken egg (energy, 111.84 kcal; carbohydrates/starch and sugars, 0.57 g; fiber, 0 g; protein, 7.44 g; total fat, 8.88 g; saturated fat, 1.97 g; sodium, 169.44 mg) + 10 g unsalted butter (energy, 77.6 kcal; carbohydrates/starches and sugars, 0 g; fiber, 0 g; protein, 0.04 g; total fat, 8.6 g; saturated fat, 5.15 g; sodium, 0.38 mg) + 165 mL black coffee brewed at 8% (energy, 13.2 kcal; carbohydrates/starches and sugars, 2.21 g; fiber, 0 g; protein, 0.89 g; total fat, 0.1 g; saturated fat, 0.02 g; sodium, 1.35 mg) + 10 g white granulated sugar (energy, 40.0 kcal; carbohydrates/starches and sugars, 9.96 g; fiber, 0 g; protein, 0.03 g; total fat, 0 g; saturated fat, 0 g; sodium, 0 mg). Total energy and nutrient profile of breakfast: energy, 517.24 kcal; carbohydrates (starches and sugars), 69.62 g; fiber, 5.6 g; protein, 13.64 g; total fat, 19.15 g; saturated fat, 7.6 g; sodium, 716.53 mg.
Morning Snack	100 mL long-life/UHT whole fluid milk (energy, 65.0 kcal; carbohydrates/starches and sugars, 7.16 g; fiber, 0 g; protein, 2.45 g; total fat, 3.05 g; saturated fat, 1.4 g; sodium, 63.8 mg) + 60 g banana (energy, 69.0 kcal; carbohydrates/starches and sugars, 15.18 g; fiber, 1.68 g; protein, 1.01 g; total fat, 0.07 g; saturated fat, 0.02 g; sodium, 0.53 mg). Total energy and nutrient profile of morning snack: energy, 134.0 kcal; carbohydrates/starches and sugars, 22.34 g; fiber, 1.68 g; protein, 3.46 g; total fat, 3.12 g; saturated fat, 1.42 g; sodium, 64.33 mg.
Lunch	100 g cooked beans served with 50% beans and 50% broth (energy, 79.0 kcal; carbohydrates/starches and sugars, 7.77 g; fiber, 6.84 g; protein, 4.69 g; total fat, 1.72 g; saturated fat, 0.28 g; sodium, 190 mg) + 250 g unsalted cooked rice (energy, 347.5 kcal; carbohydrates/starches and sugars, 70.0 g; fiber, 3.20 g; protein, 6.02 g; total fat, 3.97 g; saturated fat, 0.82 g; sodium, 4.0 mg) + 50 g green butterhead lettuce (energy, 6.5 kcal; carbohydrates/starches and sugars, 0.05 g; fiber, 1.16 g; protein, 0.84 g; total fat, 0.06 g; saturated fat, 0 g; sodium, 2.11 mg) + 50 g raw carrot (energy, 15.5 kcal; carbohydrates/starches and sugars, 2.28 g; fiber, 1.49 g; protein, 0.56 g; total fat, 0.10 g; saturated fat, 0.01 g; sodium, 5.55 mg) + 50 g cooked beef chuck eye steak (energy, 106.0 kcal; carbohydrates/starches and sugars, 0.58 g; fiber, 0.06 g; protein, 13.0 g; total fat, 5.7 g; saturated fat, 2.69 g; sodium, 116.5 mg) + 120 mL squeezed/strained orange (energy, 40.0 kcal; carbohydrates/starches and sugars, 9.10 g; fiber, traces; protein, 0.89 g; total fat, 0.08 g; saturated fat, 0 g; sodium, 0 mg). Total energy and nutrient profile of lunch: energy, 594.5 kcal; carbohydrates/starches and sugars, 89.78 g; fiber, 12.75 g; protein, 26.0 g; total fat, 11.63 g; saturated fat, 3.8 g; sodium, 318.16 mg.
Afternoon Snack	70 g Brazilian wheat bread roll (energy, 210.0 kcal; carbohydrates/starches and sugars, 41.3 g; fiber, 1.83 g; protein, 6.88 g; total fat, 1.48 g; saturated fat, 0.48 g; sodium, 476.7 mg) + 30 g Mozzarella-type cheese (energy, 96.0 kcal; carbohydrates/starches and sugars, 0.59 g; fiber, 0 g; protein, 7.14 g; total fat, 7.23 g; saturated fat, 4.08 g; sodium, 151.8 mg). Total energy and nutrient profile of afternoon snack: energy, 306.0 kcal; carbohydrates/starches and sugars, 41.89 g; fiber, 1.83 g; protein, 14.02 g; total fat, 8.71 g; saturated fat, 4.56 g; sodium, 628.5 mg.

Table A2. *Cont.*

Meal	Energy and Nutrients Conversion
Dinner	250 g cooked/unsalted/drained spaghetti-type wheat pasta (energy, 315.0 kcal; carbohydrates/starches and sugars, 65.25 g; fiber, 2.27 g; protein, 8.9 g; total fat, 1.42 g; saturated fat, 0.4 g; sodium, 4.8 mg) + 50 g cooked chicken breast (energy, 93.0 kcal; carbohydrates, 0.0 g; fiber, 0.0 g; protein, 14.85 g; total fat, 3.97 g; saturated fat, 0.89 g; sodium, 116.5 mg) + 85 g raw/natural tomato (energy, 15.3 kcal; carbohydrates/starches and sugars, 1.89 g; fiber, 1.36 g; protein, 0.89 g; total fat, 0.14 g; saturated fat, 0.01 g; sodium, 2.66 mg) + 50 g raw/natural pineapple (energy, 25 kcal; carbohydrates/starches and sugars, 5.25 g; fiber, 0.56 g; protein, 0.34 g; total fat, 0.16 g saturated fat, 0.01 g; sodium, 1.42 mg). Total energy and nutrient profile of dinner: energy, 448.3 kcal; carbohydrates/starches and sugars, 72.39 g; fiber, 4.19 g; protein, 24.98 g; total fat, 5.69 g; saturated fat, 1.31 g; sodium, 125.38 mg.
Overall	Total energy and nutrient profile of the diet: energy, 2000.0 kcal; carbohydrates/starches and sugars, 296.02 g (59% energy); fiber, 26.05 g; protein, 82.1 g (16% energy); total fat, 48.3 g (22% energy); saturated fat, 18.69 g (8.4% energy); sodium, 1852.9 mg; fruits and vegetables, 475 g; estimated free sugars *, 48.76 g (9.8% energy).

* Approximate free sugars (%) in selected sugar-containing foods in the diet: Fruits—papaya, 8%; banana, 15%; orange, 9%; pineapple, 9% [27]. Vegetables—carrot, 6%; tomato, 2% [28]. Whole milk, 5% [29]. Granulated sugar, 99.6% [15]. Sum of free sugars in the diet through consumed quantities of relevant sugar-containing foods: 4.8 g (from 60 g papaya) + 9 g (from 60 g banana) + 10.8 g (from 120 mL orange) + 4.5 g (from 50 g pineapple) + 3 g (from 50 g carrot) + 1.7 g (from 85 g tomato) + 5 g (from 100 mL whole milk) + 9.96 g (from 10 g granulated sugar) = 48.76 g.

References

1. World Health Organization (WHO). *Global Status Report on Alcohol and Health*; World Health Organization: Geneva, Switzerland, 2018.
2. Lachenmeier, D.W.; Neufeld, M.; Rehm, J. The Impact of Unrecorded Alcohol Use on Health: What Do We Know in 2020? *J. Stud. Alcohol Drugs* **2021**, *82*, 28–41. [CrossRef]
3. Laranjeira, R.; Pinsky, I.; Zaleski, M.; Caetano, R. I Levantamento Nacional Sobre Os Padrões de Consumo de Álcool Na População Brasileira. Available online: https://bvsms.saude.gov.br/bvs/publicacoes/relatorio_padroes_consumo_alcool.pdf (accessed on 8 February 2024).
4. Babor, T.F.; Casswell, S.; Graham, K.; Huckle, T.; Livingston, M.; Österberg, E.; Rehm, J.; Room, R.; Rossow, I.; Sornpaisarn, B. *Alcohol: No Ordinary Commodity: Research and Public Policy*; Oxford University Press: Oxford, UK, 2022; ISBN 978-0-19-192718-8.
5. Duailibi, S.; Laranjeira, R. Políticas Públicas Relacionadas Às Bebidas Alcoólicas. *Rev. Saúde Pública* **2007**, *41*, 839–848. [CrossRef] [PubMed]
6. Centro de informações sobre saúde e álcool (CISA). Álcool e a Saúde Dos Brasileiros: Panorama 2021. Available online: https://cisa.org.br/index.php/biblioteca/downloads/artigo/item/304-panorama2021 (accessed on 15 February 2024).
7. Brasil Decreto No 6.117, de 22 de Maio de 2007. Aprova a Política Nacional Sobre o Álcool, Dispõe Sobre as Medidas Para Redução Do Uso Indevido Do Álcool e Sua Associação Com a Violência e Criminalidade, e Dá Outras Providências. Available online: http://www.planalto.gov.br/ccivil_03/_ato2007-2010/2007/decreto/d6117.htm (accessed on 15 February 2024).
8. Laranjeira, R.; Romano, M. Consenso Brasileiro Sobre Políticas Públicas Do Álcool. *Braz. J. Psychiatry* **2004**, *26*, 68–77. [CrossRef]
9. Giles, L.; Robinson, M.; Beeston, C. *Minimum Unit Pricing (MUP) for Alcohol Evaluation. Sales-Based Consumption: A Descriptive Analysis of One-Year Post-MUP Off-Trade Alcohol Sales Data*; NHS Health Scotland: Edinburgh, UK, 2019.
10. O'Donnell, A.; Anderson, P.; Jané-Llopis, E.; Manthey, J.; Kaner, E.; Rehm, J. Immediate Impact of Minimum Unit Pricing on Alcohol Purchases in Scotland: Controlled Interrupted Time Series Analysis for 2015–18. *BMJ* **2019**, *366*, l5274. [CrossRef] [PubMed]
11. Rumgay, H.; Shield, K.; Charvat, H.; Ferrari, P.; Sornpaisarn, B.; Obot, I.; Islami, F.; Lemmens, V.E.P.P.; Rehm, J.; Soerjomataram, I. Global Burden of Cancer in 2020 Attributable to Alcohol Consumption: A Population-Based Study. *Lancet Oncol.* **2021**, *22*, 1071–1080. [CrossRef]
12. World Health Organization (WHO). No Level of Alcohol Consumption Is Safe for Our Health. Available online: https://www.who.int/europe/news/item/04-01-2023-no-level-of-alcohol-consumption-is-safe-for-our-health (accessed on 15 February 2024).
13. Associação Brasileira de Supermercados (ABRAS). Líderes de Vendas 2019. Bebidas. *SuperHiper* **2019**, *513*, 116.
14. Ministry of Health of Brazil. Dietary Guidelines for the Brazilian Population. Available online: https://bvsms.saude.gov.br/bvs/publicacoes/dietary_guidelines_brazilian_population.pdf (accessed on 15 February 2024).
15. TBCA. Tabela Brasileira de Composição de Alimentos. Versão 7.1. Available online: http://www.tbca.net.br/ (accessed on 15 February 2024).
16. *Instrução Normativa-IN Nº 75*; Agência Nacional de Vigilância Sanitária (ANVISA)/Ministry of Health: Brasília, Brazil, 8 October 2020.
17. Institute of Medicine. *Dietary Reference Intakes: The Essential Guide to Nutrient Requirements*; The National Academies Press: Washington, DC, USA, 2006.
18. World Health Organization (WHO). Healthy Diet. Available online: https://www.who.int/news-room/fact-sheets/detail/healthy-diet (accessed on 15 February 2024).
19. de Almeida, C.O.; da Costa Vilar, L.; da Silva Souza, L.F.; Reinhardt, D.H. Macedo Peso Médio Do Abacaxi No Brasil: Um Tema Em Discussão. *Bahia Agríc.* **2004**, *6*, 41–46.
20. Companhia de Entrepostos e Armazéns Gerais de São Paulo (CEAGESP). Cartilha Técnica: A Medida Das Hortaliças. Available online: https://ceagesp.gov.br/wp-content/uploads/2021/01/medidaHortalicas.pdf (accessed on 15 February 2024).
21. Ministry of Health of Brazil. Guia Alimentar Para a População Brasileira: Promovendo a Alimentação Saudável. Available online: https://bvsms.saude.gov.br/bvs/publicacoes/guia_alimentar_populacao_brasileira_2008.pdf (accessed on 5 April 2024).
22. IBGE. IBGE Releases per Capita Household Income for 2021. Available online: https://agenciadenoticias.ibge.gov.br/en/agencia-press-room/2185-news-agency/releases-en/33047-ibge-divulga-o-rendimento-domiciliar-per-capita-para-2022 (accessed on 15 February 2024).
23. IBGE. IBGE Releases Per Capita Household Income for 2020. Available online: https://agenciadenoticias.ibge.gov.br/en/agencia-press-room/2185-news-agency/releases-en/30139-ibge-divulga-o-rendimento-domiciliar-per-capita-2021 (accessed on 15 February 2024).
24. IBGE. Inflation Rises 0.73% in December, Closes 2021 with Rise of 10.06%. Available online: https://agenciadenoticias.ibge.gov.br/en/agencia-news/2184-news-agency/news/32734-inflation-rises-0-73-in-december-closes-2021-with-rise-of-10-06 (accessed on 15 February 2024).
25. IBGE. Inflation Accelerates in December and Hits 4.52% in 2020, Biggest Increase Since 2016. Available online: https://agenciadenoticias.ibge.gov.br/en/agencia-news/2184-news-agency/news/29885-inflation-accelerates-in-december-and-hits-4-52-in-2020-biggest-increase-since-2016 (accessed on 15 February 2024).
26. Pereira, E.V.S.; Oliveira, S.P.A.; Nóbrega, I.C.C.; Lachenmeier, D.W.; Araújo, A.C.P.; Telles, D.L.; Silva, M. Brazilian Vodkas Have Undetectable Levels of Ethyl Carbamate. *Quím. Nova* **2013**, *36*, 822–825. [CrossRef]

27. US Food and Drug Administration (FDA). Fruits. Nutrition Facts. Raw, Edible Weight Portion. Available online: https://www.fda.gov/food/food-labeling-nutrition/raw-fruits-poster-text-version-accessible-version (accessed on 15 February 2024).
28. US Food and Drug Administration (FDA). Vegetables. Nutrition Facts, Raw, Edible Weight Portion. Available online: https://www.fda.gov/food/food-labeling-nutrition/nutrition-information-raw-vegetables (accessed on 15 February 2024).
29. US Department of Agriculture (USDA). Milk, Whole, 3.25% Milkfat. Available online: https://fdc.nal.usda.gov/fdc-app.html#/food-details/746782/nutrients (accessed on 15 February 2024).
30. Copagaz. Quanto tempo dura um botijão de gás? Como Calcular. Available online: https://www.copagaz.com.br/blog/quanto-tempo-dura-um-botijao-de-gas/ (accessed on 8 February 2024).
31. Procon. Pesquisa de Preço Do Gás de Cozinha. 2020. Available online: https://www.joaopessoa.pb.gov.br/wp-content/uploads/2020/08/PESQUISAGAS.pdf (accessed on 2 April 2024).
32. Procon. Pesquisa de Preço Do Gás de Cozinha. 2021. Available online: https://www.joaopessoa.pb.gov.br/wp-content/uploads/2021/08/TABELAGASDECOZINHA.pdf (accessed on 2 April 2024).
33. GBD 2016 Alcohol Collaborators Alcohol Use and Burden for 195 Countries and Territories, 1990-2016: A Systematic Analysis for the Global Burden of Disease Study 2016. *Lancet* **2018**, *392*, 1015–1035. [CrossRef]
34. World Health Organization (WHO). Global Strategy to Reduce the Harmful Use of Alcohol. Available online: https://www.who.int/publications/i/item/9789241599931 (accessed on 15 February 2024).
35. Abramson, C.I.; Howard, W.; Zolna, M.; Nain, S.; Aquino, I.S.; Rocha, H.; Moraes, Z.; Page, M.M. A Price Survey Comparison of Alcoholic Beverages with the Five Basic Food Groups in Paraiba, Brazil. *J. Soc. Sci.* **2006**, *2*, 100–103. [CrossRef]
36. IBGE. Households with up to 2 Minimum Wages Spend 61% of Budget with Food, Housing. Available online: https://agenciadenoticias.ibge.gov.br/en/agencia-news/2184-news-agency/news/25637-households-with-up-to-2-minimum-wages-spend-61-of-budget-with-food-housing (accessed on 15 February 2024).
37. Plens, J.A.; Valente, J.Y.; Mari, J.J.; Ferrari, G.; Sanchez, Z.M.; Rezende, L.F.M. Patterns of Alcohol Consumption in Brazilian Adults. *Sci. Rep.* **2022**, *12*, 8603. [CrossRef] [PubMed]
38. Ministério da Agricultura, Pecuária e Abastecimento (MAPA) Resolução N° 1, de 9 de Janeiro de 2003. Available online: https://www.defesa.agricultura.sp.gov.br/legislacoes/resolucao-dipoa-1-de-09-01-2003,743.html (accessed on 5 April 2024).
39. Philippi, S.T. *Nutrição e Técnica Dietética*, 4th ed.; Manole: São Paulo, Brazil, 2019.
40. Ornellas, L.H. *Técnica Dietética: Seleção e Preparo de Alimentos*, 8th ed.; Atheneu: São Paulo, Brazil, 2013; ISBN 978-85-7454-092-4.

nutrients

MDPI

Article

Estimation of the Impact of Abdominal Adipose Tissue (Subcutaneous and Visceral) on the Occurrence of Carbohydrate and Lipid Metabolism Disorders in Patients with Obesity—A Pilot Study

Katarzyna Witczak-Sawczuk [1], Lucyna Ostrowska [1,*], Urszula Cwalina [2], Joanna Leszczyńska [1], Marta Jastrzębska-Mierzyńska [1] and Marcin Krzysztof Hładuński [3]

1 Department of Dietetics and Clinical Nutrition, Medical University of Bialystok, ul. Mieszka I 4 B, 15-054 Bialystok, Poland; katarzyna.witczak-sawczuk@umb.edu.pl (K.W.-S.)

2 Department of Biostatistics and Medical Informatics, Medical University of Bialystok, ul. Szpitalna 37, 15-295 Bialystok, Poland

3 Independent Laboratory of Molecular Imaging, Medical University of Bialystok, ul. Zurawia 71A, 15-540 Bialystok, Poland

* Correspondence: lucyna.ostrowska@umb.edu.pl

Abstract: Obesity represents a significant global public health concern. The excessive accumulation of abdominal adipose tissue is often implicated in the development of metabolic complications associated with obesity. Our study aimed to investigate the impact of particular deposits of abdominal adipose tissue on the occurrence of carbohydrate and lipid metabolism complications. We established cut-off points for visceral adipose tissue (VAT), subcutaneous adipose tissue (SAT), and the VAT/SAT ratio at which selected metabolic complications of obesity-related diseases (disorders of carbohydrate and/or lipid metabolism) occur. We conducted an observational study involving 91 subjects with first- and second-degree obesity, accounting for gender differences. Anthropometric measurements were taken, body composition analysis (BIA) was conducted, and biochemical determinations were made. Our findings suggest that commonly used parameters for assessing early metabolic risk, such as BMI or waist circumference, may overlook the significant factor of body fat distribution, as well as gender differences. Both visceral and subcutaneous adipose tissue were found to be important in estimating metabolic risk. We identified the cut-off points in women in terms of their elevated fasting glucose levels and the presence of insulin resistance (HOMA-IR: homeostasis model assessment of insulin resistance) based on SAT, VAT, and the VAT/SAT ratio. In men, cut-off points were determined for the presence of insulin resistance (HOMA-IR) based on VAT and the VAT/SAT ratio. However, the results regarding lipid disorders were inconclusive, necessitating further investigation of a larger population.

Keywords: adipose tissue; obesity; metabolic risk

1. Introduction

Obesity currently stands as a prominent worldwide public health issue. The World Health Organization defines it as a complex condition associated with the abnormal buildup of excess fat in the human body, significantly elevating the likelihood of various non-communicable diseases [1]. This condition is chronic and progressive, lacking spontaneous resolution, and is characterized by a tendency to recur [2].

Visceral fat tissue is often implicated as a key factor in the onset of metabolic complications associated with obesity [3]. This is attributed to the higher concentrations of angiotensinogen (a precursor to angiotensin) and leptin (a hormone regulating appetite) found in subcutaneous fat tissue [4,5]. In contrast, visceral fat tissue is characterized by elevated lipolytic activity, resulting in the release of significant amounts of free fatty acids (FFAs), increased gluconeogenesis, and heightened secretion of pro-inflammatory adipokines such as interleukin 6 (IL-6), resistin, visfatin, and TNF-α [5]. The current scientific findings indicate that visceral distribution of adipose tissue is associated with an increased risk of metabolic disorders, including abnormalities in carbohydrate metabolism such as insulin resistance and/or hyperglycemia. These conditions may lead to the development of type 2 diabetes, hypertension, or ischemic heart disease [6]. Consequently, visceral adipose tissue (VAT) is now acknowledged as more metabolically active and poses a greater metabolic and inflammatory risk compared to subcutaneous adipose tissue (SAT) [7–9]. However, it is essential to note that the distribution of fat tissue can vary among individuals. Additionally, subcutaneous fat tissue may exist as a superficial layer (SSAT) or a deep layer (DSAT), which shares metabolic similarities with visceral fat tissue [10].

In 2009, researchers, utilizing body scanning diagnostic techniques, illustrated the lack of consistency and predictability in the distribution of fat tissue. They observed that in a portion of the population, adipose tissue is predominantly located in the visceral area, with only limited subcutaneous presence. Conversely, another group of individuals exhibited a substantial deposit of subcutaneous fat and a minimal amount of visceral fat [11]. The reasons behind such a varied distribution of adipose tissue in the population, whether modifiable or non-modifiable, have yet to be fully understood. The author's own research has delved into an investigation of whether and to what extent individual deposits of adipose tissue influence the occurrence of disorders in carbohydrate and lipid metabolism, both in women and men.

The author's research examined the impact of individual deposits of abdominal fat tissue, including visceral and subcutaneous fat, as well as the VAT/SAT ratio, on the development of specific complications in carbohydrate and lipid metabolism. The study aimed to determine the threshold levels of visceral and subcutaneous fat tissue and the VAT/SAT ratio at which the onset of selected obesity-related complications is observed.

2. Materials and Methods

This study was the result of a research project that was registered at www.clinicaltrials.gov under the number NCT05612282; (accessed on 11 April 2022).

2.1. Ethics

The research procedure was approved by the Bioethics Committee of the Medical University of Białystok, approval numbers R-I-002/442/2015 and APK.002.528.2022. Each patient qualified for the study received detailed information about the course of the study and signed informed consent to participate in the study.

2.2. Study Principants

The observational study comprised a total of 91 individuals with obesity class I and II, based on their BMI. Among them, 64.8% were women (n = 59), and 35.2% were men (n = 32). All the participants met the complete inclusion criteria for the study, and no exclusion criteria were identified. The research project enrolled individuals of both genders, aged 20–65, with primary obesity (BMI $\geq$ 30 kg/m^2–$\leq$39.99 kg/m^2). The exclusion criteria included secondary obesity, a BMI $\geq$ 40 kg/m^2, previous surgical interventions for obesity, and having undergone other surgical procedures (at least 3 months prior). Additionally, the exclusion criteria included those with type 2 diabetes or insulin resistance (previously diagnosed or identified during therapy), hormonal disorders, hormonal contraception or hormone replacement therapy, prior oral steroid therapy, antiretroviral therapy, eating disorders, aggravated coronary heart disease, patients with pacemakers, and pregnant or lactating women.

2.3. Antropometric Parameters

The assessment of body weight involved the use of an electronic RADWAG medical scale equipped with a height meter (WPT 60/150 OW). The patients' heights were measured with a 0.1 cm margin of error, and body weight was measured with a 0.1 kg margin of error. To ensure accurate measurements, the patients were requested to remove their shoes and outer clothing.

Subsequently, the body mass index (BMI) was individually calculated for each patient by dividing their body weight, expressed in kilograms, by their height, expressed in meters squared. In accordance with the inclusion criteria, patients with a BMI ranging from $\geq$30 kg/m^2 to $\leq$39.9 kg/m^2 were deemed eligible for the study [12,13].

The waist circumference measurements were conducted using a metric tape with an accuracy of 0.5 cm. The waist circumference measurements were taken midway between the lower costal arch and the upper edge of the ilium in the mid-axillary line, and the results were expressed in centimeters [3,13].

2.4. Body Analysis

The body composition analysis utilized the bioelectrical impedance method (BIA) using a BioScan 920-2 device (Essex, UK). Each patient received information regarding the necessary criteria for study inclusion—the analysis was conducted on an empty stomach with the bladder emptied 30 min prior to the examination; a 12 h refrain from physical activity was required prior to the examination; the elimination of alcohol and caffeinated beverages from the diet 24 h before the examination was recommended; individuals with a pacemaker were excluded from participation [14].

To determine the areas of subcutaneous and visceral fat tissue, the BIA method was employed using the BioScan 920-2 device (Essex, UK), and the following measurements were estimated [14]:

- Visceral fat tissue area (cm^2) at the height of the measurement (at the navel);
- Subcutaneous fat tissue area (cm^2) at the height of the measurement (at the navel);
- VAT/SAT ratio—the ratio of visceral fat tissue to subcutaneous fat tissue.

The obtained results were processed using the Maltron BioScan 920 v1.1 software.

2.5. Biochemical Analysis

The evaluation of specific biochemical parameters for each participant was performed once at the Medical Laboratory within the University Clinical Hospital in Białystok in accordance with the established standards. Venous blood (15 mL) was collected from the antecubital vein. Following the collection, the blood underwent centrifugation to obtain serum. The concentrations of the following parameters were assessed in the blood serum: fasting glucose, fasting insulin, total cholesterol, LDL fraction cholesterol, HDL fraction cholesterol, and triglycerides. The reference values for fasting insulin concentration were set at <10 mU/mL. The fasting glucose and fasting insulin results were used to calculate the homeostasis model assessment of insulin resistance (HOMA-IR) (fasting insulin concentration (mU/mL) $\times$ fasting glucose concentration (mmol/L)/22.5). HOMA-IR values ≥ 2 indicated tissue resistance to insulin. This parameter was used to assess the occurrence of insulin resistance and, consequently, to assess the risk of developing metabolic syndrome [15]. To determine the non-HDL cholesterol fraction, the following mathematical operation was performed: total cholesterol concentration—HDL fraction cholesterol [16].

2.6. Statistical Analysis

The statistical analysis of the collected data was conducted using the STATISTICA 13.3 program (StatSoft, Kraków, Poland). The participants were categorized into groups based on their gender. The study variables were described using medians and the first and third quartiles. Given the non-normal distribution of the data, non-parametric statistical methods were employed, with the normality assessed using the Shapiro–Wilk test. Spearman's correlation coefficient was utilized to assess the relationships between quantitative variables. Cut-off points were determined for the visceral fat tissue area (evaluated at the level of the navel), subcutaneous fat tissue area (also assessed at the level of the navel), and the VAT/SAT ratio concerning all the examined biochemical parameters in the participants. The relationship between the continuous and binary variables was explored using ROC curves. The selection of the most accurate predictors involved assessing the AUC (Area Under the Curve) values.

The optimal cut-off points were identified using the tangent method and Youden's index. For all the results obtained in this study, $p < 0.05$ was considered statistically significant.

3. Results

3.1. Characteristics of the Study Group of Men and Women in Terms of Anthropometric Parameters

The research comprised 59 female and 32 male participants. The median age of the study group was 47 years for women and 42 years for men. Approximately 75% of the female participants had class I obesity, whereas among the male participants, 50% had class I obesity, and the other 50% had class II obesity. The characteristics of both the female and male participants concerning the selected anthropometric parameters and their body composition are detailed in Table 1.

Table 1. Participant characteristics.

	n	Age Me (Q1–Q3)	Body Weight Me (Q1–Q3)	BMI Me (Q1–Q3)	WC Me (Q1–Q3)	BF (kg) Me (Q1–Q3)	PBF (%) Me (Q1–Q3)	VAT (cm^2) Me (Q1–Q3)	SAT (cm^2) Me (Q1–Q3)	VAT/SAT Me (Q1–Q3)
Women	59	47.0 (39.0–57.0)	90.0 (84.5–96.7)	33.6 (32.0–35.1)	109.0 (104.0–115.0)	39.9 (35.7–43.6)	43.9 (42.2–46.2)	198.0 (148.0–262.0)	112.0 (101.0–136.0)	1.70 (1.28–2.08)
Men	32	42.0 (36.5–48.5)	115.0 (103.5–124.0)	35.2 (32.3–37.3)	120.0 (113.2–123.5)	40.2 (33.5–44.2)	34.4 (32.5–37.0)	231.5 (183.5–324.0)	113.0 (101.5–134.5)	2.09 (1.70–2.43)

BMI—body mass index; Me—median; Q1—quartile 1; Q3—quartile 3; WC—waist circumference; BF—body fat; PBF—percentage of body fat; VAT—visceral adipose tissue; SAT—subcutaneous adipose tissue; VAT/SAT—visceral-to-subcutaneous-fat ratio.

Analyzing the impact of the studied factors on the carbohydrate metabolism parameters (Table 2) revealed that in women, an increase in fasting glucose concentration correlated with higher values for age (r = 0.41, $p = 0.001$), body weight (r = 0.25, $p = 0.04$), waist circumference (r = 0.28, $p = 0.02$), total body fat (r = 0.28, $p = 0.03$), percentage of adipose tissue (r = 0.32, $p = 0.01$), visceral adipose area at the umbilicus (r = 0.26, $p = 0.04$), and subcutaneous adipose area at the umbilicus (r = 0.26, $p = 0.04$). Conversely, in men, only age significantly influenced fasting glucose (r = 0.41, $p = 0.01$). No significant effect of the studied parameters on the fasting insulin concentrations was observed in women, whereas in men, their fasting insulin concentration increased with a higher body weight (r = 0.35, $p = 0.04$), BMI (r = 0.37, $p = 0.03$), waist circumference (r = 0.35, $p = 0.04$), and total body fat (r = 0.36, $p = 0.04$). Furthermore, in women, their HOMA-IR values were significantly influenced by percentage of adipose tissue (r = 0.29, $p = 0.02$) and subcutaneous adipose area (r = 0.27, $p = 0.03$), whereas no such correlations were observed in men.

Additionally, it was noted (Table 3) that in women, the VAT area (r = −0.32, $p = 0.01$) and the VAT/SAT ratio (r = −0.32, $p = 0.01$) were associated with reduced HDL cholesterol concentrations, while an increase in triglycerides was linked to an increase in the VAT area (r = 0.26, $p = 0.04$). However, no such correlations were evident in men.

Table 2. Assessment of the correlation between age and specific anthropometric and body composition parameters among patients and carbohydrate metabolism parameters.

		Age	Body Weight	BMI	WC	BF (kg)	PBF (%)	VAT (cm^2)	SAT (cm^2)	VAT/SAT
	WOMEN									
Fasting glucose	r	0.41 *	0.25 *	0.24	0.28 *	0.28 *	0.32 *	0.26 *	0.26 *	0.16
	p	0.001	0.04	0.06	0.02	0.03	0.01	0.04	0.04	0.19
Fasting insulin	r	0.16	0.04	0.08	0.10	0.07	0.24	0.14	0.24	0.08
	p	0.21	0.74	0.52	0.40	0.56	0.06	0.27	0.06	0.52
HOMA-IR	r	0.23	0.08	0.11	0.14	0.12	0.29 *	0.18	0.27 *	0.11
	p	0.07	0.55	0.37	0.28	0.35	0.02	0.16	0.03	0.38
	MEN									
Fasting glucose	r	0.41 *	−0.26	−0.12	−0.14	−0.15	0.00	0.10	−0.10	0.07
	p	0.01	0.13	0.48	0.41	0.40	0.98	0.95	0.56	0.69
Fasting insulin	r	0.01	0.35 *	0.37 *	0.35 *	0.36 *	0.23	0.25	0.23	0.14
	p	0.93	0.04	0.03	0.04	0.04	0.20	0.16	0.18	0.43
HOMA-IR	r	0.13	0.18	0.23	0.23	0.22	0.19	0.26	0.21	0.15
	p	0.45	0.31	0.19	0.18	0.22	0.29	0.14	0.22	0.38

* $p < 0.05$,—statistically significant; BMI—body mass index; WC—waist circumference; BF—body fat; PBF—percentage of body fat; VAT—visceral adipose tissue; SAT—subcutaneous adipose tissue; VAT/SAT—visceral-to-subcutaneous-fat ratio; HOMA-IR—homeostasis model assessment of insulin resistance.

Table 3. Evaluation of the association between age and specific anthropometric parameters and body composition among patients and lipid metabolism parameters.

		Age	Body Weight	BMI	WC	BF (kg)	PBF (%)	VAT (cm^2)	SAT (cm^2)	VAT/SAT
	WOMEN									
Total cholesterol	r	0.19	−0.07	−0.01	0.05	0.02	0.12	0.08	0.05	0.05
	p	0.13	0.57	0.88	0.68	0.85	0.33	0.52	0.70	0.70
LDL-C	r	0.05	0.00	0.02	0.02	0.05	0.07	0.11	0.08	0.04
	p	0.69	0.95	0.83	0.84	0.69	0.57	0.39	0.54	0.73
HDL-C	r	−0.09	−0.12	−0.07	−0.06	−0.17	−0.20	−0.32 *	−0.12	−0.32 *
	p	0.46	0.34	0.58	0.60	0.19	0.11	0.01	0.33	0.01
Non-HDL-C	r	0.19	−0.05	0.01	0.05	0.05	0.17	0.14	0.07	0.12
	p	0.13	0.69	0.92	0.68	0.65	0.17	0.26	0.56	0.34
Triglycerydes (TGs)	r	0.16	0.06	0.11	0.12	0.13	0.18	0.26 *	0.09	0.23
	p	0.20	0.61	0.38	0.32	0.32	0.15	0.04	0.48	0.07
	MEN									
Total cholesterol	r	0.32	−0.15	−0.08	−0.04	0.01	0.12	−0.00	0.14	−0.03
	p	0.07	0.41	0.66	0.72	0.92	0.52	0.99	0.43	0.83
LDL-C	r	0.20	0.01	−0.05	0.03	0.09	0.09	0.00	0.13	−0.11
	p	0.27	0.92	0.77	0.82	0.61	0.62	0.99	0.45	0.51
HDL-C	r	−0.00	−0.21	−0.04	−0.14	−0.09	−0.05	−0.25	−0.19	−0.10
	p	0.99	0.23	0.81	0.43	0.62	0.75	0.15	0.28	0.55
Non-HDL-C	r	0.32	−0.07	−0.02	0.02	0.08	0.17	0.05	0.20	−0.03
	p	0.06	0.70	0.87	0.90	0.65	0.36	0.77	0.28	0.84
Triglycerydes (TGs)	r	0.27	−0.01	0.01	0.03	0.01	0.07	0.22	0.14	0.29
	p	0.12	0.93	0.95	0.85	0.94	0.69	0.21	0.43	0.10

* $p < 0.05$,—statistically significant; BMI—body mass index; WC—waist circumference; BF—body fat; PBF—percentage of body fat; VAT—visceral adipose tissue; SAT—subcutaneous adipose tissue; VAT/SAT—visceral-to-subcutaneous-fat ratio; LDL—low-density lipoprotein; HDL—high-density lipoprotein.

3.2. Estimation of Cut-Off Points for the Area of Visceral and/or Subcutaneous Adipose Tissue at Which Selected Parameters of Carbohydrate and/or Lipid Metabolism Occurred in Obese Participants

In the subsequent phase of the study, an effort was made to determine the cut-off values for the visceral adipose area measured at the umbilicus level beyond which disorders in selected parameters of carbohydrate and/or lipid metabolism occurred in the obese patients. Likewise, the cut-off values for the subcutaneous adipose tissue area measured at the umbilicus level and the VAT/SAT ratio were analyzed. The findings are detailed in Tables 4 and 5 and Figures 1–6.

Upon evaluating the cut-off values for visceral adipose tissue and the examined parameters among the female cohort, it was determined that the threshold for insulin resistance (HOMA-IR) was 168 cm^2, while for abnormally elevated fasting blood glucose, it was 240 cm^2. The cut-off value for visceral adipose tissue and decreased HDL cholesterol concentration was identified as 1194 cm^2, whereas for elevated serum triglycerides, it was 199 cm^2. These findings are illustrated in Figure 1.

In women, it was determined that the cut-off for the subcutaneous adipose area (as depicted in Figure 2) measured at the umbilicus was 117 cm^2 for elevated fasting glucose concentration, 111 cm^2 for a fasting insulin concentration $\geq$ 10 mU/mL, 109 cm^2 for the presence of insulin resistance (HOMA-IR), and 108 cm^2 for a reduced HDL cholesterol fraction concentration.

Table 4. VAT, SAT, and VAT/SAT ratio cut-off points at which increased values of selected carbohydrate metabolism parameters in the studied groups of women and men were detected.

	WOMEN	
VAT	SAT	V/S ratio
glucose AUC = 0.774 cut-off point = 240 cm^2	glucose AUC = 0.686 cut-off point = 117 cm^2	glucose AUC = 0.695 cut-off point = 1.55
HOMA-IR AUC = 0.682 cut-off point = 168 cm^2	insulin AUC = 0.675 cut-off point = 111 cm^2	
	HOMA-IR AUC = 0.799 cut-off point = 109 cm^2	
	MEN	
VAT	SAT	V/S ratio
insulin AUC = 0.875 cut-off point = 231 cm^2		insulin AUC = 0.850 cut-off point = 1.939
HOMA-IR AUC = 0.859 cut-off point = 168 cm^2		HOMA-IR AUC = 0.872 cut-off point = 1.876

Figure 3 illustrates the estimated threshold values for the VAT/SAT ratio in women with elevated fasting glucose levels (1.55), reduced HDL cholesterol fraction levels (1.79), and elevated serum triglycerides (1.95).

Determining the cut-off values for visceral adipose tissue and the measured parameters in the male cohort revealed that it was 231 cm^2 for a fasting insulin concentration of $\geq$10 mU/mL, 168 cm^2 for the presence of insulin resistance, and 194 cm^2 for the presence of hypertriglyceridemia. These findings are depicted in Figure 4.

Table 5. VAT, SAT, and VAT/SAT ratio cut-off points at which increased values of selected lipid metabolism parameters in the studied groups of women and men were detected.

WOMEN		
VAT	SAT	V/S Ratio
HDL-C AUC = 0.800 cut-off point = 194 cm^2	HDL-C AUC = 0.664 cut-off point = 108 cm^2	HDL-C AUC = 0.745 cut-off point = 1.79
TGs AUC = 0.716 cut-off point = 199 cm^2		TGs AUC = 0.715 cut-off point = 1.935
MEN		
VAT	SAT	V/S ratio
TGs AUC = 0.765 cut-off point = 168.50 cm^2	non-HDL-C AUC = 0.790 cut-off point = 115 cm^2	TGs AUC = 0.753 cut-off point = 1.64
	LDL—C AUC = 0.659 cut-off point = 133 cm^2	

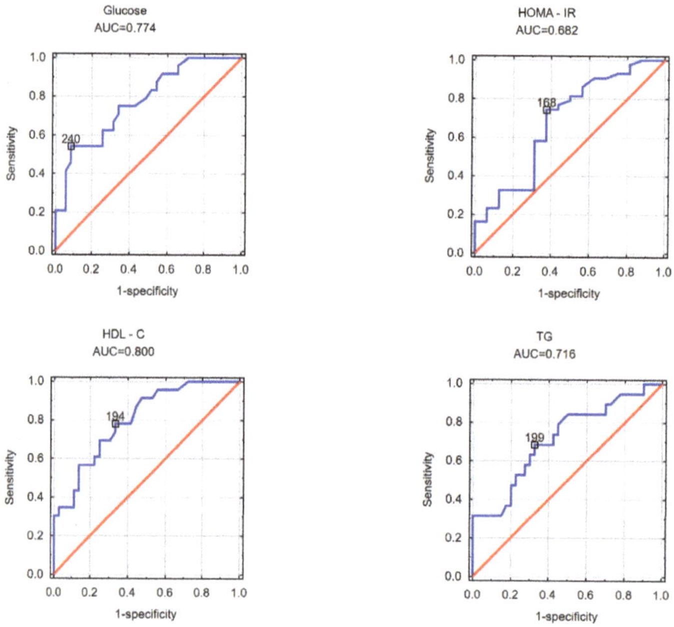

Figure 1. Cut-off points of the visceral fat tissue area estimated at the navel at which increased fasting glucose levels, increased HOMA-IR values, decreased HDL cholesterol levels, and increased triglyceride levels were observed in the study group of women.

Figure 5 displays the estimated cut-off points for the subcutaneous adipose tissue (SAT) area in men for elevated non-HDL cholesterol (115 cm^2) and for elevated LDL cholesterol fractions (133 cm^2).

In the male group, cut-off points for the VAT/SAT ratio were determined for the presence of hypertriglyceridemia (1.64), for the presence of insulin resistance (1.876), and for a fasting insulin concentration $\geq$ 10 mU/mL (1.939). These results are illustrated in Figure 6.

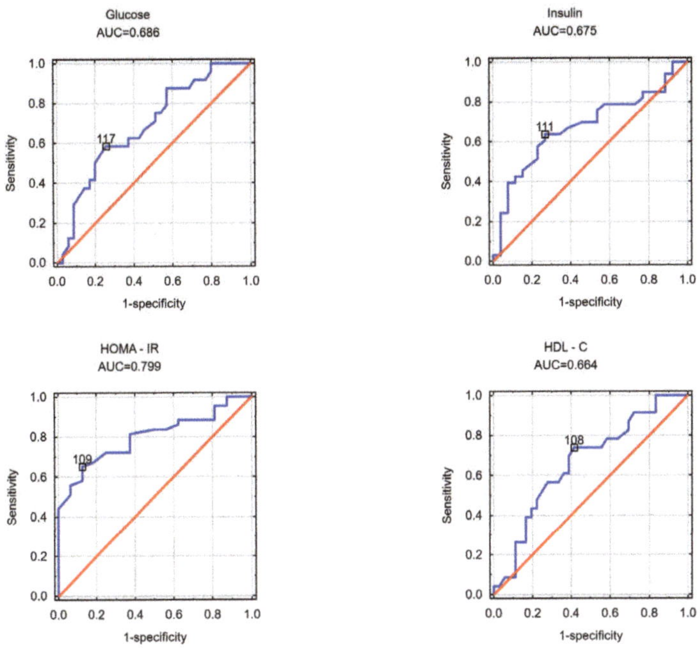

Figure 2. Illustrates the threshold values of the subcutaneous adipose area estimated at the navel, where elevated fasting glucose levels, heightened fasting insulin levels, increased HOMA-IR values, and reduced HDL cholesterol levels were observed in the female cohort.

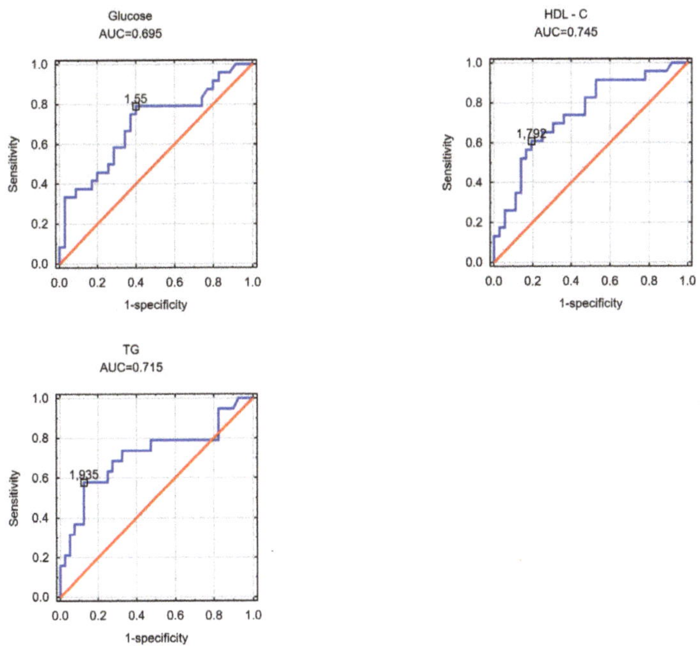

Figure 3. VAT/SAT ratio cut-off points at which increased fasting glucose levels, decreased HDL cholesterol levels and increased triglyceride levels in the study group of women were detected.

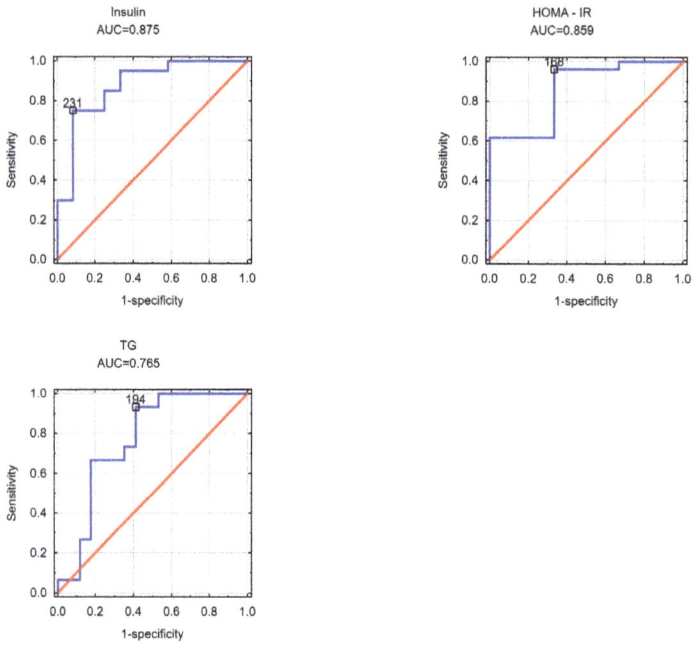

Figure 4. Cut-off points of the visceral adipose tissue area estimated at the navel at which increased fasting insulin levels, an elevated HOMA-IR index, and elevated triglyceride levels were observed in the study group of men.

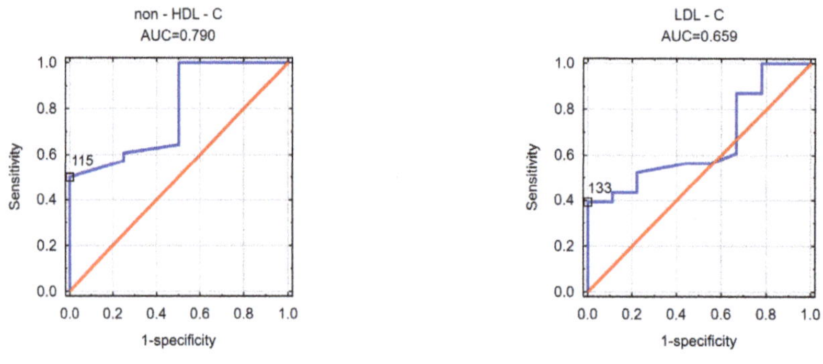

Figure 5. Cut-off points of the subcutaneous adipose tissue area estimated at the navel at which an increased non-HDL cholesterol fraction and an increased LDL cholesterol fraction were observed in the male cohort.

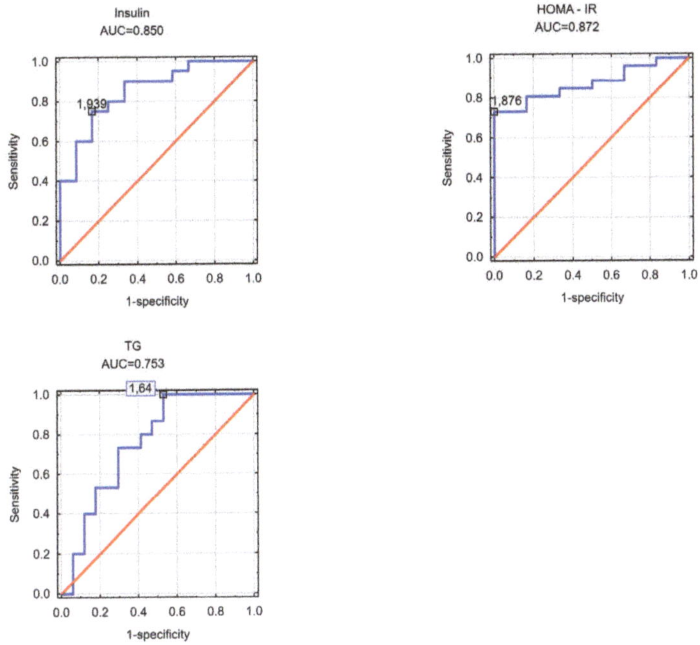

Figure 6. VAT/SAT ratio cut-off points at which increased fasting insulin concentration, elevated HOMA-IR index values, and elevated triglyceride concentrations were observed in the male cohort.

4. Discussion

Obesity presents as a significant independent risk factor for metabolic complications [17]. Central to obesity is the excessive buildup of adipose tissue due to a positive energy balance [18,19]. It is essential to recognize that adipose tissue functions as an endocrine organ, prone to significant proliferation, potentially comprising a substantial portion of human body weight, even up to 70% [20]. The surplus accumulation of adipose tissue increases the risk of chronic ailments, including cardiovascular diseases, disturbances in carbohydrate metabolism, cancer (especially gastrointestinal-related types), and joint disorders (largely attributed to mechanical stress on the joints) [18].

Until recently, obesity was categorized into gynoid and android types based on fat distribution. Gynoid obesity primarily involves fat accumulation in the gluteal–femoral region [19,21]. Conversely, android (central) obesity is characterized by abdominal fat accumulation, which is often implicated in the onset of metabolic disorders [21]. Adipose tissue located centrally is further classified into subcutaneous and visceral compartments. Visceral adipose tissue in particular has been consistently identified as a contributor to the development of metabolic complications associated with obesity [19]. Given this context, it is logical to explore the question of the factors contributing to the development of obesity-related complications, with a specific focus on the role of different adipose tissue distributions. Hence, it becomes essential to analyze abdominal adipose tissue deposits separately, distinguishing between visceral and subcutaneous fat.

The body mass index (BMI) is the most commonly utilized parameter for diagnosing obesity and in obesity-related research. However, despite its consideration of body weight and height, BMI has limitations as a predictor of metabolic disorder risk. These limitations stem from its failure to account for adipose tissue content and distribution, which are recognized as significant predictors of metabolic complications associated with obesity. While an updated version of the obesity diagnosis criteria based on BMI was introduced by the American Endocrine Societies in 2016, it primarily focused on specific complications rather than their risk factors [22]. Moreover, Stoklossa et al. observed that BMI overestimated the lean body mass in patients with a BMI > 35 kg/m^2 when using body composition assessment according to bioelectrical impedance analysis (BIA). In contrast, assessments using dual-energy X-ray absorptiometry (DXA) yielded more accurate and reliable results [23].

Waist circumference serves as a crucial parameter acknowledged by the WHO for assessing abdominal obesity and the heightened risk of developing metabolic disorders in individuals with obesity [3]. However, it is noteworthy that the standards for this parameter are rather diverse. According to the IDF, the presence of central obesity is indicated by waist circumferences $\geq$ 80 cm in women and $\geq$94 cm in men. Nevertheless, these values do not provide insight into the obesity phenotype [24]. It might be more appropriate to evaluate waist circumference based on the NCEP-ATP III criteria, which incorporate higher thresholds for women ($\geq$88 cm) and men ($\geq$102 cm) [25]. However, even with an adjustment in the reference values for waist circumference, differences in the distribution of visceral and subcutaneous fat within the abdominal cavity remain unaddressed. Therefore, while waist circumference serves as a predictive parameter for metabolic disorder development in obesity, it is prudent to seek more sensitive parameters for estimating metabolic risk in obese individuals.

Our research aimed to identify methods for assessing early metabolic risk in individuals with obesity. We sought to establish the cut-off points for visceral adipose tissue, subcutaneous adipose tissue at the umbilical level, and the VAT/SAT ratio in relation to parameters of carbohydrate and lipid metabolism. The factors contributing to the preferential accumulation of visceral adipose tissue or subcutaneous adipose tissue remain incompletely understood. Therefore, when discussing abdominal obesity and adipose tissue accumulation in the abdominal area, it is prudent to examine which adipose tissue deposits may cause predisposition to the earlier development of metabolic complications associated with obesity. This analysis includes consideration of whether visceral adipose tissue alone, subcutaneous adipose tissue alone (with particular focus on deep subcutaneous adipose tissue), or the ratio between the visceral adipose tissue and the subcutaneous adipose tissue (VAT/SAT ratio) is significant [26,27].

When analyzing the impact of adipose tissue distribution on metabolic disorders, gender is a critical factor to consider. This is particularly pertinent when evaluating parameters such as waist circumference or total body fat percentage, as well as in biochemical analyses like HDL fraction cholesterol. Gender significantly influences the assessment of the risk of specific metabolic complications and guides the selection of therapeutic approaches to the complications arising from obesity [28].

The prevailing studies in the available literature have primarily focused on establishing cut-off points for BMI or waist circumference concerning the risk of metabolic parameter abnormalities [29,30]. Additionally, certain researchers have sought cut-off points for visceral adipose tissue, indicating significant increases in the risk of metabolic complications linked to obesity [31,32]. A notable challenge in comparing these studies with our research lies in the variations in the visceral fat assessment methods (DXA, BIA, CT), leading to different units for estimating its content (cm^2, cm^3, grams). For instance, one study observed that the overall metabolic risk in postmenopausal women escalated with VAT surpassing 117.8 cm^2 [31]. Notably, an insufficient number of analyses determining cut-off points for VAT, SAT, and the VAT/SAT ratio concerning individual obesity-related disorders exists.

According to our study findings, subcutaneous adipose tissue emerges as a significant factor in assessing the risk of developing carbohydrate-related complications in women, with lower cut-off points compared to those for visceral adipose tissue. Specifically, in women, the cut-off point for elevated fasting glucose levels was 117 cm^2 for subcutaneous adipose tissue, whereas for visceral adipose tissue, it was 240 cm^2. Similarly, insulin resistance (HOMA-IR) and abnormal fasting glucose were detected at lower subcutaneous adipose tissue thresholds (109 cm^2) compared to visceral adipose tissue (168 cm^2).

Conversely, in men, visceral fat and its area seem to be associated with the onset of carbohydrate-related complications, and cut-off points for subcutaneous adipose tissue were not established. Notably, the cut-off point for visceral adipose tissue indicating the presence of insulin resistance (HOMA-IR $\geq$ 2) was identical between men and women, at 168 cm^2. The identification of the visceral adipose tissue cut-off point for insulin resistance underscores the significance of this metric in early risk assessment for obesity-related complications in men.

Conversely, for lipid disorders in women, the findings obtained require further clarification through a study involving a larger cohort. In determining the cut-off points for a decreased HDL cholesterol fraction, it was noted that the cut-off point for subcutaneous adipose tissue (108 cm^2) was lower than that for visceral adipose tissue (194 cm^2). However, it was observed that the cut-off point for visceral adipose tissue had a higher AUC (AUC = 0.800) compared to the cut-off point for subcutaneous adipose tissue (AUC = 0.664). Nevertheless, these findings do not provide conclusive evidence. For elevated triglycerides, the cut-off point for visceral adipose tissue was determined to be 199 cm^2, while no statistically significant cut-off point for elevated TGs was identified for subcutaneous adipose tissue. Similarly, in men, the results regarding lipid disorders are inconclusive. It appears that each parameter needs to be individually analyzed. Abnormal triglyceride concentrations in men seem to be associated with visceral adipose tissue accumulation (168.5 cm^2). Conversely, elevated concentrations of non-HDL cholesterol (115 cm^2) and LDL cholesterol (133 cm^2) in men may be linked to subcutaneous adipose tissue distribution. However, these analyses warrant validation in a larger cohort. The study results underscore the importance of considering gender disparities in future investigations, as men and women exhibit variations in the distribution of both subcutaneous and visceral adipose tissue. This is evident from the disparate VAT and SAT cut-off points observed in the analyzed parameters of carbohydrate and lipid disorders.

In our study design, we aimed to develop practical methods for the early detection of metabolic risk applicable in routine patient care. While dual-energy X-ray absorptiometry (DXA) is considered the gold standard for assessing total adipose tissue volume (both subcutaneous and visceral), we opted for bioelectrical impedance analysis (BIA) to evaluate total visceral adipose tissue (VAT) and subcutaneous adipose tissue (SAT) due to its practical feasibility. An important aspect of our research is the gender stratification of the study population given the variations in the total adipose tissue percentage norms and the reference values for the HDL cholesterol concentrations between men and women. However, the small sample sizes, particularly in the male subgroup (n = 32), represent a limitation of this pilot study. Nonetheless, it should be emphasized that this study serves as an initial exploration in this field.

5. Conclusions

The global prevalence of obesity underscores the need for novel, precise parameters to assess early metabolic risk in patients. Current metrics like body mass index (BMI) or waist circumference lack consideration of the adipose tissue distribution and gender disparities. Our study explored the utility of bioelectrical impedance analysis (BIA) of the subcutaneous adipose tissue at the waist height, visceral adipose tissue (VAT), and the VAT/SAT ratio in predicting carbohydrate and lipid disorders. In women, the cut-off points for elevated fasting glucose ($\geq$100 mg/dL) were determined as 117 cm^2 for SAT, 240 cm^2 for VAT, and 1.55 for the VAT/SAT ratio. For a HOMA-IR score $\geq$ 2, the cut-off points were 109 cm^2 for SAT and 168 cm^2 for VAT. Conversely, in men, only the VAT cut-off point for a HOMA-IR score $\geq$2 was established at 168 cm^2 and that for the VAT/SAT ratio at 1.876.

Regarding lipid disorders, the cut-off point for elevated triglyceride levels (>150 mg/dL) was determined to be 199 cm^2 for VAT in women and 168.5 cm^2 in men. Furthermore, the cut-off point for an elevated TG concentration relative to the VAT/SAT ratio was found to be 1.935 in women and 1.64 in men. For reduced HDL-C (<50 mg/dL), the cut-off points were established at 194 cm^2 for VAT, 108 cm^2 for SAT, and 1.79 for the VAT/SAT ratio in women. However, these findings warrant validation through larger-scale studies involving individuals with obesity.

Author Contributions: Conceptualization, K.W.-S. and L.O.; methodology, K.W-S, L.O., U.C. and M.K.H.; software, J.L. and U.C.; validation, K.W.-S. and L.O.; formal analysis, K.W.-S., L.O., U.C., M.J.-M. and J.L.; investigation, K.W.-S., L.O. and M.J.-M.; resources, K.W.-S. and L.O; data curation, K.W.-S.; writing—original draft preparation, K.W.-S., U.C. and L.O.; writing—review and editing, K.W.-S. and L.O.; visualization, K.W.-S.; supervision, L.O.; project administration, K.W.-S. and L.O.; funding acquisition, K.W.-S. and L.O. All authors have read and agreed to the published version of the manuscript.

Funding: The study was funded by the internal sources of the Medical University of Bialystok (project numbers: N/ST/MN/17/003/3316 and B.SUB.23.602).

Institutional Review Board Statement: This study was approved by the local bioethics committee of the Medical University of Białystok, Poland (R-I-002/442/2015, approved on 26 November 2015 and APK.002.528.2022, approved on 16 February 2023).

Informed Consent Statement: Informed consent was obtained from all the subjects involved in this study.

Data Availability Statement: Data are available on request due to privacy/ethics restrictions.

Acknowledgments: The authors thank the participants of the study. Trial registration: ClinicalTrials. gov. Identifier: NCT05612282. (accessed on 11 April 2022).

Conflicts of Interest: The authors declare no conflicts of interest.

References

1. World Health Organization. *WHO European Regional Obesity Report 2022*; WHO Regional Office for Europe: Copenhagen, Denmark, 2022. [CrossRef]
2. Bąk-Sosnowska, M.; Białkowska, M.; Bogdański, P.; Chomiuk, T.; Gałązka-Sobotka, M.; Holecki, M.; Jarosińska, A.; Jezierska, M.; Kamiński, P.; Kłoda, K.; et al. Zalecenia kliniczne dotyczące postępowania u chorych na otyłość 2022—Stanowisko Polskiego Towarzystwa Leczenia Otyłości. *Med. Prakt. Wyd. Specj.* **2022**, *5*, 1–87.
3. World Health Organization. *Waist Circumference and Waist-Hip Ratio: Report of a WHO Expert Consultation, Geneva, 8–11 December 2008*; World Health Organization: Geneva, Switzerland, 2011.
4. Tchkonia, T.; Thomou, T.; Zhu, Y.; Karagiannides, I.; Pothoulakis, C.; Jensen, M.D.; Kirkland, J.L. Mechanisms and Metabolic Implications of Regional Differences among Fat Depots. *Cell Metab.* **2013**, *17*, 644–656. [CrossRef] [PubMed]
5. Berry, D.C.; Stenesen, D.; Zeve, D.; Graff, J.M. The developmental origins of adipose tissue. *Development* **2013**, *140*, 3939–3949. [CrossRef] [PubMed]
6. Fox, C.S.; Massaro, J.M.; Hoffmann, U.; Pou, K.M.; Maurovich-Horvat, P.; Liu, C.Y.; Vasan, R.S.; Murabito, J.M.; Meigs, J.B.; Cupples, L.A.; et al. Abdominal visceral and subcutaneous adipose tissue compartments: Association with metabolic risk factors in the Framingham Heart Study. *Circulation* **2007**, *116*, 39–48. [CrossRef] [PubMed]
7. Song, M.-G.; Lee, H.-J.; Jin, B.-Y.; Gutierrez-Aguilar, R.; Shin, K.-H.; Choi, S.-H.; Um, S.H.; Kim, D.-H. Depot-specific differences in angiogenic capacity of adipose tissue in differential susceptibility to diet-induced obesity. *Mol. Metab.* **2016**, *5*, 1113–1120. [CrossRef] [PubMed]
8. Kwon, H.; Kim, D.; Kim, J.S. Body Fat Distribution and the Risk of Incident Metabolic Syndrome: A Longitudinal Cohort Study. *Sci. Rep.* **2017**, *7*, 10955. [CrossRef] [PubMed]
9. Lee, K.Y.; Luong, Q.; Sharma, R.; Dreyfuss, J.M.; Ussar, S.; Kahn, C.R. Developmental and functional heterogeneity of white adipocytes within a single fat depot. *EMBO J.* **2018**, *38*, e99291. [CrossRef] [PubMed]
10. Marinou, K.; Hodson, L.; Vasan, S.K.; Fielding, B.A.; Banerjee, R.; Brismar, K.; Koutsilieris, M.; Clark, A.; Neville, M.J.; Karpe, F. Structural and functional properties of deep abdominal subcutaneous adipose tissue explain its association with insulin resistance and cardiovascular risk in men. *Diabetes Care* **2014**, *37*, 821–829. [CrossRef] [PubMed]
11. Thomas, E.L.; McCarthy, J.; Fitzpatrick, J. The TOFI Phenotype. *Obes. Facts* **2009**, *2*, 1–256.
12. Brończyk-Puzoń, A.; Koszowska, A.; Bieniek, J. Podstawowe pomiary antropometryczne i pochodne wskaźniki w poradnictwie dietetycznym–część pierwsza Basic anthropometric measurements and derived ratios in dietary counseling: Part one. *Pielęgniarstwo* **2018**, *8*, 217–222. [CrossRef]
13. Walczyk, T. Anthropometric indicators of obesity. Are the new indicators a better predictor of body fat content than BMI? *J. Educ. Health Sport* **2021**, *11*, 11–23. [CrossRef]
14. *Podręcznik Użytkowania*; BioScan 920; Maltron International Ltd.: Essex, UK, 2014.

15. Vladu, I.M.; Fortofoiu, M.; Clenciu, D.; Fortofoiu, M.C.; Padureanu, R.; Radu, L.; Cojan, S.T.T.; Radulescu, P.M.; Padureanu, V. Insulin resistance quantified by the value of HOMA-IR and cardiovascular risk in patients with type 2 diabetes. *Exp. Ther. Med.* **2022**, *23*, 73. [CrossRef] [PubMed]
16. Van Deventer, H.E.; Miller, W.G.; Myers, G.L.; Sakurabayashi, I.; Bachmann, L.M.; Caudill, S.P.; Dziekonski, A.; Edwards, S.; Kimberly, M.M.; Korzun, W.J.; et al. Non-HDL cholesterol shows improved accuracy for cardiovascular risk score classification compared to direct or calculated LDL cholesterol in a dyslipidemic population. *Clin. Chem.* **2011**, *57*, 490–501. [CrossRef] [PubMed]
17. Ortega, F.B.; Lavie, C.J.; Blair, S.N. Obesity and Cardiovascular Disease. *Circ. Res.* **2016**, *118*, 1752–1770. [CrossRef] [PubMed]
18. Kinlen, D.; Cody, D.; O'Shea, D. Complications of obesity. *QJM* **2018**, *111*, 437–443. [CrossRef]
19. Blüher, M. Obesity: Global epidemiology and pathogenesis. *Nat. Rev. Endocrinol.* **2019**, *15*, 288–298. [CrossRef] [PubMed]
20. Ahmed, B.; Sultana, R.; Greene, M.W. Adipose Tissue and Insulin Resistance in Obese. *Biomed. Pharmacother.* **2021**, *137*, 111315. [CrossRef] [PubMed]
21. Forte, R.; Pesce, C.; De Vito, G.; Boreham, C.A. The Body Fat-Cognition Relationship in Healthy Older Individuals: Does Gynoid vs Android Distribution Matter? *J. Nutr. Health Aging* **2017**, *21*, 284–291. [CrossRef] [PubMed]
22. Garvey, W.T.; Mechanick, J.I.; Brett, E.M.; Garber, A.J.; Hurley, D.L.; Jastreboff, A.M.; Nadolsky, K.; Pessah-Pollack, R.; Plodkowski, R. American association of clinical endocrinologists and american college of endocrinology comprehensive clinical practice guidelines for medical care of patients with obesity. *Endocr. Pract. Off. J. Am. Coll. Endocrinol. Am. Assoc. Clin. Endocrinol.* **2016**, *22* (Suppl. S3), 1–203. [CrossRef] [PubMed]
23. Johnson Stoklossa, C.A.; Forhan, M.; Padwal, R.S.; Gonzalez, M.C.; Prado, C.M. Practical Considerations for Body Composition Assessment of Adults with Class II/III Obesity Using Bioelectrical Impedance Analysis or Dual-Energy X-Ray Absorptiometry. *Curr. Obes. Rep.* **2016**, *5*, 389–396. [CrossRef] [PubMed]
24. Alberti, K.G.; Eckel, R.H.; Grundy, S.M.; Zimmet, P.Z.; Cleeman, J.I.; Donato, K.A.; Fruchart, J.-C.; James, W.P.T.; Loria, C.M.; Smith, S.C., Jr. Harmonizing the metabolic syndrome: A joint interim statement of the international diabetes federation task force on epidemiology and prevention; national heart, lung, and blood institute; American heart association; world heart federation; international atherosclerosis society; and international association for the study of obesity. *Circulation* **2009**, *120*, 1640–1645. [CrossRef] [PubMed]
25. Expert Panel on Detection, Evaluation, and Treatment of High Blood Cholesterol in Adults. Executive summary of the third report of the National Cholesterol Education Program (NCEP) expert panel on detection, evaluation, and treatment of high blood cholesterol in adults (adult treatment panel III). *JAMA* **2001**, *285*, 2486–2497. [CrossRef] [PubMed]
26. Després, J.-P.; Lemieux, I. Abdominal obesity and metabolic syndrome. *Nat. Cell Biol.* **2006**, *444*, 881–887. [CrossRef] [PubMed]
27. Bjorntorp, P. Metabolic implications of body fat distribution. *Diabetes Care* **1991**, *14*, 1132–1143. [CrossRef] [PubMed]
28. Rochlani, Y.; Pothineni, N.V.; Mehta, J.L. Metabolic Syndrome: Does It Differ between Women and Men? *Cardiovasc. Drugs Ther.* **2015**, *29*, 329–338. [CrossRef] [PubMed]
29. Li, M.; McDermott, R.A. Using anthropometric indices to predict cardio-metabolic risk factors in Australian indigenous populations. *Diabetes Res. Clin. Pract.* **2010**, *87*, 401–406. [CrossRef] [PubMed]
30. Roriz, A.K.C.; de Oliveira, C.C.; Moreira, P.A.; Eickemberg, M.; Medeiros, J.M.B.; Sampaio, L.R. Methods of Predicting Visceral Fat in Brazilian Adults and Older Adults: A Comparison between Anthropometry and Computerized Tomography. *Arch. Latinoam. Nutr.* **2011**, *61*, 5–12. [PubMed]
31. da Rosa, S.E.; Costa, A.C.; Fortes, M.S.R.; Marson, R.A.; Neves, E.B.; Rodrigues, L.C.; Ferreira, P.F.; Filho, J.F. Cut-Off Points of Visceral Adipose Tissue Associated with Metabolic Syndrome in Military Men. *Healthcare* **2021**, *9*, 886. [CrossRef] [PubMed]
32. Hernandez-Ono, A.; Monter-Carreola, G.; Zamora-Gonzalez, J.; Cardoso-Saldana, G.; Posadas-Sanchez, R.; Torres-Tamayo, M.; Posadas-Romero, C. Association of visceral fat with coronary risk factors in a population-based sample of postmenopausal women. *Int. J. Obes.* **2002**, *26*, 33–39. [CrossRef] [PubMed]

nutrients MDPI

Article

Plant-Based Diets versus the Mediterranean Dietary Pattern and Their Socio-Demographic Determinants in the Spanish Population: Influence on Health and Lifestyle Habits

Elena Sandri [1,2], Marco Sguanci [3], Eva Cantín Larumbe [4], Germán Cerdá Olmedo [1], Lisa Ursula Werner [5], Michela Piredda [3,*] and Stefano Mancin [6]

1 Faculty of Medicine and Health Sciences, Catholic University of Valencia San Vicente Mártir, c/Quevedo, 2, 46001 Valencia, Spain; elena.sandri@ucv.es (E.S.); german.cerda@ucv.es (G.C.O.)
2 Doctoral School, Catholic University of Valencia San Vicente Mártir, c/Quevedo, 2, 46001 Valencia, Spain
3 Research Unit Nursing Science, Campus Bio-Medico di Roma University, Via Alvaro del Portillo, 21, 00128 Rome, Italy; marco.sguanci@unicampus.it
4 Faculty of Data Science, Polytechnical University of Valencia, Camí de Vera, s/n, 46022 Valencia, Spain; evacantinlarumbe@gmail.com
5 Faculty of Teaching and Science of Education, Catholic University of Valencia San Vicente Mártir, c/Quevedo, 2, 46001 Valencia, Spain; lu.werner@ucv.es
6 Department of Biomedicine and Prevention, University of Rome "Tor Vergata", Viale Montpellier, 1, 00128 Rome, Italy; stefano.mancin.84@students.uniroma2.eu
* Correspondence: m.piredda@unicampus.it; Tel.: +39-06-225-418-833

Abstract: Background: Plant-based diets are becoming more and more widespread among the Spanish population, progressively replacing the Mediterranean dietary pattern. Different studies have shown the motivations for adherence to these diets, and others have highlighted some health advantages and disadvantages. Purpose of the study: Further studies are needed to define the socio-demographic determinants that influence the choice of a plant-based diet and to study the relationship that the choice of dietary pattern has on the health and lifestyle habits of the population. Methods: A descriptive, cross-sectional study was conducted on the Spanish population. The NutSo-HH questionnaire, developed and validated by the research team, was used to gather socio-demographic, nutritional, social, and lifestyle information through non-probabilistic snowball sampling. Results: The questionnaire was completed by 22,181 Spanish citizens, of whom only 19,211 were of interest to the study. The socio-demographic variables gender, age, educational level, income level, and place of residence do not seem to influence the prevalence of a plant-based diet (n = 1638) compared to a Mediterranean diet (n = 17,573). People following a vegetarian or vegan diet have a lower BMI, and they consume less fried food, fast food, and ultra-processed dishes and fewer energy drinks or sugary beverages. They also do more exercise and sleep longer hours, smoke less, and consume alcohol less frequently. However, there seem to be more diagnosed eating disorders among people who follow a plant-based diet than those who follow a Mediterranean diet. Conclusions: People who adopt a plant-based diet tend to exhibit healthier lifestyle patterns and consume fewer foods that are detrimental to their health. However, it is essential for such dietary choices to be supervised by healthcare professionals to mitigate the risk of maladaptive behaviors evolving into eating disorders.

Keywords: vegetarian diet; vegan diet; Mediterranean diet; healthy lifestyle; survey; Spain

1. Introduction

Spain is recognized as a typical Mediterranean country, and for centuries, the Mediterranean diet has been the commonly adopted dietary pattern in the country [1]. The Mediterranean diet is characterized by a high consumption of minimally processed plant foods, such as fruits, vegetables, nuts, seeds, legumes, and whole grains. The predominant use of extra virgin olive oil as the main source of fat and the moderate consumption of dairy products, along with a variety of herbs and spices as seasonings, contributes to the diversity and richness of flavors in Mediterranean dishes. The consumption of fish, especially fish rich in omega-3 fatty acids, is recommended two to three times a week, while the consumption of red meat, processed meat, and foods high in saturated fats and added sugars is strongly limited. Wine, especially red wine, is consumed in moderation and preferably during meals, and it is considered an integral part of the Mediterranean culinary experience [2].

The health benefits of the Mediterranean diet have been extensively studied and documented in the scientific literature, and they have been associated with a longer life expectancy and a better overall quality of life [3–7]. Despite its proven benefits, it seems that in Western countries, and particularly in Spain, the Mediterranean diet is gradually being abandoned [8]. In recent years, there has been a decline in the interest among the Spanish population in the Mediterranean diet, with growing attention to other diets, such as intermittent fasting, the ketogenic diet, or a plant-based diet [9]. More and more people are adopting a plant-based diet (PBD) in all its variations [10]. The prevalence of PBD in Europe varies significantly among countries and regions, making it difficult to establish an exact percentage. Estimates typically range from 1% to 10% [11], but even these figures can vary based on cultural attitudes towards vegetarianism and veganism, the availability of vegan products, dietary habits, and socioeconomic factors [12]. In contemporary society, a growing consensus is seen among individuals, organizations, and scientists that reducing meat consumption can have positive impacts on various aspects, such as animal welfare, sustainability, and human health [13]. Behind the spread of PBDs, various motivations can be found, including the desire to improve animal welfare by reducing meat consumption [14]. By opting for plant-based diets or reducing meat consumption, people can contribute to reducing the demand for products from intensive livestock farming, potentially improving the treatment of animals. Moreover, a predominantly plant-based diet reduces the environmental impact, as PBDs tend to have a smaller ecological footprint than diets rich in animal products [15,16]. Finally, proponents of a plant-based diet argue that it has beneficial effects on human health [17]. Numerous studies have linked excessive meat consumption, especially red and processed meats, to health problems, such as heart disease [18,19], certain types of cancer [20], obesity [21], and type 2 diabetes [22]. By moderating meat consumption and incorporating more fruits, vegetables, and whole grains into the diet, people can reduce the risk of developing these health problems and improve their overall well-being. To date, there is no universally accepted definition of the term "plant-based diet". In some cases, it has been used to refer to omnivorous diets with a low content of foods of animal origin only [23]. The main categories of diets we refer to in this research are as follows: flexitarian or semi-vegetarian diets (FDs), which are mainly vegetarian with the occasional inclusion of meat or fish; vegetarian diets (VDs) (lacto-ovo-vegetarian: plant-based except for dairy products and/or eggs), and vegan diets (VGs) (100% plant-based).

In the current research landscape, there is a significant gap regarding plant-based diets. Although considerable attention has been paid to understanding the motivations behind adopting vegetarian and vegan lifestyles [24], there is a lack of studies accurately quantifying the number of individuals adhering to these dietary patterns, studying their relationship with socio-demographic determinants, and exploring the relationship with other lifestyle habits. A recent study [25] analyzing the variation in the prevalence of PBDs in the Spanish population between 2001 and 2017 and its association with lifestyle habits and health variables explored only four variables, namely physical activity, tobacco consumption, alcohol consumption, and body mass index (BMI) [25].

Study Objective

In order to integrate the available literature on the consumption of plant-based diets among the Spanish population, this study aimed to investigate the prevalence of vegetarian, vegan, and flexitarian dietary patterns compared to the Mediterranean dietary pattern in the Spanish population, to explore whether the adoption of a specific diet is influenced by socio-demographic factors (such as age, sex, level of education or income, size of town of residence, or size of region of residence), and to describe the relationship between a type of diet and social/lifestyle habits adopted in the population.

2. Materials and Methods

2.1. Study Design and Sampling

A descriptive, cross-sectional survey was conducted with adults (over 18 years of age) residing in Spain. Participants were excluded from the study if, at the time of survey completion, they had any medical condition or constraint that could impact their dietary patterns, including hospitalization or confinement.

2.2. Ethical Approval

This research adheres to the STROBE Guidelines [26] (Supplementary Materials). Approval for the study was obtained from the Research Ethics Committee of the Catholic University of Valencia under approval code UCV/2019-2020/152. Informed consent was obtained from all participants prior to their involvement in the study, and the ethical recommendations contained in the Declaration of Helsinki [27] were always followed.

2.3. Instrument

A self-designed questionnaire was utilized for data collection, comprising several sections: a diet section addressing the type of diet followed, the consumption of various food groups, and drinking habits; a section exploring the presence of diagnosed eating disorders or their symptoms; a section on physical activity and lifestyle habits relevant to health; and finally, anthropometric data such as weight, height, and socio-demographic variables. The development and psychometric testing of the instrument adhered to rigorous methodological standards and involved an expert panel, including a nutritionist, two family physicians, two psychologists, a social educator, and a communication specialist. The validation of the questionnaire included a pilot study with 53 individuals whose characteristics were similar to the target population.

2.4. Data Collection

The questionnaire was distributed utilizing non-probabilistic "snowball" sampling [28]. A Google Forms survey was created for this purpose and disseminated primarily through online channels, through which the people who helped with the dissemination shared the link to the questionnaire. Initially, the Instagram account @elretonutricional was utilized, along with the personal social networks of the researchers through WhatsApp, LinkedIn, Facebook, and Twitter and email distributions to various associations. Additionally, efforts were made to physically disseminate the questionnaire to accommodate individuals less inclined toward digital platforms. This involved posting flyers in various shops and businesses frequented by individuals with diverse socio-demographic characteristics. The data collection spanned from August 2020 to November 2021.

2.5. Variables

For nutritional analysis, we opted to utilize the IASE index (Índice de Alimentación Saludable para la población Española) [29], which was modified to create a condensed version. This adapted index assigns a maximum score of 73 points, aligning with the level of adherence to the recommendations outlined by the Spanish Society of Community Nutrition (SENC) [30]. Based on the IASE score obtained, the dietary habits of the population can be classified into three categories: 58.4 < IASE < 73: "Healthy"; 36.5 < IASE < 58.4: "Needs changes"; IASE < 36.5: "Unhealthy". Table 1 illustrates the categorization of variables utilized for the IASE.

Table 1. Conversion table from qualitative questions into quantitative questions of the IASE index.

Conversion Table Applied to IASE					
Variables	**Score**				
	10	**7.5**	**5**	**2.5**	**0**
Fruit	1 piece/portion a day, 2–4 portions a day, ≥5 portions a day				Never or rarely
Vegetables	Every day	≥5 pieces per week, 2–4 pieces a week	1 piece/ration a week		Never or rarely
Cereals	Every day	≥3 times a week	1–2 times a week		Never or rarely
Milk	Every day	≥3 times a week	1–2 times a week		Never or rarely
Medium between white and red meat	1–2 times a week	≥3 times a week		Every day	Never or very rarely
Legumes	1–2 times a week	≥3 times a week		Every day	Never or very rarely
Soft drinks	Never or rarely	Very few times (2 times maximum per month)	One glass per week	≥2 glasses per week	2 glasses every day, 3–5 glasses every day, ≥5 glasses every day
Variety	2 points if each of the daily recommendations is met, 1 point if each of the weekly recommendations is met.				

The socio-demographic variables considered were categorized as follows:

- Sex: analyzed in binary way; male and female.
- Age: categorized into four groups; young individuals (18–25 years old), young adults (26–45 years old), adults (46–65 years old), and older adults (over 65 years old).
- Level of education: basic studies (no studies, primary or secondary education, vocational training, or baccalaureate) and higher studies (bachelor's, master's, and PhD).
- Income level: low income (<2200 EUR/month per household) and medium–high income (>2200 EUR/month).
- Municipality: small municipalities (<2000 inhabitants), medium-sized towns (between 2000 and 10,000 inhabitants), and cities with more than 10,000 inhabitants.
- Place of residence: based on the different regions of Spain.

Nutritional and health habit variables not addressed in the IASE were categorized on a 4-point Likert scale (from 1 = none or low frequency to 4 = maximum frequency), while variables related to eating disorders were categorized on a 6-point Likert scale (Table 2). Exceptions were the body mass index (BMI) and minutes of exercise, which were used as numerical variables.

Table 2. Categorization of the health and lifestyle variables and the variables for eating disorders.

Variable	Category	Score
Sleeping hours	Less than 6 h	1
	Between 6 and 7 h	2
	Between 7 and 8 h	3
	More than 8 h	4
Getting up rested	Never	1
	Very seldom and sometimes	2
	Frequently and almost always	3
	Always	4
Sleep quality	0 and 1	1
	2	2
	3	3
	4 and 5	4

Table 2. *Cont.*

Variable	Category	Score
Water	Never and very rarely (2 max. per month) and 1 glass/cup/week and ≥2 glasses/cups/week	1
	2 glasses/cups or less every day	2
	3–5 glasses every day	3
	More than 5 glasses every day	4
Sugary soft drinks, coffee, and energy drinks	Never and very rarely (2 glasses max. per month)	4
	One glass per week and 2 or more glasses per week	3
	2 glasses or less every day	2
	3–5 glasses and ≥5 glasses every day	1
Juice	Never and very rarely (2 glasses max. per month)	1
	One glass per week and 2 or more glasses per week	2
	2 glasses or less every day	3
	3–5 glasses and ≥5 glasses every day	4
Fish consumption	Never or very seldom	1
	1–2 times a week	2
	≥3 times a week	3
	Every day	4
Consumption of fast food, fried, and ultra-processed dishes	Never	1
	Very seldom (2 times a month maximum)	2
	Once a week	3
	Several times a week	4
Getting drunk	Never or less than once a month	1
	Monthly	2
	Weekly	3
	Daily or almost daily	4
Alcohol consumption	Never or once a month	1
	2–4 times a month	2
	2–3 times a week	3
	4–5 times a week or every day	4
Smoking	Non-smoker	1
	Light smoker (less than 5 cigarettes per day)	2
	Moderate smoker (6–15 cigarettes per day)	3
	Severe smoker (≥16 cigarettes per day)	4
Night outings	Never and sporadically	1
	1–2 times a week	2
	≥3 times a week	3
	Every day	4
Sedentary lifestyle	<7 h	1
	7–9 h	2
	9–11 h	3
	>11 h	4
Obesophobia, no control over eating intake, concern over body image	Never	1
	Rarely	2
	Occasionally	3
	Frequently	4
	Very frequently	5
	Always	6

2.6. Data Analysis

Data were checked to identify any erroneous entries or outliers, and extreme BMI values (<14 and >40) were excluded. Descriptive and inferential statistical analyses were performed. Discrete variables were presented as absolute values and percentages, while continuous variables were expressed as means and standard deviations. The normality of the data was evaluated using the Lilliefors Test (Kolmogorov–Smirnov) at a 95% significance level [31], revealing a non-normal distribution. Consequently, Chi-2, Mann–Whitney, and Kruskal–Wallis tests [32], which are non-parametric, were employed to compare differences between categories of variables. After applying Kruskal–Wallis test, a post hoc analysis was conducted with Bonferroni correction to study pairwise comparisons. All the data analysis was carried out with Python 3.9.13 [33].

3. Results

From the total population (n = 22,181), 17,573 individuals (79.23%) reported following a Mediterranean dietary pattern, 723 (3.26%) followed a vegetarian diet, 365 (1.65%) chose a vegan diet, 550 (2.48%) defined themselves as flexitarians, and the remaining 13.38% (n = 2970) reported other types of diets (Figure 1).

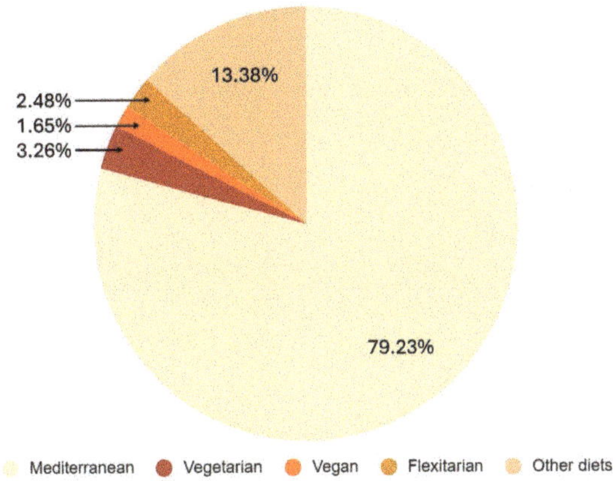

Figure 1. Distribution of the types of diet adopted (n = 22,181).

For the purpose of the study, individuals who reported following diets other than Mediterranean and plant-based diets were not included in the data analysis. Therefore, the final valid sample consisted of 19,211 individuals. Details of the sample's socio-demographic characteristics are described in Table 3.

Table 3. Sample and its socio-demographic characteristics (n = 19,211).

	Mean ± SD or n (%)
Male	3682 (19.17%)
Female	15,529 (80.83%)
Age (years)	34.49 ± 11.79
Male age	36.52 ± 13.72
Female age	34.02 ± 11.23
	Total
Education level	
Basic education	6050 (31.49%)
Higher education	13,161 (68.51%)
Income level	
Low	8370 (43.57%)
Medium–high	9220 (47.99%)
Do not know/no answer	1621 (8.44%)
Municipality	
<2000	865 (4.50%)
2000–10,000	3065 (15.95%)
>10,000	17,281 (79.54%)

The distribution of the sample's dietary behaviors according to socio-demographic variables, including gender, age, educational level, income level, and municipality of residence, showed no statistically significant differences among the analyzed groups. These findings suggest that these socio-demographic factors did not exert an influence on dietary preferences (Table 4).

Table 4. Diet prevalence according to socio-demographic groups, $n = 19{,}211$.

		Mediterranean Diet *n* (%)	Vegetarian *n* (%)	Vegan *n* (%)	Flexitarian *n* (%)	*p*-Value §
Sex	Men	3467 (94.16%)	89 (2.42%)	50 (1.36%)	76 (2.06%)	0.85
	Women	14,106 (90.84%)	634 (4.08%)	315 (2.03%)	474 (3.05%)	
Age	18–25 years old	4829 (88.22%)	325 (5.94%)	134 (2.45%)	186 (3.40%)	0.23
	26–45 years old	9190 (91.57%)	352 (3.51%)	195 (1.94%)	299 (2.98%)	
	46–65 years old	3385 (95.92%)	46 (1.30%)	36 (1.02%)	62 (1.76%)	
	>65 years old	169 (98.26%)	0 (0%)	0 (0%)	3 (1.74%)	
Education	High education	12,045 (91.52%)	487 (3.70%)	238 (1.81%)	391 (2.97%)	1.00
	Low education	5528 (91.37%)	236 (3.90%)	127 (2.10%)	159 (2.63%)	
Income	Low income	7549 (90.19%)	356 (4.25%)	204 (2.44%)	261 (3.12%)	0.92
	Medium–high income	8549 (92.72%)	293 (3.12%)	132 (1.43%)	246 (2.67%)	
Municipality	Small city	796 (92.02%)	30 (3.47%)	20 (2.31%)	19 (2.20%)	1.00
	Medium city	2800 (91.35%)	121 (3.95%)	56 (1.83%)	88 (2.87%)	
	Big city	13,977 (91.47%)	572 (3.74%)	289 (1.89%)	443 (2.90%)	

§ Chi-2 test.

The prevalence of the different diets in the Spanish regions (Figure 2a–d) was calculated by dividing the number of people following each type of diet in a region by the number of inhabitants in each region. The data reported by the National Institute of Statistics (INE) were used for this purpose. No statistically significant differences were found in the prevalence of any type of diet depending on the region (vegetarian diet $p = 0.45$; veganism $p = 0.39$; flexitarian diet $p = 0.42$; and Mediterranean diet $p = 0.36$).

Subsequently, the relationships between the four different dietary choices considered —Mediterranean, vegetarian, vegan, and flexitarian—and various health-related variables or social and lifestyle habits were explored. Statistically significant differences were observed among the groups regarding variables such as BMI ($p < 0.001$), the healthy eating index ($p < 0.001$), and unhealthy food consumption (fried food: $p < 0.001$; fast food: $p < 0.001$; and ultra-processed food: $p < 0.001$). Significant differences were also found in beverage consumption, including the frequency of sugary drink intake ($p < 0.001$) and coffee and energy drink consumption ($p < 0.001$). However, no significant differences were noted in water consumption except between the Mediterranean and Vegan diet groups ($p < 0.001$), and significant differences in fruit juice consumption were found between the Mediterranean and flexitarian groups ($p < 0.001$). Sedentary behavior did not appear to influence dietary choices, while differences in perceived health levels were significant only between the Mediterranean and vegan diet groups ($p = 0.02$), with the latter generally reporting feeling better. Regarding physical activity, differences were observed among all groups, with individuals following a plant-based diet, in all its variations, engaging in significantly more sport compared to those following a Mediterranean diet ($p < 0.001$). Regarding sleep habits, no differences were found among individuals adopting different dietary patterns in terms of sleep quality or perception, but significant differences were observed in sleep hours between those following a Mediterranean diet, vegetarians, and vegans, with the latter two groups seeming to sleep more (M versus VD: $p < 0.001$; M versus VG: $p < 0.001$). Finally, when social habits were analyzed, significant differences emerged for almost all variables: smoking ($p < 0.001$), alcohol consumption ($p < 0.001$), and nightlife ($p < 0.001$), with a tendency to adopt healthier habits for those following a plant-based diet. On the other hand, with respect to the eating disorder variables, which also showed significant differences ($p < 0.001$), these behaviors seemed to be more frequent among vegetarians and vegans than among those who follow a Mediterranean diet (Table 5). (For more detailed comparisons between the habit variables and the different dietary styles analysed, see the figures reporting the results of Dunn's tests in Appendix A).

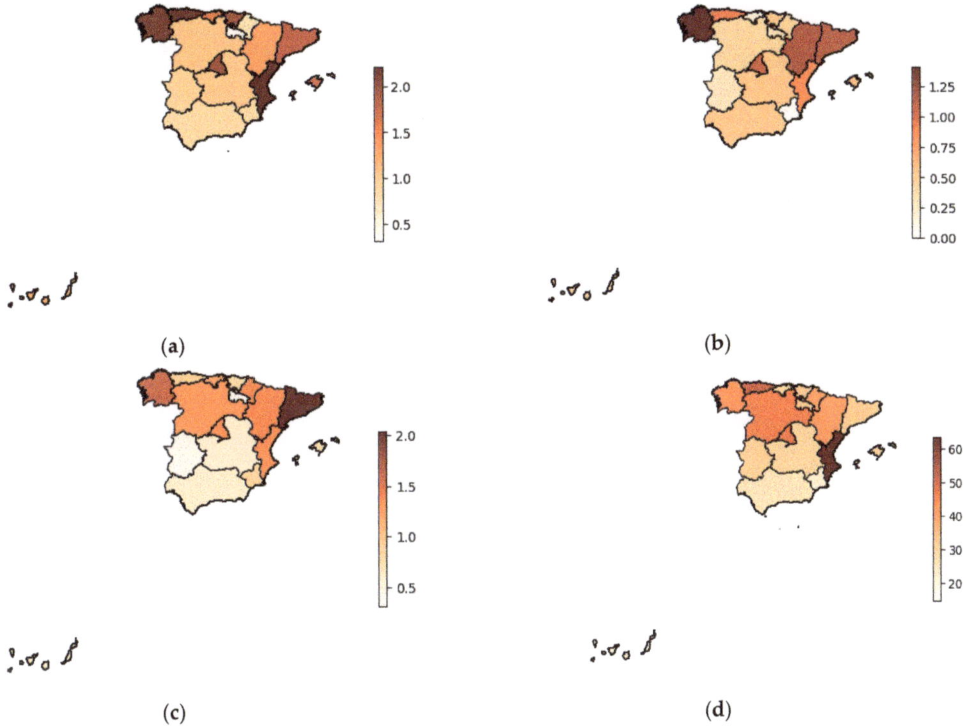

Figure 2. The prevalence of different diets in the Spanish regions: (**a**) the prevalence of vegetarianism; (**b**) the prevalence of veganism; (**c**) the prevalence of flexitarianism; and (**d**) the prevalence of the Mediterranean diet.

Table 5. Distribution of nutritional, social, and lifestyle habit variables and health variables among sample groups according to the diet followed.

Numerical Variable	Mediterranean Diet (M)	Vegetarian Diet (VD)	Vegan Diet (VG)	Flexitarian Diet (FD)	*p*-Value *
BMI	23.96 ± 4.31	22.41 ± 3.57	22.56 ± 3.6	22.64 ± 3.58	$p < 0.001$ M-VD ($p < 0.001$) M-VG ($p < 0.001$) M-FD ($p < 0.001$)
IASE	54.86 ± 9.48	50.27 ± 6.55	41.81 ± 5.85	52.97 ± 7.53	$p < 0.001$ M-VD ($p < 0.001$) M-VG ($p < 0.001$) M-FD ($p < 0.001$) VD-VG ($p < 0.001$) VD-FD ($p < 0.001$) VG-FD ($p < 0.001$)
Fried food	2.33 ± 0.81	2.01 ± 0.77	1.96 ± 0.79	1.99 ± 0.72	$p < 0.001$ M-VD ($p < 0.001$) M-VG ($p < 0.001$) M-FD ($p < 0.001$)

Table 5. *Cont.*

Numerical Variable	Mediterranean Diet (M)	Vegetarian Diet (VD)	Vegan Diet (VG)	Flexitarian Diet (FD)	*p*-Value *
Fast food	2.44 ± 0.75	2.31 ± 0.76	2.28 ± 0.76	2.18 ± 0.75	$p < 0.001$ M-VD ($p < 0.001$) M-VG ($p < 0.001$) M-FD ($p < 0.001$) VD-FD (0.01)
Ultra-processed food	2.39 ± 0.95	2.26 ± 0.91	2.13 ± 0.82	2.07 ± 0.88	$p < 0.001$ M-VD ($p < 0.001$) M-VG ($p < 0.001$) M-VD ($p < 0.001$) V-FD ($p < 0.001$)
Water	3.38 ± 0.64	3.42 ± 0.62	3.43 ± 0.60	3.49 ± 0.6	$p < 0.001$ M-VG ($p < 0.001$)
Sugary soft drinks	1.43 ± 0.69	1.24 ± 0.55	1.2 ± 0.48	1.19 ± 0.46	$p < 0.001$ M-VD ($p < 0.001$) M-VG ($p < 0.001$) M-FD ($p < 0.001$)
Juice	1.26 ± 0.55	1.20 ± 0.47	1.22 ± 0.52	1.17 ± 0.46	$p < 0.001$ M-FD ($p < 0.001$)
Coffee and energy drinks	1.72 ± 0.71	1.63 ± 0.65	1.56 ± 0.68	1.71 ± 0.66	$p < 0.001$ M-VD (0.01) M-VG ($p < 0.001$) VG-FD ($p < 0.001$)
Sedentary lifestyle	1.58 ± 0.84	1.60 ± 0.83	1.61 ± 0.87	1.66 ± 0.88	0.21 ‡
Self-perceived health	3.82 ± 0.82	3.88 ± 0.81	3.91 ± 0.92	3.89 ± 0.77	$p < 0.001$ M-VG (0.02)
Sport	144.98 ± 170.91	187.95 ± 177.32	213.99 ± 212.94	191.51 ± 180.2	$p < 0.001$ M-VD ($p < 0.001$) M-VG ($p < 0.001$) M-FD ($p < 0.001$)
Sleeping hours	2.51 ± 0.73	2.59 ± 0.72	2.55 ± 0.74	2.63 ± 0.70	$p < 0.001$ M-VD ($p < 0.001$) M-VG ($p < 0.001$)
Getting up rested	2.54 ± 0.58	2.55 ± 0.56	2.53 ± 0.63	2.53 ± 0.55	0.87 ‡
Sleep quality	3.39 ± 1.02	3.43 ± 1.01	3.38 ± 1.11	3.39 ± 0.98	0.68 ‡
Smoking	1.25 ± 0.66	1.13 ± 0.45	1.11 ± 0.39	1.11 ± 0.42	$p < 0.001$ M-VD ($p < 0.001$) M-VG ($p < 0.001$) M-FD ($p < 0.001$)
Alcohol	1.80 ± 0.89	1.58 ± 0.75	1.50 ± 0.75	1.60 ± 0.76	$p < 0.001$ M-VD ($p < 0.001$) M-VG ($p < 0.001$) M-FD ($p < 0.001$)
Getting drunk	1.06 ± 0.30	1.06 ± 0.26	1.02 ± 0.21	1.05 ± 0.25	0.04 M-VG (0.03)
Night outings	1.20 ± 0.44	1.19 ± 0.42	1.10 ± 0.32	1.19 ± 0.43	$p < 0.001$ M-VG ($p < 0.001$) VD-VG ($p < 0.001$) VG-F (0.02)
Obesophobia	3.42 ± 1.43	3.45 ± 1.42	3.40 ± 1.42	3.47 ± 1.38	0.75 ‡
No control	2.75 ± 1.29	2.82 ± 1.25	2.67 ± 1.34	2.83 ± 1.21	0.03 ‡
Body image	3.57 ± 1.28	3.68 ± 1.29	3.69 ± 1.31	3.68 ± 1.26	0.02 ‡
Diagnosed eating disorder	0.03 ± 0.16	0.07 ± 0.25	0.08 ± 0.27	0.05 ± 0.23	$p < 0.001$ M-VG ($p < 0.001$) VD-VG ($p < 0.001$) VG-FD ($p < 0.001$)

* Kruskal–Wallis test with Bonferroni correction (pairwise comparisons). ‡ No significant differences between groups.

4. Discussion

This study aimed to describe the prevalence of vegetarian, vegan, and flexitarian dietary patterns compared to the Mediterranean dietary pattern, as well as the relationship between such diets and socio-demographic factors and social/lifestyle habits in the Spanish population.

The majority of the sample (79.23%) followed a Mediterranean dietary pattern. Such a prevalence is expected for people living in a typically Mediterranean country such as Spain, which, for decades, has traditionally followed a predominantly Mediterranean diet [34]. Although the Mediterranean diet is still the predominant diet on the peninsula, more than 20% of those surveyed reported currently following another type of diet. This confirms the trend found in studies that have evidenced that Spaniards are progressively moving away from the Mediterranean dietary pattern [8,35].

Regarding the prevalence of a plant-based diet, 7.39% of the respondents stated that they chose this type of diet; more specifically, 3.26% defined themselves as vegetarians, 1.65% as vegans, and 2.48% as flexitarians. Again, these data align with those found in the literature for the European population [11], although the prevalence of veganism appears to be slightly lower than that found in a recent study [36]. Moreover, the percentage of people choosing a vegan diet is still lower than the percentage of those choosing a flexitarian or vegetarian diet, in line with previous studies [37]. It can be hypothesized that this percentage will be reversed in a few years, as several studies in Europe indicate that adherence to the vegan diet is increasing compared to adherence to the less restrictive plant-based dietary options [25,38]. There may be several reasons to explain the increasing trend of the vegan dietary pattern among the Spanish population. Two strong reasons are environmental concerns and animal welfare awareness, which are both of great interest in Western countries at present [13,14]. The vegan diet, due to its characteristics and the products it includes, reduces the environmental impact and the consumption of animals, which makes it a valid option for people who are sensitive to these issues [15,16]. Moreover, the greater availability of information on this type of diet on the internet and in networks [39], as well as the increased acceptance of vegan products among the population in recent years [40], could also favor the spread of this dietary style.

When attention was focused on the relationship between socio-demographic variables and the type of diet adopted, no significant differences were found for any of the groups explored in our sample. This suggests that the choice of one dietary style or another in Spain is not influenced by gender, age, level of education or income, or the area where a person resides. There are several possible hypotheses to explain this behavior.

On the one hand, we could highlight the democratization of health information, which may have partly leveled out the differences between population groups. In recent decades, the use of information and communication technologies (ICTs) has spread progressively in society [41]. One of the fields witnessing remarkable developments in the use of ICTs is healthcare, particularly through the emergence of eHealth. Mobile health has expanded the provision of health services via smartphones and the development of specific mobile apps, offering convenient and immediate access to a vast number of people [42,43]. Also, the increasing use of social media, which brings people from all locations and cultures into contact with each other, means that the same food habits can be adopted via imitation in very different environments [44,45]. Finally, the abundant publication on these channels of information concerning nutrition, cooking, or gastronomy can invite people to put aside more classical nutritional habits to try new types of diets, new products, or different recipes [46,47].

Another possible explanation for the lack of dependence found between dietary pattern choice and socio-demographic determinants could be that, in recent decades, particularly in Western countries, there has been a significant change in attitudes towards food and health in general. This has led to a greater awareness of different types of diets and a more widespread adoption of healthy lifestyles across the population, regardless of gender, age, educational level, income level, or place of residence [48,49].

Finally, a possible explanation can also be found in the availability and accessibility of food, which may not vary significantly between different socio-demographic groups in Spain. Industrialization and globalization have meant that, in developed countries, the range of foodstuffs on offer is very wide, and different types of products and brands can be found in a wide variety of establishments, ranging from neighborhood grocery stores to large supermarkets [50,51]. This means that almost all the population has easy and affordable access to a large variety of foods, especially basic ingredients such as fruits, vegetables, and olive oil, which are fundamental to the Mediterranean diet and to many vegetarian and vegan diets [52]. It is also worth noting that the increase in demand has led to a decrease in the cost of these products. This makes them affordable for a larger number of people, including citizens with lower incomes.

When critically analyzing the results obtained for the health and lifestyle variables with respect to the different types of diet (Table 5), regarding the dimension linked to movement and sport habits, no statistically significant differences were observed in terms of sedentary behavior. Where the differences become important is in the time devoted to sport. In the case of people who follow a Mediterranean diet, the average time spent doing sport per week was 145 min, which is slightly below the 150 min recommended by the WHO in terms of health [53]. The average weekly time spent on sports is 40–45 min more for vegetarians and flexitarians than for people who follow the Mediterranean diet, and in the case of vegans, it is even 70 min more, rising to 213 min. To determine whether there was a statistically significant difference between the followers of a plant-based diet and those who adopted a Mediterranean diet, these two groups were analyzed with the Mann–Whitney U test, which obtained a p-value < 0.001. Regular physical activity has long been proven to offer a wide range of physical, mental, and emotional health benefits, making it an important part of a healthy lifestyle. Physical activity helps burn calories and maintain a healthy weight [54]. It also contributes to fat loss and the development of lean muscle mass [55]. This strengthening of muscles and bones helps prevent muscle wasting and osteoporosis [56]. Physical exercise also strengthens the heart and improves blood circulation, thus reducing the risk of heart disease [57]. Mental and emotional health is also influenced by sport. Regular physical activity can improve cognitive function and reduce the risk of developing neurodegenerative diseases [58]. It can also improve sleep quality and help combat insomnia [59]. In addition, physical exercise releases endorphins, neurotransmitters that help reduce stress, anxiety, and depression. Achieving sporting accomplishments or simply beating one's earlier achievements in training also promotes a sense of well-being and increases self-esteem [60].

Certainly, the relationship between diet and physical activity can vary widely between individuals, and the amount of physical exercise a person undertakes may depend on a variety of factors, including their lifestyle, personal preferences, previous level of physical activity, and health goals. The results found do not allow for the establishment of a general rule that people following a vegetarian or vegan diet do more sport than those following a Mediterranean diet. However, we could hypothesize some reasons for the tendency found. Firstly, vegetarian and vegan diets are often associated with greater attention to personal well-being and to the connection between food and health. This may lead these individuals to prioritize exercise as another way to improve their health and quality of life [61]. Secondly, many people adopt a PBD for ethical reasons, such as concerns for the environment, sustainability, or animal rights. These same values could extend to taking care of one's own body, which could include regular exercise [62]. Last but certainly not least, it is worth noting that generally, people who follow a vegetarian or vegan diet often connect with a community that shares their values and goals. This community can provide support and motivation to maintain an active and healthy lifestyle, including regular exercise [63].

The difference in BMI between people who follow a traditional Mediterranean diet and those who follow a plant-based diet also stands out. In the former, the BMI is almost one and a half points higher than in the latter. These data are consistent with previous studies that have highlighted that people who follow a plant-based diet tend to have a lower body mass index (BMI) compared to those who do not. In addition, adopting a PBD also appears to be effective for weight loss [10,64]. Weight loss in people following a plant-based diet (PBD) can be attributed to the fact that, compared to the traditional Mediterranean pattern, the PBD usually involves a higher intake of fiber, polyunsaturated fats, and plant proteins, as well as a lower intake of energy, saturated fats, and animal proteins. These changes in dietary composition may contribute to more effective weight reduction in those who adopt a PBD [10]. The lower mean BMI found among the population following a plant-based diet could also be partly attributed to the fact that these people, in our sample, were more physically active than those following a Mediterranean diet. It has been shown that regular physical activity can help control weight gain or even promote weight loss [54,55].

With respect to the healthy nutrition index for the Spanish population (IASE), statistically significant differences were observed between all groups. The IASE score was lower for plant-based diets than for the Mediterranean diet and especially low (up to 13 points lower) for the vegan diet. This difference in the IASE score is explained by the fact that the IASE score is calculated on the basis of the consumption of a varied diet that includes several food families, including animal proteins such as meat and dairy products [29]. A vegan diet excludes the consumption of these foods, and therefore, the IASE score is much lower in this specific case; for this reason, the IASE score is not useful in giving us reliable information about the goodness of the diet followed.

The variables concerning the consumption of fried foods, the consumption of fast food, and the consumption of ultra-processed foods show that respondents who indicated that they followed a plant-based diet seemed to adopt healthier nutritional habits than those who followed the Mediterranean diet. Numerous studies have illustrated the detrimental health effects of fried food and ultra-processed foods [65,66], as they are often loaded with unhealthy fats, added sugars, sodium, and artificial additives while lacking essential nutrients [67]. Fried foods can pose a particular health risk. They are often high in trans fats, saturated fats, and calories. Their regular consumption has been associated with an increased risk of obesity and elevated cholesterol levels, as well as hypertension and an elevated risk of cardiovascular disease [68,69]. The regular consumption of fast food has been correlated with an increased risk of obesity, type 2 diabetes, heart disease, and certain cancers. These foods often lack the vitamins, minerals, and dietary fiber necessary for optimal health [70,71]. Ultra-processed foods often contain high levels of refined carbohydrates, unhealthy fats, added sugars, and artificial additives. The repeated consumption of such foods has been linked to weight gain, metabolic disorders, increased inflammation, and a higher incidence of chronic diseases such as obesity, type 2 diabetes, cardiovascular disease, and certain cancers [66,72].

As regards self-perceived levels of health, it seems that vegans have a more positive perception of their state of health compared to people who follow a Mediterranean diet, although the difference is not very high.

Finally, another dimension in which significant differences were found was social habits, with people following a plant-based diet in general smoking less, consuming alcohol less frequently, and tending to go out less frequently to parties and for entertainment than people following a traditional diet. These social habits are associated with a healthy lifestyle, and so the reasons that might underlie the trend found are similar to those discussed in the case of physical activity. As explained, people who follow a PBD often have a greater awareness of the impact of their habits on health [61]. Therefore, they may prioritize their personal well-being over the pursuit of momentary pleasures such as smoking, excessive drinking, or engaging in partying and fun activities. They opt for activities that promote long-term physical, mental, and emotional health. The ethical values of concern for animal welfare and the environment that normally underpin the personal choice to adopt a plant-based diet also play a role [62]. These same values can extend to other aspects of their lives, including the choice to avoid tobacco and alcohol, which can be detrimental to health and the environment.

Although most of the results show that a plant-based diet seems healthier than the Mediterranean one, we must underlie the strong and countless evidence of the benefits of the Mediterranean diet model for health and longevity. The effects of the Mediterranean diet on the prevention and treatment of cardiovascular disease are well-recognized in numerous studies [73,74], as are the positive effects on metabolic disorders [75] and some types of cancer [76].

Moreover, it is necessary to remember that a strict plant-based diet entails potential health risks. In a recent review, its correlation with the onset of physical disorders was described [77] due to a low intake of and/or a risk of deficiencies in specific nutrients that can influence bodily and mental functions. A strong incidence of mental health problems has been found in the vegan population compared to other types of diet, contributing to a lower quality of life [78,79].

Given the very limiting characteristics of this nutritional model, it is essential to consult a dietitian or nutrition professional regarding one's nutritional status and any symptoms that may appear with the aim of promptly preventing nutritional inadequacies and minimizing any negative health consequences.

Strengths and Limitations

One of the weaknesses of the study lies in the sampling technique used and in the prevalent dissemination through social media. Snowball sampling offers the advantage of reaching a large number of responses, but it may introduce a self-selection bias, as the sample collected depends on initial participants recommending other potential participants. Disseminating the survey through social media, with the support of several influential people and professionals in these fields, led to a considerable number of respondents showing an interest in nutrition and health. It is reasonable to assume that these people have above-average knowledge on the subject and that they usually strive to adopt healthier habits. An important effort was made to try to mitigate self-selection bias by also conducting a physical dissemination of the survey. To this end, several establishments throughout Spain with a diverse clientele (such as pharmacies, tobacconists, associations of citizens, etc.) were involved. Their owners were provided information about the project and asked to display posters on their premises with a QR code linking to the questionnaire so that customers in these establishments could fill out the survey if they wished to do so.

Gender bias was also observed, as about 80% of the respondents were women. There is a greater predisposition in the female public, also observed in other studies [80–83], to collaborate with these types of studies, and perhaps there is also a greater concern and sensitivity to nutrition and health issues among women than among their male counterparts. This notwithstanding, due to an awareness of the importance of achieving a balanced sample, an additional effort was made to reach more men as participants in the study, finally achieving a sample of 3682 men.

The dissemination of the sample via social networks could have introduced age-related and educational biases in the sample, leading to a greater participation rate among younger individuals and people with a higher level of education. Typically, younger people are more inclined towards and engaged with social media platforms, allocating more time to their utilization, thus enhancing their likelihood of completing the survey. A higher level of education also makes people more likely to be concerned about health and to seek information about it in various media, including social media. Our sample, with a mean age of 34 years and 68.51% of respondents with a higher education level, partially suffered from these biases. We are currently carrying out a second dissemination of the survey, trying to collect a larger sample of older, less educated, and more male respondents.

Another limitation is that the IASE healthy nutrition index is based on a varied diet comprising all food groups, including meat and meat products. For a plant-based diet and, in particular, for a vegan diet, the IASE cannot be chosen as a stand-alone indicator of the goodness of nutrition. It needs to be included in an overall picture of the consumption of other food groups and dietary habits, as we have tried to do in this study.

The undoubted strengths of the study are the very large sample size (n = 19,211), variety, and heterogeneity, as adults of all ages and educational and income levels were represented. Geographical variety was also guaranteed, as all regions of Spain were significantly represented in the sample. This made it possible to obtain reliable information on the health status and nutritional and lifestyle habits of the entire Spanish population.

5. Conclusions

People who choose to adopt a plant-based diet not only demonstrate healthier lifestyle patterns but also tend to consume a wider variety of nutrient-rich and antioxidant-rich foods. This type of diet is often associated with numerous health benefits, including a lower risk of cardiovascular diseases, obesity, and some forms of cancer. However, it is important to recognize that following a plant-based diet requires adequate planning to ensure the intake of all essential nutrients, such as proteins, vitamins, and minerals. Furthermore, it is crucial to emphasize that plant-based diets are not necessarily suitable for everyone and may require careful monitoring, especially in the initial stages of adoption. Supervision by healthcare professionals is essential to ensure that individuals maintain an optimal nutritional balance and to prevent any deficiencies or imbalances that may result from improperly planned diets.

A plant-based diet should be strictly monitored in more vulnerable groups. For instance, newborns or pregnant women can more easily experience specific micronutrient deficiencies such as a deficiency of vitamin B12, while school children or adolescents can more easily develop eating disorders. While plant-based diets offer numerous health benefits, it is important to carefully consider both the positive and negative aspects and to adopt a balanced approach to dietary choices. Further research is needed to fully understand the impacts of plant-based diets on the health and lifestyle habits of the population in order to provide more comprehensive information and support informed and healthy dietary choices.

Supplementary Materials: The following supporting information can be downloaded at: https://www.mdpi.com/article/10.3390/nu16091278/s1, STROBE checklist.

Author Contributions: E.S.: conceptualization, data curation, investigation, methodology, validation, writing—original draft, and writing—review and editing. M.S.: writing—review and editing. E.C.L.: data curation, formal Analysis, writing—review and editing. G.C.O.: conceptualization, investigation, methodology, and writing—review and editing. L.U.W.: formal analysis and writing—review and editing. M.P.: conceptualization, methodology, validation, and writing—review and editing. S.M.: conceptualization, methodology, and writing—review and editing. All authors have read and agreed to the published version of the manuscript.

Funding: This research received no external funding.

Institutional Review Board Statement: This research strictly followed the ethical principles outlined in the Declaration of Helsinki and received approval from the Ethics Research Committee of the Catholic University of Valencia (approval code UCV/2019-2020/152, 18 June 2020).

Informed Consent Statement: Prior to participating, explicit informed consent was obtained from all individuals, ensuring that they were fully informed about the study's objectives, procedures, and potential risks, and emphasizing the voluntary nature of their participation.

Data Availability Statement: The data presented in this study are available upon reasonable request from the corresponding author. The data are not publicly available due to privacy.

Acknowledgments: The authors sincerely appreciate the collaboration of all individuals who contributed to this research. Special thanks are extended to those who played a role in sharing the questionnaire and to those who devoted their time to participating in and providing responses to the survey.

Conflicts of Interest: None of the authors had any financial, personal, or professional conflict of interest in relation to the results of this study.

Appendix A

Figures A1–A8 show the results of the Dunn's Test performed for the most significant nutrition and lifestyle variables for the four population groups studied (people who followed a Mediterranean diet, respondents who adopted a vegan dietary pattern, those who preferred a vegetarian diet, and people who choose flexitarianism).

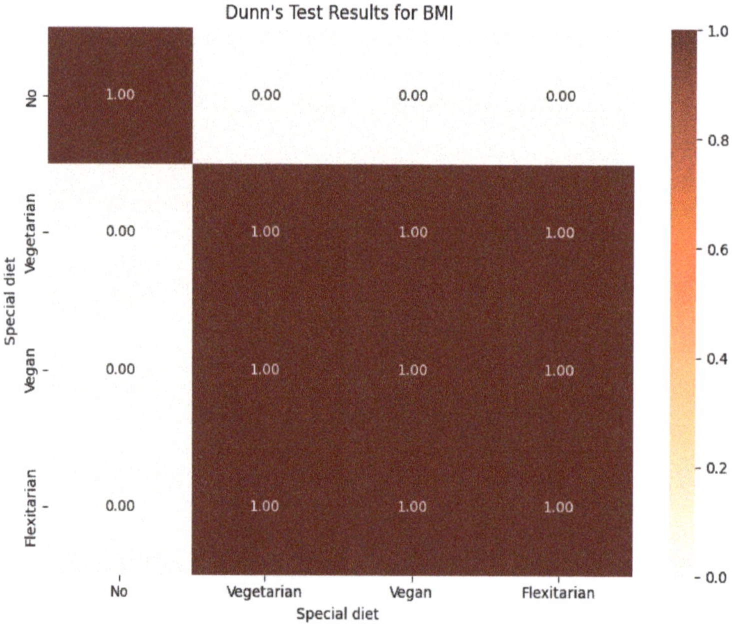

Figure A1. Dunn's test results for BMI.

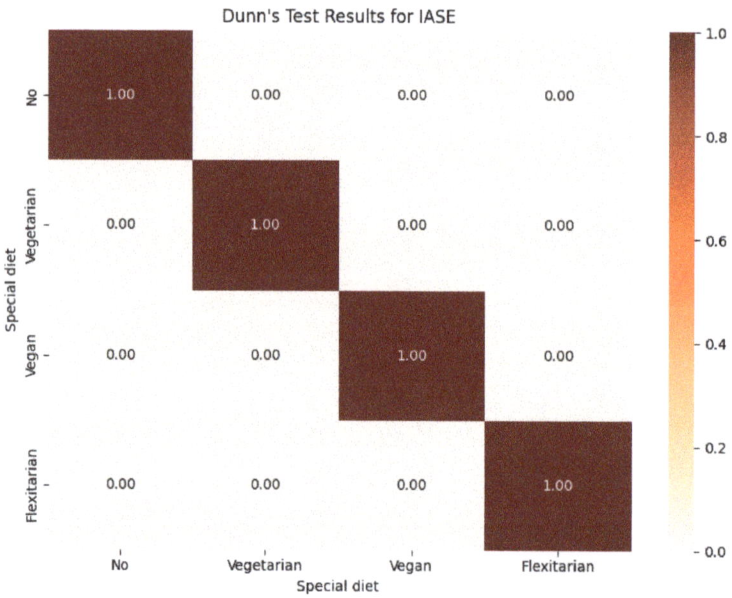

Figure A2. Dunn's test results for IASE.

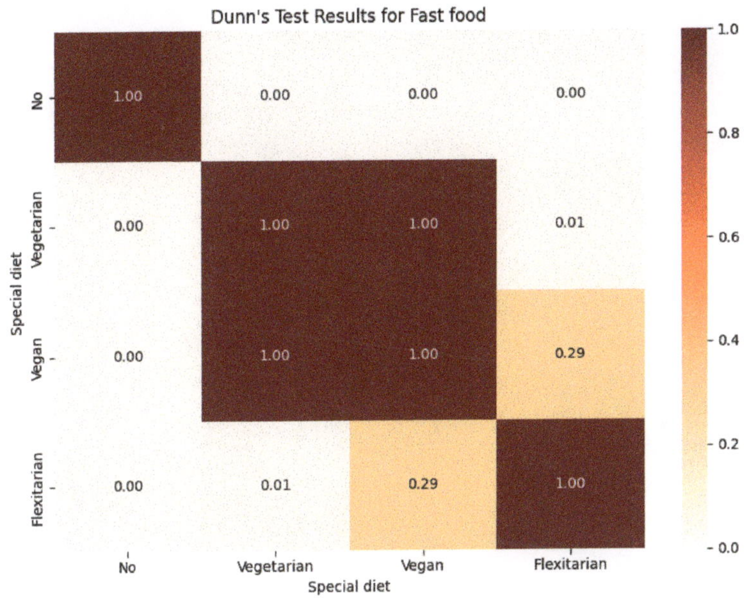

Figure A3. Dunn's test results for fast food.

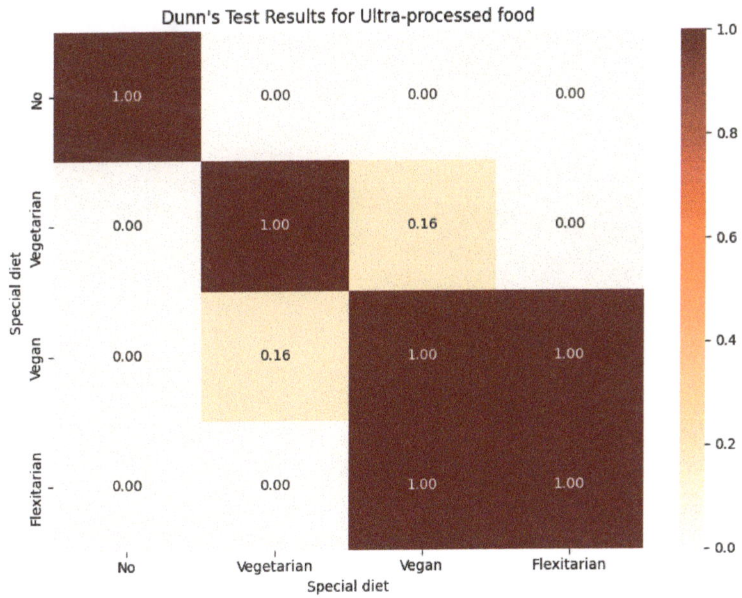

Figure A4. Dunn's test results for ultra-processed food.

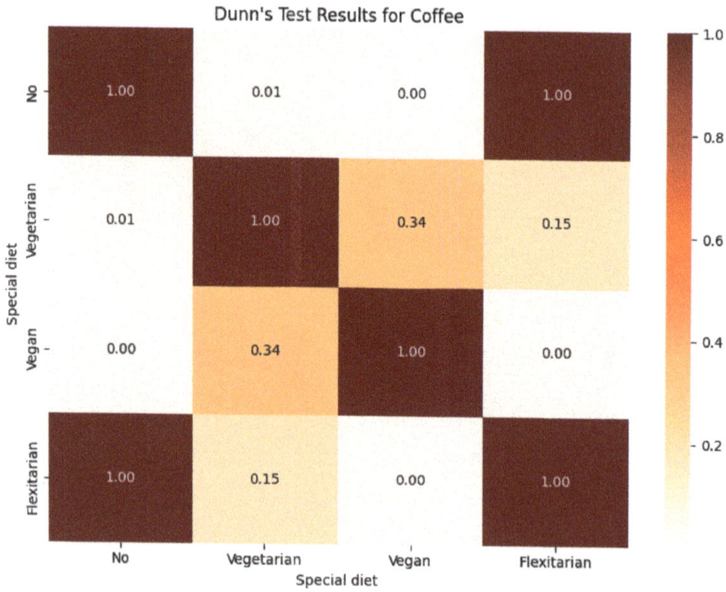

Figure A5. Dunn's test results for coffee and energy drinks.

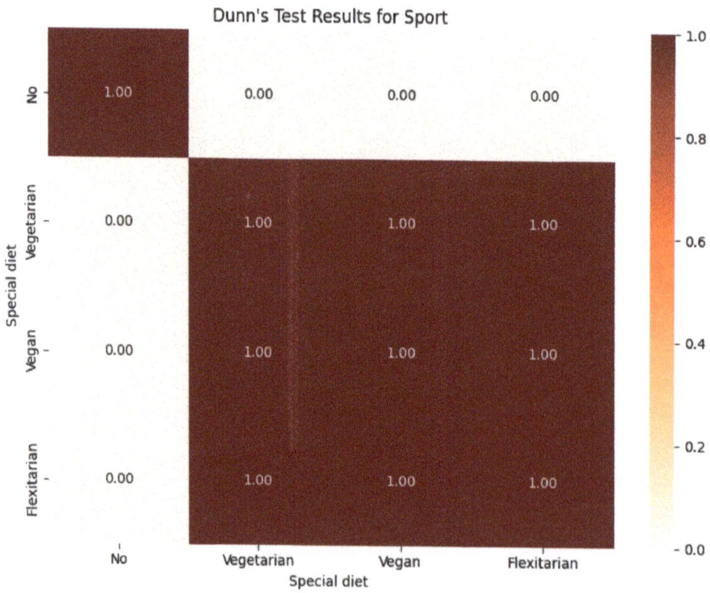

Figure A6. Dunn's test results for sport.

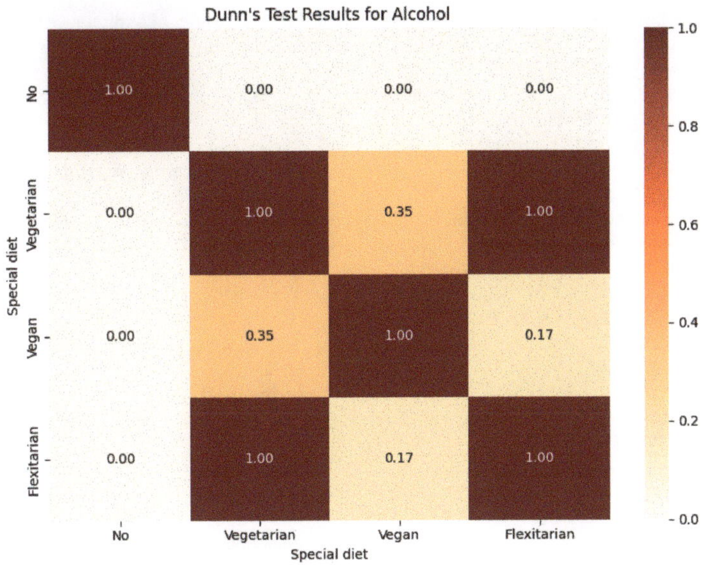

Figure A7. Dunn's test results for alcohol.

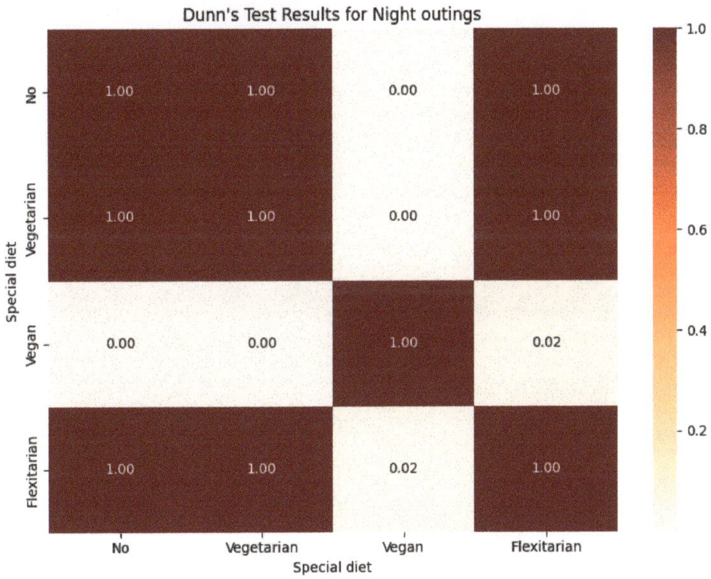

Figure A8. Dunn's test results for night outings.

References

1. Moreiras-Varela, O. The Mediterranean Diet in Spain. *Eur. J. Clin. Nutr.* **1989**, *43* (Suppl. 2), 83–87. [PubMed]
2. García-Fernández, E.; Rico-Cabanas, L.; Estruch, R.; Estruch, R.; Estruch, R.; Bach-Faig, A. Mediterranean Diet and Cardiodiabesity: A Review. *Nutrients* **2014**, *6*, 3474–3500. [CrossRef] [PubMed]
3. D'Alessandro, A.; De Pergola, G. The Mediterranean Diet: Its Definition and Evaluation of a Priori Dietary Indexes in Primary Cardiovascular Prevention. *Int. J. Food Sci. Nutr.* **2018**, *69*, 647–659. [CrossRef]
4. Dinu, M.; Pagliai, G.; Angelino, D.; Rosi, A.; Dall'Asta, M.; Bresciani, L.; Ferraris, C.; Guglielmetti, M.; Godos, J.; Del Bo, C.; et al. Effects of Popular Diets on Anthropometric and Cardiometabolic Parameters: An Umbrella Review of Meta-Analyses of Randomized Controlled Trials. *Adv. Nutr.* **2020**, *11*, 815–833. [CrossRef]

5. Godos, J.; Zappalà, G.; Bernardini, S.; Giambini, I.; Bes-Rastrollo, M.; Martinez-Gonzalez, M. Adherence to the Mediterranean Diet Is Inversely Associated with Metabolic Syndrome Occurrence: A Meta-Analysis of Observational Studies. *Int. J. Food Sci. Nutr.* **2017**, *68*, 138–148. [CrossRef] [PubMed]
6. Tosti, V.; Bertozzi, B.; Fontana, L. Health Benefits of the Mediterranean Diet: Metabolic and Molecular Mechanisms. *J. Gerontol. A Biol. Sci. Med. Sci.* **2018**, *73*, 318–326. [CrossRef] [PubMed]
7. Ventriglio, A.; Sancassiani, F.; Contu, M.P.; Latorre, M.; Di Slavatore, M.; Fornaro, M.; Bhugra, D. Mediterranean Diet and its Benefits on Health and Mental Health: A Literature Review. *Clin. Pract. Epidemiol. Ment. Health* **2020**, *16* (Suppl. 1), 156–164. [CrossRef]
8. Alemán, J.A.; Rentero, M.P.Z.; Montoro-García, S.; Mulero, J.; Garrido, A.P.; Leal, M.; Guerrero, L.; Ramos, E.; Ruilope, L.M. Adherence to the "Mediterranean Diet" in Spain and Its Relationship with Cardiovascular Risk (DIMERICA Study). *Nutrients* **2016**, *8*, 680. [CrossRef] [PubMed]
9. Modrego-Pardo, I.; Solá-Izquierdo, E.; Morillas-Ariño, C. Spanish Population Trends in Internet Searches for Information on Different Diets. *Endocrinol. Diabetes Nutr.* **2020**, *67*, 431–437. [CrossRef]
10. Tran, E.; Dale, H.F.; Jensen, C.; Lied, G.A. Effects of Plant-Based Diets on Weight Status: A Systematic Review. *Diabetes Metab. Syndr. Obes.* **2020**, *13*, 3433–3448. [CrossRef]
11. Allès, B.; Baudry, J.; Méjean, C.; Touvier, M.; Péneau, S.; Hercberg, S.; Kesse-Guyot, E. Comparison of Sociodemographic and Nutritional Characteristics between Self-Reported Vegetarians, Vegans, and Meat-Eaters from the NutriNet-Santé Study. *Nutrients* **2017**, *9*, 1023. [CrossRef] [PubMed]
12. Papier, K.; Tong, T.Y.; Appleby, P.N.; Bradbury, K.E.; Fensom, G.K.; Knuppel, A.; Perez-Cornago, A.; Schmidt, J.A.; Travis, R.C.; Key, T.J. Comparison of Major Protein-Source Foods and Other Food Groups in Meat-Eaters and Non-Meat-Eaters in the EPIC-Oxford Cohort. *Nutrients* **2019**, *11*, 824. [CrossRef] [PubMed]
13. Dakin, B.C.; Ching, A.E.; Teperman, E.; Klebl, C.; Moshel, M.; Bastian, B. Prescribing Vegetarian or Flexitarian Diets Leads to Sustained Reduction in Meat Intake. *Appetite* **2021**, *164*, 105285. [CrossRef] [PubMed]
14. Mathur, M.B.; Robinson, T.N.; Reichling, D.B.; Gardner, C.D.; Nadler, J.; Bain, P.A.; Peacock, J. Reducing Meat Consumption by Appealing to Animal Welfare: Protocol for a Meta-Analysis and Theoretical Review. *Syst. Rev.* **2020**, *9*, 3. [CrossRef] [PubMed]
15. Sabaté, J.; Soret, S. Sustainability of Plant-Based Diets: Back to the Future. *Am. J. Clin. Nutr.* **2014**, *100* (Suppl. 1), 476S–482S. [CrossRef] [PubMed]
16. Ruini, L.F.; Ciati, R.; Pratesi, C.A.; Marino, M.; Principato, L.; Vannuzzi, E. Working toward Healthy and Sustainable Diets: The "Double Pyramid Model" Developed by the Barilla Center for Food and Nutrition to Raise Awareness about the Environmental and Nutritional Impact of Foods. *Front. Nutr.* **2015**, *2*, 9. [CrossRef]
17. Orlich, M.J.; Fraser, G.E. Vegetarian Diets in the Adventist Health Study 2: A Review of Initial Findings. *Am. J. Clin. Nutr.* **2014**, *100*, 353S. [CrossRef] [PubMed]
18. Yokoyama, Y.; Nishimura, K.; Barnard, N.D.; Takegami, M.; Watanabe, M.; Sekikawa, A.; Okamura, T.; Miyamoto, Y. Vegetarian Diets and Blood Pressure: A Meta-Analysis. *JAMA Intern. Med.* **2014**, *174*, 577–587. [CrossRef] [PubMed]
19. Kahleova, H.; Levin, S.; Barnard, N.D. Vegetarian Dietary Patterns and Cardiovascular Disease. *Prog. Cardiovasc. Dis.* **2018**, *61*, 54–61. [CrossRef]
20. Tantamango-Bartley, Y.; Knutsen, S.F.; Knutsen, R.; Jacobsen, B.K.; Fan, J.; Lawrence Beeson, W.; Sabate, J.; Hadley, D.; Jaceldo-Siegl, K.; Penniecook, J.; et al. Are Strict Vegetarians Protected against Prostate Cancer? *Am. J. Clin. Nutr.* **2016**, *103*, 153–160. [CrossRef]
21. Ivanova, S.; Delattre, C.; Karcheva-Bahchevanska, D.; Benbasat, N.; Nalbantova, V.; Ivanov, K. Plant-Based Diet as a Strategy for Weight Control. *Foods* **2021**, *10*, 3052. [CrossRef] [PubMed]
22. Kim, M.-H.; Bae, Y.-J. Comparative Study of Serum Leptin and Insulin Resistance Levels Between Korean Postmenopausal Vegetarian and Non-Vegetarian Women. *Clin. Nutr. Res.* **2015**, *4*, 175. [CrossRef] [PubMed]
23. Key, T.J.; Papier, K.; Tong, T.Y.N. Plant-Based Diets and Long-Term Health: Findings from the EPIC-Oxford Study. *Proc. Nutr. Soc.* **2022**, *81*, 190–198. [CrossRef] [PubMed]
24. Radnitz, C.; Beezhold, B.; DiMatteo, J. Investigation of Lifestyle Choices of Individuals Following a Vegan Diet for Health and Ethical Reasons. *Appetite* **2015**, *90*, 31–36. [CrossRef] [PubMed]
25. Acevedo Cantero, P.; Ortega Santos, C.P.; López-Ejeda, N. Vegetarian Diets in Spain: Temporal Evolution through National Health Surveys and Their Association with Healthy Lifestyles. *Endocrinol. Diabetes Nutr.* **2023**, *70* (Suppl. 2), 1–8. [CrossRef] [PubMed]
26. von Elm, E.; Altman, D.G.; Egger, M.; Pocock, S.J.; Gøtzsche, P.C.; Vandenbroucke, J.P. The Strengthening the Reporting of Observational Studies in Epidemiology (STROBE) Statement: Guidelines for Reporting Observational Studies. *J. Clin. Epidemiol.* **2008**, *61*, 344–349. [CrossRef] [PubMed]
27. World Medical Association Declaration of Helsinki: Ethical Principles for Medical Research Involving Human Subjects. *JAMA* **2013**, *310*, 2191–2194. [CrossRef]
28. Biernacki, P.; Waldorf, D. Snowball Sampling: Problems and Techniques of Chain Referral Sampling. *Sociol. Methods Res.* **1981**, *10*, 141–163. [CrossRef]
29. AI, N.N.; Moncada R., O. Quality of the Spanish Diet According to the Healthy Eating Index. *Nutr. Hosp.* **2011**, *26*, 330–336.
30. Grupo Colaborativo de la Sociedad Española de Nutrición Comunitaria (SENC) Guías Alimentarias Para La Población Española; La Nueva Pirámide de La Alimentación Saludable. *Nutr. Hosp.* **2016**, *33*, 1–48.

31. Massey, F.J. The Kolmogorov-Smirnov Test for Goodness of Fit. *J. Am. Stat. Assoc.* **1951**, *46*, 68. [CrossRef]
32. McKight, P.E.; Najab, J. Kruskal-Wallis Test. In *The Corsini Encyclopedia of Psychology*; John Wiley & Sons: Hoboken, NJ, USA, 2010; Volume 1. [CrossRef]
33. Welcome to Python.Org. Available online: https://www.python.org/ (accessed on 12 March 2024).
34. Rodriguez Artalejo, F.; Banegas, J.R.; Graciani, M.A.; Hernández Vecino, R.; Rey Calero, J. Food and Nutrient Consumption in Spain in the Period 1940-1988. Analysis of Its Consistency with the Mediterranean Diet. *Med. Clin.* **1996**, *106*, 161–168.
35. Herrera-Ramos, E.; Tomaino, L.; Sánchez-Villegas, A.; Ribas-Barba, L.; Gómez, S.F.; Wärnberg, J.; Osés, M.; González-Gross, M.; Gusi, N.; Aznar, S.; et al. Trends in Adherence to the Mediterranean Diet in Spanish Children and Adolescents across Two Decades. *Nutrients* **2023**, *15*, 2348. [CrossRef] [PubMed]
36. Going Plant-Based: The Rise of Vegan and Vegetarian Food | Euromonitor. Available online: https://go.euromonitor.com/sb-packaged-food-210330-rise-vegan-vegetarian-food.html (accessed on 12 March 2024).
37. Lantern | Estudios: The Green Revolution 2019. Available online: https://www.lantern.es/papers/the-green-revolution-2019 (accessed on 12 March 2024).
38. Aavik, K. *Contesting Anthropocentric Masculinities through Veganism: Lived Experiences of Vegan Men*; Palgrave Macmillan: Cham, Switzerland, 2023; pp. 1–256. [CrossRef]
39. Pilař, L.; Kvasničková Stanislavská, L.; Kvasnička, R. Healthy Food on the Twitter Social Network: Vegan, Homemade, and Organic Food. *Int. J. Environ. Res. Public Health* **2021**, *18*, 3815. [CrossRef]
40. Anusha Siddiqui, S.; Bahmid, N.A.; Mahmud, C.M.M.; Boukid, F.; Lamri, M.; Gagaoua, M. Consumer acceptability of plant-, seaweed-, and insect-based foods as alternatives to meat: A critical compilation of a decade of research. *Crit. Rev. Food Sci. Nutr.* **2023**, *63*, 6630–6651. [CrossRef] [PubMed]
41. Wahl, H.W.; Gerstorf, D. A Conceptual Framework for Studying COntext Dynamics in Aging (CODA). *Dev. Rev.* **2018**, *50*, 155–176. [CrossRef]
42. Atlas of EHealth Country Profiles: The Use of EHealth in Support of Universal Health Coverage. Available online: https://www.who.int/publications/i/item/9789241565219 (accessed on 12 March 2024).
43. Big Data En Salud Digital | Universo Abierto. Available online: https://universoabierto.org/2023/01/19/big-data-en-salud-digital/ (accessed on 12 March 2024).
44. Kucharczuk, A.J.; Oliver, T.L.; Dowdell, E.B. Social Media's Influence on Adolescents' Food Choices: A Mixed Studies Systematic Literature Review. *Appetite* **2022**, *168*, 105765. [CrossRef]
45. Bartelmeß, T.; Godemann, J. Exploring the Linkages of Digital Food Communication and Analog Food Behavior: A Scoping Review. *Int. J. Environ. Res. Public Health* **2022**, *19*, 8990. [CrossRef]
46. Rogers, A.; Wilkinson, S.; Downie, O.; Truby, H. Communication of Nutrition Information by Influencers on Social Media: A Scoping Review. *Health Promot. J. Austr* **2022**, *33*, 657–676. [CrossRef]
47. Klassen, K.M.; Douglass, C.H.; Brennan, L.; Truby, H.; Lim, M.S.C. Social Media Use for Nutrition Outcomes in Young Adults: A Mixed-Methods Systematic Review. *Int. J. Behav. Nutr. Phys. Act.* **2018**, *15*, 70. [CrossRef]
48. Mingay, E.; Hart, M.; Yoong, S.; Hure, A. Why We Eat the Way We Do: A Call to Consider Food Culture in Public Health Initiatives. *Int. J. Environ. Res. Public Health* **2021**, *18*, 11967. [CrossRef] [PubMed]
49. Nisbett, N.; Harris, J.; Headey, D.; van den Bold, M.; Gillespie, S.; Aberman, N.L.; Adeyemi, O.; Aryeetey, R.; Avula, R.; Becquey, E.; et al. Stories of Change in Nutrition: Lessons from a New Generation of Studies from Africa, Asia and Europe. *Food Secur.* **2023**, *15*, 133. [CrossRef] [PubMed]
50. Machín, L.; Curutchet, M.R.; Gugliucci, V.; Vitola, A.; Otterbring, T.; de Alcantara, M.; Ares, G. The Habitual Nature of Food Purchases at the Supermarket: Implications for Policy Making. *Appetite* **2020**, *155*, 104844. [CrossRef] [PubMed]
51. Amit, S.K.; Uddin, M.M.; Rahman, R.; Islam, S.M.R.; Khan, M.S. A Review on Mechanisms and Commercial Aspects of Food Preservation and Processing. *Agric. Food Secur.* **2017**, *6*, 51. [CrossRef]
52. Ziso, D.; Chun, O.K.; Puglisi, M.J. Increasing Access to Healthy Foods through Improving Food Environment: A Review of Mixed Methods Intervention Studies with Residents of Low-Income Communities. *Nutrients* **2022**, *14*, 2278. [CrossRef] [PubMed]
53. World Health Organization. *Global Recommendations on Physical Activity for Health*; WHO Library Cataloguing-in-Publication: Geneva, Switzerland, 2010; pp. 1–58.

54. Swift, D.L.; McGee, J.E.; Earnest, C.P.; Carlisle, E.; Nygard, M.; Johannsen, N.M. The Effects of Exercise and Physical Activity on Weight Loss and Maintenance. *Prog. Cardiovasc. Dis.* **2018**, *61*, 206–213. [CrossRef] [PubMed]
55. Kolnes, K.J.; Petersen, M.H.; Lien-Iversen, T.; Højlund, K.; Jensen, J. Effect of Exercise Training on Fat Loss—Energetic Perspectives and the Role of Improved Adipose Tissue Function and Body Fat Distribution. *Front. Physiol.* **2021**, *12*, 737709. [CrossRef]
56. Hong, A.R.; Kim, S.W. Effects of Resistance Exercise on Bone Health. *Endocrinol. Metab.* **2018**, *33*, 435–444. [CrossRef] [PubMed]
57. Nystoriak, M.A.; Bhatnagar, A. Cardiovascular Effects and Benefits of Exercise. *Front. Cardiovasc. Med.* **2018**, *5*, 135. [CrossRef]
58. Bonanni, R.; Cariati, I.; Tarantino, U.; D'arcangelo, G.; Tancredi, V. Physical Exercise and Health: A Focus on Its Protective Role in Neurodegenerative Diseases. *J. Funct. Morphol. Kinesiol.* **2022**, *7*, 38. [CrossRef]
59. Xie, Y.; Liu, S.; Chen, X.J.; Yu, H.H.; Yang, Y.; Wang, W. Effects of Exercise on Sleep Quality and Insomnia in Adults: A Systematic Review and Meta-Analysis of Randomized Controlled Trials. *Front. Psychiatry* **2021**, *12*, 664499. [CrossRef] [PubMed]
60. Mahindru, A.; Patil, P.; Agrawal, V. Role of Physical Activity on Mental Health and Well-Being: A Review. *Cureus* **2023**, *15*, 33475. [CrossRef] [PubMed]
61. Alnasser, A.; Alomran, N. The Motivations and Practices of Vegetarian and Vegan Saudis. *Sci. Rep.* **2023**, *13*, 9742. [CrossRef] [PubMed]
62. Hopwood, C.J.; Bleidorn, W.; Schwaba, T.; Chen, S. Health, Environmental, and Animal Rights Motives for Vegetarian Eating. *PLoS ONE* **2020**, *15*, e0230609. [CrossRef]
63. Reuber, H.; Muschalla, B. Dietary Identity and Embitterment among Vegans, Vegetarians and Omnivores. *Health Psychol. Behav. Med.* **2022**, *10*, 1038. [CrossRef]
64. Turner-McGrievy, G.; Mandes, T.; Crimarco, A. A Plant-Based Diet for Overweight and Obesity Prevention and Treatment. *J. Geriatr. Cardiol.* **2017**, *14*, 369. [CrossRef]
65. Fuhrman, J. The Hidden Dangers of Fast and Processed Food. *Am. J. Lifestyle Med.* **2018**, *12*, 375. [CrossRef]
66. Pagliai, G.; Dinu, M.; Madarena, M.P.; Bonaccio, M.; Iacoviello, L.; Sofi, F. Consumption of Ultra-Processed Foods and Health Status: A Systematic Review and Meta-Analysis. *Br. J. Nutr.* **2021**, *125*, 308–318. [CrossRef]
67. Maldonado-Pereira, L.; Barnaba, C.; de Los Campos, G.; Medina-Meza, I.G. Evaluation of the Nutritional Quality of Ultra-Processed Foods (Ready to Eat + Fast Food): Fatty Acids, Sugar, and Sodium. *J. Food Sci.* **2022**, *87*, 3659–3676. [CrossRef]
68. Cahill, L.E.; Pan, A.; Chiuve, S.E.; Sun, Q.; Willett, W.C.; Hu, F.B.; Rimm, E.B. Fried-Food Consumption and Risk of Type 2 Diabetes and Coronary Artery Disease: A Prospective Study in 2 Cohorts of US Women and Men. *Am. J. Clin. Nutr.* **2014**, *100*, 667–675. [CrossRef]
69. Qin, P.; Zhang, M.; Han, M.; Liu, D.; Luo, X.; Xu, L.; Zeng, Y.; Chen, Q.; Wang, T.; Chen, X.; et al. Fried-food consumption and risk of cardiovascular disease and all-cause mortality: A meta-analysis of observational studies. *Heart* **2021**, *107*, 1567–1575. [CrossRef]
70. Tengiz, Z.M.; Oraman, Y. The Evaluation of the Students' Attitudes and Behavior towards Fast Food Consumption. In *Foodbalt 201, proceedings of the 13th Baltic Conference on Food Science and Technology: Food. Nutrition. Well-Being*; Latvia University of Life Sciences and Technologies: Jelgava, Latvia, 2019; pp. 232–237. [CrossRef]
71. Azizi Fard, N.; De Francisci Morales, G.; Mejova, Y.; Schifanella, R. On the Interplay between Educational Attainment and Nutrition: A Spatially-Aware Perspective. *EPJ Data Sci.* **2021**, *10*, 18. [CrossRef]
72. Elizabeth, L.; Machado, P.; Zinöcker, M.; Baker, P.; Lawrence, M. Ultra-Processed Foods and Health Outcomes: A Narrative Review. *Nutrients* **2020**, *12*, 1955. [CrossRef]
73. Dinu, M.; Pagliai, G.; Casini, A.; Sofi, F. Mediterranean Diet and Multiple Health Outcomes: An Umbrella Review of Meta-Analyses of Observational Studies and Randomised Trials. *Eur. J. Clin. Nutr.* **2018**, *72*, 30–43. [CrossRef]
74. Sofi, F.; Abbate, R.; Gensini, G.F.; Casini, A. Accruing Evidence on Benefits of Adherence to the Mediterranean Diet on Health: An Updated Systematic Review and Meta-Analysis. *Am. J. Clin. Nutr.* **2010**, *92*, 1189–1196. [CrossRef]
75. Sofi, F.; Macchi, C.; Abbate, R.; Gensini, G.F.; Casini, A. Mediterranean Diet and Health Status: An Updated Meta-Analysis and a Proposal for a Literature-Based Adherence Score. *Public Health Nutr.* **2014**, *17*, 2769–2782. [CrossRef]
76. Schwingshackl, L.; Hoffmann, G. Does a Mediterranean-Type Diet Reduce Cancer Risk? *Curr. Nutr. Rep.* **2016**, *5*, 9–17. [CrossRef]
77. Bakaloudi, D.R.; Halloran, A.; Rippin, H.L.; Oikonomidou, A.C.; Dardavesis, T.I.; Williams, J.; Wickramasinghe, K.; Breda, J.; Chourdakis, M. Intake and Adequacy of the Vegan Diet. A Systematic Review of the Evidence. *Clin. Nutr.* **2021**, *40*, 3503–3521. [CrossRef]
78. Matta, J.; Czernichow, S.; Kesse-Guyot, E.; Hoertel, N.; Limosin, F.; Goldberg, M.; Zins, M.; Lemogne, C. Depressive Symptoms and Vegetarian Diets: Results from the Constances Cohort. *Nutrients* **2018**, *10*, 1695. [CrossRef]
79. Lavallee, K.; Zhang, X.C.; Michelak, J.; Schneider, S.; Margraf, J. Vegetarian Diet and Mental Health: Cross-Sectional and Longitudinal Analyses in Culturally Diverse Samples. *J. Affect. Disord.* **2019**, *248*, 147–154. [CrossRef]
80. Sun, Y.H. Health concern, food choice motives, and attitudes toward healthy eating: The mediating role of food choice motives. *Appetite* **2008**, *51*, 42–49. [CrossRef] [PubMed]
81. Karam, J.; Haddad, C.; Sacre, H.; Serhan, M.; Salameh, P.; Jomaa, L. Financial Wellbeing and Quality of Life Among a Sample of the Lebanese Population: The Mediating Effect of Food Insecurity. *Front. Nutr.* **2022**, *9*, 906646, Erratum in *Front. Nutr.* **2022**, *9*, 1029025. [CrossRef]

82. Urhan, M.; Okut Aysin, E. Nutritional and health behaviour predictors of the weight gain during the COVID-19 pandemic. *Eur. J. Nutr.* **2022**, *61*, 2993–3002. [CrossRef] [PubMed]
83. Ferrara, M.; Langiano, E.; Falese, L.; Diotaiuti, P.; Cortis, C.; De Vito, E. Changes in Physical Activity Levels and Eating Behaviours during the COVID-19 Pandemic: Sociodemographic Analysis in University Students. *Int. J. Environ. Res. Public Health* **2022**, *19*, 5550. [CrossRef] [PubMed]

nutrients

MDPI

Article

Analysis of Malnutrition among Children under Five Years across Contrasting Agroecosystems of Northwest Ethiopia: Application of Structural Equation Modeling

Biruk Yazie Wubetie [1,2,*], Atsushi Tsunekawa [3], Nigussie Haregeweyn [4], Mitsuru Tsubo [3], Zerihun Nigussie [2], Taye Minichil Meshesha [1,5] and Takeshi Abe [4]

1 The United Graduate School of Agricultural Sciences, Tottori University, 4-101 Koyama-Minami, Tottori 680-8553, Japan
2 College of Agriculture and Environmental Sciences, Bahir Dar University, Bahir Dar P.O. Box 5501, Ethiopia
3 Arid Land Research Center, Tottori University, 1390 Hamasaka, Tottori 680-0001, Japan
4 International Platform for Dryland Research and Education, Tottori University, 1390 Hamasaka, Tottori 680-0001, Japan
5 School of Civil and Water Resources Engineering, Debre Markos Institute of Technology, Debre Markos University, Debre Markos P.O. Box 269, Ethiopia
* Correspondence: birukyazie@gmail.com

Abstract: Child malnutrition remains a public health challenge in developing countries, but a comprehensive understanding of its burden and its determinants in specific local contexts is generally lacking. This study examined the prevalence of malnutrition and its determinants among children aged <5 years across contrasting agroecosystems in northwest Ethiopia. A community-based cross-sectional study involving 400 respondents was employed. Data were collected through semi-structured questionnaires and anthropometric measurements, complemented with focus group discussions and key informant interviews. The direct and indirect effects of the determinants of malnutrition were examined using structural equation modeling (SEM). The overall prevalence of child malnutrition, measured using the Composite Index of Anthropometric Failure, was 49%, with notable variation across agroecosystems (from 36.1% [midland with red soil] to 59% [lowland and valley fragmented]). Disease experience had significant positive direct effects on malnutrition. Dietary intake had negative and significant total (direct and indirect) effects on malnutrition, partially mediated through disease experience. Serial mediation in SEM analysis revealed significant indirect relationships between malnutrition and food security, feeding and care practices, household environment, health services, maternal diet, maternal empowerment, household wealth, and nutrition-sensitive agricultural practices. In conclusion, child malnutrition was highly prevalent and higher among children in the lowland and valley fragmented agroecosystem, characterized by unfavorable agro-climatic conditions, lower wealth status, poor health services access, and higher disease (particularly malaria) exposure. This study demonstrates the dynamics and multifaceted nature of malnutrition, highlighting the importance of considering geographical differences when planning interventions for childhood malnutrition and its determinants.

Keywords: child malnutrition; dietary intake; structural equation modeling; dryland; Ethiopia

1. Introduction

Malnutrition remains a significant global public health challenge despite concerted global efforts to enhance child nutrition. As of 2022, the statistics reveal a distressing reality: globally, over one-fifth of children aged <5 years were stunted (amounting to 148.1 million children), and 45 million children were affected by wasting [1]. Even more alarming is the fact that approximately 5.2 million children aged <5 years died due to malnutrition-related complications, with nearly half of these fatalities attributed to malnutrition [1]. The prevalence of malnourished children is disproportionately concentrated in Asia and Africa, with these regions bearing the brunt of the crisis. For instance, by 2020, more than half of all stunted and more than two-thirds of all wasted children aged <5 years lived in Asia, and two of every five stunted and more than one-quarter of all wasted children aged <5 years lived in Africa [2].

Echoing the global trend, child malnutrition remains a pressing public health issue in Ethiopia. The latest Ethiopian Demographic and Health Survey (EDHS) underscores this reality, revealing that 38% of children aged <5 years across Ethiopia are stunted, with an alarming 46% of children aged <5 years in the Amhara region being stunted. In addition, approximately 24% and 10% of these children are underweight and wasted, respectively [3]. The ramifications of child malnutrition are profound, accounting for approximately 28% of child mortality, 16% of primary school repetition, an 8% reduction in the workforce, and an annual economic cost of ETB 55.5 billion, equivalent to approximately 16.5% of the country's gross domestic product [4].

Addressing the burden of child malnutrition requires a comprehensive understanding of its determinants within specific contexts, including at the individual, household, community, region, and environmental levels [5]. The framework conceptualized by the United Nations International Children's Emergency Fund (UNICEF) identifies three types of determinants of malnutrition: basic, underlying, and immediate [6]. Empirical studies conducted globally confirm that a child's dietary intake and disease experiences constitute immediate causes of malnutrition [7–11]. Similarly, studies conducted in various developing countries, including Ethiopia, highlight the significant association between child malnutrition and underlying determinants such as food security, feeding and care practices, health services, and household environments (water, sanitation, and hygiene) [7,8,10–27]. In addition, these studies also highlight the significant role of basic factors, such as maternal education, media exposure, training, nutrition-sensitive agricultural practices, agroecosystem characteristics, and household wealth in child malnutrition.

The Ethiopian government has demonstrated a strong commitment to addressing child malnutrition, as evidenced by the formulation of numerous multisectoral programs, policies, and initiatives since 2008. These include the National Nutrition Program (NNP-I and NNP-II), Nutrition-Sensitive Agriculture (NSA) policy, Seqota Declaration, National Nutrition Policy and Strategy, and the recently developed Food-Based Dietary Guideline [28,29]. However, despite these efforts, child malnutrition persists in Ethiopia, particularly in the Amhara region, where nearly half of all children aged <5 years are reported to be stunted [3]. This underscores the need for further research to provide us with a comprehensive understanding of the prevalence of child malnutrition and its determinants.

Although previous studies have provided valuable insights into child malnutrition, significant research gaps remain, particularly with regard to the effects of agriculture and agroecosystem characteristics on child malnutrition, which are often overlooked in the existing literature. In addition, methodological advances are warranted to better capture the complex and multifaceted nature of malnutrition determinants [30]. To this end, we used structural equation modeling (SEM) techniques in the present study, leveraging the UNICEF conceptual framework, to analyze the hierarchical relationships between malnutrition and its determinants. Unlike conventional regression analysis, SEM offers a more nuanced understanding of these relationships by allowing for the measurement of latent variables and their direct and indirect effects on malnutrition. Furthermore, this study used the Composite Index of Anthropometric Failure (CIAF) to comprehensively assess the prevalence of child malnutrition, thereby mitigating the risk of underestimation associated with conventional single anthropometric indicators [31].

The aims of the present study were to comprehensively examine the prevalence of malnutrition and to explore its determinants among children aged <5 years in northwest Ethiopia. The findings hold significant implications for stakeholders involved in nutrition-sensitive and nutrition-specific intervention programs, facilitating a nuanced understanding of spatial variations across agroecosystems. Therefore, targeting and working on <5 years children is a great window of opportunity to tackle the intergenerational impact of malnutrition.

Conceptual Framework

Drawing upon UNICEF's conceptual framework and prior studies conducted in developing countries [6,32,33], this study adapts a conceptual framework tailored towards the Ethiopian context. The framework delineates the determinants and consequences of child malnutrition, operating across multiple levels of causation, from broad socioeconomic and environmental factors to immediate child-level factors. At its core, the framework distinguishes between basic, underlying, and immediate factors hypothesized to impact child malnutrition directly and indirectly, as shown in Figure 1. Immediate causes, such as exposure to disease and inadequate dietary intake, are identified as primary instigators of malnutrition in children. However, factors within each child's household (e.g., insufficient access to food, poor maternal and child feeding practices, inadequate health services, and poor household environment encompassing issues like lack of safe water and sanitation) are recognized as proximal determinants significantly affecting the immediate causes of malnutrition. These household-level determinants represent proximal context indirectly affecting a child's nutritional status. Beyond the household level, broader social factors encompassing socioeconomic status and environmental conditions are identified as distal causes, exerting their influence by shaping the quality and quantity of the resources available within households. Consequently, factors operating at the societal level are deemed as basic or root causes underlying child malnutrition.

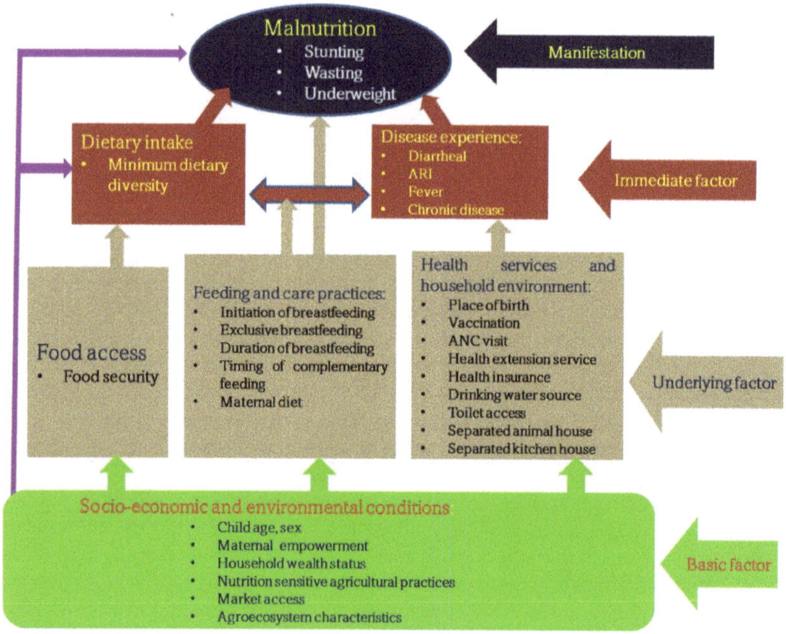

Figure 1. Modified conceptual framework on determinants associated with child malnutrition [6].

2. Materials and Methods

2.1. Study Area

The Chemoga watershed in the northwest part of Ethiopia is located within the Upper Blue Nile Basin (Figure 2), a region characterized by its diverse topography, ranging from highlands to lowlands. The Chemoga watershed is approximately 300 km northwest of

Addis Ababa, the capital of Ethiopia, and covers a considerable land area with varying climatic and ecological conditions. The area is predominantly characterized by contrasting agroecosystems with diverse agricultural practices (Table 1), with altitudes ranging from 800 m above sea level (asl) in the lowlands and valley fragmented to higher peaks in the hilly and mountainous highlands (4200 m asl). The Chemoga watershed plays a vital role in the hydrology of the region, ultimately contributing to the flow of the Blue Nile River. Human activities, such as crop cultivation, livestock grazing, and settlement, are prevalent throughout the watershed, including along steep slopes, exerting pressure on the natural environment and contributing to land degradation [34]. Livelihoods in the area primarily rely on a mixed farming system integrating both crop cultivation and the rearing of livestock. Overall, the Chemoga watershed serves as an important ecological and hydrological component of the Upper Blue Nile Basin, playing a crucial role in sustaining local livelihoods and biodiversity.

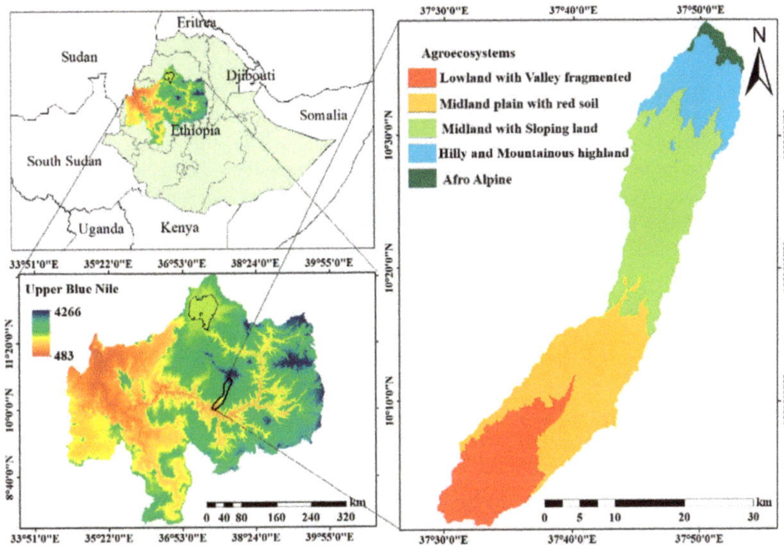

Figure 2. Maps showing the location of the study area.

Table 1. General characteristics of the agroecosystems in Chemoga watershed.

Agroecosystem [A]	Mean Annual Temperature (°C)	Mean Annual Rainfall (mm)	Altitude (m asl)	Farming System
AEZ-1	15.7–27.4	996.29	800–1400	Sorghum–maize–teff
AEZ-2	10.4–22.7	1251.10	1400–2400	Wheat–maize–teff
AEZ-3	10–22	1282.40	2400–2800	Wheat–barley
AEZ-4	8.8–21.2	1399.30	2800–3800	Potato–barley
AEZ-5	5.4–18.1	1434.5	3800–4200	Choke protected area

Rainfall and temperature data averaged over 1983–2018 from the Ethiopian Metrological Agency. [A] Locations of the different agroecosystem zones (AEZs) are shown in Figure 2. AEZ-1, lowland with valley fragmented; AEZ-2, midland plain with red soils; AEZ-3, midland with sloping land; AEZ-4, hilly and mountainous highland; AEZ-5, afro alpine. Sources: own survey and [35].

2.2. Study Design and Sampling Procedures

The present study employed a cross-sectional study design and strategically used a multi-stage sampling method, with agroecosystem typology serving as a key stratification parameter. Initially, the Chemoga watershed was delineated with five distinct agroecosystems that covered three districts, namely Sinan, Gozamin, and Baso Liben. Subsequently, four representative kebeles (the smallest administrative units in Ethiopia, each classified according to their unique agroecosystem characteristics) were randomly chosen from four agroecosystems within three districts in the Chemoga watershed, namely Sinan (AEZ-3, AEZ-4), Gozamin (AEZ-1, AEZ-2), and Baso Liben (AEZ-1, AEZ-2). Since there are no human settlements within the afro-alpine agroecosystem (AEZ-5), it has been excluded from the sample selection process. In collaboration with local health extension workers, households with children aged <5 years were identified in the selected kebeles using the health post's records as the sampling frame. Then, using a systematic random sampling approach, child–mother pairs were selected, with sample sizes allocated proportionately based on the number of children aged <5 years in each of the kebele. In cases where an individual mother had more than one child aged <5 years, one child was randomly selected for inclusion in the study.

The determination of the sample size adhered to the established formula for a single population proportion, ensuring appropriateness and rigor in the sampling process:

$$n = \frac{(Z_{\alpha/2})^2 \times \mathrm{p(q)}}{\mathrm{d}^2}$$

where n is the required sample size, $Z_{\alpha/2}$ is the upper point of $\alpha/2$ (which has a value of 1.96 in the standard normal distribution with a 95% confidence level), p is the prevalence of the outcome of interest and was assumed to be 50% because there have been no previous studies in the area, q is calculated as $(1-\mathrm{p})$, and d is the desired precision (5%). To achieve the desired precision level, a 5% non-response rate was considered. Finally, the study included 404 pairs of children aged <5 years along with their mothers.

2.3. Data Collection Methods

The study used a detailed household survey and anthropometric assessments involving 404 children aged <5 years with their mothers. The survey was conducted in June and July 2023. Data were collected through semi-structured questionnaires and anthropometric measurements. This was complemented with a focus group discussion and key informant interviews. The survey covered comprehensive information at various levels (child, maternal, household, and community), encompassing data on socioeconomic conditions, food security, dietary diversity, and relevant agricultural practices. The survey was administered by trained health and agricultural extension workers who were well acquainted with the sampled kebeles. The survey was closely supervised by the first author (BYW). To facilitate smooth administration, data collectors underwent a day-long training session. The survey was enriched with insights from key informant interviews, involving health and agricultural extension workers, alongside field observations.

2.4. Data Measurement

2.4.1. Food Security

Food security status was assessed using the Household Food Insecurity Access Scale (HFIAS), a validated tool used in various developing countries [36]. This tool consists of nine standard generic questions addressing a household's experiences over the past month across three domains of food insecurity: (i) anxiety and uncertainty regarding food availability, including worries about whether the household would have enough to eat; (ii) limitations in the variety and preferences of food accessed; and (iii) insufficient food intake in terms of meal sizes and their frequencies.

2.4.2. Dietary Diversity

Each child's mother was asked about the foods that she and her child had eaten and the beverages they had consumed in the past 24 h. This study used the Food and Agriculture Organization of the United Nations (FAO) guideline, which measures dietary diversity across seven food groups for children and ten food groups for women (WDDS).

Dietary diversity scores (DDSs) for children and women were calculated by summing the number of food groups consumed in the 24 h prior to the survey [37,38].

2.4.3. Anthropometric Measurements

Anthropometric data were obtained by measuring children's weight and height. Weight measurements in children were obtained without footwear and with minimal clothing, using the recommended UNICEF weighing scale to the nearest 0.1 kg. In cases where children refused to be weighed, their mothers would carry them and stand on the scale; the child's weight was then determined by subtracting the mother's weight from the combined weight of the mother and child. Scales were calibrated before weighing each child using a fixed 2 kg mass. For children who could stand independently, height was measured, without footwear, to the nearest 0.1 cm using a standard calibrated standing height board. Children were positioned against the standing board, ensuring that five body parts (heels, bat, buttocks, shoulders, and back of the head) touched the board. A measuring tape was fixed to the board, and the child stood with their head comfortably erect, aligning the lower border of the eye's orbit with the external canal of the ear. Measurements were taken using a horizontally held thin wooden board by touching the top of the head. For children who could not stand independently, length measurements were taken to the nearest 0.1 cm by using a length board fixed with measuring tape and equipped with a headpiece and elongated foot piece. During the measurement, the child's head touched the headpiece, and their heels were in contact with the foot piece. The hands remained relaxed throughout the measuring process. For each child, three consecutive measurements of weight and height/length were obtained, with the average of the three measurements used in the final analysis. The age of the child, in months, was determined from the date of birth (as reported by the mother) to the day of data collection.

2.5. Data Quality Assurance

Data quality was ensured through a meticulous design of the questionnaire and data collection process. Data collectors and supervisors underwent training on both data collection procedures and ethical considerations. A pre-test survey was conducted on 5% of households with similar backgrounds outside the targeted watershed to validate and tailor the questionnaire to local conditions. This iterative process validated the questionnaire and allowed for the customization of instruments. Supervisors checked on a daily basis to ensure completeness and consistency. In addition, the principal investigator (BYW) monitored the overall quality of the data collection as well as thorough entry, and proper management of all the data before the final analysis.

2.6. Data Management and Analysis

Data were managed using SPSS version 28 (IBM Inc., Armonk, NY, USA). The data were then exported to Stata version 17 (Stata Corp, College Station, TX, USA) for further analysis by a combination of descriptive (percentage, mean, standard deviation [SD]) and inferential (chi-squared test, *t*-test, one-way analysis of variance [ANOVA]) statistics. The study primarily used SEM to measure the direct and indirect effects of risk factors on child malnutrition using SPSS AMOS version 29. In addition, a logistic regression model was used to analyze the direct influence of immediate factors only on child malnutrition. A household's wealth index was computed through principal component analysis based on the main assets owned by the households (as shown in the Supplementary Materials). Standard deviation for the Z-score was computed for height-for-age, weight-for-age, and weight-for-height indices by comparison against the median of the World Health Organization (WHO) standards using the Emergency Nutrition Assessment (ENA) and WHO Anthro plus version 1.0.4 software.

2.7. Structural Equation Modeling

The hierarchical, complex, and interconnected nature of the determinants associated with child malnutrition requires a model that is capable of incorporating and estimating a set of equations simultaneously. This study used the SEM model, considering multiple levels (basic, underlying, immediate), with each level representing variables influencing one another that are treated as a dependent or response variable, as shown in the conceptual framework (Figure 1). SEM combines the statistical elements of multiple regression, confirmatory factor analysis, and path analysis [39]. This analysis was performed using AMOS version 29 software. It examines complex models with both measured and unmeasured variables (latent variables), allowing for the inclusion of endogenous, exogenous, and mediator variables. Unlike path analysis, SEM entertains latent variables alongside observed variables [39]. Mediation analysis was performed to predict the indirect effect of determinants on child malnutrition. In the context of the SEM framework, mediation is categorized as either full or partial [40]. Mediators can further be classified as single or multiple, single when only one variable lies in the causal pathway between exogenous and endogenous variables, and multiple when more than one mediator operates concurrently at the same stage in the structural model (termed "serial" or "sequential" mediation) [40]. Multigroup SEM analysis was conducted to estimate the effects on the structural model across different groups, offering insights into possible variations in relationships among variables across these groups.

SEM has two parts: a measurement model and a structure model. In the present study, model fitness for both models was determined using the goodness-of-fit index (GFI), comparative fit index (CFI), root mean square error of approximation (RMSEA), and standardized root mean squared residual (SRMR) [41]. Before running SEM, confirmatory factor analysis was performed to verify the model's fit by excluding items with low factor loading. The measurement model was validated through reliability and validity assessments prior to the evaluation of causal relationships among variables in the structural model. The reliability test reflects the internal consistency of the observed variables through composite reliability, whereas validity examines the extent to which the indicator or a measure accurately reflects its constructs. Therefore, construct reliability and validity were determined using composite reliability (CR) and average variance extracted (AVE). The maximum likelihood estimation procedure was used in the model analysis. The estimation of the indirect effects used the product-of-coefficients test, whereas total effects were obtained by summing the direct and indirect effects, using bootstrap techniques to determine the level of significance. The Bayesian analysis method addressed missing data with the assumption of missing completely at random. Standardized and unstandardized coefficients, and their exponential (odds ratio), were used to estimate the direct, indirect, and total effects of predictors on child malnutrition. Ultimately, statistical significance was declared when $p < 0.05$. Generally, SEM provided a comprehensive analysis of the complex relationships influencing child malnutrition.

2.8. Operational Definitions and Key Variables of The Study

Malnutrition, as conceptualized in this study, encompasses various manifestations of undernutrition, namely stunting, wasting, and underweight. These conditions collectively contribute to a state of malnutrition, which is assessed through the CIAF, categorizing individuals into malnourished and not malnourished groups.

The CIAF represents a comprehensive metric that evaluates malnutrition by combining multiple anthropometric failure indicators, including stunting, wasting, and underweight into a single index. It provides a more holistic measure of nutritional status than individual indicators alone.

The main variables in this study are derived from the UNICEF conceptual framework, with some modification by customization to the Ethiopian context. Therefore, by reviewing the related literature, the key basic, underlying, and immediate factors are identified and included in the final model. For the sake of SEM analysis and interpretation in AMOS software, some multiple categorical measured variables, such as education, vaccination, wealth index, and agroecosystems, were changed to dummy categories (Table 2).

Table 2. Description and measurement of predictor variables.

Variable	Indicators	Measurement	Level
Latent variable			
Women empowerment	Education level	1, can read and write; 0, otherwise	Basic factors
	Nutrition related training taken	1, yes; 0, otherwise	
	Media exposure	1, yes; 0, otherwise	
NSA practices	Home gardening	1, good practice; 0, poor practice	
	Livestock in TLU	Number of livestock in TLU	
Feeding and care practices	Initiation of BF	1, started within 1 h; 0, otherwise	Underlying factors
	Exclusive BF	1, yes; 0, otherwise	
	Initiation of CF	1, started on time; 0, otherwise	
Household environment	Toilet availability	1, yes; 0, otherwise	
	Kitchen house	1, separated from living quarters; 0, otherwise	
	Animal house	1, separated from living quarters; 0, otherwise	
Health services	Vaccination	1, fully vaccinated; 0, otherwise	
	ANC visit	1, ≥4 visit; 0, otherwise	
	Health insurance	1, they have; 0, otherwise	
	Extension service	Number of contacts per year	
Disease experience	Diarrheal disease	1, experienced it; 0, otherwise	Immediate factor
	Fever	1, experienced it; 0, otherwise	
	ARI	1, experienced it; 0, otherwise	
	Chronic illness	1, experienced it; 0, otherwise	
Observed variables			
Wealth status	Wealth index	1, rich; 0, poor	Basic
Food access	Food security	1, food secure; 0, food insecure	Underlying
Maternal diet	Minimum WDDS	1, ≥5 food groups; 0, otherwise	Underlying
Child dietary intake	Minimum CDDS	1, ≥4 food groups; 0, otherwise	Immediate
Agroecosystem	AEZ	1, AEZ-2,3,4; 0, AEZ-1	Basic
Malnutrition	CIAF	1, malnourished; 0, otherwise	Outcome

AEZ, agroecosystem zone; ANC, antenatal care; ARI, acute respiratory infection; BF, breastfeeding; CDDS, dietary diversity score for children; CF, complementary feeding; CIAF, Composite Index of Anthropometric Failure; NSA, nutrition-sensitive agricultural practices; TLU, Tropical Livestock Unit; WDDS, dietary diversity score for women.

2.9. Ethical Considerations

Before data collection, ethical approval was obtained from the Department of Rural Development and Agricultural Extension, College of Agriculture and Environmental Sciences, Bahir Dar University. During the survey, an official letter was sent to all districts to obtain permission for data collection. Verbal consent was obtained from all study participants before the commencement of the data collection. The data obtained from each study participant was kept confidential.

3. Results

3.1. Basic Sociodemographic Characteristics

Of the final 400 children aged <5 years included in the study (99% response rate), approximately 54% were boys and about 46% were girls (Table S1). The mean age of the children stood at 23 months, while the mean age of the mothers was 34 years. A significant majority (~95%) of mothers were married. Only 18% of the mothers had basic literacy skills; furthermore, only 10.3% had had the opportunity to participate in formal education (Table S1). Approximately one-quarter of the mothers received training pertaining to child nutrition, covering essential aspects such as infant and child feeding practices, and overall health awareness. Of note, 40% of the mothers were equal decision makers in their households, particularly on significant matters. Approximately two-thirds of the households fell within the bracket of poor to middle wealth, indicative of the prevalent economic challenges faced by the studied communities (Table S1).

3.2. Food Security, Dietary Diversity, and Feeding Practices

As presented in Table 3, most children (61%) in this study were from food-insecure households. Most children (~90%) were exclusively breastfed up to 6 months of age, and approximately 92% were breastfed within 1 h of birth. However, nearly half the children (46%) were not introduced to complementary feeding within the recommended time of 6 months. For children, the mean(±SD) child DDS was 3.62 ± 1.03 (out of seven standard food groups), and only 43.5% achieved the minimum DDS (four or more food groups) in the 24 h prior to the survey. The number of children achieving minimum DDS differs significantly between the malnourished and normal nutritional status groups (Table 3). For the mothers, the mean minimum DDS was 4.45 ± 0.84 (out of 10 standard food groups), and approximately 40% met the minimum DDS (five or more food groups; Table 3).

Table 3. Household food security, maternal and child diet, and their feeding practices.

Variables	Malnutrition (%)			x^2
	Yes	No	Total	
Household food security status				
Food insecure	38.3	22.5	60.8	48.30 **
Food secure	10.8	28.5	39.3	
Exclusive breastfeeding				
No	6.0	4.5	10.5	1.25
Yes	43.0	46.5	89.5	
Initiation of breastfeeding				
Not within 1 h of birth	6.0	2.0	8.0	9.41 **
Within 1 h of birth	43.0	49.0	92.0	
Initiation of complementary feeding				
Not timely	24.0	21.5	45.5	1.88
Timely started	25.0	29.5	54.5	
Minimum child DDS				
Not achieved	37.4	19.1	56.5	55.25 **
Achieved	11.5	32.0	43.5	
Minimum maternal DDS				
Not achieved	28.2	31.8	60.0	3.68 *
Achieved	22.8	17.3	40.0	

* $p < 0.05$, ** $p < 0.01$; DDS, dietary diversity score.

As shown in Figure 3, starch staples (e.g., grains, roots, and tubers) formed a significant component of the daily diet, with approximately 85% of children and all mothers reporting the consumption of starch staples within the 24 h period preceding the survey. Legumes and nuts, as well as other fruits and vegetables (particularly onions), were the most frequently consumed food groups, whereas both children and mothers consumed notably less animal-based foods and vitamin A-rich fruits and vegetables (see Figure 3). There was a linear relationship between children and their respective mothers in the distribution of food group consumption (Figure 3C), although the primary focus of the comparisons was to determine intrahousehold variations in dietary intake due to possible misconceptions about child feeding habits in rural families.

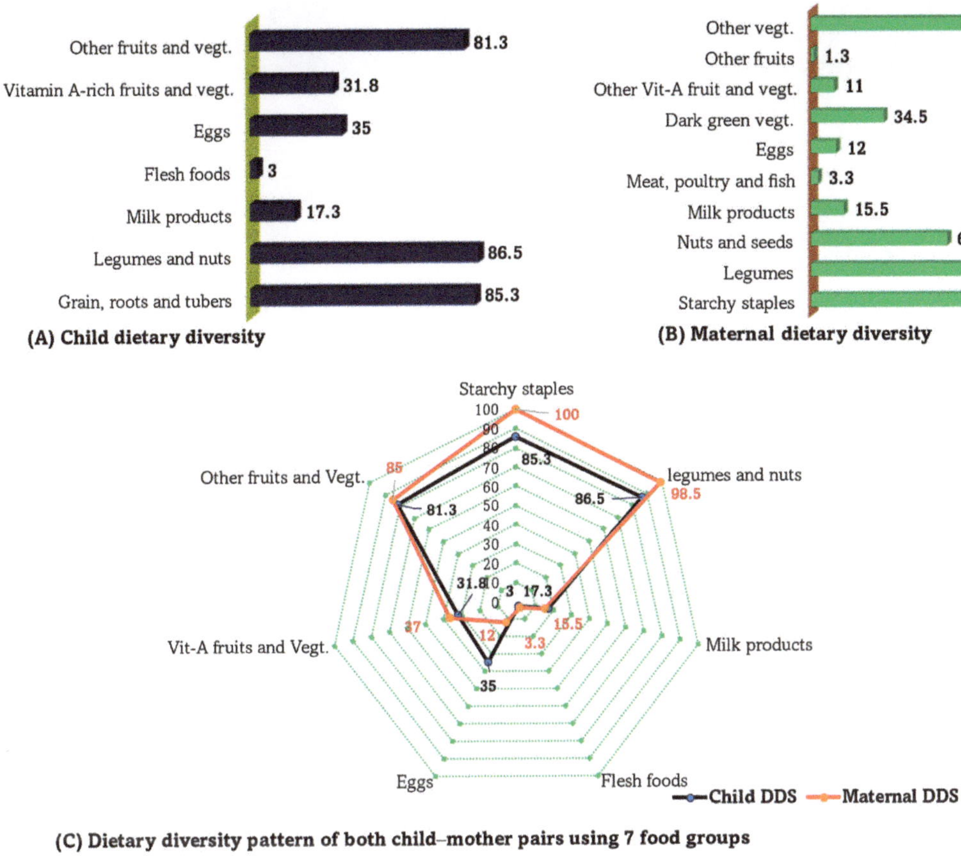

Figure 3. (**A**,**B**) Minimum dietary diversity among children (**A**) and mothers (**B**). (**C**) Consumption patterns among children and mothers based on 7 food groups.

3.3. Home Gardening as a Nutrition-Sensitive Agricultural Practice

The home gardening practices among the surveyed households were limited in scope. Approximately 10% of households cultivated micronutrient-rich fruits and vegetables, specifically dark green leafy and Vitamin A-rich varieties (Figure S1). Conversely, there was a relatively robust production of animal-based foods, although actual consumption remained constrained. The assessment of home gardening practices, based on the home gardening index derived through principal component analysis, revealed that approximately 30% of households had a higher level of engagement in home gardening activities aimed at enhancing both food security and household income (Figure S1).

3.4. Household Environment, Health Services, and Children's Disease Experiences

Regarding water, sanitation, and hygiene within households, slightly more than half (53.4%) of households had access to piped drinking water (Table 4). Furthermore, over three-quarters of households had their own toilets, separate kitchens, and animal housing that was detached from their primary living quarters. Approximately 69.5% of mothers adhered to the recommended minimum number of antenatal care (ANC) visits during pregnancy; however, approximately 27.5% of children included in the study were delivered at home without professional assistance. Nearly four of five children had received complete vaccinations. On average, the mothers of the surveyed children had had interactions with health extension workers twice in the previous year (Table 4). In addition, slightly over four-fifths of households had availed themselves of health insurance services. However, instances of fever and diarrheal diseases were reported for approximately one-fifth of children (Table 4).

Table 4. Household environment and health service utilization and disease experiences.

Variables	Indicators	Responses	Malnutrition (%)			x^2
			Yes	No	Total	
Household environment	Water source	Not pipe	21.1	25.6	46.6	2.19
		Pipe water	28.1	25.3	53.4	
	Toilet access	Open field	10.3	6.0	16.3	6.15 *
		Own toilet	38.8	45.0	83.8	
	kitchen house	Not separate	5.0	2.5	7.5	4.05 *
		Separate	44.0	48.5	92.5	
	Animal housing	Not separate	8.0	7.8	15.8	0.10
		Separate from living quarters	41.0	43.3	84.3	
Health services	ANC follow-up	<4 times	16.8	13.8	30.5	2.46
		≥4 times	32.3	37.3	69.5	
	Place of birth	Home	15.8	11.8	27.5	4.16 *
		Health institution	33.3	39.3	72.5	
	Child vaccination	Not at all	1.3	1.3	2.5	4.09 *
		Partially vaccinated	10.8	7.2	18.0	
		Fully vaccinated	37.0	42.5	79.5	
	Health insurance	No	10.8	8.3	19.0	2.16
		Yes	38.3	42.8	81.0	
	No. of health extension contact in past 12 months [A]		2.02 ± 2.4	2.9 ± 2.5		t = −3.69 **
Disease experiences	Diarrhea	No	36.5	46.3	82.8	18.4 **
		Yes	12.5	4.8	17.3	
	ARI	No	46.0	49.5	95.5	2.35
		Yes	3.0	1.5	4.5	
	Fever	No	37.8	44.8	82.5	7.93 **
		Yes	11.3	6.3	17.5	
	Chronic disease	No	41.8	49.0	90.8	14.08 **
		Yes	7.2	2.0	9.3	

[A] Data are given as the mean ± SD. * $p < 0.05$, ** $p < 0.01$. ANC, antenatal care; ARI, acute respiratory infection.

3.5. Prevalence of Stunting, Wasting, and Underweight and Overall CIAF

The height-for-age, weight-for-age, and weight-for-height indices (stunting, underweight, and wasting, respectively) were compared with a WHO standardized normal distribution curve, which has a mean of zero and an SD of one. As indicated in Table 5, approximately 39% of children aged <5 years in this study have experienced stunting, with approximately 6% classified as severely stunted. The overall mean (± SD) of the height-for-age Z-score was −1.34 ± 0.35, with statistical analysis (ANOVA F = 2.43, $p = 0.065$) suggesting that there is no significant difference in mean scores for children across the four distinct agroecosystems (Figure 4A). The prevalence of wasting (weight for height) and underweight (height for age) was 9.5% and 11.5%, respectively, with approximately 1% of children experiencing severe forms of these conditions.

Table 5. Prevalence (%) of malnutrition based on Z-scores.

Forms of Malnutrition	Severity of Malnutrition		All Children (Z-Score < −2)	Mean ± SD Z-Score
	Moderate (Z-Score −2 to −3)	Severe (Z-Score < −3)		
Stunting (HAZ)	32.8 (22.0–43.6)	6.3 (3.4–9.2)	39.1 (30.3–47.9)	−1.34 ± 0.35
Wasting (WHZ)	8.4 (4.6–14.4)	1.1(0.4–2.1)	9.5 (4.6–14.4)	0.21 ± 0.49
Underweight (WAZ)	10.2 (5.2–15.2)	1.3 (0.3–2.2)	11.5 (5.7–17.2)	−0.51 ± 0.23
	CIAF		49	

Unless indicated otherwise, data show the percentage of children in each group, with 95% confidence intervals given in parentheses. CIAF, Composite Index of Anthropometric Failure; HAZ, height-for-age Z-score; WAZ, weight-for-age Z-score; WHZ, weight-for-height Z-score.

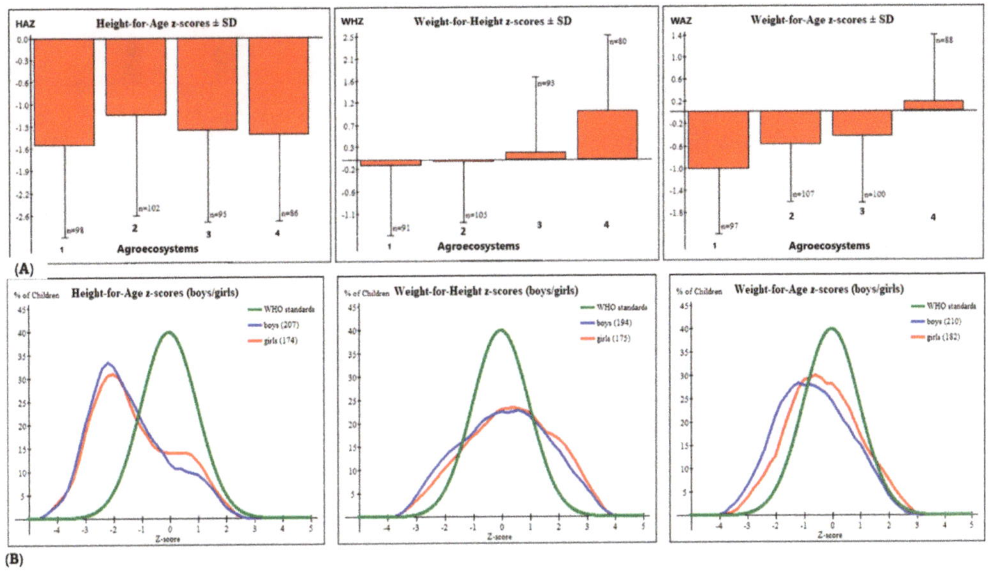

Figure 4. (**A**) Mean (±SD) height-for-age (HAZ), weight-for-height (WHZ), and weight-for-age (WAZ) Z-scores across agroecosystems. (**B**) Prevalence of stunting (HAZ), wasting (WHZ), and underweight (WAZ) in the study area compared with World Health Organization (WHO) standards.

The ANOVA test revealed significant differences in the mean Z-scores for both weight-for-height (F = 21.36, $p < 0.001$) and height-for-age (F = 17.54, $p < 0.001$) indices across the agroecosystems.

Based on the CIAF, nearly half the children in the study were malnourished. Of these, slightly less than one-third (31.5%) were stunted or had a short stature (Figure 5). Approximately 10% of children had double anthropometric failures (both stunting and either wasting or underweight simultaneously), whereas 2% had triple anthropometric failures (stunting, wasting, and underweight concurrently). Chi-squared analysis revealed statistically significant differences in the distribution of malnourished children across various AEZs ($\chi^2 = 24.84$; $p < 0.001$). Notably, the prevalence of malnutrition was higher in the lowland and valley fragmented agroecosystem (AEZ-1).

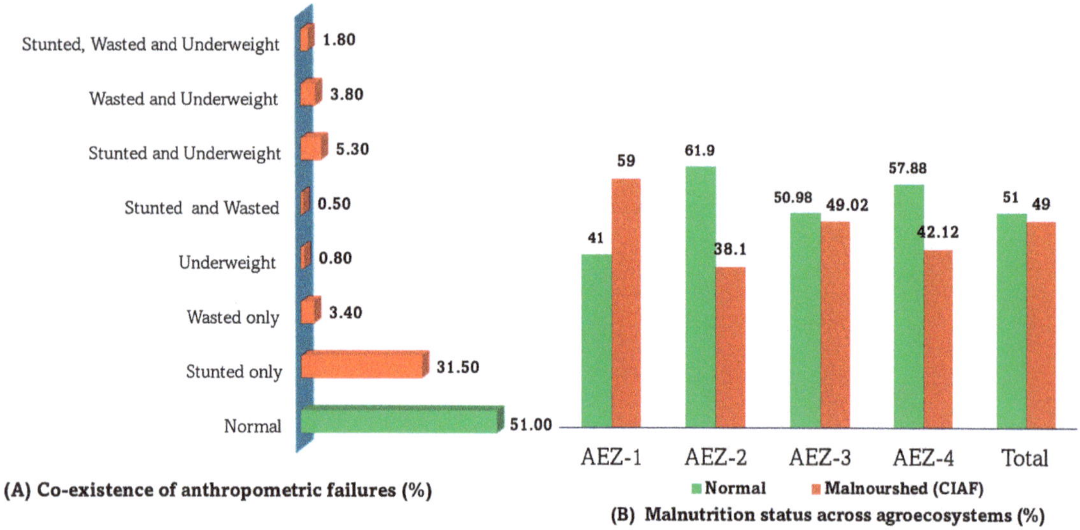

Figure 5. (**A**) Burden of the coexistence of indices of anthropometric failure among children. (**B**) Prevalence and distribution of overall malnutrition across agroecosystem zones (AEZ).

3.6. Determinants Associated with Child Malnutrition

SEM analysis was conducted at both the measurement and structural levels. The path diagram in Figure 6 illustrates detailed hypothetical relationships between exogenous and endogenous variables.

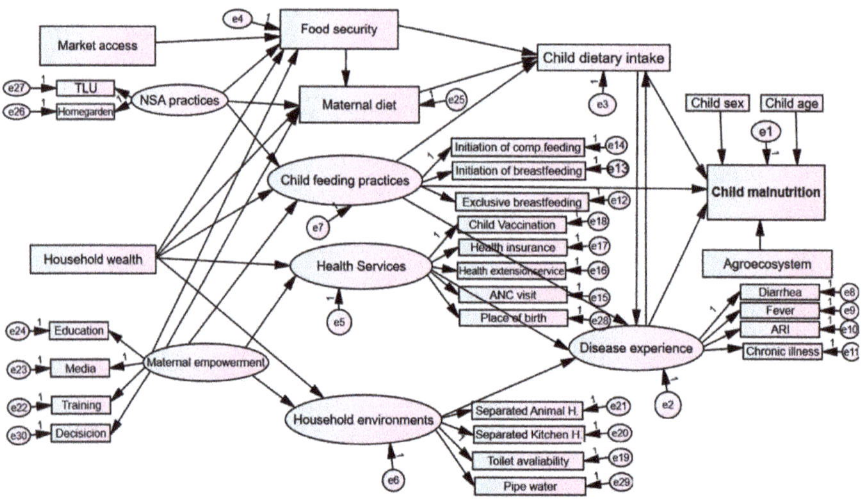

Figure 6. Conceptual structural equation modeling and its hypothesized path diagram. Circles in the SEM diagram indicate latent exogenous and endogenous variables, whereas rectangles represent observed or measured exogenous and endogenous variables. Arrows between circles and rectangles indicate the paths and relationship between variables, as denoted by their coefficients. 1 refers to fixed loading. ANC, antenatal care; ARI, acute respiratory infection; comp, complementary; NSA, nutrition-sensitive agriculture; TLU, livestock size by Tropical Livestock Unit; Decision, decision making; Media, media exposure.

3.6.1. Measurement Model

Confirmatory factor analysis was used to test the measurement model. During this process, factor loadings for each item within every construct were examined, and items with low factor loadings were excluded. The fitness of the measurement model was assessed based on the CFI, with a threshold of ≥0.9, and the SRMR, with a threshold of <0.08. Construct reliability was evaluated using the CR, with a threshold of ≥0.7. The validity of the constructs was assessed through the AVE, with a threshold of ≥0.5. As indicated in Table 6, all the values met their respective acceptance thresholds, indicating that the constructs were reliable and valid, and the measurement model adequately fit the data. The anticipated outcome for the chi-square test of model fitness was non-significant. However, it was indeed significant as expected, due to its sensitivity to sample size during model testing.

Table 6. Reliability and validity tests of constructs and model fit statistics for the measurement model.

Constructs/Latent Variables	No. Items	CR	AVE	CFI	SRMR	x^2 (p Value)
NSA practices	2	0.71	0.58	0.99	0.01	58.55 (0.01)
Maternal empowerment	3	0.78	0.56	0.99	0.023	76.77 (0.001)
Feeding and care practice	3	0.70	0.45	0.99	0.01	60.14 (0.001)
Household environment	3	0.77	0.53	0.98	0.001	190.33 (0.001)
Health services	4	0.76	0.50	0.99	0.01	49.4 (0.001)
Diseases experience	4	0.80	0.51	0.94	0.05	21.25 (0.001)

AVE, average variance extracted; CFI, comparative fit index; CR, composite reliability; NSA, nutrition-sensitive agriculture; SRMR, standardized root mean squared residual.

3.6.2. Structural Model

The fitness of the structural model was evaluated using several indices (Table 7). The GFI yielded a value of 0.91, slightly surpassing the acceptable range of >0.9. The CFI returned a value of 0.78, falling below the desired threshold of >0.9. The RMSEA was calculated at 0.082, slightly exceeding the acceptable range of <0.08. However, the Chi-square divided by the degrees of freedom yielded a value of 3.71, which falls within the acceptable range of 3–5. Given these results, the model required modification to ensure that all the model fit statistics fell within their acceptable ranges. Therefore, model modifications were made iteratively until all indices met the criteria for a satisfactory fit. This process aimed to enhance the overall fitness of the structural model and improve its validity for the dataset under investigation. The model is very complex and involves more measured variables, which makes it difficult to be more fitted; however, the model is still good enough to predict the data. The main intention of SEM analysis is to verify a theoretical hypothesis rather than solely enhance a model's goodness-of-fit. Pursuing improvements in fitness alone may result in inappropriate model configuration. Consequently, the model may fail to accurately represent reality, thus diminishing the persuasive power of the researcher's argument.

Table 7. Model fitness indices for the modified structural model.

Indices	x^2	df	x^2/df	RMSEA	CFI	GFI
Structural model	867.90	234	3.71	0.082	0.75	0.91
Acceptable range	-	-	3–5	<0.08	>0.9	>0.9

CFI, comparative fit index; GFI, goodness-of-fit index; RMSEA, root mean square error of approximation.

3.6.3. Direct Effects of Structural Model

Figure 7 shows the finalized structural model following the re-specification of the conceptual model, incorporating adjustments based on modification indices to enhance the model's fit. Table 8 provides insights into the direct effects within the model. Child dietary intake was found to have a significant negative direct effect on children's malnutrition (β = −0.295, Exp(B) = 0.75, p = 0.001), indicating that an increase in dietary intake is associated with a decrease in the likelihood of malnutrition. Conversely, disease experiences as a risk factor had a significant positive effect on children's malnutrition (β = 0.306, Exp(B) = 1.36, p = 0.009), suggesting that experiencing disease increases the likelihood of malnutrition.

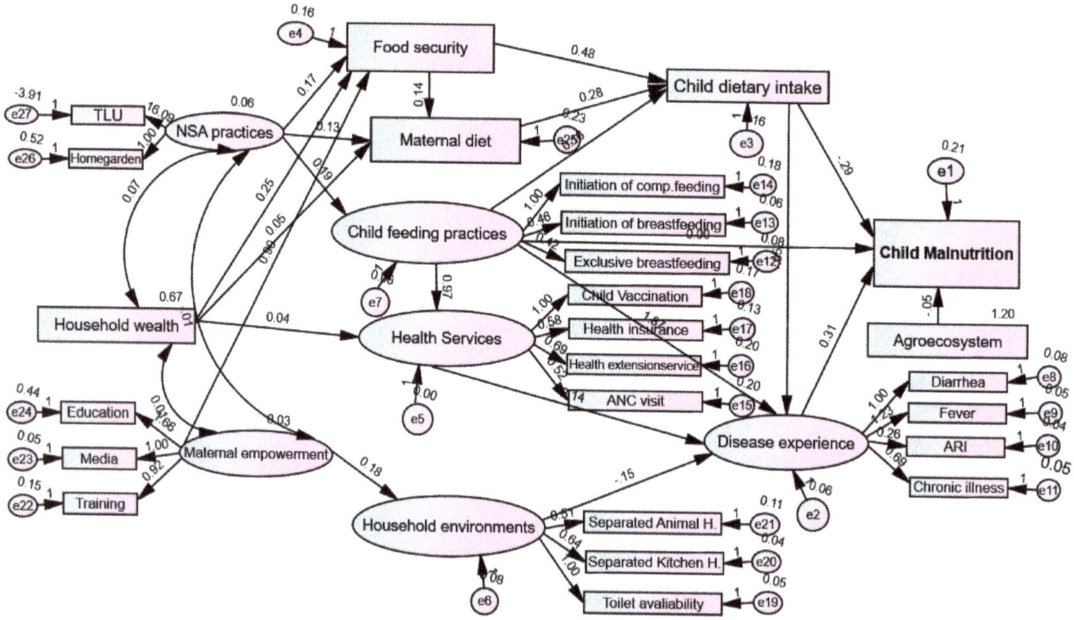

Figure 7. Direct effect estimates of modified SEM and its output paths diagram. Circles in the SEM diagram indicate latent exogenous and endogenous variables, whereas rectangles represent observed or measured exogenous and endogenous variables. Arrows between circles and rectangles indicate the paths and relationship between variables, as denoted by their coefficients. ANC, antenatal care; ARI, acute respiratory infection; comp, complementary; NSA, nutrition-sensitive agriculture; TLU, livestock size by Tropical Livestock Unit; Decision, decision making; Media, media exposure.

Furthermore, the model confirmed that agroecosystems had a significant negative effect on children's malnutrition status (β = −0.051, Exp(B) = 0.60, p = 0.015), indicating that children in the lowland and valley fragmented agroecosystem (AEZ-1) were at higher risk of malnutrition than children in other agroecosystems. To keep the length of this paper to a minimum, the path estimates towards the other endogenous variables shown in Table 8 are not discussed further. However, the full direct effect results of the SEM analysis with regression path coefficients are provided (Table 8; Figure 7). To see the effect of agroecosystem variation on child malnutrition, binary logistic regression was conducted by controlling or adjusting for other immediate factors that are shown in the conceptual framework. Using AEZ-1 as the reference group, the adjusted odds ratios for the likelihood of being malnourished were 0.424 (p = 0.027) in AEZ-2, 0.609 (p = 0.207) in AEZ-3, and 0.274 (p = 0.001) in AEZ-4 (Table S2).

Table 8. Standardized and unstandardized estimates for direct effects on structural model.

Direct Effect Paths			S (β)	β	S.E.	Exp(B)	*p*
Child malnutrition	←	Child dietary intake	−0.295	−0.295	0.048	0.75	0.001
	←	Feeding and care practice	−0.001	−0.059	0.130	0.55	0.647
	←	Agroecosystem zone	−0.113	−0.051	0.021	0.60	0.015
	←	Disease experience	0.151	0.306	0.118	1.36	0.009
Child dietary intake	←	Food security	0.475	0.478	0.041	1.61	0.001
	←	Maternal diet	0.278	0.282	0.041	1.33	0.001
	←	Feeding and care practice	0.082	0.158	0.100	1.17	0.115
Disease experience	←	Household environment	−0.182	−0.155	0.056	0.86	0.006
	←	Child dietary intake	−0.104	−0.051	0.028	0.95	0.068
	←	Feeding and care practice	1.958	1.865	1.137	6.46	0.101
	←	Health services	−2.172	−2.14	1.51	0.12	0.063
Food security	←	NSA practices	0.084	0.172	0.086	1.19	0.046
	←	Wealth status	0.422	0.254	0.029	1.29	0.001
	←	Maternal empowerment	0.262	0.903	0.216	2.47	0.001
Maternal diet	←	Wealth status	0.089	0.053	0.035	1.05	0.125
	←	Food security	0.145	0.144	0.055	1.15	0.009
	←	NSA practices	0.064	0.13	0.09	1.14	0.148
Feeding and care practice	←	NSA	0.174	0.186	0.066	1.20	0.005
Household environment	←	Maternal empowerment	0.144	0.177	0.124	1.19	0.155
Health services	←	Wealth status	0.138	0.042	0.021	1.04	0.049
	←	Feeding and care practice	0.99	0.970	0.168	2.64	0.001

NSA, nutrition-sensitive agriculture policy; S (β), standardized coefficient; Exp(B), exponential of coefficient, ←, refers to the direction of effect paths.

3.6.4. Indirect and Total Effects in the Mediation Analysis of the Structural Model

Serial mediation analysis was applied because the mediators have a kind of hierarchal or sequential nature (Figure 7). Therefore, the serial mediation analysis, detailed in Table 9, elucidated several significant pathways, contributing to the relationship between various factors and child malnutrition. Maternal empowerment had a negative and significant direct effect on malnutrition ($\beta = -0.06$, Exp(B) = 0.94, $p = 0.012$). This effect was fully mediated via food security, maternal diet, household environment, minimum child dietary diversity, and child disease experiences. Similarly, the effects of NSA practices ($\beta = -0.03$, Exp(B) = 0.97, $p = 0.038$) and household wealth status ($\beta = -0.12$, Exp(B) = 0.89, $p = 0.001$) on malnutrition were fully mediated and significantly negative, indicating no direct effect. Food security, maternal diet, household environment, and health service utilization were identified as underlying causes of malnutrition, with only indirect and significantly negative effects on child malnutrition (Table 9). Child feeding and care practices were considered as both underlying and immediate causes of malnutrition, with no significant direct effect ($\beta = -0.001$, Exp(B) = 0.99, $p = 0.995$), but a negative and significant indirect effect ($\beta = -0.059$, Exp(B) = 0.941, $p = 0.045$) mediated by dietary intake and child disease experiences. Child dietary intake (minimum dietary diversity) had a partially mediated effect on malnutrition via disease experiences, with a significant total effect. In addition, the SEM output confirmed that agroecosystem and disease had a fully unmediated significant relationship with malnutrition.

Detailed standardized coefficients for indirect and total effects resulting from mediation analysis within the entire structural model are provided in Tables S3 and S4, respectively.

Table 9. Mediation effects (standardized) on child malnutrition in the structural model.

Exogenous Variables	Direct Effect		Indirect Effect		Total Effect		Mediation Analysis
	β	Exp(B)	B	Exp(B)	β	Exp(B)	
NSA practices	–	–	−0.03	0.97 *	−0.03	0.97 *	Full mediation
Maternal Empowerment	–	–	−0.06	0.94 *	−0.06	0.94 *	Full mediation
Wealth status	–	–	−0.12	0.88 **	−0.12	0.88 *	Full mediation
Agroecosystem	−0.11	0.89 *	–	–	−0.11	0.89 *	Not applicable
Food security	–	–	−0.16	0.85 **	−0.16	0.85 **	Full mediation
Maternal diet	–	–	−0.09	0.91 **	−0.09	0.91 **	Full mediation
Health services	–	–	−0.33	0.72 **	−0.33	0.72 **	Full mediation
Household environment	–	–	−0.03	0.97 *	−0.03	0.97 *	Full mediation
Child feeding and care	−0.001	0.99	−0.059	0.94 *	−0.06	0.94	Full mediation
Child dietary diversity	−0.30	0.74 **	−0.02	0.98 *	−0.32	0.73 **	Partial mediation
Disease experiences	0.15	1.16 **	–	–	0.15	1.16 **	Not applicable

* $p < 0.05$, ** $p < 0.01$; NSA, nutrition-sensitive agriculture.

3.6.5. Agroecosystem-Based Multigroup SEM Analysis

In this study, a multigroup SEM analysis was conducted to compare two distinct groups, resulting in the formation of four binary groups: AEZ-1 vs. other AEZs (AEZ-2, -3, -4); AEZ-2 vs. other AEZs; AEZ-3 vs. other AEZs; and AEZ-4 vs. other AEZs. Figure 8 presents the structural model, wherein each parameter is uniquely named across the groups, with 'a' and 'b' followed by group numbers representing the relationships between the variables. The comparison analysis, facilitated by the chi-squared difference test ($x^2 = 108.53$, $p < 0.001$), revealed a significant difference between AEZ-1 and other AEZs when contrasting the structural weights constrained model with the unconstrained model-free model. However, although this test indicated a significant difference in the group overall, it did not pinpoint where specific paths in the model differed.

Further examination revealed that specific paths, such as b1_1, b9_1, b10_1, b14_1, and a11_1, exhibited significant differences between AEZ-1 and other AEZs (Figure 8; Table 10). Overall, the comparison between the overall structural weight model and the unconstrained model demonstrated significant differences, implying variations in the effects of paths between AEZ-1 and other AEZs. However, the chi-squared difference test did not reveal significant differences in the structural model weights between AEZ-2 and other AEZs ($\chi^2 = -420.38$), AEZ-3 and other AEZs ($\chi^2 = -403.492$), and AEZ-4 and other AEZs ($\chi^2 = -671.56$).

In the multigroup SEM analysis, each structural relationship was individually constrained to determine if specific relationships differed across the groups. The results of constraining the relationship 'a11_1' revealed a significant chi-squared difference ($\chi^2 = 6.412$, $p < 0.01$), indicating that the effects of disease on malnutrition vary significantly between children living in AEZ-1 and those living in other AEZs. Furthermore, the model results showed significant chi-square difference tests in the specific relationship paths of the constrained "b1_1 ($\chi^2 = 12.589$, $p < 0.01$), b9_1 ($\chi^2 = 16.69$, $p < 0.01$), b10_1 ($\chi^2 = 3.32$ *), and b14_1 ($\chi^2 = 48.04$, $p < 0.01$)" between children living in AEZ-1 and those living in other AEZs. However, there were no significant differences between these two groups in the remaining paths in the structural model, despite the overall structural model showing significant differences between the two groups (Figure 8; Table 10).

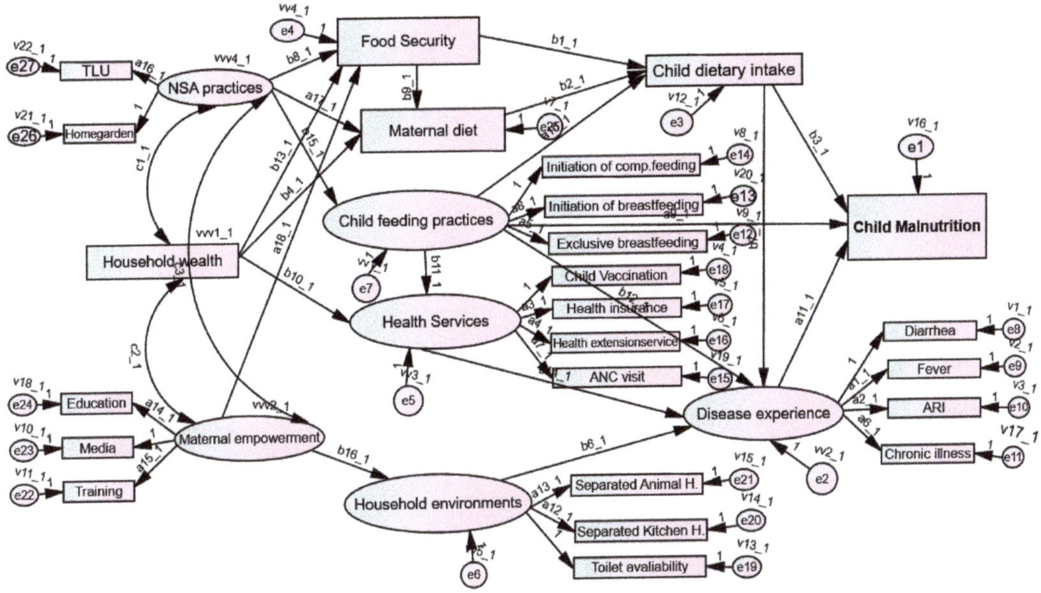

Figure 8. Path diagram for multigroup SEM analysis between agroecosystem zone (AEZ)-1 and other AEZs. Circles in the SEM diagram indicate latent exogenous and endogenous variables, whereas rectangles represent observed or measured exogenous and endogenous variables. Arrows between circles and rectangles indicate the paths and relationship between variables, as denoted by their coefficients. ANC, antenatal care; ARI, acute respiratory infection; comp, complementary; NSA, nutrition-sensitive agriculture; TLU, livestock size by Tropical Livestock Unit; Decision, decision making; Media, media exposure.

Table 10. Agroecosystem as moderator in the multigroup SEM analysis.

Specific Relationship Paths		Group				Model Comparison (x^2-Difference Test)
		AEZ-1		Other AEZs		
		β	Exp(B)	β	Exp(B)	
Malnutrition	←Child dietary intake	−0.14	0.87	−0.31	0.73 **	−19.47
	←Feeding and care practice	−0.03	0.97	−0.70	0.50	−19.83
	←Disease experience	3.04	20.91 **	0.295	1.34 **	6.412 **
Child dietary intake	←Food security	0.22	1.25 **	0.57	1.77 **	12.59 **
	←Maternal diet	0.41	1.51 **	0.21	1.23 **	2.93
	←Feeding and care practice	0.01	1.01	0.66	1.93	−19.96
Disease experience	←Household environment	0.04	1.04	0.001	1.01	0.34
	←Child dietary intake	−0.79	0.45	−0.03	0.76	−19.75
	←Feeding and care practice	0.01	1.01	−1.81	0.16	−16.41
	←Health services	−1.46	0.23 *	−0.83	0.44	48.04 **
Food security	←Wealth status	0.27	1.30 **	0.30	1.35 **	0.384
	←Maternal empowerment	0.03	1.03	0.91	2.48 **	1.814
Maternal diet	←Wealth status	0.140	1.15 **	0.07	1.08	1.17
	←Food Security	0.23	1.26 **	0.21	1.23 **	16.69 **
	←NSA	−0.15	0.86	0.001	1.001	1.50

Table 10. *Cont.*

Specific Relationship Paths		Group				Model Comparison (x^2-Difference Test)
		AEZ-1		Other AEZs		
		β	Exp(B)	β	Exp(B)	
Feeding and care practice	←NSA	−0.14	0.87	−0.002	0.99	0.80
Household environment	←Maternal empowerment	−0.01	0.99	0.29	1.34 **	1.53
Health services	←Wealth status	0.15	1.16 *	−0.03	0.97	3.32 *
	←Feeding and care practice	0.007	1.01	−0.05	0.95	−12.81
Overall model comparison (structural weight model vs. unconstrained model)						108.14 **

* $p < 0.05$, ** $p < 0.01$; AEZ, agroecosystem zone; NSA, nutrition-sensitive agriculture.

4. Discussion

In this study, we investigated the prevalence of child malnutrition. Among children aged <5 years in this study, approximately 39% were stunted (i.e., short stature for their age). This figure aligns closely with the national prevalence of stunting reported in the latest EDHS of 38%. However, it is of note that the prevalence of stunting in this study was slightly lower than that reported specifically for the Amhara region of 46% [3]. The difference between our findings and those for the Amhara region could be attributed to the wider geographical coverage of the latter, encompassing significant spatial variations in the environment and agricultural productivity. Such discrepancies in environmental conditions and agricultural productivity may give rise to diverse socioeconomic conditions, which, in turn, could influence the prevalence of child malnutrition. The prevalence of wasting and underweight in this study was lower than the national averages reported in the EDHS of 10% and 24%, respectively [3], as well as lower than those reported for the Tigray region of northern Ethiopia [42]. These findings suggest that stunting, representing a chronic form of malnutrition, is the predominant anthropometric failure affecting children in the Chemoga watershed.

In addition, we found a high prevalence of CIAF in this study, with approximately half the children experiencing some form of anthropometric failure. The prevalence of CIAF surpassed that of single conventional indices of anthropometric failure, such as stunting, wasting, and underweight. Significant variations in the prevalence of CIAF were observed across the four AEZs in the study. The highest prevalence of CIAF was reported in the lowland and valley fragmented agroecosystem (AEZ-1), whereas the lowest was recorded among children from AEZ-2 (midland with red soil). The higher prevalence of child malnutrition in AEZ-1 is consistent with findings reported previously [9,24,43–45], and it may be due to unfavorable agroecosystem conditions, resulting in lower agricultural productivity and weak socio-economic status. Of note, a lower proportion of children from the hilly and mountainous highland agroecosystem (AEZ-4) were malnourished. This could be attributed to their dietary practices, characterized by the high consumption of potatoes, which are high in calories, as a staple food. Moreover, the environmental advantages of cold temperatures in AEZ-4 may contribute to the maintenance of better health conditions among children, as suggested by previous studies [20,46]. However, this stands in stark contrast to the lower prevalence reported in AEZ-4 in previous studies [24,44], underscoring the complex interplay among environmental factors, dietary practices, and nutritional outcomes across different AEZs. A possible reason for the apparent discrepancy could be differences in how children's nutritional status was assessed: unlike the previous studies, which used a conventional single index of anthropometric failure, we used CIAF in the present study. This finding provides significant insights into specific geographic variations in child malnutrition, offering advantages in identifying the neediest subpopulations and allocating scare resources for further nutrition-sensitive and nutrition-specific interventions not only in the study area, but also in other similar environments [8].

In this study, we used SEM to investigate causal relationship between various determinants (including basic, underlying, and immediate factors) and child malnutrition. Our analysis revealed negative and statistically significant direct and indirect effects of child dietary intake on malnutrition. Specifically, the odds ratio for the total effect (combining direct and indirect effects) of minimum dietary diversity on malnutrition was 0.75. This implies that with each unit increase in a child's DDS, the odds of experiencing malnutrition decrease by 0.75 units. In simpler terms, achieving minimum dietary diversity is associated with a notable 25% reduction in the relative risk of malnutrition. This underscores the significance of dietary diversity in mitigating the likelihood of malnutrition among children. Furthermore, our analysis revealed that the effect of dietary diversity on malnutrition was partially mediated through the exposure of children to diseases. This suggests that adequate diversification in a child's diet, encompassing foods from at least four of the seven food groups, as recommended by the FAO [37], could enhance nutrient adequacy, subsequently lowering children's susceptibility to diseases and thereby reducing the risk of malnutrition. However, it is concerning that more than half of the children in this study failed to meet the minimum DDS, particularly lacking in the consumption of animal-based foods and fruits and vegetables. This finding echoes the findings of prior studies conducted not only in Ethiopia [8,24,47] but also across Sub-Saharan Africa [12,32] and in countries like South Africa [48] and Ghana [49], highlighting the challenge of improving nutritional status without ensuring adequate dietary diversity among children in the region.

Our analysis also revealed a direct and significant positive effect of disease experiences on malnutrition. Specifically, the unmediated effect of disease exposure on malnutrition was quantified with an odds ratio, indicating that for each unit increase in a child's exposure to disease, the odds of being malnourished increase by 1.36 units. Consequently, children experiencing disease are more likely to suffer from malnutrition compared with their healthier counterparts. This finding aligns with prior research, including reports from the EDHS [3] and UNICEF [50], and studies conducted in northwest Ethiopia [13]. It underscores the detrimental impact of various diseases on children's nutritional status, which can be attributed to factors such as loss of appetite, the malabsorption of nutrients, and overall malfunctioning of metabolic processes.

In parallel with this descriptive result regarding child malnourishment, SEM and binary logistic regression analysis were conducted to measure the influence of agroecosystem characteristics on child malnutrition. The result of these analyses confirmed that agroecosystem is significantly associated with malnutrition based on logistic regression output, compared with a child from the lowland and valley fragmented agroecosystem (AEZ-1), where the risk of being malnourished was reduced by 42% and 27% for children from the midland with red soil (AEZ-2) and hilly and mountainous highland (AEZ-4) agroecosystems, respectively (Supplementary Table S1). Studies from the Amhara region in Ethiopia [24] and from Indonesia [11] and Ecuador [51] provide evidence of the effects of agroecosystem and agroecology on an individual's nutritional status.

Based on logistic regression output, the risk of being malnourished was reduced by 42% and 27% for a child from midland with plain lands and from hilly and mountainous highland agroecosystems, respectively, compared with a child from the lowland and valley fragmented agroecosystem zone (Supplementary Table S1). Evidence from Amhara region, Ethiopia [24], Indonesia [11], and Ecuador [51] also indicated the influence of agroecosystem and agroecology on individual's nutritional status. The higher risk of malnutrition in AEZ-1 could be related to higher climate change vulnerability and the resulting lower agricultural productivity and socioeconomic status compared with the midland with red soil agroecosystem (AEZ-2) [35].

Similarly, when comparing children in AEZ-1 to those in AEZ-4, the observed variations in nutritional status could be due to differences in dietary habits. In AEZ-4, potatoes are a staple calorie-rich food consumed daily, potentially leading to additional weight gain and an increase in anthropometric indices. Another factor contributing to differences between AEZ-1 and AEZ-4 could be the environmental conditions. AEZ-4 is characterized by cold temperatures, which could provide an advantage for maintaining health compared with AEZ-1; in AEZ-1, children are exposed to higher temperatures and may be more susceptible to heat stress, which aggravates the burden of child malnutrition. This is supported by findings of studies conducted in Ethiopia [20] and Uganda [52]. Moreover, in multigroup SEM analysis used to investigate differences in path coefficients across AEZs in which agroecosystem was used as a moderator variable after being recategorized into four dichotomous groups, the Chi-squared test for the whole structural model across all groups was only significant for the first group (AEZ-1 vs. others [AEZ-2, -3, and -4]). Further analyses were performed for AEZ-1 vs. others to identify differences in specific path coefficients, in addition to the whole structural model. This analysis highlighted specific entry points for further nutrition-sensitive and -specific interventions to reduce the burden of childhood malnutrition.

In this study, childcare and feeding practices, treated as a latent variable, were hypothesized to have direct and indirect effects on child malnutrition. However, SEM analysis indicated insignificant direct effects of child feeding practices on malnutrition, thus not supporting our prior hypothesis. In contrast, previous studies conducted in Ethiopia [7,8,13,53], Nigeria [54], and India [55] demonstrated an effect of child feeding practices, particularly breastfeeding and complementary feeding, on child nutritional status using various regression analyses other than SEM. Despite the lack of a direct effect, the indirect effects of care and feeding practices on malnutrition in the present study were statistically significant and negative. These indirect effects were mediated through a child's dietary intake and disease. Children who initiated breast feeding within 1 h of birth were exclusively breastfed up to 6 months of age and who were introduced to semisolid and solid complementary food in a timely manner were less likely to have a history of illness and inadequate dietary diversity. Consequently, this led to a reduced risk of childhood malnutrition.

Household food security is a key underlying determinant of malnutrition [56,57]. Mediation analysis in the present study revealed that household food security had a significant negative indirect effect on child malnutrition. Children from food-secure households were less likely to be malnourished than children from food-insecure households. When a child is from a food-secure household, the relative risk of being malnourished is decreased by 15% compared with a child from a food-insecure household. This finding is supported by the findings of a study in Indonesia that used SEM analysis [11].

The household environment, particularly factors related to water, sanitation, and hygiene, plays a pivotal role in influencing child malnutrition. As per our prior hypothesis, the result of the SEM analysis confirmed a negative and statistically significant indirect effect of household environment on malnutrition through the mediator of disease experience. In this study, a child from a healthy household environment (i.e., with their own toilet, separated kitchen facilities, and housing animals separately) was less likely to be malnourished compared with children from less ideal household environments. This finding aligns with that of studies conducted in Ethiopia [58] and Indonesia [11] using SEM analysis, as well as other studies conducted in Ethiopia [7,59], Nigeria [54], and India [55]. A potential explanation for the role of the household environment in child malnutrition is that an unhealthy household environment could facilitate the rapid spread of infectious diseases. This result emphasizes the need to address not only direct determinants of nutrition but also broader household environmental determinants, through which their impact is indirectly manifested [60].

In the SEM analysis, treating health services as a 'latent variable' provides a comprehensive understanding of their influence on child malnutrition. Considering child vaccination status, ANC visits, household health insurance, and health extension services as components to measure the latent construct 'health services' emerge as a vital strategy in the broader effort to combat child malnutrition. In the present study, the effect of health services on child malnutrition was negative and statistically significant and was fully mediated through disease experience. This aligns with previous studies conducted in Ethiopia [59,61] and Indonesia [11] and suggests that ensuring adequate health services utilization can play a crucial role in improving child health and consequently reducing the prevalence of malnutrition.

The findings of this study underscore the crucial influence of maternal empowerment and maternal diet in the complex framework of child malnutrition. In addition to working on a child directly, it is important to ensure the empowerment of mothers alongside addressing their dietary needs. The path coefficient in the SEM analysis revealed that the indirect effect of maternal diet on child malnutrition was negative and statistically significant. A child's mother who achieved the minimum of five of the ten food groups in a population can be used as a proxy indicator for better micronutrient adequacy [62]. Other studies have also consistently shown an association between inadequate maternal dietary diversity and an increased likelihood of child malnutrition [58,60,62,63]. This may be due to the influence of a mother's cultural preferences, adherence to food taboos, limitations regarding food access, and economic constraints, ultimately affecting a child's dietary diversity and their nutritional outcome. This dual approach of targeting both children and their mothers are pivotal in devising a comprehensive strategy to improve child nutrition.

Similarly, SEM analysis revealed that maternal empowerment significantly influenced malnutrition at as far distance as the basic factors. When a mother's empowerment was increased by one unit, the likelihood of her child being malnourished was reduced by 0.94 units, or their risk of malnutrition decreased by 6%. This may be attributed to empowered mothers being more likely to have high decision-making power in the household regarding child food and health care services. This finding aligns with the results of community-based cross-sectional studies conducted in Ethiopia [24,33] and Tanzania [16], as well as the findings of a systematic review study [64]; collectively, the results of these studies showed that maternal empowerment serves as a distant basic determinant of child nutrition, encompassing aspects such as education level, media exposure, and decision making power regarding a child's health and nutrition.

Household wealth was found to have significant negative indirect effects on malnutrition. According to serial mediation analysis, when the wealth index increased by 1 unit, the odds of malnutrition among children decreased by 0.88 units. In this study, children from poor households were more likely to experience any forms of malnutrition than children from rich households. The effect of household wealth was fully mediated, and the hypothesis in the conceptual structural model is supported. This finding is supported by other studies [11,12,22,32,33,54,65–67].

Most importantly, this study indicated that the probability of a child being malnourished was significantly lower among children from households who practiced better NSA, which was measured in this study as home gardening practices and livestock production. The effects of NSA practices on child malnutrition were indirect and fully mediated via underlying and immediate factors. These findings are consistent with some previous studies [19,68,69]. The likely explanation for the finding is that NSA practices play a crucial role in addressing the problem of food insecurity (the physical and economic accessibility of food) at a household level, which is one of the key underlying determinants of child malnutrition. In subsistence rural families, NSA practices, particularly home gardening, allow families to cultivate a variety of fruits and vegetables, as well as animal-based foods, which promotes a diverse and nutritious diet for children. This diversity ensures that children receive the essential micronutrients necessary for their growth and development [28].

5. Conclusions

In the present study, the prevalence of child malnutrition across four agroecosystems in northwest Ethiopia was unacceptably high. The prevalence of child malnutrition varied spatially and was particularly high among children residing in the lowland and valley fragmented agroecosystem compared with other areas. Furthermore, a high proportion of both children and their mothers did not meet the required minimum dietary diversity, in particular, the consumption of animal-based foods and fruits and vegetables was limited. SEM analysis was used as a robust analytical tool to address the hierarchical nature of risk factors of child malnutrition. The SEM analysis confirmed the direct effect of immediate factors and uncovered the indirect effects of basic and underlying determinants for child malnutrition by adapting the modified version of UNICEF's conceptual framework for malnutrition. Based on the results of the SEM analysis, disease experience and minimum dietary diversity have significant direct effects on child malnutrition, whereas the direct effects of childcare and feeding practices were not statistically significant. Underlying factors such as health service utilization, household environment, feeding practices, household food security, and minimum maternal dietary diversity, as well as basic factors such as household wealth, maternal empowerment, and NSA practices, had significant indirect effects on child malnutrition. The holistic analytical approach used in this study allowed for a more comprehensive understanding of the dynamics and multifaceted nature of malnutrition, providing valuable insights into the implementation of sustainable and targeted nutrition-sensitive and specific-interventions. Based on our findings, we also recommend considering geographical differences in the burden of childhood malnutrition when planning interventions.

Supplementary Materials: The following supporting information can be downloaded at: https://www.mdpi.com/article/10.3390/nu16081208/s1, Table S1: Socio-demographic and economic characteristics of the respondents; Table S2: Binary logistic regression analysis output of direct effect of immediate factors on malnutrition; Table S3: Standardized indirect effect of structural model; Table S4: Standardized total effect of structural model; Figure S1: Home gardening practices as nutrition-sensitive agricultural practices in the households by percentage.

Author Contributions: B.Y.W.: conceptualization, methodology, investigation, data curation, software, data analysis, writing original draft, visualization; A.T., N.H. and M.T.: conceptualization, methodology, investigation, resources, writing review and editing, supervision, project admission, fund acquisition; Z.N.: methodology, writing review and editing; T.M.M.: methodology, writing review and editing. T.A.: methodology, writing review and editing. All authors have read and agreed to the published version of the manuscript.

Funding: This research work was supported by the Science and Technology Research Partnership for Sustainable Development (SATREPS, grant number JPMJSA1601) and the Ministry of Education, Culture, Sports, Science and Technology (MEXT) of Japan.

Institutional Review Board Statement: Before data collection, ethical clearance was obtained from the ethical review committee of the Rural Development and Agricultural Extension Department, Bahir Dar University (RDAE/71/023, 15 June 2023). An official letter was sent to all districts to obtain permission for data collection.

Informed Consent Statement: Informed consent was obtained from all subjects involved in the study.

Data Availability Statement: The data presented in this study are available on request to the corresponding author.

Acknowledgments: The authors acknowledge the support of SATREPS and MEXT. The authors are grateful to all supervisors and data enumerators for their assistance in house-to-house data collection. The authors are also grateful to all mothers for their willingness to devote their time to provide the required data.

Conflicts of Interest: The authors declare no conflicts of interest.

References

1. FAO; IFAD; UNICEF; WFP; WHO. *The State of Food Security and Nutrition in the World 2023: Urbanization, Agrifood Systems Transformation and Healthy Diets across the Rural–Urban Continuum*; FAO: Rome, Italy, 2023. [CrossRef]
2. UNICEF/WHO/WORLD Bank Levels and Trends in Child Malnutrition UNICEF/WHO/World Bank Group Joint Child Malnutrition Estimates Key Findings of the 2021 Edition. World Health Organization (WHO). 2021. Available online: https://www.who.int/publications/i/item/9789240025257 (accessed on 13 March 2024).
3. Central Statistical Agency (CSA) [Ethiopia] and ICF. Demographic and Health Survey 2016. *Int. Food Res. J.* **2016**, *18*, 659–665.

4. African Union Commission. *Cost of Hunger in Ethiopia: The Social and Economic Impact of Child Undernutrition in Ethiopia Summary Report; Ethiopian Health and Nutrition research Institute, Addis Ababa.* 2013. Available online: https://documents.wfp.org/stellent/groups/public/documents/newroom/wfp263405.pdf?_ga=2.63063785.774106612.1713402049-1002408942.1694654416 (accessed on 13 March 2024).
5. Black, M.M.; Lutter, C.K.; Trude, A.C.B. All children surviving and thriving: Re-envisioning UNICEF's conceptual framework of malnutrition. *Lancet Glob. Health* **2020**, *8*, e766–e767. [CrossRef] [PubMed]
6. UNICEF. *Strategy for Improved Nutrition of Children and Women in Developing Countries*; The Management of Multilateral Organizations: New York, NY, USA, 1990.
7. Abebe, Z.; Haki, G.D.; Baye, K. Child feeding style is associated with food intake and linear growth in rural Ethiopia. *Appetite* **2017**, *116*, 132–138. [CrossRef] [PubMed]
8. Ahmed, K.Y.; Agho, K.E.; Page, A.; Arora, A.; Ogbo, F.A. Mapping geographical differences and examining the determinants of childhood stunting in Ethiopia: A bayesian geostatistical analysis. *Nutrients* **2021**, *13*, 2104. [CrossRef] [PubMed]
9. Alemu, Z.A.; Ahmed, A.A.; Yalew, A.W.; Simanie, B. Spatial variations of household food insecurity in East Gojjam Zone, Amhara Region, Ethiopia: Implications for agroecosystem-based interventions. *Agric. Food Secur.* **2017**, *6*, 36. [CrossRef]
10. Danso, F.; Appiah, M.A. Prevalence and associated factors influencing stunting and wasting among children of ages 1 to 5 years in Nkwanta South Municipality, Ghana. *Nutrition* **2023**, *110*, 111996. [CrossRef] [PubMed]
11. Manongga, S.P.; Yutomo, L. Determinant Factors of Malnutrition in Papuan Children Under Five Years: Structural Equation Model Analysis. *Indones. J. Multidiscip. Sci.* **2023**, *2*, 2379–2394. [CrossRef]
12. Baye, K.; Laillou, A.; Chitweke, S. Socio-economic inequalities in child stunting reduction in sub-Saharan Africa. *Nutrients* **2020**, *12*, 253. [CrossRef] [PubMed]
13. Bayih, M.T.; Arega, Z.; Motbainor, A. Nutritional status of 6–59 months of age children is not significantly varied between households with and without home gardening practices in Zege, northwest Ethiopia, 2020: Community based comparative study. *BMC Pediatr.* **2022**, *22*, 221. [CrossRef]
14. Christian, A.K.; Atiglo, D.Y.; Okyere, M.A.; Obeng-Dwamena, A.; Marquis, G.S.; Jones, A.D. Women's empowerment, children's nutritional status, and the mediating role of household headship structure: Evidence from sub-Saharan Africa. *Matern. Child Nutr.* **2023**, *19*, e13520. [CrossRef]
15. Corsi, D.J.; Mejía-Guevara, I.; Subramanian, S.V. Improving household-level nutrition-specific and nutrition-sensitive conditions key to reducing child undernutrition in India. *Soc. Sci. Med.* **2016**, *157*, 189–192. [CrossRef] [PubMed]
16. Debela, B.L.; Gehrke, E.; Qaim, M. Links between Maternal Employment and Child Nutrition in Rural Tanzania. *Am. J. Agric. Econ.* **2021**, *103*, 812–830. [CrossRef]
17. Derso, E.A.; Campolo, M.G.; Alibrandi, A. The Causes and Factors Associated with Infant Mortality Rate in Ethiopia: The Application of Structural Equation Modelling. *Children* **2023**, *10*, 397. [CrossRef] [PubMed]
18. Dewey, K.G. Reducing stunting by improving maternal, infant and young child nutrition in regions such as South Asia: Evidence, challenges and opportunities. *Matern. Child Nutr.* **2016**, *12*, 27–38. [CrossRef] [PubMed]
19. Hirvonen, K.; Headey, D. Can governments promote homestead gardening at scale? Evidence from Ethiopia. *Glob. Food Secur.* **2018**, *19*, 40–47. [CrossRef] [PubMed]
20. Randell, H.; Grace, K.; Bakhtsiyarava, M. Climatic conditions and infant care: Implications for child nutrition in rural Ethiopia. *Popul. Environ.* **2021**, *42*, 524–552. [CrossRef] [PubMed]
21. Sharma, I.K.; Di Prima, S.; Essink, D.; Broerse, J.E.W. Nutrition-Sensitive Agriculture: A Systematic Review of Impact Pathways to Nutrition Outcomes. *Adv. Nutr.* **2021**, *12*, 251–275. [CrossRef] [PubMed]
22. Abate, K.H.; Belachew, T. Chronic Malnutrition Among Under Five Children of Ethiopia May Not Be Economic. A Systematic Review and Meta-Analysis. *Ethiop. J. Health Sci.* **2019**, *29*, 265–277. [CrossRef]
23. Ahmed, A.S.; Ahmed, T.; Roy, S.K.; Alam, N.; Hossain, M.I. Determinants of undernutrition in children under 2 years of age from Rural Bangladesh. *Indian Pediatr.* **2012**, *49*, 821–824. [CrossRef]
24. Alemu, Z.A.; Ahmed, A.A.; Yalew, A.W.; Birhanu, B.S.; Zaitchik, B.F. Individual and community level factors with a significant role in determining child height-for-age Z score in East Gojjam Zone, Amhara Regional State, Ethiopia: A multilevel analysis. *Arch. Public Health* **2017**, *75*, 27. [CrossRef]
25. Alemu, G.; Shigute, Z.; Mebratie, A.; Sparrow, R.; Bedi, A.S. On the functioning of community-based health insurance schemes in rural Ethiopia. *Soc. Sci. Med.* **2023**, *345*, 115739. [CrossRef]
26. Arriola, K.R.J.; Ellis, A.; Webb-Girard, A.; Ogutu, E.A.; McClintic, E.; Caruso, B.; Freeman, M.C. Designing integrated interventions to improve nutrition and WASH behaviors in Kenya. *Pilot Feasibility Stud.* **2020**, *6*, 10. [CrossRef] [PubMed]
27. Ayele, B.A.; Tiruneh, S.A.; Ayele, A.A.; Zemene, M.A.; Chanie, E.S.; Hailemeskel, H.S. Prevalence and determinants of overweight/obesity among under-five children in sub-Saharan Africa: A multilevel analysis. *BMC Pediatr.* **2022**, *22*, 585. [CrossRef] [PubMed]
28. Baxter, R.; Hastings, N.; Law, A.; Glass, E.J. Fill the nutrient Gap. *Anim. Genet.* **2008**, *39*, 561–563. [CrossRef] [PubMed]
29. Federal Government of Ethiopia, Ministry of Health EPHI. *Ethiopia: Food-Based Dietary Guidelines–2022*; Ethiopian Public Health Institute: Addis Ababa, Ethiopia, 2022; p. 108.

30. Mattes, R.D.; Rowe, S.B.; Ohlhorst, S.D.; Brown, A.W.; Hoffman, D.J.; Liska, D.J.; Feskens, E.J.M.; Dhillon, J.; Tucker, K.L.; Epstein, L.H.; et al. Valuing the Diversity of Research Methods to Advance Nutrition Science. *Adv. Nutr.* **2022**, *13*, 1324–1393. [CrossRef] [PubMed]
31. Nandy, S.; Svedberg, P. The Composite Index of Anthropometric Failure (CIAF): An Alternative Indicator for Malnutrition in Young Children. In *Handbook of Anthropometry: Physical Measures of Human Form in Health and Disease*; Preedy, V.R., Ed.; Springer: New York, NY, USA, 2012; pp. 127–137. [CrossRef]
32. Aboagye, R.G.; Seidu, A.A.; Ahinkorah, B.O.; Arthur-Holmes, F.; Cadri, A.; Dadzie, L.K.; Hagan, J.E.; Eyawo, O.; Yaya, S. Dietary diversity and undernutrition in children aged 6–23 months in sub-saharan africa. *Nutrients* **2021**, *13*, 3431. [CrossRef] [PubMed]
33. Fenta, H.M.; Zewotir, T.; Muluneh, E.K. Spatial data analysis of malnutrition among children under-five years in Ethiopia. *BMC Med. Res. Methodol.* **2021**, *21*, 232. [CrossRef] [PubMed]
34. Meshesha, M.T.; Tsunekawa, A.; Haregeweyn, N.; Tsubo, M.; Fenta, A.A.; Berihun, M.L.; Arega, M.; Setargie, T.A.; Kassa, S.B. Agroecology-based land use/land cover change detection, prediction and its implications for land degradation: A case study in the Upper Blue Nile Basin. *Int. Soil Water Conserv. Res.* **2024**, *12*, 1–12. [CrossRef]
35. Simane, B.; Benjamin, Z.; Mutlu, O. Agroecosystem analysis of the choke mountain watersheds, Ethiopia. *Sustainability* **2013**, *5*, 592–616. [CrossRef]
36. Coates, J.; Swindale, A.; Bilinsky, P. *Household Food Insecurity Access Scale (HFIAS) for Measurement of Food Access: Indicator Guide*; Version 3; The Food and Nutrition Technical Assistance: Washington, DC, USA, 2007.
37. FAO. *Guidelines for Measuring Household and Individual Dietary Diversity*; FAO Nutrition and Consumer Protection Division with support from the EC/FAO Food Security Information for Action Programme and the Food and Nutrition Technical Assistance (FANTA) Project; FAO: Rome, Italy, 2007.
38. Swindale, A.; Bilinsky, P. *Household Dietary Diversity Score (HDDS) for Measurement of Household Food Access: Indicator Guide (Version 2)*; The Food and Nutrition Technical Assistance: Washington, DC, USA, 2006.
39. Harris, J.E.; Gleason, P.M. Application of Path Analysis and Structural Equation Modeling in Nutrition and Dietetics. *J. Acad. Nutr. Diet.* **2022**, *122*, 2023–2035. [CrossRef]
40. MacKinnon, D.P.; Krull, J.L.; Lockwood, C.M. Equivalence of the mediation, confounding and suppression effect. *Prev. Sci.* **2000**, *1*, 173–181. [CrossRef]
41. Hair, J.F.; Black, W.C.; Babin, B.J.; Anderson, R. *Multivariate Data Analysis*, 7th ed.; Pearson: New York, NY, USA, 2010.
42. Gebretsadik, G.G.; Abraha, M.; Bereket, T.; Hailemariam, F.; Gebrearegay, F.; Hagos, T.; Assefa, M.; Berhe, K.; Gebregziabher, H.; Adhanu, A.K.; et al. Prevalence and multi-level factors associated with acute malnutrition among children aged 6–59 months from war affected communities of Tigray, Northern Ethiopia, 2021: A cross-sectional study. *Confl. Health* **2023**, *17*, 10. [CrossRef]
43. Deaconu, A.; Berti, P.R.; Cole, D.C.; Mercille, G.; Batal, M. Agroecology and nutritional health: A comparison of agroecological farmers and their neighbors in the Ecuadorian highlands. *Food Policy* **2021**, *101*, 102034. [CrossRef]
44. Zaitchik, B.F.; Simane, B.; Habib, S.; Anderson, M.C.; Ozdogan, M.; Foltz, J.D. Building Climate Resilience in the Blue Nile/Abay Highlands: A Role for Earth System Sciences. *Int. J. Environ. Res. Public Health* **2012**, *9*, 435–461. [CrossRef]
45. Wubetie, B.Y.; Tsunekawa, A.; Haregeweyn, N.; Tsubo, M.; Nigussie, Z.; Meshesha, T.M. An agroecosystem-based multilevel analysis of household dietary diversity and its linkage with agricultural production diversification in the Upper Blue Nile Basin, Ethiopia. *Environ. Dev.* **2024**, accepted.
46. Randell, H.; Gray, C.; Grace, K. Stunted from the start: Early life weather conditions and child undernutrition in Ethiopia. *Soc. Sci. Med.* **2020**, *261*, 113234. [CrossRef]
47. Molla, A.; Egata, G.; Getacher, L.; Kebede, B.; Sayih, A.; Arega, M.; Bante, A. Minimum acceptable diet and associated factors among infants and young children aged 6–23 months in Amhara region, Central Ethiopia: Community-based cross-sectional study. *BMJ Open* **2021**, *11*, e044284. [CrossRef]
48. Modjadji, P.; Molokwane, D.; Ukegbu, P.O. Dietary diversity and nutritional status of preschool children in north west province, south africa: A cross sectional study. *Children* **2020**, *7*, 174. [CrossRef] [PubMed]
49. Frempong, R.B.; Annim, S.K. Dietary diversity and child malnutrition in Ghana. *Heliyon* **2017**, *3*, e00298. [CrossRef] [PubMed]
50. UNICEF. *UNICEF Conceptual Framework on Maternal and Child Nutrition*; Nutr. Child Dev. Sect. Program Gr 3 United Nations Plaza: New York, NY, USA, 2021; pp. 2–3. Available online: www.unicef.org/nutrition (accessed on 13 March 2024).
51. Deaconu, A.; Berti, P.R.; Cole, D.C.; Mercille, G.; Batal, M. Market foods, own production, and the social economy: How food acquisition sources influence nutrient intake among Ecuadorian farmers and the role of agroecology in supporting healthy diets. *Sustainability* **2021**, *13*, 4410. [CrossRef]
52. Amondo, E.I.; Nshakira-Rukundo, E.; Mirzabaev, A. The effect of extreme weather events on child nutrition and health. *Food Secur.* **2023**, *15*, 571–596. [CrossRef]
53. Gebremedhin, S.; Baye, K.; Bekele, T.; Tharaney, M.; Asrat, Y.; Abebe, Y.; Reta, N. Predictors of dietary diversity in children ages 6 to 23 mo in largely food-insecure area of South Wollo, Ethiopia. *Nutrition* **2017**, *33*, 163–168. [CrossRef] [PubMed]
54. Ogbo, F.A.; Agho, K.E.; Page, A. Determinants of suboptimal breastfeeding practices in Nigeria: Evidence from the 2008 demographic and health survey. *BMC Public Health* **2015**, *15*, 259. [CrossRef] [PubMed]
55. Dhami, M.V.; Ogbo, F.A.; Osuagwu, U.L.; Ugboma, Z.; Agho, K.E. Stunting and severe stunting among infants in India: The role of delayed introduction of complementary foods and community and household factors. *Glob. Health Action* **2019**, *12*, 1638020. [CrossRef]

56. FAO; IFAD; UNICEF; WFP; WHO. *The State of Food Security and Nutrition in the World 2018: Building Climate Resilience for Food Security and Nutrition*; FAO: Rome, Italy, 2018.
57. Wubetie, B.Y.; Mekonen, T.K. Undernutrition and associated factors among lactating mothers in rural Yilmana Densa District, Northwest Ethiopia: A community-based cross-sectional study. *Food Sci. Nutr.* **2022**, *11*, 1383–1393. [CrossRef] [PubMed]
58. Takele, K.; Zewotir, T.; Ndanguza, D. A combined model of child malnutrition and morbidity in Ethiopia using structural equation models. *Sci. Rep.* **2023**, *13*, 471. [CrossRef]
59. Mekonnen, H. Malnutrition and its Correlates among Rural Primary School Children of Fogera District, Northwest Ethiopia. *J. Nutr. Disord. Ther.* **2013**, *12*, 002. [CrossRef]
60. Black, R.E.; Victora, C.G.; Walker, S.P.; Bhutta, Z.A.; Christian, P.; de Onis, M.; Ezzati, M.; Grantham-McGregor, S.; Katz, J.; Martorell, R.; et al. Maternal and child undernutrition and overweight in low-income and middle-income countries. *Lancet* **2013**, *382*, 427–451. [CrossRef] [PubMed]
61. Ma'Alin, A.; Birhanu, D.; Melaku, S.; Tolossa, D.; Mohammed, Y.; Gebremicheal, K. Magnitude and factors associated with malnutrition in children 6–59 months of age in Shinille Woreda, Ethiopian Somali regional state: A cross-sectional study. *BMC Nutr.* **2016**, *2*, 44. [CrossRef]
62. FAO. *Minimum Dietary for Women*; FAO: Rome, Italy, 2021; pp. 1–176. [CrossRef]
63. Farah, A.M.; Endris, B.S.; Gebreyesus, S.H. Maternal undernutrition as proxy indicators of their offspring's undernutrition: Evidence from 2011 Ethiopia demographic and health survey. *BMC Nutr.* **2019**, *5*, 17. [CrossRef]
64. Santoso, M.V.; Kerr, R.B.; Hoddinott, J.; Garigipati, P.; Olmos, S.; Young, S.L. Role of Women's Empowerment in Child Nutrition Outcomes: A Systematic Review. *Adv. Nutr.* **2019**, *10*, 1138–1151. [CrossRef] [PubMed]
65. Kassie, G.W.; Workie, D.L. Determinants of under-nutrition among children under five years of age in Ethiopia. *BMC Public Health* **2020**, *20*, 399. [CrossRef] [PubMed]
66. Bahru, B.A.; Jebena, M.G.; Birner, R.; Zeller, M. Impact of Ethiopia's productive safety net program on household food security and child nutrition: A marginal structural modeling approach. *SSM-Popul. Health* **2020**, *12*, 100660. [CrossRef] [PubMed]
67. Tesfaw, L.M.; Woya, A.A. Potential mediators of the link between wealth index and anthropometric indices of under-five children in Ethiopia. *Front. Public Health* **2022**, *10*, 981484. [CrossRef] [PubMed]
68. Selepe, M.; Hendriks, S. The impact of home gardens on pre-schoolers nutrition in Eatonside in the Vaal Triangle, South Africa. *Afr. J. Hosp. Tour. Leis.* **2014**, *3*, 1–14.
69. Cabalda, A.B.; Rayco-Solon, P.; Solon, J.A.A.; Solon, F.S. Home Gardening Is Associated with Filipino Preschool Children's Dietary Diversity. *J. Am. Diet. Assoc.* **2011**, *111*, 711–715. [CrossRef]

nutrients

MDPI

Article

Is Obesity a Cause for Shame? Weight Bias and Stigma among Physicians, Dietitians, and Other Healthcare Professionals in Poland—A Cross-Sectional Study

Alicja Baska [1,2,*,†], Karolina Świder [3,†], Wojciech Stefan Zgliczyński [1,2], Karolina Kłoda [4,5], Agnieszka Mastalerz-Migas [5,6] and Mateusz Babicki [5,6]

1 Department of Lifestyle Medicine, School of Public Health, Centre of Postgraduate Medical Education, 01-813 Warsaw, Poland; wzgliczynski2@cmkp.edu.pl
2 Polish Society of Lifestyle Medicine, 00-382 Warsaw, Poland
3 NZOZ Biogenes, 53-224 Wroclaw, Poland; karolina.swider.pl@gmail.com
4 MEDFIT Karolina Kłoda, 70-240 Szczecin, Poland; wikarla@gazeta.pl
5 Scientific Section of the Polish Society of Family Medicine, 51-141 Wroclaw, Poland; agnieszka.migas@gmail.com (A.M.-M.); ma.babicki@gmail.com (M.B.)
6 Department of Family Medicine, Wroclaw Medical University, 50-367 Wroclaw, Poland
* Correspondence: alicja.baska@cmkp.edu.pl
† These authors contributed equally to this work.

Abstract: Weight bias and weight stigma pose significant challenges in healthcare, particularly affecting obesity management practices and patient care quality. Our study evaluates their prevalence and impact among healthcare professionals in Poland. Using the Fat Phobia Scale and custom questions, we surveyed 686 professionals via Computer-Assisted Web Interview (CAWI). Results reveal a moderate level of explicit weight bias (mean score: 3.60 ± 0.57), with significant variations across professional groups: physicians (3.70 ± 0.48), dietitians (3.51 ± 0.48), and others (3.44 ± 0.77). Common feelings towards individuals with obesity include willingness to help (57.0%) and compassion (37.8%), yet 29.9% perceive obesity as shameful. The results also vary depending on the respondent's sex or BMI. These findings underscore the need for evidence-based interventions to mitigate weight stigma and enhance understanding of obesity among healthcare professionals.

Keywords: weight bias; stigma; obesity; overweight; healthcare professionals

1. Introduction

Weight bias is described as the presence of negative weight-related attitudes, belief assumptions, and judgments held about people living in large bodies [1]. It encompasses three constructs: prejudice (as a negative evaluation of a social group/individual), stereotyping (convictions about the etiology and/or maintenance of obesity), and discrimination (actions or behaviors) [2]. The frequent examples of weight bias include attributing the following to individuals with obesity: laziness, lack of willpower, low level of intelligence, a lack of moral character, bad hygiene, and unattractiveness [3]. The World Obesity Federation distinguishes weight (or obesity) stigma from weight bias as its manifestation, defined as discriminatory acts and ideologies targeted towards individuals because of their weight and size [3]. Weight stigma can manifest as negative comments directed at people with obesity, reinforcement of harmful stereotypes in the media, and environmental factors, such as medical settings that may not adequately accommodate individuals with obesity.

There is a mounting body of evidence that demonstrates how weight bias and stigma pose a significant challenge to the effective treatment and prevention of obesity. This challenge stems from their detrimental impact on health and their widespread prevalence, including in healthcare settings [4]. In the "Joint international consensus statement for ending stigma of obesity" published in Nature Medicine in 2020 [5], it was concluded that weight stigma has significant adverse effects on both mental and physical health. Weight-based stigma is associated with increased risks of depressive symptoms, anxiety, substance use, and social isolation, as well as reduced self-esteem and heightened stress levels [5]. A 2018 systematic review found that obesity stigma is positively linked to various health indicators, including conditions such as obesity itself and diabetes, as well as physiological markers like cortisol and C-reactive protein level and oxidative stress [6]. This underscores the far-reaching impact of weight stigma on health outcomes. Additionally, there is evidence suggesting that individuals who experience weight-based stigma are less likely to adopt healthy behaviors, such as engaging in physical activity and maintaining a healthy diet. This, in turn, heightens the risk of exacerbating obesity [7]. Moreover, patients with obesity may encounter barriers in accessing appropriate healthcare, not only in relation to obesity but also for other health conditions and preventive care, such as cancer screenings. These barriers include experience of previous stigma from healthcare professionals, feelings of embarrassment, guilt, or fear related to the equipment not being able to accommodate individuals with obesity [8]. It is also important to emphasize that the assumption that obesity is a matter of choice and can be reversed through voluntary decisions, such as 'eating less and moving more', not only harms the individuals affected but also has implications for public health and research [5]. The impact of this assumption is visible, for example, in public campaigns and policies that tend to overlook environmental and societal factors that play a major role in the epidemic of obesity, which in turn can further perpetuate obesity stigma among individuals [9].

The most recent Canadian Adult Obesity Clinical Practice Guidelines published in 2020 included weight bias, stigma, and discrimination for the first time in its history [1]. These issues were addressed in a separate initial chapter "in recognition of emerging and compelling evidence that they represent a significant challenge to practice and policy". The primary recommendation in the Canadian guidelines calls for healthcare providers to assess their attitudes and beliefs regarding obesity and consider how these attitudes and beliefs may influence care delivery (Level 1a; Grade A). Various measures are available to assess weight bias, validated and widely used in research, including the Fat Phobia Scale (FPS), the Antifat Attitudes Test (AFAT), the Antifat Attitudes Scale (AFAS), and others [10], sometimes in combination.

Weight bias has been reported among healthcare professionals of different professions, including primary care physicians, nurses, dietitians, and medical students worldwide. One study examining weight stigma among women who were overweight and obese found that as much as 53% of them experienced inappropriate comments from their physicians, who ranked as the second most common source of weight stigma (out of 20 different sources). Participants reported similar experiences with nurses (46%) and dietitians (37%) [11]. It is known that weight bias in healthcare settings reduces the quality of care, impacting not only obesity management practices but also the patient–healthcare professional relationship, consequently affecting patients' engagement in healthcare services [12,13].

In 2022, the Polish Society for the Treatment of Obesity published guidelines that also included a chapter on countering discrimination and stigmatization of patients with obesity [14], followed by the release of the "Charter of Rights for Patients with Obesity" [15]. Despite these developments, scientific research on the prevalence and characteristics of weight bias among healthcare professionals in Poland has been limited, and most of the few studies available only used non-validated, custom questionnaires, making the results difficult to compare and evaluate. As a response to this gap, our research group, comprised of representatives from the Scientific Section of the Polish Society of Family Medicine in collaboration with the Centre of Postgraduate Medical Education and the Polish Society and Lifestyle Medicine, embarked on a study focusing on weight stigma and fat phobia in Poland using the Fat Phobia Scale (FPS) combined with a custom questionnaire. This article represents the second part of our research, with the first part primarily investigating weight bias among the general public [16]. Therefore, the aim of this study was to evaluate the level of weight bias and stigma among healthcare professionals (physicians, dietitians, and others) in Poland.

2. Materials and Methods

The study was conducted using a Computer-Assisted Web Interview (CAWI). The data was collected from April to July 2023. Prior to completing the questionnaire, participants were presented with information about the research aim and methodology and were required to provide informed consent. The data collection process ensured full anonymity; no personal data was collected.

The survey was distributed among Polish resident doctors attending obligatory specialization courses organized by the Centre of Postgraduate Medical Education as well as via social media platforms, including Facebook and Instagram, specifically targeting medical professionals, such as groups for medical doctors who require confirmation of a medical license. An invitation to complete the questionnaire was also shared via newsletters of the Polish Society of Family Medicine and the Polish Society of Lifestyle Medicine.

The research tool was an online questionnaire prepared in Polish via Google Forms. It consisted of four sections. The first section collected information on the characteristics of the respondents (gender, age, place of residence, weight, height, and profession). The respondents were also asked to indicate the frequency of contact with people living with obesity. The second part used the Fat Phobia Scale (FPS), examining explicit weight bias. The scale consists of 14 pairs of adjectives (positive/negative) designed to characterize a person with obesity, using a five-point Likert scale. The total scale score was obtained by summing the scores from each question and dividing by 14 (the number of scale items), resulting in a value ranging from 1 to 5. A higher score on the scale indicates a greater level of fat phobia. According to the scale design, a score of 2.5 indicates a neutral attitude. Scores above this value suggest a negative attitude, while scores below indicate a positive attitude. A score of 4.40 or above indicates a high level of fat phobia, while a score of 3.6 is seen as an indication of an average amount of fat phobia. The internal consistency of the tool was found to be 0.893 [17]. The FPS was translated into Polish by a certified bilingual team member. It was then independently back-translated into English by two medical professionals proficient in English. The original FPS was verified against the back translations, and no significant differences were found. The third section included custom questions assessing the level of stigma, describing the feelings of the respondents when in contact with people with obesity (for example, the likelihood of dating, hiring, entrusting a child in their care, and befriending a person with obesity). The fourth section comprised custom questions concerning knowledge about obesity. These questions aimed to verify whether respondents perceived obesity as a chronic disease and whether they could identify the BMI category for diagnosing obesity (single-choice questions). The questions also assessed their knowledge of obesity causes, effective forms of treatment, and obesity-related conditions (multiple-choice questions). The custom questions in both sections were developed by our multidisciplinary team of authors, drawing on their many years of expertise in obesity treatment, public health, medical education, medical communications, patient advocacy, and extensive literature review.

Statistical Analysis

The analysis was carried out using Statistica 13.0 by StatSoft (Cracow, Poland). The analyzed variables were of qualitative and quantitative nature. The normal distribution was assessed using the Shapiro–Wilk test. Basic descriptive statistics were applied, including percentages, means, and standard deviations. The comparison of qualitative variables was conducted using the chi-square test. For quantitative variables, non-parametric tests such as the Mann–Whitney U test or the Kruskal–Wallis Test were used. The degree of correlation between quantitative variables was evaluated using the Spearman correlation test. The significance level was assumed at 0.05.

3. Results

3.1. Characteristics of the Study Group

The study involved 686 healthcare professionals, including 404 physicians (58.7%), 117 dietitians (17.0%), and 167 individuals representing other medical professions (24.3%). The latter group included 42 nurses (6.1%), 22 physiotherapists (3.2%), 12 pharmacists (1.7%), 12 dentists (1.7%), 3 paramedics (0.6%), and 76 people other than those listed (11.0%). The average age of the respondents was 34.6 ± 7.7 years. The majority were females (88.1%) and residents of large cities (69.9%). The majority of respondents exhibited a normal BMI (60.5%). Notably, there were significant differences in the prevalence of overweight and obesity among different members of the studied group, with physicians recording rates of 18.6% and 17.3%, dietitians 10.3% and 4.2%, and other health professionals 26.4% and 18.6%, respectively. A detailed overview of the characteristics of the study group is presented in Table 1.

Table 1. Characteristics of the study participants.

Analyzed Variables		Studied Group N(%)/M ± SD	Healthcare Professional			*p*
			Physicians (%)/M ± SD	Dieticians (%)/M ± SD	Others (%)/M ± SD	
Sex	Female	606 (88.1)	348 (86.1)	111 (94.9)	147 (88.0)	0.134 *
	Male	82 (11.9)	56 (13.9)	6 (5.1)	20 (12.0)	
	Other	0 (0.0)	0 (0.0)	0 (0.0)	0 (0.0)	
Age (years)		34.6 ± 7.7	34.7 ± 6.9	31.6 ± 6.7	36.4 ± 9.3	**0.005 #**
Weight (kg)		69.7 ± 16.9	70.5 ± 16.6	62.2 ± 10.9	73.2 ± 19.4	**<0.001 #**
Height (cm)		168.6 ± 7.4	168.7 ± 7.5	167 ± 6.7	168.7 ± 7.6	0.503 #
BMI (kg/m^2)		24.5 ± 5.4	24.7 ± 5.3	22.1 ± 3.3	25.6 ± 6.3	**<0.001 #**
BMI	Underweight	35 (5.1)	16 (4.0)	9 (7.7)	10 (6.0)	**<0.001 ***
	Normal weight	416 (60.5)	243 (60.1)	91 (77.8)	82 (49.0)	
	Overweight	131 (19.0)	75 (18.6)	12 (10.3)	44 (26.4)	
	Obesity	106 (15.4)	70 (17.3)	5 (4.2)	31 (18.6)	
Place of residence	Rural area	69 (10.0)	32 (7.9)	15 (12.8)	22 (13.2)	**0.001 ***
	Town of up to 20,000 inhabitants	39 (5.7)	16 (4.0)	4 (3.4)	19 (11.4)	
	City of 20,000–100,000 inhabitants	99 (14.4)	51 (12.6)	23 (19.7)	25 (15.0)	
	City of 100,000–500,000 inhabitants	144 (20.9)	89 (22.0)	22 (18.8)	33 (19.8)	
	City of over 500,000 inhabitants	337 (49.0)	216 (53.5)	53 (45.3)	68 (40.6)	
Healthcare professional	Physicians	404 (58.7)	-	-	-	-
	Dieticians	117 (17.0)	-	-	-	
	Others	167 (24.3)	-	-	-	

M—mean, SD—Standard deviation, N—number, kg—kilograms, cm—centimeters, BMI—body mass index, # Kruskal–Wallis H Test, * Chi-squared test, Significant effects (<0.05) are marked in bold.

3.2. Fat Phobia Scale (FPS)

In the examination of the FPS scale, respondents achieved an average score of 3.60 ± 0.57, suggesting an average level of fat phobia [17]. The highest scores were recorded for the assessment of "dislikes food/likes food" (4.13 ± 0.89) and "undereats/overeats" (4.09 ± 0.87). Conversely, the lowest scores were noted for the comparisons "weak/strong" (3.00 ± 0.86) and "lazy/industrious" (3.16 ± 1.68).

When comparing the level of fat phobia among various groups of healthcare professionals, physicians scored higher on all the individual items and exhibited the highest level of explicit weight bias (3.70 ± 0.48), surpassing that of both dietitians (3.51 ± 0.48) and a group comprising other healthcare professionals (3.44 ± 0.77). Both the group of dietitians and the group of other healthcare professionals demonstrated a below-average level of fat phobia ($p < 0.001$). A detailed analysis of the FPS scale scores can be found in Table 2.

Table 2. Analysis of the FPS (Fat Phobia Scale) scores considering individual questions and distinguishing between doctors, dieticians, and other respondents.

FPS Pair of Adjectives	Studied Group M ± SD	Healthcare Professionals			
		Physicians M ± SD	Dieticians M ± SD	Others M ± SD	p #
Total score	3.60 ± 0.57	3.70 ± 0.48	3.51 ± 0.48	3.44 ± 0.77	**<0.001**
Lazy/industrious	1.68 ± 0.08	3.29 ± 0.75	2.98 ± 0.67	2.96 ± 1.09	**<0.001**
No willpower/has willpower	3.16 ± 0.97	3.71 ± 0.79	3.56 ± 0.85	3.46 ± 1.09	**0.028**
Attractive/unattractive	3.68 ± 0.91	3.80 ± 0.83	3.39 ± 0.96	3.57 ± 1.14	**0.002**
Good self-control/poor self-control	3.81 ± 0.81	3.93 ± 0.72	3.80 ± 0.80	3.53 ± 1.06	**<0.001**
Fast/slow	3.67 ± 0.92	3.77 ± 0.79	3.55 ± 0.94	3.54 ± 1.14	**0.048**
Having endurance/having no endurance	3.45 ± 0.93	3.57 ± 0.78	3.43 ± 0.96	3.16 ± 1.09	**<0.001**
Active/inactive	3.57 ± 0.91	3.73 ± 0.86	3.41 ± 0.87	3.31 ± 1.13	**<0.001**
Weak/strong	3.00 ± 0.86	3.09 ± 0.74	2.86 ± 0.90	2.89 ± 1.05	**0.008**
Self-indulgent/self-sacrificing	3.41 ±0.97	3.50 ± 0.88	3.27 ± 0.97	3.32 ± 1.15	**0.032**
Dislikes food/likes food	4.13 ± 0.89	4.18 ± 0.86	4.04 ± 0.95	4.06 ± 0.89	0.164
Shapeless/shapely	3.46 ± 1.04	3.56 ± 0.94	3.10 ± 1.12	3.45 ± 1.17	**<0.001**
Undereats/overeats	4.09 ± 0.87	4.21 ± 0.81	3.95 ± 0.97	3.90 ± 0.91	**0.002**
Insecure/secure	3.76 ± 0.93	3.65 ± 0.92	3.83 ± 0.88	3.38 ± 1.05	**0.001**
Low self-esteem/high self-esteem	3.76 ± 0.93	3.79 ± 0.89	3.94 ± 0.89	3.57 ± 1.00	**0.004**

Items 3, 4, 5, 6, 7, 10, and 12 scored as follows: 1 2 3 4 5; Items 1, 2, 8, 9, 11, 13, and 14 scored as follows: 5 4 3 2 1. Fat Phobia Scale (FPS) score of the overweight vignette was from 1 = positive attributes to 5 = negative attributes. M—mean, SD—Standard deviation, # Kruskal–Wallis H Test, Significant effects (<0.05) are marked in bold.

It was also demonstrated that a negative correlation exists between the FPS score and the likelihood of engaging in various social interactions with people with obesity. The strongest association was observed for the probability of going on a date with an individual living with obesity. A detailed analysis of the correlation between the FPS score and social interactions with individuals with obesity is presented in Table 3.

Table 3. The analysis of correlation between the FPS score and the likelihood of social interactions with individuals with obesity.

	Probability							
	Employment of a Person with Obesity		Going on a Date with a Person with Obesity		Entrusting the Care of Your Children to a Person with Obesity		Befriending a Person with Obesity	
	r	*p*	r	*p*	r	*p*	r	*p*
FPS total score	−0.151	**<0.001**	−0.310	**<0.001**	−0.202	**<0.001**	−0.122	**0.001**

Significant effects (<0.05) are marked in bold.

3.3. *Custom Questions Assessing the Level of Stigmatisation*

In analyzing custom questions evaluating the perception of patients with obesity, it was found that 94.2% of medical professionals believe that people with obesity are not inherently worse than those with normal weight. Moreover, 70.1% indicated that obesity is not a reason for shame. However, a notable 74.6% of respondents expressed the view that individuals with obesity are less attractive than those with normal body weight. This perception varied, with 80.0% of physicians holding this belief compared to 66.6% of dietitians and 67.0% of other medical professionals ($p < 0.001$). Furthermore, when assessed on a 10-point scale, the likelihood of going on a date with a person with obesity received the lowest score of 4.47 ± 2.89 compared to other social interactions, while befriending a person with obesity emerged as the most probable (8.91 ± 1.94).

Among the respondents, the most prevalent feelings accompanying interactions with individuals living with obesity included the willingness to help (on average, 57.0% of respondents), kindness (47.4%), and compassion (37.8%). The least frequent were contempt (2.6%), mercy (8.6%), and reluctance (8.7%). Notably, differences between the two homogenous groups were observed. In comparison to dietitians, physicians seemed to experience less kindness (44.3% vs. 64.9%, $p < 0.001$), liking/affection (20.1% vs. 31.6%, $p = 0.023$), and willingness to help (63.6% vs. 70.9%, $p < 0.001$), while expressing more impatience (14.9% vs. 2.6%, $p < 0.001$), reluctance (10.6% vs. 2.6%; $p = 0.009$), and discomfort in contact (13.9 vs. 7.7). However, physicians also demonstrated more compassion (42.1% vs. 35.0%, $p = 0.012$). When asked to provide their opinion on whether individuals living with obesity face discrimination using a 10-point scale, respondents provided an average score of 7.62 ± 2.27. There were no major differences between different healthcare professionals' groups. A detailed overview of the custom questions related to obesity stigma is presented in Table 4.

Table 4. Custom questions assessing the level of stigmatization of patients with obesity.

Analyzed Variables		Studied Group N(%)/M ± SD	Healthcare Professionals			*p*
			Physicians (%)/M ± SD	Dieticians (%)/M ± SD	Others (%)/M ± SD	
Are people with obesity worse than people with normal weight?	Definitely yes	5 (0.7)	4 (1.0)	0 (0.0)	1 (0.6)	**0.011** *
	Yes	11 (1.6)	4 (1.0)	3 (2.5)	4 (2.4)	
	Rather yes	24 (3.5)	12 (3.0)	1 (0.9)	11 (6.7)	
	Rather no	78 (11.3)	46 (11.4)	10 (8.6)	22 (13.1)	
	No	231 (33.6)	152 (37.6)	30 (25.6)	49 (29.3)	
	Definitely no	339 (49.3)	186 (46.0)	73 (62.4)	80 (47.9)	

Table 4. *Cont.*

Analyzed Variables		Studied Group N(%)/M ± SD	Healthcare Professionals			
			Physicians (%)/M ± SD	Dieticians (%)/M ± SD	Others (%)/M ± SD	p
Are people with obesity less attractive than people with normal weight?	Definitely yes	99 (14.4)	60 (14.9)	11 (9.4)	28 (16.7)	**<0.001 ***
	Yes	141 (20.5)	86 (21.3)	17 (14.5)	38 (22.8)	
	Rather yes	273 (39.7)	177 (43.8)	50 (42.7)	46 (27.5)	
	Rather no	83 (12.1)	43 (10.6)	14 (12.0)	26 (15.6)	
	No	59 (8.6)	26 (5.4)	13 (11.1)	20 (12.0)	
	Definitely no	33 (4.7)	12 (3.0)	12 (10.3)	9 (5.4)	
Would you hire a person with obesity as an employer?	Definitely yes	175 (25.5)	102 (25.3)	32 (27.4)	41 (24.6)	**<0.001 ***
	Yes	312 (45.3)	204 (50.4)	45 (38.5)	63 (37.7)	
	Rather yes	151 (21.9)	81 (20.1)	22 (18.8)	48 (28.7)	
	Rather no	38 (5.5)	12 (3.0)	12 (10.3)	14 (8.4)	
	No	7 (1.1)	2 (0.5)	4 (3.3)	1 (0.6)	
	Definitely no	5 (0.7)	3 (0.7)	2 (1.7)	0 (0.0)	
Is obesity a cause for shame?	Definitely yes	14 (2.0)	9 (2.2)	1 (0.9)	4 (2.4)	**<0.001 ***
	Yes	36 (5.2)	28 (6.9)	1 (0.9)	7 (4.2)	
	Rather yes	156 (22.7)	99 (24.6)	14 (12.0)	43 (25.8)	
	Rather no	195 (28.3)	116 (28.7)	27 (23.0)	52 (31.1)	
	No	185 (26.9)	108 (26.7)	40 (34.2)	37 (22.1)	
	Definitely no	102 (14.9)	44 (10.9)	34 (29.0)	24 (14.4)	
On a scale of 1 to 10, how likely is it in your case?						
Employment of a person with obesity		8.11 ± 2.29	8.34 ± 2.08	7.81 ± 2.46	7.79 ± 2.59	**0.039 #**
Going on a date with a person with obesity		4.47 ± 2.89	4.36 ± 2.87	4.42 ± 2.83	4.78 ± 2.98	0.315 #
Entrusting the care of your children to a person with obesity		7.88 ± 2.43	7.93 ± 2.30	7.88 ± 2.57	7.75 ± 2.67	0.847 #
Befriending a person with obesity		8.91 ± 1.94	8.94 ± 1.80	9.07 ± 1.88	8.75 ± 2.29	0.479 #
People with obesity are discriminated against in Poland		7.62 ± 2.27	7.52 ± 2.28	7.52 ± 2.26	7.94 ± 2.25	**0.038 #**
Feelings accompanying interactions with individuals living with obesity						
Mercy		59 (8.6)	34 (8.4)	9 (7.7)	16 (9.6)	0.841 *
Reluctance		60 (8.7)	43 (10.6)	3 (2.6)	14 (8.4))	**0.009 ***
Contempt		18 (2.6)	11 (2.7)	0 (0.0)	7 (4.2)	**0.022 ***
Kindness		326 (47.4)	179 (44.3)	76 (64.9)	71 (42.5)	**<0.001 ***
Discomfort in contacts		85 (12.4)	56 (13.9)	9 (7.7)	20 (12.0)	0.173 *
Liking/affection		162 (23.5)	81 (20.1)	37 (31.6)	44 (26.4)	**0.023 ***
Impatience		71 (10.3)	60 (14.9)	3 (2.6)	8 (4.8)	**<0.001 ***
Indifference		133 (19.3)	72 (17.8)	20 (17.1)	41 (24.6)	0.155 *
Compassion		260 (37.8)	170 (42.1)	41 (35.0)	49 (29.3)	**0.012 ***
Willingness to help		392 (57.0)	257 (63.6)	83 (70.9)	52 (31.1)	**<0.001 ***

M—mean, SD—Standard deviation, N—number, # Kruskal–Wallis H Test, * Chi-squared test, Significant effects (<0.05) are marked in bold.

3.4. Other Factors Influencing the Perception of Weight Stigma

3.4.1. Sex

The results indicate that female medical professionals notice higher levels of discrimination against individuals living with obesity in Poland (7.81 vs. 6.23, $p < 0.001$). They are also more inclined to engage in positive social interactions with these individuals (dating, befriending, employing, or childcare provision). Female healthcare professionals report feeling more kindness (49.3% vs. 33.3%, $p = 0.016$) and affection (24.6% vs. 14.8%, $p = 0.029$) while experiencing less contempt (2.0% vs. 7.4%, $p = 0.048$) and indifference (17.3% vs. 34.6%, $p < 0.001$) in interactions with individuals living with obesity. For the remaining 6 out of 10 feelings (mercy, reluctance, discomfort, impatience, compassion, and willingness to help), similar trends were observed, although the differences between male and female respondents were not found to be statistically significant. Similarly, no significant difference in FPS scores between the two sexes was found.

3.4.2. Respondents' Body Mass Index

Individuals meeting the obesity criteria reported the highest scores when asked about the incidence of discrimination against people living with obesity. Similarly, they also obtained the highest scores in assessing the likelihood of positive social interactions with people living with obesity (dating, befriending, employing, or childcare provision). Healthcare professionals with a BMI indicating obesity report feeling more kindness and compassion than healthcare professionals with a normal BMI while experiencing less reluctance. For the remaining 7 out of 10 feelings (mercy, contempt, discomfort, affection, impatience, indifference, and willingness to help), similar trends were observed, although the differences between respondents with underweight, normal BMI, overweight, and obesity were not found to be statistically significant. Similarly, only slight differences were observed in FPS scores: the respondents with obesity had the lowest FPS score (3.50) compared to respondents with overweight (3.61), normal weight (3.61), and underweight (3.61). These differences, though, were not statistically significant.

3.4.3. Place of Residence

No statistically significant differences were identified based on the place of residence.

Detailed results analyzing the impact of demographic variables and respondents' BMI are presented in Tables 5 and 6.

Table 5. Analysis of the differences in the FPS total score and engagement in positive social interactions by demographic and weight.

Analyzed Variables		FPS Total Score		Probability of Employment of a Person with Obesity		Probability of Going on a Date with a Person with Obesity		Probability of Entrusting the Care of Your Children to a Person with Obesity		Probability of Befriending a Person with Obesity		People with Obesity Are Discriminated in Poland	
		M ± SD	p	M ± SD	p	M ± SD	p	M ± SD	p	M ± SD	p	M ± SD	p
Sex	Female	3.59 ± 0.57	0.204 *	8.29 ± 2.20	<0.001 *	4.67 ± 2.88	<0.001 *	7.99 ± 2.39	<0.001 *	9.01 ± 1.88	<0.001 *	7.81 ± 2.11	<0.001 *
	Male	3.69 ± 0.58		6.81 ± 2.57		2.94 ± 2.49		7.02 ± 2.63		8.23 ± 2.30		6.23 ± 2.89	
BMI	Underweight	3.62 ± 0.66	0.674 #	7.69 ± 1.95	0.046 #	3.57 ± 2.25	<0.001 #	7.20 ± 2.29	0.001 #	9.11 ± 1.28	0.497 #	8.00 ± 1.98	<0.001 #
	Normal weight	3.61 ± 0.53		8.08 ± 2.36		3.93 ± 2.71		7.83 ± 2.49		8.85 ± 2.00		7.34 ± 2.32	
	Overweight	3.61 ± 0.68		8.12 ± 2.14		4.64 ± 2.73		7.79 ± 2.34		8.91 ± 2.00		7.73 ± 2.24	
	Obesity	3.55 ± 0.60		8.42 ± 2.30		6.69 ± 2.86		8.38 ± 2.32		9.14 ± 1.83		8.48 ± 1.99	

M—mean, SD—Standard deviation, # Kruskal–Wallis Test, * Mann–Whitney U, FPS—Fat Phobia Scale, Significant effects (<0.05) are marked in bold.

Table 6. Analysis of associations between feelings accompanying interactions with individuals living with obesity and demographic and weight characteristics.

Feelings Accompanying Interactions with Individuals Living with Obesity	Sex *n* (%)			BMI *n* (%)				
	Male	Female	*p*	Underweight	Normal Weight	Overweight	Obesity	*p*
Mercy	9 (11.1)	50 (8.3)	0.657 *	4 (11.4)	38 (9.1)	10 (7.6)	7 (6.6)	0.752 *
Reluctance	12 (14.8)	48 (7.9)	0.114 *	2 (5.7)	44 (10.6)	12 (9.2)	2 (1.9)	**0.013** *
Contempt	6 (7.4)	12 (2.0)	**0.048** *	1 (2.9)	10 (2.4)	4 (3.1)	3 (2.8)	0.987 *
Kindness	27 (33.3)	299 (49.3)	**0.016** *	18 (51.4)	190 (45.7)	55 (42.0)	63 (59.4)	**0.037** *
Discomfort in contacts	13 (16.1)	72 (11.9)	0.521 *	6 (17.1)	53 (12.7)	20 (15.3)	6 (5.7)	0.101 *
Liking/affection	12 (14.8)	149 (24.6)	**0.029** *	7 (20.0)	95 (22.8)	31 (23.7)	29 (27.4)	0.748 *
Impatience	12 (14.8)	59 (9.8)	0.367 *	2 (5.7)	47 (11.3)	16 (12.2)	6 (5.7)	0.238 *
Indifference	28 (34.6)	105 (17.3)	**<0.001** *	5 (14.3)	85 (20.4)	28 (21.4)	15 (14.2)	0.381 *
Compassion	25 (30.9)	235 (38.8)	0.283 *	6 (17.1)	152 (36.5)	56 (42.8)	46 (43.4)	**0.017** *
Willingness to help	42 (51.9)	349 (57.6)	0.353 *	24 (68.6)	237 (57.0)	72 (55.0)	59 (55.7)	0.529 *

BMI—body mass index; N—number; * Chi-squared test; Significant effects (<0.05) are marked in bold.

3.5. Level of Knowledge about Obesity

In the analysis of questions aimed at assessing the level of knowledge about obesity, it was found that 98.5% of medical professionals acknowledge obesity as a chronic disease requiring treatment, while only 84.7% correctly identify the BMI category for diagnosing obesity. Regarding the reasons for obesity development, respondents most commonly selected excessive calorie intake (98.8%), lack of physical activity (94.3%), or complications from certain medications (91.0%). Notably, 26.5% of respondents incorrectly identified hyperthyroidism as a cause of obesity, with the majority from the group of other medical professionals (58.1%).

When it comes to effective treatment methods, the most frequently chosen answer was regular physical activity (97.5%), followed by pharmacological treatment (87.1%) and bariatric surgery (85.6%). Substantial differences were observed among various respondent groups. Physicians significantly favored pharmacological treatment (93.6%) and bariatric surgery (93.1%) as effective treatments, in contrast to dietitians (75.2%, 75.2%) and other health professionals (79.6%, 74.9%). Surprisingly, 4.1% of respondents considered fasting as an effective form of obesity treatment, with higher percentages among other medical professionals (6.6%) and physicians (4.0%), but only one dietician (0.9%).

Among the most commonly indicated obesity-related conditions, respondents frequently chose hypertension (98.7%), decreased exercise tolerance (98.7%), diabetes (98.4%), depression (98.4%), and hormonal disorders (95.9%). Less frequently mentioned complications included deterioration of hair and/or nail growth (74.7%) and gout (71.7%). Only 63.5% of respondents (65.6% physicians, 77.8% dietitians, and 48.5% representatives of other medical professions) acknowledged that obesity can contribute to the development of dementia.

A detailed overview of the level of knowledge distinguishing between different groups of healthcare professionals is presented in Table 7.

Table 7. A detailed overview of the level of knowledge about obesity.

Analysed Variables		Studied Group N(%)	Healthcare Professionals			p *
			Physicians (%)/M ± SD	Dieticians (%)/M ± SD	Others (%)/M ± SD	
Obesity	is a chronic disease that requires treatment	678 (98.5)	400 (99.0)	114 (97.4)	164 (98.2)	0.501 *
	is a disease that does not require treatment	2 (0.3)	1 (0.3)	0 (0.0)	1 (0.6)	
	is not a chronic disease	8 (1.2)	3 (0.7)	3 (2.6)	2 (1.2)	
BMI criterion for the diagnosis of obesity	≥25	41 (6.0)	7 (1.7)	6 (5.1)	28 (16.8)	**<0.001** *
	≥27.5	39 (5.7)	16 (4.0)	2 (1.7)	21 (12.6)	
	≥30	583 (84.7)	367 (90.8)	108 (92.3)	108 (64.6)	
	≥29	25 (3.6)	14 (3.5)	1 (0.9)	10 (6.0)	
Causes of obesity	Lack of physical activity	649 (94.3)	386 (95.5)	110 (94.0)	153 (91.6)	0.198 *
	Excessive calorie supply	680 (98.8)	404 (100.0)	116 (99.2)	160 (95.8)	**<0.001** *
	Certain chronic diseases, e.g., diabetes	494 (71.8)	271 (67.1)	76 (65.0)	147 (88.0)	**<0.001** *
	Hyperthyroidism	182 (26.5)	58 (14.4)	27 (23.1)	97 (58.1)	**<0.001** *
	Effects of certain drugs, e.g., steroids and antipsychotics	626 (91.0)	375 (92.8)	96 (82.1)	155 (92.8)	**0.003** *
Effective form of obesity treatment	Bariatric surgery	589 (85.6)	376 (93.1)	99 (75.2)	125 (74.9)	**<0.001** *
	Pharmacological treatment	599 (87.1)	378 (93.6)	88 (75.2)	133 (79.6)	**<0.001** *
	Regular physical activity	671 (97.5)	397 (98.3)	113 (96.6)	161 (96.4)	0.332 *
	Starvation	28 (4.1)	16 (4.0)	1 (0.9)	11 (6.6)	**0.032** *
Obesity complications	Poorer exercise tolerance/fatigue	679 (98.7)	404 (100.0)	115 (98.3)	160 (95.8)	**<0.001** *
	Hypertension	679 (98.7)	401 (99.3)	117 (100.0)	161 (96.4)	**0.012** *
	Diabetes mellitus	677 (98.4)	403 (99.8)	116 (99.2)	158 (94.6)	**<0.001** *
	Hormonal disorders	660 (95.9)	396 (98.0)	115 (98.3)	149 (89.2)	**<0.001** *
	Female menstrual disorders	639 (92.9)	394 (97.5)	108 (92.3)	137 (82.0)	**<0.001** *
	Decrease in libido	641 (93.2)	387 (95.8)	112 (95.7)	142 (85.0)	**<0.001** *
	Deterioration of hair and/or nail growth	514 (74.7)	308 (76.2)	96 (82.1)	110 (65.9)	**0.005** *
	Depression	677 (98.4)	401 (99.3)	117 (100.0)	159 (95.2)	**0.002** *
	Future dementia	437 (63.5)	265 (65.6)	91 (77.8)	81 (48.5)	**<0.001** *
	Gout	493 (71.7)	315 (78.0)	99 (84.6)	79 (47.3)	**<0.001** *

Significant effects (<0.05) are marked in bold, * Chi-squared test.

4. Discussion

While weight stigma manifests across multiple settings, healthcare settings require special consideration due to their critical role in caring for and treating individuals' physical and mental health.

Healthcare professionals, participants in our study, attained an average Fat Phobia Scale (FPS) score of 3.60 ± 0.57, indicating an average level of fat phobia. Our analysis revealed discernible variations among different medical professions, with physicians exhibiting the highest weight bias (FPS = 3.70), followed by dietitians (FPS = 3.51) and other healthcare professionals (FPS = 3.44). These findings suggest a moderate level of fat phobia among Polish doctors and a comparatively lower level among other healthcare professionals. To our knowledge, weight bias has not been extensively explored in Poland, and no study has previously examined its extent among healthcare professionals using validated tools. However, a 2020 study in Poland found that 82.6% of patients with obesity experienced inappropriate behaviors, often attributed to healthcare professionals [18]. Additionally, a recent Polish study reported that 48.4% of respondents witnessed discriminatory behaviors of medical staff toward patients with obesity [19].

Weight bias among healthcare professionals in Poland appears to surpass that of professionals in other countries. A large multinational study published in 2020, encompassing over 1,500 healthcare professionals from 77 countries, estimated the FPS score among healthcare professionals to be 3.40 [20], while a 2021 systematic review and meta-analysis—based on five studies utilizing the FPS—estimated a mean FPS score of 3.48. Notably, dietitians demonstrated the lowest explicit weight bias with a score of 3.37, slightly lower than their counterparts in Poland (3.51). In contrast, physicians in Poland exhibited a similar level of explicit weight bias compared to general practitioners in Germany (3.70) [19].

Although weight bias has been reported in multiple studies among representatives of various medical professions, including physicians (e.g., general practitioners [21] or professionals engaged in the management of obesity [22], dietitians [23], nurses [24], and physical therapists [25]), to the best of our knowledge, no other study has specifically compared weight bias among different healthcare professionals using the FPS. However, such a comparison was made among UK trainee dietitians, doctors, nurses, and nutritionists [26]. Interestingly, in contrast to our study, no significant differences in FPS scores between physicians- and dietitians-to-be were found. Nonetheless, their scores were higher than the mean FPS score for all healthcare professionals summarized in the aforementioned meta-analysis and higher than those of the population of healthcare professionals in Poland.

In conjunction with the Fat Phobia Scale, numerous studies worldwide have employed various tools, including the Antifat Attitudes Scale [27] and the Attitudes Towards Obese Persons Scale [25,28], to investigate explicit weight bias among healthcare professionals. Additionally, multiple studies utilizing custom questionnaires and various methods aim to provide valuable insights for a better understanding of the potential consequences of this phenomenon [22]. For example, a study involving medical students presented sample presentations of clinical cases, revealing that patients with obesity were often described as less attractive and compliant compared to patients with normal weight [29]. Similarly, in a study comparing the reactions of physicians, doctors reported feeling more negatively toward patients who were overweight and suggested they would spend less time with them [30]. Among nurses, between 5.9% and 24.3% reported feeling repulsed by individuals living with obesity [31], while 34.6% to 47.7% reported experiencing discomfort when caring for patients with obesity [32]. In our analysis, we attempted to identify the feelings accompanying healthcare professionals in interactions with individuals living with obesity as another way of quantifying weight bias. It revealed that, on average, 29.9% of health professionals in Poland identify obesity as a cause for shame, 19.4% of them experience indifference in contact with people with obesity, 12.4% feel discomfort, and 10.3% express impatience. On the other hand, on average, 57.0% feel a willingness to help, 47.4% show kindness, and 37.8% show compassion.

These biases are reflected in patient experiences, with patients reporting disrespectful, patronizing, insensitive, and/or contemptuous treatment from healthcare professionals [33]. A study conducted in Poland revealed that patients with obesity often experience different forms of improper behavior, including unpleasant, judgmental comments (81%), disdainful remarks (77%), and disgruntled grimaces (68%). They also admitted feeling blamed for carrying excess weight (73%).

Findings from all these studies, spanning as far back as 1989, consistently affirm the enduring existence of weight bias within the healthcare professional community [10] as a problem requiring urgent action [5]. Poland is no exception, especially considering that the levels of weight stigma appear to be mildly higher than in other studied populations.

The assessment of weight bias often involves an exploration of contributing factors. As multiple studies conducted among healthcare professionals highlighted the relevance of the respondents' own BMI, in our analysis, we also looked into the correlation between respondents' self-reported BMI and attitudes towards individuals living with obesity. We found that healthcare professionals with a BMI indicating obesity scored the highest in the question regarding the incidence of discrimination against people with obesity in Poland. They also often experienced more kindness and compassion and less reluctance in interactions with individuals with obesity compared to respondents with normal BMI. These differences were not reflected in the level of weight bias assessed by the Fat Phobia Scale. This contrasts with several studies where higher self-reported BMI was predictive of lower fat phobia, including studies conducted among physicians [34], health professionals specializing in obesity [22], and trainees [26].

Our study also revealed significant differences in weight bias and attitudes across genders. The female respondents declared experiencing more kindness and affection while less contempt and indifference in interactions with people living with obesity compared to men. They were also more likely to engage in positive social interactions and seemed to be more sensitive to noticing discrimination. Several studies have investigated gender differences in weight bias, consistently highlighting lower bias in women. A 2012 study [34] involving a substantial sample of medical doctors in the US (nearly 2300) revealed that females exhibited less implicit and explicit bias. Similarly, two studies conducted among general practitioners in Germany [21] and Canada [35] found that female physicians held fewer negative attitudes than their male counterparts. Another study involving healthcare professionals from over 70 countries [20] reported similar trends. However, a study focusing on healthcare professionals specializing in obesity [22] reported that women expressed significantly stronger implicit bias than men, while measures of explicit weight bias did not show an association with gender. Likewise, in our study, explicit weight bias measured by FPS did not exhibit significant differences between genders.

Numerous studies also propose that age serves as yet another significant factor influencing the level of weight bias. This connection was identified in the previously mentioned study conducted among healthcare professionals specializing in obesity [22]. Additionally, a similar correlation is hinted at by the findings in studies involving German general practitioners and those conducted among medical and nutrition students [21,26]. However, in our study, the analysis of age's impact on weight bias among healthcare professionals in Poland was constrained by the homogeneity of our respondent group. Consequently, the determination of whether age indeed influences weight bias in this specific population remains uncertain. Further research with a more diverse and experienced participant pool is warranted to provide more comprehensive insights.

In addition to evaluating healthcare professionals' attitudes, our study also assessed respondents' knowledge of the disease. An overwhelming 98.5% of medical professionals acknowledge obesity as a disease. Comparatively, in a similar study conducted recently in Sweden among primary care physicians, 91% of respondents recognized obesity as a disease [36].

One question revealed a significant difference between the various groups of our respondents who pertained to effective treatment methods. Physicians overwhelmingly favored pharmacological treatment and bariatric surgery, with 93.6% and 93.1% of them, respectively, indicating these as effective treatment methods in a multiple-answer question. This contrasts notably with the findings from the Swedish study, where over half of the respondents (58%) did not believe that pharmacological treatment was effective. An explanation of these differences might be attributed to the time of data collection: the Swedish study was conducted in 2021, a period when pharmacological treatment might not have been as widely accessible and commonly used, and not all currently available and registered drugs were readily available in Sweden at that time.

Similarly, a 2020 study involving over 1500 healthcare professionals from nearly 80 countries shed light on perceptions regarding effective treatment methods. In a single-answer question asking respondents to indicate the most effective treatment for severe obesity, 61% chose bariatric surgery, while 37% believed that lifestyle interventions (diet and exercise—16%, psychological support and behavior modification—21%) were more effective [20]. To the best of our knowledge, this study is one of the two studies conducted in Poland that compare knowledge on obesity among different healthcare professionals. The earlier study, published in 2023 [37], had a smaller group of 184 respondents and substantially differed in the composition of the study group, including 52.2% of physicians, 20.7% of nurses, and 19.0% of physiotherapists compared to 58.7% of physicians, 17.0% of dietitians, and 24.3% of other healthcare professionals (including nurses, physiotherapists, pharmacists, dentists, and paramedics). Interestingly, no statistically significant differences in knowledge were observed among representatives of different medical professions in that study, in contrast to our research, where several such correlations were found. While both studies observed similar knowledge levels regarding BMI criteria for recognizing obesity (84.7% in our study vs. 89.1% in the previous study), the results concerning methods of treatment cannot be directly compared. This discrepancy arises from the fact that data for the previous study were collected from January 2019 to September 2020, when currently available methods of pharmacological treatment were unavailable. Thus, our study appears to be the only recent investigation assessing perceptions of effective obesity treatment methods among healthcare professionals in Poland.

The authors acknowledge the inherent limitations associated with the methodology employed in this study, particularly regarding the chosen data collection methods. However, leveraging online platforms and social media substantially aids in reaching a diverse audience across Poland. The utilization of an anonymous Internet survey format might encourage more candid responses, especially given the sensitivity of the subject matter, although it does not exclude the social desirability bias. The analyzed sample does not represent the entire population of healthcare professionals in Poland, emphasizing the need for future studies to provide a more comprehensive understanding of the topic. What is more, this cross-sectional study does not provide information on the evolution of the results over time.

The results indicate that constant monitoring of the level of fat phobia and weight stigma among healthcare professionals is necessary. Conducting such surveys may have the added value of increasing awareness of the challenge of attitudes towards patients with excess body weight and thus may positively influence the effectiveness of the treatment process.

5. Conclusions

The results of this study reveal a moderate level of weight stigma among healthcare professionals in Poland as well as highlight gaps in knowledge about obesity. Given the well-documented negative impact of weight stigma on healthcare quality, it is imperative to implement evidence-based interventions aimed at enhancing the knowledge, skills, and competencies of health professionals. These interventions should include educating professionals about uncontrollable and non-modifiable causes of obesity, improving communication skills, integrating patient perspectives into educational programs, and fostering self-assessment of attitudes and internalized weight bias.

6. Recommendations

We strongly advocate for utilizing these findings to inform institutions, scientific societies responsible for healthcare professional training, and public health entities in Poland. By expanding and leveraging these results through further research in this field, effective, evidence-based interventions can be developed to combat weight bias and stigma and enhance understanding of obesity among healthcare professionals. This collaborative effort will ultimately contribute to improving healthcare delivery and promoting equitable treatment for individuals affected by obesity.

Author Contributions: Conceptualization, K.Ś., K.K., A.B., and M.B.; methodology, K.Ś., K.K., A.B., and M.B.; validation K.Ś., W.S.Z., K.K., A.B., A.M.-M., and M.B.; formal analysis, M.B.; investigation, K.Ś., K.K., A.B., and M.B.; resources, K.Ś.; data curation, K.Ś., K.K., A.B., and M.B.; writing—original draft preparation, K.Ś., W.S.Z., K.K., A.B., and M.B.; writing—review and editing, K.Ś., W.S.Z., K.K., A.B., A.M.-M., and M.B.; visualization, A.B.; supervision, A.M.-M.; project administration, K.Ś., W.S.Z., K.K., A.B., A.M.-M., and M.B.; funding acquisition, A.B. and W.S.Z. All authors have read and agreed to the published version of the manuscript.

Funding: Center of Postgraduate Medical Education, Warsaw, Poland.

Institutional Review Board Statement: The study was conducted in accordance with the Declaration of Helsinki and approved by the Bioethics Committee of the Medical University of Wroclaw (approval number: KB 222/2023N, approval date: 31 August 2023).

Informed Consent Statement: Informed consent was obtained from all subjects involved in the study upon filling in the questionnaire.

Data Availability Statement: The database used in this study is available upon request. The data are not publicly available due to privacy restrictions.

Acknowledgments: We would like to express our appreciation to Dorota Komar and Damian Parol for their support in recruiting participants for this study by granting access to their social media networks.

Conflicts of Interest: The authors declare no conflicts of interest.

References

1. Kirk, S.F.; Ramos-Salas, X.; Alberga, A.S.; Russell-Mayhew, S. *Canadian Adult Obesity Clinical Practice Guidelines: Reducing Weight Bias in Obesity Management, Practice and Policy*; Obesity Canada: Edmonton, AB, Canada, 2020.
2. Lee, M.; Ata, R.N.; Brannick, M.T. Malleability of weight-biased attitudes and beliefs: A meta-analysis of weight bias reduction interventions. *Body Image* **2014**, *11*, 251–259. [CrossRef]
3. Weight Stigma | World Obesity Federation. Available online: https://www.worldobesity.org/what-we-do/our-policy-priorities/weight-stigma (accessed on 27 October 2023).
4. Tomiyama, A.J.; Carr, D.; Granberg, E.M.; Major, B.; Robinson, E.; Sutin, A.R.; Brewis, A. How and why weight stigma drives the obesity "epidemic" and harms health. *BMC Med.* **2018**, *16*, 123. [CrossRef]
5. Rubino, F.; Puhl, R.M.; Cummings, D.E.; Eckel, R.H.; Ryan, D.H.; Mechanick, J.I.; Nadglowski, J.; Ramos Salas, X.; Schauer, P.R.; Twenefour, D.; et al. Joint international consensus statement for ending stigma of obesity. *Nat. Med.* **2020**, *26*, 485–497. [CrossRef]
6. Wu, Y.K.; Berry, D.C. Impact of weight stigma on physiological and psychological health outcomes for overweight and obese adults: A systematic review. *J. Adv. Nurs.* **2018**, *74*, 1030–1042. [CrossRef] [PubMed]
7. Sutin, A.R.; Stephan, Y.; Terracciano, A. Weight Discrimination and Risk of Mortality. *Psychol. Sci.* **2015**, *26*, 1803. [CrossRef] [PubMed]
8. Graham, Y.; Hayes, C.; Cox, J.; Mahawar, K.; Fox, A.; Yemm, H. A systematic review of obesity as a barrier to accessing cancer screening services. *Obes. Sci. Pract.* **2022**, *8*, 715. [CrossRef] [PubMed]
9. Ruddock, H.K.; Orwin, M.; Boyland, E.J.; Evans, E.H.; Hardman, C.A. Obesity Stigma: Is the 'Food Addiction' Label Feeding the Problem? *Nutrients* **2019**, *11*, 2100. [CrossRef] [PubMed]
10. Lawrence, B.J.; Kerr, D.; Pollard, C.M.; Theophilus, M.; Alexander, E.; Haywood, D.; O'connor, M. Weight bias among health care professionals: A systematic review and meta-analysis. *Obesity* **2021**, *29*, 1802–1812. [CrossRef]
11. Puhl, R.M.; Brownell, K.D. Confronting and coping with weight stigma: An investigation of overweight and obese adults. *Obesity* **2006**, *14*, 1802–1815. [CrossRef]
12. Alberga, A.S.; McLaren, L.; Russell-Mayhew, S.; Von Ranson, K.M. Canadian Senate Report on Obesity: Focusing on Individual Behaviours versus Social Determinants of Health May Promote Weight Stigma. *J. Obes.* **2018**, *2018*, 8645694. [CrossRef] [PubMed]
13. Mensinger, J.L.; Tylka, T.L.; Calamari, M.E. Mechanisms underlying weight status and healthcare avoidance in women: A study of weight stigma, body-related shame and guilt, and healthcare stress. *Body Image* **2018**, *25*, 139–147. [CrossRef]
14. Bąk-Sosnowska, M.; Białkowska, M.; Bogdanski, P.; Chomiuk, T.; Gałązka-Sobotka, M.; Holecki, M.; Jarosińska, A.; Jezierska-Kazberuk, M.; Kamiński, P.; Kłoda, K.; et al. *Kliniczne Dotyczące Postępowania u Chorych na Otyłość 2022—Stanowisko Polskiego Towarzystwa Leczenia Otyłości*; PTLO: Poznan, Poland, 2022.
15. Karta Praw Chorego na Otyłość—O Czym Informuje? | PSoO. Available online: https://ootylosci.pl/karta-praw-chorego-na-otylosc/ (accessed on 27 October 2023).

16. Świder, K.; Baska, A.; Babicki, M.; Mastalerz-Migas, A.; Kłoda, K. Weight stigma and fat phobia in Poland—Attitudes towards people living with obesity and the level of knowledge about obesity among the social media internet respondents and medical professionals. *Front. Nutr.* **2023**, *10*, 1287783. [CrossRef]
17. Bacon, J.G.; Scheltema, K.E.; Robinson, B.E. Fat phobia scale revisited: The short form. *Int. J. Obes. Relat. Metab. Disord. J. Int. Assoc. Study Obes.* **2001**, *25*, 252–257. [CrossRef]
18. Sobczak, K.; Leoniuk, K.; Rudnik, A. Experience of Polish Patients with Obesity in Contacts with Medical Professionals. *Patient Prefer. Adherence* **2020**, *14*, 1683. [CrossRef] [PubMed]
19. Sobczak, K.; Leoniuk, K. Attitudes of Medical Professionals Towards Discrimination of Patients with Obesity. *Risk Manag. Healthc. Policy* **2021**, *14*, 4169. [CrossRef]
20. O'Keeffe, M.; Flint, S.W.; Watts, K.; Rubino, F. Knowledge gaps and weight stigma shape attitudes toward obesity. *Lancet Diabetes Endocrinol.* **2020**, *8*, 363–365. [CrossRef]
21. Schwenke, M.; Luppa, M.; Pabst, A.; Welzel, F.D.; Löbner, M.; Luck-Sikorski, C.; Kersting, A.; Blüher, M.; Riedel-Heller, S.G. Attitudes and treatment practice of general practitioners towards patients with obesity in primary care. *BMC Fam. Pract.* **2020**, *21*, 169. [CrossRef]
22. Schwartz, M.B.; Chambliss, H.O.N.; Brownell, K.D.; Blair, S.N.; Billington, C. Weight Bias among Health Professionals Specializing in Obesity. *Obes. Res.* **2003**, *11*, 1033–1039. [CrossRef] [PubMed]
23. Diversi, T.M.; Hughes, R.; Burke, K.J. The prevalence and practice impact of weight bias amongst Australian dietitians. *Obes. Sci. Pract.* **2016**, *2*, 456–465. [CrossRef]
24. Robstad, N.; Westergren, T.; Siebler, F.; Söderhamn, U.; Fegran, L. Intensive care nurses' implicit and explicit attitudes and their behavioural intentions towards obese intensive care patients. *J. Adv. Nurs.* **2019**, *75*, 3631–3642. [CrossRef]
25. Elboim-Gabyzon, M.; Attar, K.; Peleg, S. Weight Stigmatization among Physical Therapy Students and Registered Physical Therapists. *Obes. Facts* **2020**, *13*, 104–116. [CrossRef] [PubMed]
26. Swift, J.A.; Hanlon, S.; El-Redy, L.; Puhl, R.M.; Glazebrook, C. Weight bias among UK trainee dietitians, doctors, nurses and nutritionists. *J. Hum. Nutr. Diet. Off. J. Br. Diet. Assoc.* **2013**, *26*, 395–402. [CrossRef] [PubMed]
27. Setchell, J.; Watson, B.; Jones, L.; Gard, M.; Briffa, K. Physiotherapists demonstrate weight stigma: A cross-sectional survey of Australian physiotherapists. *J. Physiother.* **2014**, *60*, 157–162. [CrossRef] [PubMed]
28. Wang, Y.; Ding, Y.; Song, D.; Zhu, D.; Wang, J. Attitudes toward obese persons and weight locus of control in Chinese nurses: A cross-sectional survey. *Nurs. Res.* **2016**, *65*, 125–131. [CrossRef] [PubMed]
29. Wigton, R.S.; McGaghie, W.C. The effect of obesity on medical students' approach to patients with abdominal pain. *J. Gen. Intern. Med.* **2001**, *16*, 262–265. [CrossRef]
30. Hebl, M.R.; Xu, J. Weighing the care: Physicians' reactions to the size of a patient. *Int. J. Obesity* **2001**, *25*, 1246–1252. [CrossRef]
31. Bagley, C.R.; Conklin, D.N.; Isherwood, R.T.; Pechiulis, D.R.; Watson, L.A. Attitudes of Nurses toward Obesity and Obese Patients. *Sage J.* **1989**, *68 Pt 1*, 954. [CrossRef]
32. Maroney, D.; Golub, S. Nurses' attitudes toward obese persons and certain ethnic groups. *Percept. Mot. Ski.* **1992**, *75*, 387–391. [CrossRef]
33. Alberga, A.S.; Edache, I.Y.; Forhan, M.; Russell-Mayhew, S. Weight bias and health care utilization: A scoping review. *Prim. Health Care Res. Dev.* **2019**, *20*, e116. [CrossRef]
34. Sabin, J.A.; Marini, M.; Nosek, B.A. Implicit and Explicit Anti-Fat Bias among a Large Sample of Medical Doctors by BMI, Race/Ethnicity and Gender. *PLoS ONE* **2012**, *7*, e48448. [CrossRef]
35. Alberga, A.S.; Nutter, S.; MacInnis, C.; Ellard, J.H.; Russell-Mayhew, S. Examining Weight Bias among Practicing Canadian Family Physicians. *Obes. Facts* **2019**, *12*, 632–638. [CrossRef] [PubMed]
36. Carrasco, D.; Thulesius, H.; Jakobsson, U.; Memarian, E. Primary care physicians' knowledge and attitudes about obesity, adherence to treatment guidelines and association with confidence to treat obesity: A Swedish survey study. *BMC Prim. Care* **2022**, *23*, 208. [CrossRef] [PubMed]
37. Mojkowska, A.; Sobczak, K.; Leoniuk, K.; Henzler, M.; Jackowski, M. Medical or Common Knowledge? Knowledge of Medical Professionals on Obesity Diagnosis Criteria and Treatment. *Obes. Facts* **2023**, *16*, 216–223. [CrossRef] [PubMed]

nutrients

MDPI

Article

Consumption of Tap Water and Sociodemographic-Associated Characteristics: A Nationwide Cross-Sectional Study

Jacopo Dolcini [1,*], Manuela Chiavarini [1], Elisa Ponzio [1], Giorgio Firmani [1], Marcello Mario D'Errico [1] and Pamela Barbadoro [1,2,*]

[1] Department of Biomedical Sciences and Public Health, Section of Hygiene, Preventive Medicine and Public Health, Polytechnic University of the Marche Region, 60131 Ancona, Italy; m.chiavarini@staff.univpm.it (M.C.); e.ponzio@staff.univpm.it (E.P.); g.firmani@pm.univpm.it (G.F.); m.m.derrico@staff.univpm.it (M.M.D.)

[2] Centre of Obesity, Marche Polytechnic University, Via Tronto 10a, 60126 Ancona, Italy

* Correspondence: j.dolcini@staff.univpm.it (J.D.); p.barbadoro@staff.univpm.it (P.B.)

Abstract: Safe water is a global public health concern amid increasing scarcity and pollution. Bottled water production and consumption contribute to these problems. This study examines tap water consumption in Italy, assessing associated sociodemographic factors and related health outcomes such as obesity and self-perceived health status. Data from the Italian National Statistics Institute's "Aspects of daily life" survey (N = 45,597) were analyzed. Covariates included education, age, gender, economic status, region, concerns about waste and climate change, consumption of carbonated drinks excluding water, alcohol consumption, consumption of vegetables, consumption of snacks, body mass index, and self-perceived health status. Bivariate analyses and mixed-effect logistic regression models explored the associations. People who drink tap water made up 19,674, with a higher prevalence in people aged 45 to 59 old, people with a graduate/post-graduate degree diploma, with optimal economic resources, people concerned about waste production and climate change, and those coming from the north-east regions of Italy. Underweight people showed a higher prevalence of TW consumption as well as those who less than occasionally drank carbonated drinks, drank alcohol, consumed vegetables more than once a day and snacks less than once a week, dairy products more than once a day, sweet less than once a week, cured meat less than once a week, and chicken meat less than once a week, those with no consumption of sheep meat, consumption of beef meat less than once a week and consumption of pork meat less than once a week, and those with a satisfactory level of perceived health status. Regressions showed that all other age classes are less likely to drink tap water than people younger than 20 years old. The category with "inadequate" economic resources is more likely to consume tap water. Low educational classes show a low likelihood of consuming tap water as well as islands. A concern about waste production and climate change is associated with an increased likelihood of consuming tap water. Tap water consumption was negatively associated with obesity but not with a satisfactory self-perceived health status. Insights from this study can inform public health strategies.

Keywords: safe water; public health; sociodemographic characteristics; environmental health; health outcomes

1. Introduction

Drinking safe water is a critical public health element worldwide. Improved water supply and sanitation, and better management of water resources, can boost countries' economic growth and can contribute greatly to poverty reduction [1]. Anyway, in the next future, the availability of safe water could be a worldwide issue [2,3]. Environmental challenges such as climate change and extreme events, water scarcity, and pollution are increasingly becoming a global concern [4–6]. Many studies have shown how the production and consumption of bottled water (BW) are contributors to these problems [3,4]. Others have shown how tap water (TW) would be preferable due to the high environmental impact of bottle manufacturing [7]. Moreover, increasing evidence has shown a higher level of exposure to microplastics from BW versus TW [8], increasing concerns about possible human health effects from its consumption. Nowadays, in many countries, there is the possibility to have access to cheap and safe potable TW, but BW consumption has been increasing globally [9]. Recently, there has been a growing interest in investigating possible reasons for preferring TW or BW. Some of them have focused attention on health and safety concerns about TW [8,9], while others on organoleptic properties [10–12]. The European region has diverse TW consumption patterns between and within countries, with the highest share of TW intake observed in northern Europe [13]. Moreover, different sociodemographic characteristics associated with TW or BW consumption have been investigated, delineating a complex scenario [14]; in particular, gender differences have been highlighted, with women drinking more BW [13–15] since women seem to perceive TW riskier but at the same time, they have more general environmental awareness [16,17]. Moreover, ethnicity and culture, as well as self-perceived health status and diet choices are among the key drivers of TW and city dwellers tend to drink less TW, with the lowest consumption observed at restaurants and the highest in people's homes [13,18]. Other studies have found that the consumption of TW was higher at higher incomes [19] while age showed conflicting results, with older people drinking more TW than others in some areas while the opposite is true in others [20,21]. Regarding education, some studies showed that individuals with higher education are less likely to drink bottled water as their primary source of water [20] and general lower educational attainment showed a higher prevalence of TW avoidance among adults and children [14]. Additionally, research shows that free access to safe and acceptable drinking water may be beneficial in reducing sugary drinks [22] and also it has an important role in weight reduction, body fat reduction, and appetite suppression and it may be useful in the prevention of overweight and obesity [23,24], but the equation with health outcomes may be complicated by complex scenarios where in some regions TW consumption may be influenced by increased exposure to actual and perceived risk of endocrine-disrupting compounds [25].

The aim of this study is to evaluate the consumption of TW and its association with selected sociodemographic characteristics and dietary habits at a nationwide level in Italy.

Moreover, we evaluated the possible association between TW consumption and health-related outcomes, particularly focusing on self-perceived health status and an obese Body Mass Index.

2. Materials and Methods

(i) Design, Data Source, and Participants

Information on tap and BW consumption was obtained from the multi-purpose survey on families' "Aspects of daily life", carried out by the Italian National Statistics Institute (ISTAT) [26]. The survey is carried out on a yearly basis in a representative sample of the Italian population and is part of the integrated system of multipurpose surveys on families aimed at detecting a plurality of behavioral dimensions and segments of daily life. The questionnaire is standardized, and the survey is carried out by a sequential CAWI/PAPI mixed-mode technique [26] and it has been used in several studies [27,28]. We analyzed data coming from the 2021 edition of the survey, including 45,597 subjects and 20,000 families. In this specific case, the populations for the current surveys were identified by the Italian National Statistics Institute within the set of municipalities, which was divided into two subsets: municipalities with larger demographic size constituted a separate stratum and were defined as Self-Representative (SR); the remaining municipalities were defined as Non Self-Representative (NSR) and were divided, based on demographic size, into strata of equal breadth. From these strata, the sample municipalities (two for each stratum) were selected with probabilities proportional to their size. For each of the municipalities involved in the survey (SR and NSR), a cluster sampling was carried out: the clusters—the families—were randomly selected from the registry list, and all the members belonging to the actual family were surveyed. The minimum number of sample families for each municipality was set to 24. The families were selected for each sample municipality from the theoretical sample selected for the Master Sample for each family included in the sample, and the characteristics under investigation of all actual members belonging to the same family were recorded. The size of the theoretical sample in terms of families, set at the national level primarily based on cost and operational criteria, was approximately 24,000 families. The number of involved sample municipalities should not exceed 900, to allow for effective control and supervision. The allocation of the sample of families and municipalities, among the various regions, was therefore calculated by adopting a compromise criterion to ensure both the reliability of estimates at the national level and that of estimates within each of the territorial domains [26].

(ii) Variables

The following variables were included in the analyses: educational level (graduate/postgraduate degree, high school diploma, middle school diploma, primary school diploma/none), age (<20 years old, 20–44 years old, 45–59 years old, 60–74 years old, ≥75 years old), gender (males/females), economical resources in last 12 months (1 = inadequate, 2 = scarce, 3 = adequate, and 4 = optimal), geographical area of residency (north-west, north-east, center, south, the islands), concern about waste production (yes/no), concern about climate change (yes/no), consumption of carbonated drinks excluding water (1 = more than 1 L/day, 2 = between ½/1 L day, 3 = less than ½ L, 4 = less than occasionally, 5 = occasionally, 6 = no use), alcohol consumption (1 = yes, 0 = no), consumption of vegetables (1 = more than once a day, 2 = once a day, 3 = sometimes a week, 4 = less than once a week, 5 = never), consumption of snacks (1 = more than once a day, 2 = once a day, 3 = sometimes a week, 4 = less than once a week, 5 = never), body mass index (BMI; 1 = underweight (<18.5 kg/m^2), 2 = normal (18.5–24.99 kg/m^2), 3 overweight (25.00–29.99 kg/m^2, 4 = obese (>30.00 kg/m^2), self-perceived health status (1 = satisfactory, 0 = not satisfactory), and consumption of dairy products, sweet, cured meat, chicken meat, sheep meat, beef meat, and pork meat (1 = more than once a day, 2 = once a day, 3 = sometimes a week, 4 = less than once a week, 5 = never).

(iii) Ethical Considerations

Ethical review and approval were waived for this study since we utilized data from the Italian Health Interview Survey, a routine initiative conducted by the Italian National Institute of Statistics according to national guidelines. As a national institute operating under legal mandates, ethical approval is not mandated for nationwide surveys. The data underwent anonymization and aggregation by ISTAT, ensuring privacy, and were subsequently made publicly accessible for research purposes. Informed consent was obtained from all subjects involved in the study.

(iv) Statistical Analysis

Bivariate analyses were performed to study the association of TW consumption with relevant variables using chi-square tests. Logistic regression models were built to adjust for confounders and to evaluate the factors independently associated with TW consumption (1, if TW consumption is present; 0 if not). The Hosmer–Lemeshow test was used to evaluate the goodness of fit of the model. Regarding health outcomes, we considered self-perceived health status satisfaction level (dichotomized in two levels: 1 = satisfactory, 0 = not satisfactory) and BMI (dichotomized in two levels: 1 = obese, 0 = not obese). The level of significance was set to 0.05. Analyses were performed with STATA, version 15 (Stata Corp., College Station, TX, USA).

3. Results

(i) Bivariate analysis

Among the selected sample, people who usually drink TW were 19,674, representing 43.15% (95% confidence interval, CI 42.69–43.60). In terms of prevalence, bivariate analysis (Table 1) highlighted a higher prevalence of TW consumption in people aged 45 to 59 years old (N = 4942, 25.12%, p-value < 0.05) with no statistically significant differences among males and females. People with a graduate/post-graduate degree diploma showed the highest prevalence of consumption (N = 3111, 48.56%, p-value < 0.05) as well as people with optimal economic resources (N = 356, 50%, p-value < 0.05). Considering concern for environmental issues, our sample showed a higher prevalence of people consuming TW among those that were concerned about waste production (N = 7963, 44.21%, p-value < 0.05) and among those that were concerned about climate change (N = 9586, 44.66%, p-value < 0.05). Regarding the Geographical Area of Residency, there was a higher prevalence of TW consumption in the north-east regions of Italy (N = 5966, 64.98%, p-value < 0.05). Underweight people showed higher prevalence of TW consumption (N = 509, 46.27% p-value < 0.05), as well as those who drank less than occasionally carbonated drinks (N = 1932, p-value < 0.05); drank alcohol (N = 12,519, 44.66%, p-value < 0.05); consumed vegetables more than once a day (N = 3584, 46.83%, p-value < 0.05), snacks less than once a week (N = 7265, 45.10%, p-value = 0.05), dairy products more than once day (N = 910, 48.74, p-value < 0.05); sweets less than once a week (N = 7372, 43.68%, p-value = 0.25), cured meat less than once a week (N = 5363, 44.58%, p-value < 0.05), and chicken meat less than once a week (N = 3393, 48.5%, p-value < 0.05); never consumed sheep meat (N = 9126 45.78%, p-value < 0.05); consumed beef meat less than once a week (N = 6470 47.15%, p-value < 0.05) and consumed pork meat less than once a week (N = 7690, 44.99%, p-value < 0.05). Regarding perceived health status, the highest prevalence of TW consumption was shown from those with a satisfactory level (N = 14,323, 44.03%, p-value < 0.05).

Table 1. Distribution of the proportion of people drinking TW according to selected personal characteristics.

Variables		N	% of People Drinking TW	*p*-Value
Sex	Males	9524	43.28	0.58
	Females	10,150	43.02	
Age class (years)	<20	3142	15.97	0.00
	20–44	4577	23.26	
	45–59	4942	25.12	
	60–74	4298	21.85	
	≥75	2715	13.80	
Educational level	Graduate/Post-Graduate degree	3111	48.56	0.00
	High school diploma	6640	43.55	
	Middle school diploma	4874	41.19	
	Primary school diploma/none	4013	41.52	
Economical resources in the last 12 months	Optimal	356	50.00	0.00
	Adequate	13,545	43.76	
	Scarce	5103	41.24.	
	Inadequate	670	42.92	
Concern about waste production	No	11,711	42.45	0.00
	Yes	7963	44.21	
Concern about climate change	No	10,088	41.8	0.00
	Yes	9586	44.66	
Geographical Area of residency	North-West	4712	46.21	0.00
	North-East	5966	64.98	
	Center	3649	41.63	
	South	4482	35.8	
	The Islands	857	17.45	

Table 1. *Cont.*

Variables		N	% of People Drinking TW	*p*-Value
BMI	Normal	8571	43.94	0.00
	Underweight	509	46.27	
	Overweight	5869	42.90	
	Obese	1974	40.66	
Carbonated drink consumption (excluding water)	More than 1 L/day	170	40.57	0.00
	From 1/2 L to 1 L/day	482	43.19	
	Less than 1/2 L day	1241	40.68	
	Occasionally	6103	41.89	
	Less than occasionally	1932	45.87	
	No/never	7897	44.96	
Alcohol consumption	No	5618	40.89	0.00
	Yes	12,519	44.66	
Consumption of vegetables	More than once a day	3584	46.83	0.00
	Once a day	6645	44.43	
	Sometimes a week	6968	41.80	
	Less than once a week	1349	39.20	
	Never	643	39.30	
Consumption of snacks	More than once a day	186	41.24	0.00
	Once a day	731	42.65	
	Sometimes a week	4276	40.71	
	Less than once a week	7265	45.10	
	Never	6616	43.50	
Self-perceived health status	Not satisfactory	3088	41.05	0.00
	Satisfactory	14,323	44.03	
Consumption of dairy products	More than once a day	910	48.74	0.00
	Once a day	3585	46.82	
	Sometimes a week	11,065	43.00	
	Less than once a week	2737	39.90	
	Never	874	40.26	
Consumption of sweets	More than once a day	445	40.20	0.25
	Once a day	2062	43.08	
	Sometimes a week	7119	43.34	
	Less than once a week	7372	43.68	
	Never	2135	43.37	
Consumption of cured meat	More than once a day	363	43.21	0.01
	Once a day	1450	43.23	
	Sometimes a week	9668	42.59	
	Less than once a week	5363	44.58	
	Never	1972	43.27	
Consumption of chicken meat	More than once a day	325	37.57	0.00
	Once a day	1650	40.77	
	Sometimes a week	13,074	42.38	
	Less than once a week	3393	48.5	
	Never	734	46.66	
Consumption of sheep meat	More than once a day	148	44.44	0.00
	Once a day	396	41.08	
	Sometimes a week	3796	38.6	
	Less than once a week	5600	43.34	
	Never	9126	45.78	

Table 1. *Cont.*

Variables		N	% of People Drinking TW	*p*-Value
Consumption of beef meat	More than once a day	183	39.7	0.00
	Once a day	798	42.33	
	Sometimes a week	10,206	41.14	
	Less than once a week	6470	47.15	
	Never	1462	44.74	
Consumption of pork meat	More than once a day	166	43.34	0.00
	Once a day	587	41.16	
	Sometimes a week	7535	41.69	
	Less than once a week	7690	44.99	
	Never	3118	43.97	

(ii) Logistic regression for TW consumption

Multilevel regression analysis predicting the level of one of the dependent variables, which was the presence of TW consumption (1 = presence of TW consumption), showed that (Table 2) all age classes from 20 to 74 years old were less likely to drink TW than people younger than 20 years old but only two classes reached statistical significance (20–44 OR = 0.75, C.I. 0.65–0.88, 45–59 OR = 0.85, C.I. 0.73–0.99). Our model highlights also how the level of schooling may influence TW consumption. Compared to the highest level of education (graduate/post-graduate), other educational classes showed a low likelihood of consuming TW, with a statically significant level (High School diploma OR = 0.8, C.I. 0.75–0.85, Middle School Diploma OR = 0.71, C.I. 0.66–0.77, Elementary school diploma/none OR = 0.69, C.I. 0.63–0.76). Regarding the Geographical Area of residence, we did observe statically significant differences among different regions, with increased consumption in the north-west (baseline) and north-east (OR = 2.13, C.I. 1.99–2.27) and less consumption in the center (OR = 0.85, C.I. 0.8–0.91), south (OR = 0.67, C.I. 0.63–0.72) and the islands (OR 0.25, C.I. 0.22–0.27). In our model, we also considered some variables associated with attention to environmental issues. A concern about waste production was associated with an increased likelihood of consuming TW (OR = 1.09, C.I. 1.04–1.14). A similar trend of likelihood was shown for concern for climate change but was not statistically significant (OR = 1.05, C.I. 1.00–1.1). Looking at eating habits, TW consumption was associated with alcohol consumption (OR = 1.11, C.I. 1.05–1.17), with the lowest classes of sweet consumption ("less than once a week" OR = 1.22 C.I. 1.03–1.45, "never" 1.27 C.I. 1.06–1.52) and the lowest classes of chicken and beef meat (respectively "less than once a week" OR = 1.45 C.I. 1.16–1.81, "never" OR = 1.33 C.I. 1.04–1.70; "less than once a week" OR = 1.67 C.I. 1.13–2.45, "never" OR = 1.58 C.I. 1.06–2.33). Regarding dairy products and sheep meat consumption, all decreasing classes of consumption showed a low likelihood of TW consumption being statically significant.

Table 2. Factors associated with TW consumption at logistic regression analysis. Hosmer–Lemeshow test 0.43.

Variables		OR	CI 95%	*p*-Value
Age	<20	1		
	20–44	0.75	0.65–0.88	0.00
	45–59	0.85	0.73–0.99	0.04
	60–74	0.86	0.73–1.00	0.06
	≥75	0.95	0.80–1.12	0.53

Table 2. *Cont.*

Variables		OR	CI 95%	*p*-Value
Educational level	Graduate/Post-graduate degree	1		
	High School diploma	0.8	0.75–0.85	0.00
	Middle school diploma	0.71	0.66–0.77	0.00
	Primary school diploma/none	0.69	0.63–0.76	0.00
Concern about waste production	No	1		
	Yes	1.09	1.04–1.14	0.00
Geographical Area of residency	North-West	1		
	North-East	2.13	1.99–2.27	0.00
	Center	0.85	0.80–0.91	0.00
	South	0.67	0.63–0.72	0.00
	The Islands	0.25	0.22–0.27	0.00
Alcohol consumption	No	1		
	Yes	1.11	1.05–1.17	0.00
Dairy Products	More than once a day	1		
	Once a day	0.87	0.77–0.99	0.03
	Sometimes a week	0.77	0.68–0.87	0.00
	Less than once a week	0.66	0.58–0.75	0.00
	Never	0.71	0.61–0.83	0.00
Sweet	More than once a day	1		
	Once a day	1.09	0.91–1.30	0.36
	Sometimes a week	1.18	1.00–1.40	0.05
	Less than once a week	1.22	1.02–1.44	0.02
	Never	1.27	1.06–1.52	0.00
Chicken Meat	More than once a day	1		
	Once a day	1.07	0.86–1.34	0.54
	Sometimes a week	1.20	0.97–1.49	0.09
	Less than once a week	1.45	1.16–1.81	0.00
	Never	1.33	1.04–1.70	0.03
Sheep Meat	More than once a day	1		
	Once a day	0.62	0.40–0.96	0.03
	Sometimes a week	0.60	0.39–0.90	0.01
	Less than once a week	0.59	0.39–0.89	0.01
	Never	0.54	0.36–0.82	0.00
Beef Meat	More than once a day	1		
	Once a day	1.67	1.12–2.49	0.01
	Sometimes a week	1.41	0.96–2.08	0.08
	Less than once a week	1.67	1.13–2.45	0.01
	Never	1.58	1.06–2.33	0.02

(iii) Logistic regression for perceived health status

We then performed a multilevel regression analysis predicting the level one of the dependent variables, the presence of satisfactory self-perceived health status (1 = satisfactory perceived health status), with perceived health status as the main outcome (Table 3). One possible variable that was independently associated, the consumption of tap water, showed no statistically significant association (OR = 1.05, C.I. 0.99–1.11) with satisfactory perceived health status. This perception showed a decreasing trend of likelihood with age increase, and it reached statistical significance among all different age classes (20–44, OR = 0.65, C.I. 0.49–0.88; 45–59, OR = 0.34, C.I. 0.25–0.45; 60–74, OR = 0.21, C.I. 0.16–0.28; $\geq$75 OR = 0.12, C.I. 0.08–0.15). The same decreasing trend was found regarding lower levels of education, but only people with a middle school diploma (OR = 0.90, C.I. 0.81–0.99) and with an elementary school diploma/no diploma (OR = 0.66, C.I. 0.59–0.74) reached statistical significance. A low likelihood of a satisfactory perceived health status was found also with a decreasing availability of economic resources in the last 12 months, particularly for people who declared few (OR = 0.51, C.I. 0.39–0.66) and insufficient resources (OR = 0.33, C.I. = 0.25–0.45). Again, self-perceived health status was worse in the central, southern and island regions (OR = 0.88, C.I. 0.8–0.96; OR = 0.8, C.I. 0.73–0.87; OR = 0.73, C.I. 0.66–0.81), as well as in underweight (OR = 1.47, C.I. 1.23–1.75) and overweight people (OR = 1.32, C.I. 1.10–1.58) with respect to normal-weight subjects. Regarding the presence of alcohol consumption, it was found to be positively associated with perceived health status (OR = 1.32, C.I. 1.24–1.41). Considering the consumption of vegetables, the likelihood of association with a satisfactory perceived health status showed opposite trends since the lower the consumption of vegetables, the lowest odds of association, and this was significant for "sometimes a week" (OR = 0.88, C.I. 0.81–0.96), "less than once a week" (OR = 0.74, C.I. 0.65–0.84) and "never" (OR = 0.72, C.I. 0.6–0.88). Regarding the consumption of sweets, compared with those who declared consumption "more than once a day", the likelihood of association with a satisfactory perceived health status showed the highest odds of associations, with a statistical significance among all classes of consumption ("Sometimes a week" OR = 1.32 C.I. 1.07–1.62; Less than once a week OR = 1.26 C.I. 1.03–1.55). Again, considering the consumption of cured meat, the likelihood of association with a satisfactory perceived health status showed the highest odds of associations, with a statistical significance all among decreasing classes of consumption ("Once a day" OR = 1.45 C.I. 1.12–1.87, "Sometimes a week" OR = 1.31 C.I. 1.03–1.66; "Less than once a week" OR = 1.30 C.I. 1.02–1.66).

Table 3. Factors associated with a satisfactory self-perceived health status at logistic regression analysis. Hosmer–Lemeshow test 0.08.

Variables		OR	95% CI	*p*-Value
Sex	Males	1		
	Females	0.83	0.78–0.88	0.00
Age	<20	1		
	20–44	0.65	0.49–0.88	0.00
	45–59	0.34	0.25–0.45	0.00
	60–74	0.21	0.16–0.28	0.00
	≥75	0.12	0.08–0.15	0.00
Educational level	Graduate/Post-graduate degree	1		
	High School diploma	0.96	0.87–1.05	0.38
	Middle school diploma	0.90	0.81–0.99	0.05
	Elementary school diploma/none	0.66	0.59–0.74	0.00
Economical resources in the last 12 months	Optimal	1		
	Adequate	1.01	0.78–1.31	0.94
	Scarce	0.51	0.39–0.66	0.00
	Inadequate	0.33	0.25–0.45	0.00
Concern about waste production	No	1		
	Yes	1.07	1.01–1.13	0.03
Geographical Area of residency	North-West	1		
	North-East	1.03	0.94–1.13	0.56
	Center	0.88	0.8–0.96	0.00
	South	0.8	0.73–0.87	0.00
	Islands	0.73	0.66–0.81	0.00
BMI	Normal	1		
	Underweight	1.47	1.23–1.75	0.00
	Overweight	1.32	1.10–1.58	0.00
	Obese	0.88	0.73–1.06	0.18
Alcohol consumption	No	1		
	Yes	1.32	1.24–1.41	0.00

Table 3. *Cont.*

Variables		OR	95% CI	*p*-Value
Consumption of vegetables	More than once a day	1		
	Once a day	0.95	0.87–1.03	0.19
	Sometimes a week	0.88	0.81–0.96	0.00
	Less than once a week	0.74	0.65–0.84	0.00
	Never	0.72	0.6–0.88	0.001
Sweet	More than once a day	1		
	Once a day	1.11	0.90–1.38	0.33
	Sometimes a week	1.32	1.07–1.62	0.00
	Less than once a week	1.26	1.03–1.55	0.03
	Never	1.04	0.84–1.28	0.75
Cured Meat	More than once a day	1		
	Once a day	1.45	1.12–1.87	0.00
	Sometimes a week	1.31	1.03–1.66	0.03
	Less than once a week	1.30	1.02–1.66	0.03
	Never	1.23	0.95–1.59	0.11

(iv) Logistic regression for obesity

We then performed a multilevel regression analysis with obesity as the main outcome (Table 4) and possible variables that were independently associated with it: consumption of TW showed a statistically significant low likelihood association (OR = 0.93, C.I. 0.87–0.99) with being obese. The obese status also showed an increasing trend of likelihood with aging, and it reached statistical significance among all different age classes (20–44 years, OR = 2.44, C.I. 1.68–3.55; 45–59, OR = 4.36, C.I. 3.01–6.33; 60–74, OR = 5.70, C.I. 3.92–8.29; ≥75 OR = 3.93, C.I. 2.68–5.78). The same trend was found regarding lower levels of education, which was statistically significant for high school diplomas (OR = 1.53, C.I. 1.36–1.71), middle school diplomas (OR = 1.78, C.I. 1.57–2.00), and elementary school diploma/none diploma (OR = 2.18, C.I. 1.89–2.50). An increasing trend of association for being obese in southern parts of Italy, compared to northern ones, was found but only the south geographical area reached a statically significant association (OR = 1.33, C.I. 1.21–1.47). A satisfactory perceived health status was negatively associated with the likelihood of being obese (OR = 0.63, C.I. 0.59–0.68) as well as alcohol consumption (OR = 0.83, C.I. 0.78–0.91). Considering the consumption of sweets, a low likelihood of an obese BMI was associated with lowest classes of consumption ("Once a day" OR = 0.71 C.I. 0.55–0.90, "Sometimes a week" OR = 0.77 C.I. 0.61–0.97). Regarding the consumption of carbonated drinks (excluding water), compared to those who declared themselves as consuming more than 1 L per day, all other subjects showed a negative association trend with being obese with the "never" consumption class, which reached statistical significance (OR = 0.67 C.I. 0.48–0.93).

Table 4. Factors associated with obese BMI at logistic regression analysis. Hosmer–Lemeshow test 0.71.

Variables		OR	CI 95%	*p*-Value
Tap Water consumption	No	1		
	Yes	0.93	0.87–0.99	0.05
Sex	Males	1		
	Females	0.79	0.73–0.84	0.00

Table 4. *Cont.*

Variables		OR	CI 95%	p-Value
Age	<20	1		
	20–44	2.44	1.68–3.55	0.00
	45–59	4.36	3.01–6.33	0.00
	60–74	5.70	3.92–8.29	0.00
	≥75	3.93	2.68–5.78	0.00
Educational level	Graduate/Post-graduate			
	High School diploma	1.53	1.36–1.71	0.00
	Middle school diploma	1.78	1.57–2.00	0.00
	Primary school diploma/none	2.18	1.89–2.50	0.00
Geographical Area of residence	North-West	1		
	North-East	1.10	0.99–1.23	0.06
	Center	0.97	0.88–1.08	0.63
	South	1.33	1.21–1.47	0.00
	The Islands	1.12	0.99–1.27	0.08
Alcohol consumption	No	1		
	Yes	0.84	0.78–0.91	0.00
Self-perceived health status	Not Satisfactory	1		
	Satisfactory	0.63	0.59–0.68	0.00
Carbonated drinks consumption (excluding water)	More than 1 L/day	1		
	From 1/2 L to 1 L/day	0.73	0.5–1.06	0.1
	Less than 1/2 L day	0.90	0.64–1.27	0.55
	Occasionally	0.86	0.62–1.19	0.37
	Less than occasionally	0.73	0.52–1.03	0.07
	No/never	0.67	0.48–0.93	0.02
Sweet	More than once a day	1		
	Once a day	0.71	0.55–0.90	0.00
	Sometimes a week	0.77	0.61–0.97	0.03
	Less than once a week	0.84	0.67–1.06	0.14
	Never	0.85	0.67–1.09	0.20

4. Discussion

Safe drinking water represents a worldwide major concern because of several factors, such as pollution and climate change, that are heavily impacting human health all around the globe, in particular among residents of developing countries. Impacts on surface water and groundwater resources and water-related illnesses are increasing, especially under changing climate scenarios such as diversity in rainfall patterns, increasing temperature, flash floods, severe droughts, heat waves, and heavy precipitation [29]. Recently, a link between health and environmental impacts and drinking water choices has been shown, since it has been estimated that the environmental impact of BW is 1400–3500 percent higher than TW [30]. On the other hand, BW consumption has sharply increased in recent years worldwide [31], and, interestingly, the recent increase in BW use globally has been driven by an increase in demand in low- and middle-income countries (LMICs), despite parallel increases in access to piped water in some countries [32]. To better understand these trends, it is extremely important to study possible variables associated with increased trap water consumption that can allow policy decision-makers to take adequate actions. Our study fits in this context, since we investigated several demographic and socioeconomic variables that can be associated with increased consumption of TW. Unlike other studies [13,15], our regression model did not observe a statistically significant association of TW consumption with gender; on the other hand, regarding age, the younger the age classes were less likely to be TW consumers, in particular people aged 20–44 years old. This result agrees with other studies [14]. Interestingly, lower levels of schooling compared to the graduate/post-graduate level showed a reduced frequency of TW consumption and this is partially in disagreement with other findings [33]. It is possible that in our country, people with higher levels of schooling have an increased awareness about the safety and importance of consuming TW also for environmental issues, as testified by our result in terms of the presence of concern about waste production, since we found a statistically significant association of increased likelihood of TW consumption for this variable. So, generally speaking, an increased level of knowledge may be associated with increased awareness and environmentally friendly behaviors. It must be highlighted that concern for climate change showed a similar trend, but it did not reach statistical significance in terms of association with TW consumption, indicating a complex scenario in terms of knowledge of environmental issues by the general population. An important consideration regards the Geographical area of residency: in the regression model, we observed a statistically significant difference among different geographical areas and we found a decreasing trend of TW consumption from North to South, particularly evident on the islands where there is the lowest likelihood of TW consumption. This result may be explained by the lower presence of natural water sources between the northern and the southern parts of Italy, especially for islands like Sicily and Sardinia where water is particularly scarce [34]. Looking at heating habits, TW consumption was shown to be associated with more healthy habits like a lower consumption of sweets, chicken and beef meat, possibly reflecting subjects' awareness of a balanced healthy diet associated with consumption of non-bottled water.

Looking at health outcomes, we focused on the perceived health status declared by subjects and we studied the possible association with a positive attitude and consumption of TW together with other variables included in the logistic model. Even if TW consumption showed an increased likelihood of association with a satisfactory perceived health status, the association did not reach statistical significance. On the other hand, other variables showed a coherent association, in agreement also with studies conducted by others, since the likelihood of perceiving a satisfactory health status decreases with age [35], with underweight or overweight/obese BMI classes [36], with lower availability of economic resources [37] and lower levels of education [38,39]. Moreover, we found a worsening perception of own health status from North to south, as found by others [40,41]. Also, the consumption of vegetables showed interesting trends, with a low likelihood of a satisfactory perceived health status associated with a lower consumption of vegetables, which reached statical significance for the lowest classes (identified as "less than once a week" and "never"). These results are in accordance with other studies [42,43]. Consumption of sweets and cured meat both showed a higher association with a satisfactory perceived health status, associated with lower consumption classes [44,45]. Taken together, these considerations may allow us to speculate that the model proposed describes quite accurately the reality of variables independently associated with a satisfactory perceived health level, including the consumption of TW, which showed a positive likelihood of association even if not statically significant.

Looking at BMI, we found that the consumption of TW showed a possible protective effect towards being obese. This could be explained by the fact that individuals who preferred to consume TW were more likely to have both a healthier lifestyle and a lower consumption of refined, carbonated, and sugary beverages [22,46], which are responsible for weight gain [47], cardiovascular issues [48], diabetes [49] and overall poorer glycemic control [50]. Also, this model showed coherent associations with other independent variables, that were confirmed by other studies, since we found an increased likelihood of being obese with aging [51,52], with a lower educational level [52,53], for subjects with a geographical area of residency in the southern parts of Italy [54], with sweet consumption [45] and also with the consumption of carbonated drinks [47].

To our knowledge, this is the first study in Italy to take into consideration the consumption of TW and possible associated sociodemographic variables and health outcomes, such as perceived health status and BMI. Moreover, our data covered a nationwide sample of thousands of subjects, and interviews and data collection were conducted under rigorous methodological methods, since they were carried out by ISTAT-trained personnel.

Nevertheless, some limitations should be acknowledged. Given the nature of this study, as a prevalence study rather than a longitudinal one, certain details regarding individuals' dietary habits might have lacked precision. This is testified, for example, by the absence of the exact amount of TW consumption, which could have been more informative about water attitudes. Also, we did not have specific information on possible specific pathological conditions that could have been associated with the consumption of TW, but only aggregated variables, like the perceived health status, which we used in our models. Moreover, all data must be considered declarative, generating a possible declarative or recall bias in our sample. Lastly, it is important to note that the official language of ISTAT, the government institution conducting the survey, is Italian. The survey administration was not declared in other languages, which may have resulted in a selection bias. This bias could have excluded individuals, even residents in Italy, who did not fully understand the Italian language.

5. Conclusions

Taken together, our data show very informative results that can be very useful in terms of public health. For example, increasing education about the importance of TW consumption may improve this aspect among those lower-educated people who do not drink TW, maybe due to misleading beliefs about its safety, and at the same time increase a probably low self-awareness about the importance of plastic-free water consumption towards environmental issues that are related to BW production and distribution. Moreover, the increasing number of people accessing safe TW can be considered as a "One Health" approach, since through the administration of a fundamental health element and right such as free drinkable water, a nation can obtain important results on other several aspects like environmental issues and economic and social equality. Interestingly, some diet patterns may influence or be associated with TW consumption, as highlighted by our results. TW water can also influence health outcomes, both perceived and objective ones: we decided to focus on two general aspects of health outcomes, i.e., perceived health status and BMI, based on the availability of our data. Regarding BMI, according to already-existing studies, we investigated the association of TW consumption and an obese BMI, since numerous studies in the literature have explored enhancements of water consumption in relationships with cardiovascular diseases such as diabetes, hypertension, and obesity. Even if underweight could have been investigated, the representative sample with this condition in our population was too low and this BMI class is less frequent and problematic in developed countries like Italy. A possible further investigation could include more specific health outcomes such as specific chronic diseases and the consumption of TW, maybe with dedicated cross-sectional and longitudinal investigations. This approach may help health policymakers to better design health promotion campaigns and prevention strategies aimed at reducing health inequalities, which may be obtained also through the promotion of TW consumption.

Author Contributions: Conceptualization, J.D. and P.B.; formal analysis J.D.; data curation J.D., M.C., E.P. and G.F.; writing—original draft preparation, J.D. and P.B.; writing—review and editing, J.D., M.C., E.P., G.F. and P.B.; supervision, P.B. and M.M.D. All authors have read and agreed to the published version of the manuscript.

Funding: This research received no external funding.

Institutional Review Board Statement: Ethical review and approval were waived for this study due to the following reasons: The study exclusively utilizes data from the Italian Health Interview Survey, a routine initiative conducted by the Italian National Institute of Statistics according to national guidelines. As a national institute operating under legal mandates, ethical approval is not mandated for nationwide surveys. The data undergo anonymization and aggregation by ISTAT, ensuring privacy, and are subsequently made publicly accessible for research purposes.

Informed Consent Statement: Informed consent was obtained from all subjects involved in the study.

Data Availability Statement: The data undergo anonymization and aggregation by ISTAT and are subsequently made publicly accessible for research purposes at the following link: https://www.istat.it/it/archivio/129956 (access on 12 December 2023).

Conflicts of Interest: The authors declare no conflicts of interest.

References

1. WHO. Drinking-Water. Available online: https://www.who.int/news-room/fact-sheets/detail/drinking-water (accessed on 5 June 2023).
2. Boretti, A.; Rosa, L. Reassessing the projections of the World Water Development Report. *npj Clean Water* **2019**, *2*, 15. [CrossRef]
3. World Water Development Report 2018 | UN-Water. Available online: https://www.unwater.org/publications/world-water-development-report-2018 (accessed on 26 February 2024).
4. du Plessis, A. Current and Future Water Scarcity and Stress. In *Water as an Inescapable Risk: Current Global Water Availability, Quality and Risks with a Specific Focus on South Africa*; Springer: Berlin/Heidelberg, Germany, 2019; pp. 13–25. [CrossRef]
5. Cole, M.; Lindeque, P.; Halsband, C.; Galloway, T.S. Microplastics as contaminants in the marine environment: A review. *Mar. Pollut. Bull.* **2011**, *62*, 2588–2597. [CrossRef]
6. Free, C.M.; Jensen, O.P.; Mason, S.A.; Eriksen, M.; Williamson, N.J.; Boldgiv, B. High-levels of microplastic pollution in a large, remote, mountain lake. *Mar. Pollut. Bull.* **2014**, *85*, 156–163. [CrossRef] [PubMed]
7. Horowitz, N.; Frago, J.; Mu, D. Life cycle assessment of bottled water: A case study of Green2O products. *Waste Manag.* **2018**, *76*, 734–743. [CrossRef]
8. Danopoulos, E.; Twiddy, M.; Rotchell, J.M. Microplastic contamination of drinking water: A systematic review. *PLoS ONE* **2020**, *15*, e0236838. [CrossRef]
9. Arnold Emily and Larsen Janet. Plan B Updates-51: Bottled Water-Pouring Resources Down the Drain | EPI. Available online: https://www.earth-policy.org/plan_b_updates/2006/update51 (accessed on 6 June 2023).
10. Geerts, R.; Vandermoere, F.; Van Winckel, T.; Halet, D.; Joos, P.; Steen, K.V.D.; Van Meenen, E.; Blust, R.; Borregán-Ochando, E.; Vlaeminck, S.E. Bottle or tap? Toward an integrated approach to water type consumption. *Water Res.* **2020**, *173*, 115578. [CrossRef] [PubMed]
11. Debbeler, L.J.; Gamp, M.; Blumenschein, M.; Keim, D.; Renner, B. Polarized but illusory beliefs about tap and bottled water: A product- and consumer-oriented survey and blind tasting experiment. *Sci. Total Environ.* **2018**, *643*, 1400–1410. [CrossRef] [PubMed]
12. Ballantine, P.W.; Ozanne, L.K.; Bayfield, R. Why Buy Free? Exploring Perceptions of Bottled Water Consumption and Its Environmental Consequences. *Sustainability* **2019**, *11*, 757. [CrossRef]
13. World Health Organization. Increased Drinking-Water Consumption Brings Gains for Health and the Environment. Available online: https://www.who.int/europe/news/item/19-03-2020-increased-drinking-water-consumption-brings-gains-for-health-and-the-environment (accessed on 26 February 2024).
14. Rosinger, A.Y.; Young, S.L. In-Home Tap Water Consumption Trends Changed Among U.S. Children, but Not Adults, between 2007 and 2016. *Water Resour. Res.* **2020**, *56*, e2020WR027657. [CrossRef]
15. Doria, M.F. Bottled water versus tap water: Understanding consumers' preferences. *J. Water Health* **2006**, *4*, 271–276. [CrossRef]
16. Saylor, A.; Prokopy, L.S.; Amberg, S. What's wrong with the tap? Examining perceptions of tap water and bottled water at Purdue University. *Environ. Manag.* **2011**, *48*, 588–601. [CrossRef] [PubMed]
17. Anadu, E.C.; Harding, A.K. Risk Perception and Bottled Water Use. *J. Am. Water Works Assoc.* **2000**, *92*, 82–92. [CrossRef]
18. Juba, O.S.; Tanyanyiwa, V.I. Perceptions on the use of bottled water in restaurants in Harare's Central Business District (CBD). *Phys. Chem. Earth Parts A/B/C* **2018**, *105*, 239–246. [CrossRef]
19. Vieux, F.; Maillot, M.; Rehm, C.D.; Barrios, P.; Drewnowski, A. Trends in tap and bottled water consumption among children and adults in the United States: Analyses of NHANES 2011–16 data. *Nutr. J.* **2020**, *19*, 10. [CrossRef] [PubMed]
20. Dupont, D.; Adamowicz, W.L.; Krupnick, A. Differences in water consumption choices in Canada: The role of socio-demographics, experiences, and perceptions of health risks. *J. Water Health* **2010**, *8*, 671–686. [CrossRef] [PubMed]
21. Spicer, N.; Parlee, B.; Chisaakay, M.; Lamalice, D. Drinking Water Consumption Patterns: An Exploration of Risk Perception and Governance in Two First Nations Communities. *Sustainability* **2020**, *12*, 6851. [CrossRef]
22. Moreno, G.D.; Schmidt, L.A.; Ritchie, L.D.; McCulloch, C.E.; Cabana, M.D.; Brindis, C.D.; Green, L.W.; Altman, E.A.; Patel, A.I. A cluster-randomized controlled trial of an elementary school drinking water access and promotion intervention: Rationale, study design, and protocol. *Contemp. Clin. Trials* **2021**, *101*, 106255. [CrossRef] [PubMed]
23. Laja García, A.I.; Moráis-Moreno, C.; Samaniego-Vaesken, M.L.; Puga, A.M.; Partearroyo, T.; Varela-Moreiras, G. Influence of Water Intake and Balance on Body Composition in Healthy Young Adults from Spain. *Nutrients* **2019**, *11*, 1923. [CrossRef] [PubMed]
24. Vij, V.A.K.; Joshi, A.S. Effect of excessive water intake on body weight, body mass index, body fat, and appetite of overweight female participants. *J. Nat. Sci. Biol. Med.* **2014**, *5*, 340. [CrossRef]
25. Wee, S.Y.; Aris, A.Z.; Yusoff, F.M.; Praveena, S.M.; Harun, R. Drinking water consumption and association between actual and perceived risks of endocrine disrupting compounds. *npj Clean Water* **2022**, *5*, 25. [CrossRef]

26. ISTAT. Aspects of Daily Life: Public Use micro.stat Files. Available online: https://www.istat.it/en/archivio/129959 (accessed on 31 October 2023).
27. Dolcini, J.; Ponzio, E.; Campanati, A.; D'Errico, M.M.; Barbadoro, P. Gender, Socioeconomic and Health Characteristics Associated to Dermatological visits in Italy: Secondary Analysis of a National Cross-Sectional Survey. *Dermatology* **2023**, *239*, 1013–1018. [CrossRef] [PubMed]
28. Dolcini, J.; Ponzio, E.; D'Errico, M.M.; Barbadoro, P. Socioeconomic differences in dietary habits in Italy before and during COVID-19 pandemic: Secondary analysis of a nationwide cross-sectional study. *BMC Public Health* **2024**, *24*, 153. [CrossRef] [PubMed]
29. Ahmed, T.; Zounemat-Kermani, M.; Scholz, M. Climate Change, Water Quality and Water-Related Challenges: A Review with Focus on Pakistan. *Int. J. Environ. Res. Public Health* **2020**, *17*, 8518. [CrossRef] [PubMed]
30. Villanueva, C.M.; Garfí, M.; Milà, C.; Olmos, S.; Ferrer, I.; Tonne, C. Health and environmental impacts of drinking water choices in Barcelona, Spain: A modelling study. *Sci. Total Environ.* **2021**, *795*, 148884. [CrossRef]
31. Rodwan, J.G. Bottled Water 2017. *Staying Strong: US and International Developments and Statistics*. 2018. Available online: https://www.bottledwater.org/wp-content/uploads/2020/03/BMC2016_BWR_StatsArticle.pdf (accessed on 2 August 2023).
32. Cohen, A.; Ray, I. The global risks of increasing reliance on bottled water. *Nat. Sustain.* **2018**, *1*, 327–329. [CrossRef]
33. Kuok, K.K.; Chiu, P.C. Indigenous drinking-water consumption pattern of residents in Kuching city: Results of a pilot study. *J. Water Sanit. Hyg. Dev.* **2018**, *8*, 817–824. [CrossRef]
34. Fresh Water Resources-Italy-Climatechangepost.com. Available online: https://www.climatechangepost.com/italy/fresh-water-resources/ (accessed on 2 August 2023).
35. Giacomozzi, C.; Palmieri, L.; Gargiulo, L.; Noce, C.L.; Iannucci, L.; Di Lonardo, A.; Vannucchi, S.; Onder, G.; Colivicchi, F.; Giampaoli, S.; et al. The Perceived Health Status from Young Adults to Elderly: Results of the MEHM Questionnaire within the CUORE Project Survey 2008–2012. *Int. J. Environ. Res. Public Health* **2020**, *17*, 6160. [CrossRef]
36. Narciso, J.; Croome, N. How does body mass index impact self-perceived health? A pan-European analysis of the European Health Interview Survey Wave 2. *BMJ Nutr. Prev. Health* **2022**, *5*, 235. [CrossRef] [PubMed]
37. Cialani, C.; Mortazavi, R. The effect of objective income and perceived economic resources on self-rated health. *Int. J. Equity Health* **2020**, *19*, 196. [CrossRef]
38. Faresjö, T.; Rahmqvist, M. Educational level is a crucial factor for good perceived health in the local community. *Scand. J. Public Health* **2010**, *38*, 605–610. [CrossRef]
39. Shaaban, A.N.; Martins, M.R.O.; Peleteiro, B. Factors associated with self-perceived health status in Portugal: Results from the National Health Survey 2014. *Front. Public Health* **2022**, *10*, 879432. [CrossRef] [PubMed]
40. Toth, F. How health care regionalisation in Italy is widening the North–South gap. *Health Econ. Policy Law* **2014**, *9*, 231–249. [CrossRef]
41. Bruzzi, S.; Ivaldi, E.; Santagata, M. Measuring Regional Performance in the Italian NHS: Are Disparities Decreasing? *Soc. Indic. Res.* **2022**, *159*, 1057–1084. [CrossRef] [PubMed]
42. Hrezova, E.; Bobak, M.; Capkova, N.; Stefler, D.; Pikhart, H. Low fruit and vegetable intake is associated with poor self-rated health in the Czech part of the HAPIEE study. *Nutr. Health* **2021**, *29*, 269–276. [CrossRef] [PubMed]
43. Goodwin, D.K.; Knol, L.L.; Eddy, J.M.; Fitzhugh, E.C.; Kendrick, O.W.; Donahue, R.E. The Relationship between Self-Rated Health Status and the Overall Quality of Dietary Intake of US Adolescents. *J. Am. Diet. Assoc.* **2006**, *106*, 1450–1453. [CrossRef] [PubMed]
44. Libera, J.; Iłowiecka, K.; Stasiak, D. Consumption of processed red meat and its impact on human health: A review. *Int. J. Food Sci. Technol.* **2021**, *56*, 6115–6123. [CrossRef]
45. Gillespie, K.M.; Kemps, E.; White, M.J.; Bartlett, S.E. The Impact of Free Sugar on Human Health—A Narrative Review. *Nutrients* **2023**, *15*, 889. [CrossRef] [PubMed]
46. Reese, A.C.; Burgos-Gil, R.; Cleary, S.D.; Lora, K.; Rivera, I.; Gittelsohn, J.; Seper, S.; Monge-Rojas, R.; Colón-Ramos, U. Use of a Water Filter at Home Reduces Sugary Drink Consumption among Parents and Toddlers in Predominantly Hispanic Community: Results From the Water Up!@ Home Intervention Trial. *J. Acad. Nutr. Diet* **2023**, *123*, 41. [CrossRef]
47. González-Morales, R.; Canto-Osorio, F.; Stern, D.; Sánchez-Romero, L.M.; Torres-Ibarra, L.; Hernández-López, R.; Rivera-Paredez, B.; Vidaña-Pérez, D.; Ramírez-Palacios, P.; Salmerón, J.; et al. Soft drink intake is associated with weight gain, regardless of physical activity levels: The health workers cohort study. *Int. J. Behav. Nutr. Phys. Act.* **2020**, *17*, 60. [CrossRef]
48. Narain, A.; Kwok, C.S.; Mamas, M.A. Soft drinks and sweetened beverages and the risk of cardiovascular disease and mortality: A systematic review and meta-analysis. *Int. J. Clin. Pract.* **2016**, *70*, 791–805. [CrossRef]
49. Torres-Ibarra, L.; Rivera-Paredez, B.; Hernández-López, R.; Canto-Osorio, F.; Sánchez-Romero, L.M.; López-Olmedo, N.; González-Morales, R.; Ramírez, P.; Salmerón, J.; Barrientos-Gutiérrez, T. Regular consumption of soft drinks is associated with type 2 diabetes incidence in Mexican adults: Findings from a prospective cohort study. *Nutr. J.* **2020**, *19*, 126. [CrossRef] [PubMed]
50. de Moraes, M.M.; Mediano, M.F.F.; de Souza, R.A.G.; Moura, A.S.; da Veiga, G.V.; Sichieri, R. Discouraging soft drink consumption reduces blood glucose and cholesterol of Brazilian elementary students: Secondary analysis of a randomized controlled trial. *Prev. Med.* **2017**, *100*, 223–228. [CrossRef] [PubMed]
51. Hales, C.M.; Carroll, M.D.; Fryar, C.D.; Ogden, C.L. NCHS Data Brief No. 360. February 2020. Available online: https://www.cdc.gov/nchs/products/databriefs/db360.htm (accessed on 19 January 2024).

52. Donfrancesco, C.; Profumo, E.; Noce, C.L.; Minutoli, D.; Di Lonardo, A.; Buttari, B.; Vespasiano, F.; Vannucchi, S.; Galletti, F.; Onder, G.; et al. Trends of overweight, obesity and anthropometric measurements among the adult population in Italy: The CUORE Project health examination surveys 1998, 2008, and 2018. *PLoS ONE* **2022**, *17*, e0264778. [CrossRef] [PubMed]
53. Monteiro, C.A.; Conde, W.L.; Popkin, B.M. Independent Effects of Income and Education on the Risk of Obesity in the Brazilian Adult Population. *J. Nutr.* **2001**, *131*, 881S–886S. [CrossRef]
54. Gallus, S.; Odone, A.; Lugo, A.; Bosetti, C.; Colombo, P.; Zuccaro, P.; La Vecchia, C. Overweight and obesity prevalence and determinants in Italy: An update to 2010. *Eur. J. Nutr.* **2013**, *52*, 677–685. [CrossRef]

nutrients

MDPI

Article

Exploring Diet and Nutrient Insufficiencies across Age Groups: Insights from a Population-Based Study of Brazilian Adults

Mauro Fisberg [1,2,*], Lais Duarte Batista [3], Agatha Nogueira Previdelli [4], Gerson Ferrari [4] and Regina Mara Fisberg [3]

[1] Centro de Excelência em Nutrição e Dificuldades Alimentares (CENDA), Instituto Pensi, Fundação José Luiz Egydio Setúbal, Hospital Infantil Sabará, São Paulo 01227-200, Brazil
[2] Department of Pediatrics, Federal University of São Paulo, São Paulo 04023-062, Brazil
[3] Department of Nutrition, School of Public Health, University of São Paulo, São Paulo 01246-904, Brazil; laisduarte@usp.br (L.D.B.); rfisberg@usp.br (R.M.F.)
[4] Faculty of Health Sciences, Universidad Autónoma de Chile, Providencia 7500912, Chile; agatha.usp@gmail.com (A.N.P.); gersonferrari08@yahoo.com.br (G.F.)
* Correspondence: mauro.fisberg@gmail.com

Abstract: Assessing dietary inadequacies can contribute to understanding the nutritional vulnerabilities of a country. This study aimed to investigate nutrient intakes and micronutrient inadequacies in the Brazilian adult population, with an interest in different age subgroups. We conducted a cross-sectional study with 1812 individuals aged 19 to 65 years from a population-based study with a representative sample of Brazilian adults. Dietary intake was assessed by two 24 h food recalls, and the probabilities of inadequate intake were estimated using the Dietary Reference Intake targets. Adequate macronutrient intake was over 99% for proteins, 84.7% for carbohydrates, and 80.7% for total fats. There was a high probability of inadequacy (above 90%) for vitamins D and E, but vitamin D inadequacy was very similar between the sexes. In contrast, vitamin E was more likely to be inadequately consumed among women. A high probability of inadequacies (above 85%) of calcium and magnesium were found in the population, regardless of age group. Except for iron, the probability of an inadequacy of other minerals increased with age. The results showed a relevant proportion of nutrient inadequacies, with those most at risk being women and older individuals, helping with the better targeting and monitoring of public-health policies that address nutritional problems in the population.

Keywords: dietary intake; micronutrients; nutrition surveys; public health

1. Introduction

Diet is an important aspect of human health, providing essential nutrients for growth, development, and lifelong health [1]. Suboptimal dietary patterns and inadequate nutrient intakes are associated with several non-communicable diseases (NCDs), such as high blood pressure, obesity, micronutrient deficiencies, and type 2 diabetes, contributing to morbidity and mortality worldwide [2]. In 2017, dietary risk factors accounted for 22% of total adult mortality, highlighting its relevant role as a modifiable risk behavior to promote health [3].

Diet-related health consequences result from a nutritional imbalance in the intake of macronutrients, vitamins, and minerals. High energy, sodium, saturated fat, and refined carbohydrate intakes are usually risk factors for many NCDs [4]. Additionally, deficiencies in calcium, iron, dietary fiber, vitamin D, and other micronutrients are a public-health concern based on their demonstrated role in the maintenance of bodily functions [5].

Studies evaluating nutrient deficiencies usually focus on children, adolescents, and pregnant or lactating women because these deficiencies are most common among these groups [6,7]. However, to promote health and prevent inadequacies, it is essential to meet individuals' nutrient requirements for all age groups [8]. Inadequate diets in adults can have negative consequences for individuals and society, contributing to the development of diseases, decreased quality of life, human development deficits, economic productivity loss, and increased health costs [8,9]. In addition, the burden of diseases tends to be higher in the elderly than in other age groups [10]. Therefore, from a public-health point of view, preventing nutritional inadequacies in stages before the onset of the disease is a strategy that can contribute to overcoming this problem.

In Brazil, like in other low- and middle-income countries, obesity and diet-related chronic diseases co-exist with undernutrition, indicating the double burden of malnutrition [11,12]. There is a high prevalence of overweight and obesity but also of critical micronutrient deficiencies affecting many individuals in the country. More than half of the population is overweight [2], while dietary surveys have shown a high prevalence of inadequate intakes of calcium, sodium, magnesium, vitamins A, E, D, and pyridoxine [13].

Furthermore, access to robust dietary intake data is central to nutrition epidemiology and policy applications, but it has been a persistent limitation in nutrition research [14,15]. Major obstacles include the considerable efforts and expenses required in dietary data assessment, especially at a population level, which may lead to data scarcity. Thus, providing information to estimate the burden of disease risk and dietary inadequacies or excesses among the sexes and age subgroups can contribute to understanding the nutritional vulnerabilities of a country and its population [16]. Noteworthily, investigations of dietary intake and inadequacies at the population level provide an assessment of the country's diet, which may contribute to public policies aimed at improving nutritional status and preventing chronic diseases. Therefore, this study aimed to investigate energy and nutrient intakes and the prevalence of micronutrient inadequacies in the Brazilian adult population and was particularly interested in differences in age and subgroups.

2. Materials and Methods

2.1. Study Design and Settings

This is a descriptive, cross-sectional study with data from the Brazilian Study of Nutrition and Health (EBANS), a population-based study with a representative sample of individuals aged 15 to 65 years [17] and residents of the urban area of the five macro-regions of Brazil. The EBANS provides data from the Brazilian population to the Latin American Nutrition and Health Study (ELANS) [18], a multicenter study aimed at assessing individuals' nutritional status, physical activity, and food intake in eight Latin American countries. Data collection occurred between October 2014 and July 2015 in two home visits at least eight days apart.

2.2. Subjects and Sample Size

The cities included in the study were selected by systematic random sampling. The urban conglomerates were chosen systematically, and smaller cities were randomly selected based on population density. Within the conglomerates, the Primary Sampling Units (PSUs), represented by municipalities, districts, and residential areas, and the Secondary Sampling Units (SSUs), defined as the census sectors, were randomly selected. In each SSU, the households were selected systematically, and the interviewer went through each residential block in a clockwise direction, with a sampling interval of three homes. Within the households, the selection of individuals was controlled by quotas, respecting the selection criteria of half the individuals with the closest birthday and the other half with the most distant birthday from the interview date. If selected, participants from the same house could be included in the study sample only if they were from different age strata (e.g., adolescents vs. adults). Because we did not include adolescents in this study, the sample only contained individuals from different households. The overall rationale, design, and study sampling were previously described by Fisberg et al. [17], and the final sample of the EBANS included 2000 participants. The present study focused only on the adult life stage, including data of individuals aged 19 to 65 years, of both sexes, with a final sample size of 1812 respondents. Pregnant and lactating women and people with inborn errors of metabolism were not included. Figure 1 illustrates the sampling flowchart for the study (Figure 1).

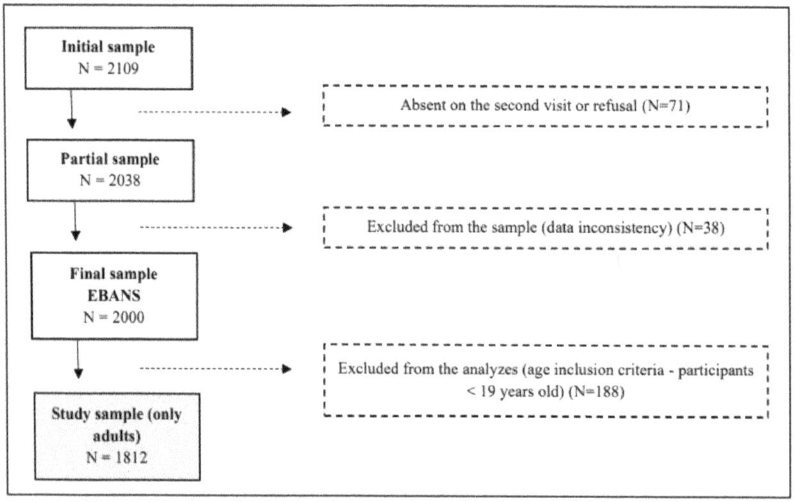

Figure 1. Study flowchart. Adapted from Fisberg et al., 2019 [17].

2.3. *Dietary Intake Assessment*

Dietary food intake was assessed by two 24-h food recalls (24 HRs) (one at each home visit), representing both weekdays and weekends. The 24 HRs were applied following the standardized procedures by the Multiple Pass Method (MPM) to minimize data-collection errors and with the support of a photo album of portion sizes and utensils to improve the accuracy of the data [19]. Nutritional values were obtained using the Nutrition Data System for Research (NDSR software, 2014 version, NCC, University of Minnesota, Minneapolis, MN, USA), and the agreement was compared with the values of Brazilian food composition tables [20]. Nutritional values in the database were corrected if the concordance rate was not between 80% and 120% with corresponding foods in the Brazilian food composition tables. To do so, the researchers (nutritionists) developed statistical routines to replace the original value with the correct one. Mixed dishes and/or Brazilian preparations not in the NDSR software database were added as recipes, matching the nutrient composition for the Brazilian context. Total daily intake values below 800 kcal/day or above 4000 kcal/day suggested errors in collection or data entry, so the 24 HRs were revised, and the nutritionists made the necessary corrections [21]. The Multiple Source Method (MSM) statistical modeling software [22] was used to estimate the usual intake of nutrients at both population and individual levels.

Macronutrient adequacy was compared to the Acceptable Macronutrient Distribution Range (AMDR), which includes the lower and upper limits of the recommendation for each macronutrient. The AMDR ranges, applicable for both sexes, are between 45 and 65% of the total energy intake from carbohydrates, 20–35% of the total energy intake of total fat, and 10–35% of the total energy intake of protein [23]. Total fiber and saturated fats intakes were evaluated considering the cutoffs proposed by the World Health Organization (WHO) [24,25], which recommends a minimum amount of 25 g per day of total fiber for both men and women and less than 10% of the individual's total energy intake from saturated fats. For added sugar, we used the Dietary Guidelines for Americans 2020–2025 [26] because WHO guidelines consider recommendations for free sugar but not added sugar [27]. It recommends an intake below 10% of total energy intake from added sugar. To estimate the probability of an inadequate intake of vitamins and minerals, we used the Dietary Reference Intake (DRI) intake targets proposed by the Institute of Medicine (IOM) [23].

The distribution of the usual nutrient intake was compared to the estimated average requirement (EAR), which considers the specific needs of each sex and age group, to obtain the probability of inadequacy for each age range. The EAR represents the average value of the estimated daily intake to meet the needs of half (50%) of the individuals in the population. It is noteworthy that there is no established EAR value for choline. Therefore, we used adequate intake (AI) to evaluate its ingestion. If the individual's intake is higher than AI, it is most likely that the intake is adequate. We calculated the proportion of individuals with an intake greater than the AI values in the population to determine the probability of adequacy for this nutrient [28].

The participants also reported the use of any type of nutritional supplement, providing the name of the product (when possible) or its main components (e.g., omega 3, vitamin D, or iron, etc.).

2.4. Sociodemographic and Anthropometric Measurements

A trained team obtained anthropometric measurements in duplicate during the first home visit following standardized protocols. Body weight and height were measured using a Sanny® portable scale (Sanny®, São Paulo, Brazil) with a precision of 0.1 kg and a portable Sanny® stadiometer with a precision of 0.1 cm, respectively. The nutritional status was classified based on the body mass index (BMI), according to the cutoff points established by the WHO for individuals above 19 years [29]. Excess weight included those in the overweight or obesity category (people with BMI $\geq$ 25 kg/m^2). The participants self-reported sociodemographic data: age, sex, and educational and socioeconomic levels. The interviewer filled in regional information. Socioeconomic status was classified into three levels, according to the Brazilian Economic Classification Criteria: high (classes A1, A2, and B1), medium (classes B2 and C1), and low (classes C2, D, and E) [30].

We applied the long version of the International Physical Activity Questionnaire (IPAQ) [31] on the second home visit to determine the individual's physical activity level, using the last seven days as a reference. The long-form IPAQ has been validated internationally to assess total physical activity in individuals from 12 countries with Spearman's correlation coefficients ranging from 0.46 to 0.96 [32]. Participants were categorized as active ($\geq$150 min/week) or insufficiently active (<150 min/week) using moderate-to-vigorous physical activity guidelines as defined by the WHO [33]. Details on IPAQ data have been published elsewhere [34,35].

2.5. Statistical Analysis

Participants' characteristics were summarized for the general population and stratified by sex and age strata, presented as absolute and relative frequencies. The age-range categories were chosen based on the different life stages of the DRI recommendations [23]. Thus, for comparison among age groups, this study considered younger adults as individuals between 19 and 30 years old; middle-aged adults, between 31 and 50; and older adults, aged 51 to 65. The chi-square test was used to investigate the association between the categorical variables of interest among the different age groups and between sexes. The distribution of continuous variables was checked for normality using the Kolmogorov–Smirnov test to apply the appropriate parametric or non-parametric tests. We applied the Kruskal–Wallis test with Dunn post hoc pairwise multiple comparisons to investigate differences in the distribution of continuous variables. Nutrient intakes and distribution were described by means, medians, standard deviation (SD), and interquartile ranges (IQR). The prevalence of adequate intakes for each nutrient of interest (e.g., macronutrients, fiber, added sugar, and saturated fats) was calculated considering the proportion of individuals within, below, or above recommendations. The probability of inadequacy in micronutrient intakes was calculated using the z-score (using the Z-standard curve) of the mean intake of the population and the EAR of each nutrient, using the equation [36]: $Z = (EAR - mean)/SD$. All statistical analyses were performed in SPSS software (version 16 for Windows, SPSS Inc., Chicago, IL, USA) with a significance level of 5% (p-value < 0.05).

3. Results

The study included 1812 adults aged 19–65 (54.3% female). Participants' characteristics are shown in Table 1. Most of the population was in the middle or low-income strata and had at least a secondary education (high school). There was also a high frequency of people who studied only up to middle school (complete or incomplete), especially among older adults (aged between 51 and 65 years old). In the three age groups, the proportion of women with a low socioeconomic level was higher than men. However, the association among age groups and socioeconomic status was only significant in women ($p = 0.033$) and not in men ($p = 0.099$). Only 8.3% of the general population had a high socioeconomic level, compared to 45.1% and 46.6% in the medium and low levels, respectively (considering all age groups).

The results suggested an association between excess weight (BMI $\geq$ 25 kg/m^2) and the different age groups in the general population and between the sexes ($p < 0.001$). The population had a high prevalence of excess weight, which was even higher with aging. In younger adults (19–30 years), excess weight affected 48% of the population, while in older adults (51–65 years), this prevalence reached 74.5%. This relation between excess weight with age occurred in both sexes, but the excess weight was higher among men than women only for older adults (75.5% vs. 73.9%).

Considering the IPAQ, only 41.3% of the population (considering all age groups together) reported sufficient physical activity, and the proportion of active men was higher than women (46.7% vs. 36.8%). In both sexes, the age group of older adults (51 to 65 years) had the highest percentages of insufficiently active individuals. Still, the association between physical activity and age groups was only significant in women ($p = 0.010$). Only 93 respondents reported using some nutritional supplement, representing just over 5% of the population, with women representing almost twice as many men among those who reported it. However, no association was found between the use of supplements with different age groups.

Table 2 presents the energy and macronutrient-intake distributions across age groups. As expected, men reported a higher energy intake than women in all age groups, but in both sexes, the energy report was lower as the individuals got older ($p < 0.001$). Compared to the AMDR, the mean contribution to the total energy intake (%EI) of all three macronutrients (carbohydrates, proteins, and total fats) was within the recommended range for all age groups. In the present study, a higher proportion of participants met the recommendations for proteins, with over 99% consuming it within the AMDR. For carbohydrates and total fats, the percentages were 84.7% and 80.7%, respectively. However, there is a pattern of more people consuming carbohydrates below the AMDR (13.6%) than above (1.7%), which is the inverse for total fats, with more people consuming them above than below the AMDR (17.6% vs. 1.7%) (Table S1).

Women presented a higher carbohydrate intake than men in all age groups ($p < 0.001$), and a higher total fat ($p = 0.006$) and saturated fat ($p = 0.003$) intake for those in the middle-aged group (31–50 years old). Across age stages, the absolute value of protein consumption decreased with age, with data showing a daily mean intake of 84.3 g, 78.9 g, and 69.9 g, respectively, for young (19–30 years old), middle-aged (31–50 years old), and older adults (51–65 years old). However, older individuals tended to present a higher contribution to %EI from protein than younger and middle-aged adults ($p < 0.001$). Eicosapentaenoic fatty acid (EPA) intake was also higher in older adults compared to younger adults ($p < 0.001$), but DHA intake did not differ among age groups.

Table 1. Sociodemographic, nutritional status, physical activity level, and supplement use of Brazilian adults in the EBANS study, stratified by sex and age group. Brazil, 2015.

	Total Population (N = 1812)							Male (N = 828)							Female (N = 984)						
	Age Strata (Years)							Age Strata (Years)							Age Strata (Years)						
	19–30		31–50		51–65			19–30		31–50		51–65			19–30		31–50		51–65		
	N	%	N	%	N	%	p-Value	N	%	N	%	N	%	p-Value	N	%	N	%	N	%	p-Value
	573	**32.0**	**851**	**47.0**	**388**	**21.0**		**295**	**16.0**	**394**	**22.0**	**139**	**8.0**		**278**	**15.0**	**457**	**25.0**	**249**	**14.0**	
Education level																					
None to middle school	196	23.8	380	46.2	247	30.0		95	32.2	178	45.2	86	61.9		101	36.3	202	44.2	161	64.7	
High school	345	60.2	372	43.7	104	26.8	**<0.001**	185	62.7	172	43.7	38	27.3	**<0.001**	160	57.6	200	43.8	66	26.5	**<0.001**
College/university degree	32	5.6	99	11.6	37	9.5		15	5.1	44	11.2	15	10.8		17	6.1	55	12.0	22	8.8	
Socioeconomic status																					
High	44	7.7	78	9.2	31	8.0		26	8.8	33	8.4	13	9.4		18	6.5	45	9.9	18	7.2	**0.033**
Middle	269	47.0	402	47.2	143	36.9	**0.003**	157	53.2	200	50.8	55	39.6	0.099	112	40.3	202	44.2	88	35.3	
Low	260	45.4	371	43.6	214	55.2		112	38.0	161	40.9	71	51.1		148	53.2	210	46.0	143	57.4	
Excess weight																					
BMI < 25 kg/m^2	298	52.0	303	35.6	99	25.5	**<0.001**	156	52.9	148	37.6	34	24.5	**<0.001**	142	51.1	155	33.9	65	26.1	**<0.001**
BMI ≥ 25 kg/m^2	275	48.0	548	64.4	289	74.5		139	47.1	246	62.4	105	75.5		136	48.9	302	66.1	184	73.9	
PAL (IPAQ)																					
Insufficiently active	300	54.4	462	56.6	233	62.1	0.058	131	46.1	210	54.8	75	55.2	0.058	169	63.1	252	58.1	158	66.1	**0.010**
Active	252	45.7	355	43.5	142	37.9		153	53.9	173	45.2	61	44.9		99	36.9	182	41.9	81	33.9	
Supplement use																					
No	488	85.2	722	84.8	318	82.0		257	87.1	345	87.6	115	82.7		231	83.1	377	82.5	203	81.5	
Yes	26	4.5	42	4.9	25	6.4	0.624	11	3.7	14	3.6	9	6.5	0.558	15	5.4	28	6.1	16	6.4	0.986
Not informed	59	10.3	87	10.2	45	11.6		27	9.2	35	8.9	15	10.8		32	11.5	52	11.4	30	12.1	

p-value: Chi-square test. BMI: Body Mass Index. PAL: Physical-Activity Level. IPAQ: International Physical Activity Questionnaire.

Table 2. Energy intake and macronutrient distributions reported by Brazilian adults in the EBANS study, stratified by sex and age group. Brazil, 2015.

Nutrient Intake	Total Population (n = 1812)					K–Wallis	Male (n = 828)					Female (n = 984)					K–Wallis
	Mean	SD	P25	P50	P75	p-Value *	Mean	SD	P25	P50	P75	Mean	SD	P25	P50	P75	p Value **
Energy (kcal)																	
19–30 years	1978	623	1564	1888	2275	**<0.001 a,b,c**	2252	651	1824	2162	2523	1687	430	1366	1691	1921	**<0.001 e,f,h,i,j,k,l**
31–50 years	1830	576	1417	1753	2151		2088	594	1690	2034	2416	1609	458	1278	1564	1866	
51–65 years	1566	464	1230	1511	1844		1827	474	1493	1810	2077	1420	389	1147	1341	1648	

Table 2. *Cont.*

Nutrient Intake	Total Population (n = 1812)					K–Wallis	Male (n = 828)					Female (n = 984)					K–Wallis
	Mean	SD	P25	P50	P75	*p*-Value *	Mean	SD	P25	P50	P75	Mean	SD	P25	P50	P75	*p* Value **
Carbohydrates (% EI)																	
19–30 years	50.78	6.65	46.76	51.16	55.05	0.103	49.89	6.71	45.19	49.94	54.54	51.72	6.46	47.98	52.01	55.91	**<0.001 j,k,l**
31–50 years	50.13	6.61	45.76	50.29	54.71		49.30	6.76	44.81	49.62	53.67	50.84	6.4	46.59	50.67	55.33	
51–65 years	50.35	7.25	46.06	50.81	54.79		48.64	6.82	44.27	48.96	53.21	51.30	7.31	46.98	51.64	56.14	
Proteins (% EI)																	
19–30 years	17.26	3.31	15.09	16.97	19.15	**0.001 b,c**	17.58	3.42	15.38	17.11	19.6	16.92	3.15	14.9	16.77	18.7	**<0.001 e,f**
31–50 years	17.53	3.37	15.18	17.21	19.46		17.51	3.33	15.35	17.21	19.58	17.54	3.41	15.11	17.21	19.32	
51–65 years	18.11	3.54	15.72	17.81	19.92		18.64	3.57	16.37	18.61	20.28	17.82	3.5	15.45	17.31	19.69	
Total fats (% EI)																	
19–30 years	30.18	4.91	27.32	30.08	33.37	0.383	29.89	4.78	27.22	30.02	33.22	30.48	5.03	27.37	30.38	33.6	**0.006 k**
31–50 years	29.8	5.25	26.74	30.05	33.12		28.99	5.46	25.92	29.47	32.68	30.5	4.96	27.46	30.45	33.81	
51–65 years	29.7	5.38	26.43	29.83	33.31		29.3	5.25	25.94	29.71	32.88	29.93	5.46	26.7	30.25	33.54	
Saturated fats (% EI)																	
19–30 years	9.95	1.99	8.69	9.9	11.33	0.274	9.85	1.9	8.62	9.93	11.25	10.06	2.07	8.75	9.87	11.55	**0.003 k**
31–50 years	9.84	2.13	8.47	9.7	11.23		9.57	2.22	8.16	9.47	10.91	10.08	2.03	8.73	9.9	11.39	
51–65 years	9.81	2.17	8.35	9.8	11.1		9.58	2.05	8.25	9.58	10.93	9.93	2.23	8.53	9.94	11.27	
Unsaturated fats (% EI)																	
19–30 years	7.61	1.87	6.27	7.52	8.76	0.319	7.46	1.82	6.19	7.5	8.51	7.77	1.92	6.47	7.57	8.94	0.093
31–50 years	7.45	1.86	6.31	7.39	8.47		7.26	1.82	6.13	7.33	8.36	7.61	1.87	6.47	7.4	8.68	
51–65 years	7.41	1.79	6.26	7.31	8.43		7.31	1.65	6.19	7.39	8.26	7.47	1.86	6.27	7.31	8.62	
EPA (mg)																	
19–30 years	11.81	8.42	7.51	10.5	13.32	**<0.001 a,b**	10.98	7.19	7.18	9.56	13.02	12.68	9.49	8.58	11.27	13.64	**<0.001 e,j,k**
31–50 years	12.8	8.22	8.34	11.08	14.57		12.19	8.51	7.9	10.31	13.75	13.32	7.94	9.21	11.74	15.27	
51–65 years	13.49	10.73	8.55	11.58	14.67		12.93	8.31	8.47	11.06	14.7	13.8	11.87	8.96	11.92	14.67	
DHA (mg)																	
19–30 years	48.16	33.58	29.41	40.23	54.51	0.187	49.46	37.06	29.41	40.69	55.86	46.79	29.43	29.28	39.19	54.1	0.550
31–50 years	51.05	36.38	29.81	40.93	58.58		51.72	36.33	30.02	41.1	58.63	50.48	36.46	29.71	40.62	57.73	
51–65 years	50.4	39.84	28.28	39.26	57.41		52.03	35.75	26.2	38.68	64.18	49.49	42	29.25	39.31	53.35	

SD: Standard deviation. % EI: Nutrient intake as a percentage of total energy intake. EPA: Eicosapentaenoic fatty acid. DHA: Docosahexaenoic fatty acid. * Kruskal–Wallis test with post hoc pairwise comparisons: analysis to evaluate the differences among age groups in the overall population: (a) significant differences between age groups 19–30 years and 31–50 years; (b) significant differences between age groups 19–30 years and 51–65 years; (c) significant differences between age groups 31–50 years and 51–65 years. ** Kruskal–Wallis test with post hoc pairwise comparisons: analysis to evaluate the differences between sexes and the three age groups: (d) significant differences between age groups 19–30 years and 31–50 years among men; (e) significant differences between age groups 19–30 years and 51–65 years among men; (f) significant differences between age groups 31–50 years and 51–65 years among men; (g) significant differences between age groups 19–30 years and 31–50 years among women; (h) significant differences between age groups 19–30 years and 51–65 years among women; (i) significant differences between age groups 31–50 years and 51–65 years among women; (j) significant differences between 19 to 30 years (male) vs. 19 to 30 years (female); (k) significant differences between 31 and 50 years (male) vs. 31 and 50 years (female); (l) significant differences between 51 and 65 years (male) vs. 51 and 65 years (female).

Table 3 shows the prevalence of inadequacy in total fiber, added sugar, and saturated fat intake. More than 80% of Brazilian adults had a fiber intake below the recommendation, regardless of age group. This scenario was even worse in women, with the prevalence of inadequacy exceeding 90%. While for women, the prevalence of inadequacy was higher in younger adults, decreasing in the older age group, this relationship was inverse for men, with an increase in inadequacy over age groups. However, these differences were not significant.

Table 3. Prevalence of inadequacy in total fiber, added sugar, and saturated fat intake in Brazilian adults, stratified by sex and age group. Brazil, 2015.

Nutrient	Total Population (n = 1812)			Male (n = 828)			Female (n = 984)		
	n	%	*p*-Value	n	%	*p*-Value	n	%	*p*-Value
Total fiber (g)		**<25 g/day**			**<25 g/day**			**<25 g/day**	
Total—19–65 years	1508	83.22		580	70.05		928	94.31	
19–30 years	463	80.8	0.062	197	66.78	0.170	266	95.68	0.354
31–50 years	709	83.31		278	70.56		431	94.31	
51–65 years	336	86.6		105	75.54		231	92.77	
Added sugar (% EI)		**>10% of EI**			**>10% of EI**			**>10% of EI**	
Total—19–65 years	1121	61.87		453	54.71		668	67.89	
19–30 years	404	70.51	$p < 0.001$	184	62.37	$p < 0.001$	220	79.14	$p < 0.001$
31–50 years	523	61.46		212	53.81		311	68.05	
51–65 years	194	50		57	41.01		137	55.02	
Saturated fat (%EI)		**>10% of EI**			**>10% of EI**			**>10% of EI**	
Total—19–65 years	814	44.92		346	41.79		468	47.56	
19–30 years	273	47.64	0.225	143	48.47	0.014	130	46.76	0.940
31–50 years	366	43.01		148	37.56		218	47.7	
51–65 years	175	45.1		55	39.57		120	48.19	

p-value: Chi-square test. % EI: Nutrient intake as a percentage of total energy intake.

There was also a high prevalence of individuals consuming added sugar above the recommended value, and overconsumption was even greater in women compared to men. In both sexes, people aged 19 to 30 years had the highest frequencies of excessive intake of added sugar, while the lowest values were observed among adults aged 51 to 65 ($p < 0.001$). On the other hand, saturated fat intake above the recommendations decreased with age for men ($p = 0.014$), but there were no significant differences among age groups for women ($p = 0.940$). In terms of proportion, women presented a higher prevalence of excess saturated fat intake than men in middle-aged and older-adult age groups.

Tables 4 and 5 present the distribution and the probabilities of inadequate intakes of vitamins and minerals in the population. The results showed a high probability of inadequacy (above 90%) for vitamins D and E. Vitamin D inadequacy was very similar between the sexes, but vitamin E was more likely to be inadequately consumed among women. Vitamin A also exceeds 53% of inadequacy among men (in all age groups) and 46% among women. Furthermore, the probability of adequacy of choline in the population was very low, reaching 10% only among men in the age group of 19 to 30 years. For the remaining age groups, choline adequacy is around 6%, with the worst-case scenario among older adults.

Thiamine (vitamin B1) showed the best results, with the lowest probabilities of inadequacy in the population. However, some important differences between age groups were noted, such as the significant increase in the inadequacy of thiamine and pyridoxine, especially in men, between young and older adults. While in the first age group, the inadequacy of thiamine did not reach 6%, in older adults, this value was close to 20%. In women, pyridoxine ranged from an inadequacy of 22.1% (among young adults) to 48.4% in older adults.

Regarding minerals, a high probability of inadequacies of calcium and magnesium was found in the population. Except for iron, the probability of inadequacies of the other minerals increased with age. In addition, iron inadequacy in women was higher than in men in all age groups.

Table 4. Distribution and probabilities of inadequate vitamin intakes in Brazilian adults, stratified by sex and age group. Brazil, 2015.

Micronutrient	Brazil (n = 1812)		Male (n = 828)				Female (n = 984)			
	Mean	SD	Mean	SD	EAR	Inadequacy (%)	Mean	SD	EAR	Inadequacy (%)
Vitamin A (mcg)										
19–30 years	554.51	590.02	567.77	706.99	625	53.19%	540.43	433.56	500	46.41%
31–50 years	547.55	459.15	557.57	497.32	625	55.57%	538.91	423.85	500	46.41%
51–65 years	527.48	461.74	560.79	503.24	625	55.17%	508.88	436.81	500	49.20%
Vitamin C (mg)										
19–30 years	90.52	84.76	90.04	90.16	75	43.25%	91.03	78.80	60	34.83%
31–50 years	91.56	79.72	90.19	84.13	75	42.86%	92.74	75.78	60	33.36%
51–65 years	98.00	83.26	94.88	82.79	75	40.52%	99.74	83.63	60	31.56%
Vitamin D (mcg)										
19–30 years	3.54	2.16	3.79	2.27	10	99.69%	3.28	2.00	10	99.88%
31–50 years	3.32	1.85	3.52	1.96	10	99.95%	3.16	1.73	10	99.87%
51–65 years	3.12	1.73	3.24	1.72	10	99.99%	3.05	1.73	10	99.46%
Vitamin E (mg)										
19–30 years	7.40	2.73	8.03	2.86	12	91.77%	6.72	2.43	12	98.50%
31–50 years	7.06	2.91	7.74	3.22	12	90.66%	6.47	2.48	12	98.71%
51–65 years	6.55	2.61	7.41	3.09	12	93.06%	6.07	2.15	12	99.70%
Thiamin (mg)										
19–30 years	1.62	0.51	1.82	0.52	1.0	5.82%	1.42	0.42	0.9	10.93%
31–50 years	1.60	0.57	1.78	0.58	1.0	9.01%	1.45	0.52	0.9	14.23%
51–65 years	1.50	0.66	1.76	0.90	1.0	19.77%	1.36	0.41	0.9	13.14%
Riboflavin (mg)										
19–30 years	1.38	0.47	1.52	0.50	1.1	19.77%	1.23	0.39	0.9	20.05%
31–50 years	1.30	0.45	1.43	0.47	1.1	24.20%	1.18	0.39	0.9	23.27%
51–65 years	1.17	0.37	1.33	0.41	1.1	28.77%	1.08	0.32	0.9	28.43%
Pyridoxine (mg)										
19–30 years	1.74	0.72	2.01	0.80	1.1	12.17%	1.46	0.47	1.1	22.06%
31–50 years	1.67	0.70	1.95	0.78	1.1	13.79%	1.43	0.50	1.1	25.14%
51–65 years	1.49	0.65	1.80	0.82	1.4	31.21%	1.32	0.45	1.3	48.40%
Vitamin B12 (mcg)										
19–30 years	4.41	2.38	4.97	2.57	2.0	12.30%	3.82	2.01	2.0	18.14%
31–50 years	4.26	2.34	4.76	2.58	2.0	14.23%	3.83	2.01	2.0	18.14%
51–65 years	3.87	1.63	4.71	1.95	2.0	8.23%	3.41	1.19	2.0	11.70%
Choline *						**Prob. Adeq. (%)**				**Prob. Adeq. (%)**
19–30 years	337.85	123.23	387.9	132.47	550 *	10.51%	284.74	85.042	425 *	6.12%
31–50 years	325.45	113.15	370.34	118.32	550 *	6.60%	286.75	92.497	425 *	6.78%
51–65 years	295.85	98.167	351.12	107.99	550 *	2.28%	265	76.691	425 *	4.02%

SD: Standard deviation. EAR: Estimated Average Requirement. Inadequacy (%) expresses the probability of inadequacy based on EAR values for each micronutrient. * AI—Adequate intake. For choline, the probability of adequacy is estimated based on AI values (EAR is not available).

Table 5. Distribution and probabilities of inadequate mineral intakes in Brazilian adults, stratified by sex and age group. Brazil, 2015.

Micronutrient	Brazil (n = 1812)		Male (n = 828)				Female (n = 984)			
	Mean	SD	Mean	SD	EAR	Inadequacy (%)	Mean	SD	EAR	Inadequacy (%)
Calcium (mg)										
19–30 years	470.80	244.02	509.13	265.31	800	86.42%	430.12	212.21	800	95.91%
31–50 years	451.66	239.22	463.56	219.30	800	93.70%	441.40	254.94	800	92.07%
51–65 years	424.57	204.40	454.31	213.32	800	95.73%	407.98	197.75	1000	99.86%
Iron (mg)										
19–30 years	12.36	4.18	14.20	4.18	6.0	2.50%	10.40	3.17	8.10	23.27%
31–50 years	11.36	4.11	13.22	4.38	6.0	4.95%	9.75	3.05	8.10	29.46%
51–65 years	9.98	3.27	11.77	3.02	6.0	2.81%	8.98	2.97	5.00	9.01%
Magnesium (mg)										
19–30 years	216.45	71.79	246.95	77.02	330	85.99%	184.09	48.01	255	93.06%
31–50 years	211.69	69.51	240.75	73.45	350	93.19%	186.64	54.77	265	92.36%
51–65 years	199.76	62.56	228.55	65.74	350	96.78%	183.69	54.58	265	93.19%
Zinc (mg)										
19–30 years	12.40	5.33	14.53	6.04	9.4	19.77%	10.13	3.15	6.8	14.46%
31–50 years	11.51	4.48	13.29	4.87	9.4	21.19%	9.97	3.43	6.8	17.88%
51–65 years	10.41	4.05	12.29	3.95	9.4	23.27%	9.36	3.71	6.8	24.51%

SD: Standard deviation. EAR: Estimated Average Requirement. Inadequacy (%) expresses the probability of inadequacy based on EAR values for each micronutrient.

4. Discussion

This study evaluated energy and nutrient intakes in the Brazilian adult population, investigating differences between sexes and age subgroups. We have also estimated the probability of inadequate intakes of vitamins and minerals in the population. In summary, the results showed many nutrient inadequacies relevant to public health, with a worse scenario among women and older people. There was a high consumption of saturated fat and added sugar and a low adequacy in fiber intake. Additionally, many vitamins and minerals were consumed below the recommendations, resulting in a high probability of inadequacy in the population.

In previous studies, men consumed slightly more calories from protein than women, while women reported more energy from carbohydrates [37]. However, Araujo et al. [38] found a mean energy contribution lower from total fats (about 27%) and higher from carbohydrates (about 55%) than in our research. Our results also showed a decrease in energy intake and calories from total and saturated fats with the advance of age. A possible explanation for this reduction in fat intake with age may be associated with the occurrence and diagnosis of chronic non-communicable diseases, especially cardiovascular diseases, which are more frequent in older people [10]. Usually, with the diagnosis, there are recommendations for changes in lifestyle or the restriction of some food groups, especially fats. This can lead to modifications in the dietary patterns of these individuals, with a reduction in fats, which may also impact energy intake. It may also be related to the decrease in added sugar consumption across age groups because of the diagnosis of type 2 diabetes, which recommends reducing or substituting sugar intake with sweeteners [39]. One factor that might also contribute to these differences in energy intake across ages and between the sexes is the misreporting of energy intake. Older people and women tend to under-report their energy intake more than others [40].

Although the mean percentages of macronutrient contribution to total energy intake were within the AMDR, it is important to mention some limitations, since AMDR considers the distribution of macronutrients within the total caloric intake. Therefore, the distribution may be within the adequate range even when energy intake is inadequate (both above and below). In addition, the AMDR for proteins is quite broad, considering values between 10 and 35% of energy intake to be adequate [23]. However, the health effects of a diet with 10% proteins compared to one with 35% may differ, but still, both would be considered adequate protein intakes by the AMDR.

Most of the population was in the lower categories of education and socioeconomic level, which are relevant in studies that assess nutritional inadequacies and health [41]. These measures are directly associated with the individual's purchasing power and household food availability, contributing to nutrient intake and adequacy. Especially in lower-income countries, studies show a positive association between the level of education and healthy food choices [42,43].

Most of the population does not meet the requirements for fiber, with worse results for women. Fruits and vegetables, which are important sources of fiber, contribute to a low percentage of the total fiber intake in the population (Table S2), which might justify its low intake. Like in other studies in the Brazilian population, the top three foods that contribute to fiber intake are beans, rice, and bread [44].

EPA and DHA intake varies a lot among studies, and there needs to be a consensus on the recommended dosage for the general population or healthy individuals. However, in our sample, the intake of these two fatty acids was below previous studies. Lu et al. [45] investigated omega-3 fatty acids in the body composition of women with polycystic ovary syndrome and found a mean intake of EPA and DHA of 19.8 mg/day and 18.1 mg/day, respectively. On the other hand, Carballo-Casla et al. [46], investigating fish consumption by Spanish people over 60 years of age, found a much higher mean intake for both fatty acids (EPA—260 mg and DHA—500 mg). Previous studies suggest that doses of 2 to 4 g of EPA/DHA daily can lower triglyceride levels by 25 to 30% [47]. Thus, the Brazilian Cardiology Society suggests that this dose (2–4 g per day) or even higher doses may be recommended only for severe hypertriglyceridemia. However, the actual EPA and DHA intake in the population represents less than 10% of these values. These differences, especially compared to the Spanish context, may be partially attributed to the population's dietary habits and patterns. Mediterranean countries usually present higher eating frequencies of healthy fats, fish, and omega-3 food sources than Western countries [48]. In Brazil, on the other hand, the dietary intake of polyunsaturated fatty acids is below the recommendations [49]. Major food groups that contribute to its intake, such as fish, the primary food source of EPA and DHA, represent less than 1% of the total energy intake [50]. Evidence that evaluates EPA and DHA intakes is still scarce in Brazil.

We observed a high probability of inadequate intake of vitamins E, D, calcium, and magnesium, with most inadequacies increasing with age. Also, choline adequacy was low in both sexes and even worse in older adults. The most significant difference between the sexes was observed in their iron intake, the micronutrient with the lowest probability of inadequacy in the population. The results are in accordance with previous studies in Brazil and may be related to dietary aspects and public policies in the country. Araujo et al. [38] and Verly Junior et al. [13] also found an inadequate prevalence of over 90% for vitamin D, E, and calcium when evaluating micronutrient intakes in Brazilian adults. The authors also found less than 5% of inadequacy in iron intake in men.

Important calcium food sources, such as milk, yogurt, cheese, fish, and seafood are scarcely consumed by the population [50]. Additionally, the high inadequacy of vitamin D may be explained by the established recommended reference values, considering mainly the US population, assuming little or no sun exposure [51]. This scenario may not be applicable in countries with a predominantly tropical climate, like Brazil, where most of the vitamin D requirement can be met by synthesis from sun exposure. A previous study with a representative sample of São Paulo, the city with the largest population in Brazil, found an inadequate vitamin D intake in nearly 100% of the population. However, serum levels were adequate in almost half of the population [52]. Thus, the EAR for vitamin D in Brazil may be overestimated.

Whole grains are more commonly consumed by women, which may explain the differences between the sexes in inadequacies of B vitamins [53]. In a recent investigation that simulated the effect of replacing refined cereals with whole grains, one of the adverse effects would be the reduction of niacin, riboflavin, pyridoxine, and folate, which could be associated with grain processing [54]. It may also be related to the differences in iron inadequacy between the sexes, which is notably higher in women (in all age groups) than in men. Due to the specific needs associated with the menstrual period, the EAR for iron for adult women is higher than for men, which may increase the magnitude of this difference in the inadequacy of this mineral. After mandatory wheat and corn flour enrichment with iron and folic acid, bread, pasta, and biscuits are the main food sources contributing to these two micronutrients. These are foods commonly restricted in women's diets due to the perception of their association with weight gain [55].

Nevertheless, this study is not without limitations. Dietary data collection is subject to bias and errors. Although this study assessed food intake using two 24 HRs and adjusted it to estimate the usual intake, especially evaluating micronutrients, this number of collections may not be sufficient to reflect its actual intake. Additionally, only the nutrient intake from food sources was considered in the analysis. However, a robust data collection and analysis methodology was applied to minimize these errors, and the reported supplement use was very low in the population. Furthermore, we had to adopt international cut-off values because the Dietary Guidelines for the Brazilian Population [56] only present qualitative but not quantitative recommendations for evaluating nutrient adequacies. However, even though the cut-offs were not developed specifically for the Brazilian population, these recommendations are based on robust scientific reviews of the current body of evidence commonly related to health and disease risk. Additionally, this study only collected data in the urban areas of the country. However, in 2015, only 14% of the Brazilian population lived in rural areas, according to the World Bank [57]. Thus, a strength of the study is the dietary assessment at the populational level, with a representative sample of Brazilian adults living in urban areas, which can provide information about the nutritional diagnosis for most of the country.

5. Conclusions

The present study comprehensively provides information on macro and micronutrient inadequacies and excessive intakes in Brazilian adults. Substantial inadequate nutrient intakes were verified among the population, with those most at-risk being women and older individuals. The results showed a relevant scenario of nutrient inadequacies with public-health concerns, such as fiber, added sugar, vitamin D and E, choline, calcium, and magnesium, which should be addressed through governmental policies, programs, and interventions in the clinical practice of health care professionals. Promoting the consumption of adequate and micronutrient-rich foods, strengthening food fortification, and nutritional supplementation, particularly for groups at risk, are valuable strategies that might help to alleviate these inadequacies, which can improve the population's nutritional status and, ultimately, the individuals' quality of life. These findings may contribute to identifying subgroups in the population that are vulnerable to inadequate nutrient intake, to target better and monitor public health policies, and to assist in reducing nutritional problems in the population.

Supplementary Materials: The following supporting information can be downloaded at: https://www.mdpi.com/article/10.3390/nu16050750/s1, Table S1: Macronutrient intake in adults in the urban areas of Brazil, 2015.; Table S2: Top 10 food sources contributing to nutrient total intake in adults in the urban areas of Brazil, 2015.

Author Contributions: Conceptualization, M.F. and R.M.F.; methodology, M.F. and R.M.F.; validation, G.F., L.D.B. and A.N.P.; formal analysis, A.N.P.; resources, M.F., G.F. and R.M.F.; writing—original draft preparation, L.D.B.; writing—review and editing, L.D.B.; project administration, M.F.; funding acquisition, M.F. All authors have read and agreed to the published version of the manuscript.

Funding: The EBANS was partially supported by a scientific grant from the Coca-Cola Company and different grants and support from the Instituto Pensi/Hospital Infantil Sabara. Reckitt Brasil supported the publication of this paper. There are no specific grant numbers associated with the process.

Institutional Review Board Statement: The study was conducted in accordance with the Declaration of Helsinki and approved by the Research Ethics Committee of Hospital Infantil Sabará—Jose Luiz Egydio Setúbal Foundation (protocol code 31670314.8.0000.5567 on 17 June 2014). The Western Institutional Review Board, Inc. also approved the ELANS protocol on 22 June 2015 (Study number: 1145835).

Informed Consent Statement: Written informed consent was obtained from all subjects involved in the study.

Data Availability Statement: Data is available upon reasonable request. It is not publicly available due to confidentiality/ethical restrictions. Data can be available through the EBANS institutional board for researchers who meet the criteria for access to confidential data. For data requests, please contact: Instituto PENSI (PENSI Institute) Ave. Angelica 2071, 2nd floor. Sao Paulo, Brazil. 01221-200. Phone: +55-11-2526-2525. Email: pesqeasy@pensi.org.br.

Acknowledgments: We thank Irina Kovalskys, for her support in all protocol phases of the ELANS project. We want to thank Reckitt Brazil, through Medical Affairs Nutrition, for their support in the publication of this paper. To the whole group of the ELANS project, our deepest gratitude.

Conflicts of Interest: The authors declare no conflicts of interest. The funders had no role in the design of the study; in the collection, analyses, or interpretation of data; in the writing of the manuscript; or in the decision to publish the results.

References

1. Wilson, N.; Blakely, T.; Foster, R.H.; Hadorn, D.; Vos, T. Prioritizing risk factors to identify preventive interventions for economic assessment. *Bull. World Health Organ.* **2012**, *90*, 88–96. [CrossRef] [PubMed]
2. Felisbino-Mendes, M.S.; Cousin, E.; Malta, D.C.; Machado, Í.E.; Ribeiro, A.L.P.; Duncan, B.B.; Schmidt, M.I.; Silva, D.A.S.; Glenn, S.; Afshin, A.; et al. The burden of non-communicable diseases attributable to high BMI in Brazil, 1990–2017: Findings from the Global Burden of Disease Study. *Popul. Health Metr.* **2020**, *18*, 18. [CrossRef] [PubMed]
3. Afshin, A.; Sur, P.J.; Fay, K.A.; Cornaby, L.; Ferrara, G.; Salama, J.S.; Mullany, E.C.; Abate, K.H.; Abbafati, C.; Abebe, Z.; et al. Health effects of dietary risks in 195 countries, 1990–2017: A systematic analysis for the Global Burden of Disease Study 2017. *Lancet* **2019**, *393*, 1958–1972. [CrossRef] [PubMed]
4. Oikonomou, E.; Psaltopoulou, T.; Georgiopoulos, G.; Siasos, G.; Kokkou, E.; Antonopoulos, A.; Vogiatzi, G.; Tsalamandris, S.; Gennimata, V.; Papanikolaou, A.; et al. Western Dietary Pattern Is Associated with Severe Coronary Artery Disease. *Angiology* **2018**, *69*, 339–346. [CrossRef] [PubMed]
5. Mujica-Coopman, M.F.; Brito, A.; López de Romaña, D.; Ríos-Castillo, I.; Cori, H.; Olivares, M. Prevalence of Anemia in Latin America and the Caribbean. *Food Nutr. Bull.* **2015**, *36*, S119–S128. [CrossRef] [PubMed]
6. Galani, Y.J.H.; Orfila, C.; Gong, Y.Y. A review of micronutrient deficiencies and analysis of maize contribution to nutrient requirements of women and children in Eastern and Southern Africa. *Crit. Rev. Food Sci. Nutr.* **2022**, *62*, 1568–1591. [CrossRef] [PubMed]
7. Bailey, R.L.; Pac, S.G.; Fulgoni, V.L.; Reidy, K.C.; Catalano, P.M. Estimation of Total Usual Dietary Intakes of Pregnant Women in the United States. *JAMA Netw. Open* **2019**, *2*, e195967. [CrossRef]
8. Bai, Y.; Herforth, A.; Masters, W.A. Global variation in the cost of a nutrient-adequate diet by population group: An observational study. *Lancet Planet Health* **2022**, *6*, e19–e28. [CrossRef]
9. Perez-Escamilla, R.; Bermudez, O.; Buccini, G.S.; Kumanyika, S.; Lutter, C.K.; Monsivais, P.; Victora, C. Nutrition disparities and the global burden of malnutrition. *BMJ* **2018**, *361*, k2252. [CrossRef]
10. Jura, M.; Kozak, L.P. Obesity and related consequences to ageing. *Age* **2016**, *38*, 23. [CrossRef]
11. Wegmüller, R.; Bentil, H.; Wirth, J.P.; Petry, N.; Tanumihardjo, S.A.; Allen, L.; Williams, T.N.; Selenje, L.; Mahama, A.; Amoaful, E.; et al. Anemia, micronutrient deficiencies, malaria, hemoglobinopathies and malnutrition in young children and non-pregnant women in Ghana: Findings from a national survey. *PLoS ONE* **2020**, *15*, e0228258. [CrossRef] [PubMed]
12. Popkin, B.M.; Corvalan, C.; Grummer-Strawn, L.M. Dynamics of the double burden of malnutrition and the changing nutrition reality. *Lancet* **2020**, *395*, 65–74. [CrossRef] [PubMed]
13. Verly, E., Jr.; Marchioni, D.M.; Araujo, M.C.; Carli, E.D.; de Oliveira, D.C.R.S.; Yokoo, E.M.; Sichieri, R.; Pereira, R.A. Evolução da ingestão de energia e nutrientes no Brasil entre 2008–2009 e 2017–2018. *Rev. De Saúde Pública* **2021**, *55* (Suppl. S1), 1–22. [CrossRef] [PubMed]
14. Micha, R.; Coates, J.; Leclercq, C.; Charrondiere, U.R.; Mozaffarian, D. Global Dietary Surveillance: Data Gaps and Challenges. *Food Nutr. Bull.* **2018**, *39*, 175–205. [CrossRef]
15. Miller, V.; Singh, G.M.; Onopa, J.; Reedy, J.; Shi, P.; Zhang, J.; Tahira, A.; Morris, M.L.S.; Marsden, D.P.; Kranz, S.; et al. Global Dietary Database 2017: Data availability and gaps on 54 major foods, beverages, and nutrients among 5.6 million children and adults from 1220 surveys worldwide. *BMJ Glob. Health* **2021**, *6*, e003585. [CrossRef]
16. Simone, P.; Carolina, B.; Ty, B.; Pia, J.A.; Sabri, B.; Ling, C.; Anali, G.; Tue, C.; Arnold, D.; Selma, K.G.; et al. Estimating national and subnational nutrient intake distributions of global diets. *Am. J. Clin. Nutr.* **2022**, *116*, 551–560. [CrossRef]
17. Fisberg, M.; Kovalskys, I.; Previdelli, A.N.; Zimberg, I.Z.; Del'Arco, A.P.W.T.; Ferrari, G.L.D.M. Brazilian Study of Nutrition and Health (EBANS)—Brazilian data of ELANS: Methodological opportunities and challenges. *Rev. Da Assoc. Méd. Bras.* **2019**, *65*, 669–677. [CrossRef]
18. Fisberg, M.; Kovalskys, I.; Gomez, G.; Rigotti, A.; Cortes, L.Y.; Herrera-Cuenca, M.; Yepez, M.C.; Pareja, R.G.; Guajardo, V.; Zimberg, I.Z.; et al. Latin American Study of Nutrition and Health (ELANS): Rationale and study design. *BMC Public Health* **2015**, *16*, 93. [CrossRef]
19. Moshfegh, A.J.; Rhodes, D.G.; Baer, D.J.; Murayi, T.; Clemens, J.C.; Rumpler, W.V.; Paul, D.R.; Sebastian, R.S.; Kuczynski, K.J.; Ingwersen, L.A.; et al. The US Department of Agriculture Automated Multiple-Pass Method reduces bias in the collection of energy intakes. *Am. J. Clin. Nutr.* **2008**, *88*, 324–332. [CrossRef] [PubMed]
20. Universidade de São Paulo (USP). Food Research Center (FoRC). Versão 6.0. 2017. Tabela Brasileira de Composição de Alimentos (TBCA). Available online: https://www.tbca.net.br/ (accessed on 8 February 2024).
21. Kovalskys, I.; Fisberg, M.; Gómez, G.; Rigotti, A.; Cortés, L.Y.; Yépez, M.C.; Pareja, R.G.; Herrera-Cuenca, M.; Zimberg, I.Z.; Tucker, K.L.; et al. Standardization of the Food Composition Database Used in the Latin American Nutrition and Health Study (ELANS). *Nutrients* **2015**, *7*, 7914–7924. [CrossRef] [PubMed]
22. Harttig, U.; Haubrock, J.; Knüppel, S.; Boeing, H. The MSM program: Web-based statistics package for estimating usual dietary intake using the Multiple Source Method. *Eur. J. Clin. Nutr.* **2011**, *65*, S87–S91. [CrossRef]
23. IOM/Food and Nutrition Board. *Dietary Reference Intakes for Energy, Carbohydrate, Fiber, Fat Fatty Acids, Cholesterol, Protein, and Amino Acids (Macronutrients)*; National Academics Press: Washington, DC, USA, 2005.
24. World Health Organization. *Saturated Fatty Acid and Trans-Fatty Acid Intake for Adults and Children*; WHO guideline: Geneva, Switzerland, 2023.

25. World Health Organization. *Carbohydrate Intake for Adults and Children*; WHO guideline: Geneva, Switzerland, 2023.
26. U.S. Department of Agriculture and U.S. Department of Health and Human Services. *Dietary Guidelines for Americans, 2020–2025*, 9th ed.; U.S. Department of Agriculture and U.S. Department of Health and Human Services: Washington, DC, USA, 2020.
27. WHO. World Health Organization. *Guideline: Sugars Intake for Adults and Children*; WHO: Geneva, Switzerland, 2015.
28. Marchioni, D.M.L.; Slater, B.; Fisberg, R.M. Aplicação das Dietary Reference Intakes na avaliação da ingestão de nutrientes para indivíduos. *Rev. De Nutr.* **2004**, *17*, 207–216. [CrossRef]
29. WHO—World Health Organization. *WHO Consultation on Obesity: Preventing and Managing the Global Epidemic*; WHO: Geneva, Switzerland, 1998.
30. Kamakura, W.; Mazzon, J.A. Critérios de estratificação e comparação de classificadores socioeconômicos no Brasil. *Rev. De Adm. De Empresas* **2016**, *56*, 55–70. [CrossRef]
31. Matsudo, S.; Araújo, T.; Marsudo, V.; Andrade, D.; Andrade, E.; Braggion, G. Questionário Internacional de Atividade Física (IPAQ): Estudo de validade e reprodutibilidade no Brasil. *Rev. Bras. Ativ. Fís. Saúde* **2012**, *6*, 5–18.
32. Craig, C.L.; Marshall, A.L.; Sjöström, M.; Bauman, A.E.; Booth, M.L.; Ainsworth, B.E.; Pratt, M.; Ekelund, U.L.F.; Yngve, A.; Sallis, J.F.; et al. International Physical Activity Questionnaire: 12-Country Reliability and Validity. *Med. Sci. Sports Exerc.* **2003**, *35*, 1381–1395. [CrossRef] [PubMed]
33. Bull, F.C.; Al-Ansari, S.S.; Biddle, S.; Borodulin, K.; Buman, M.P.; Cardon, G.; Carty, C.; Chaput, J.P.; Chastin, S.; Chou, R.; et al. World Health Organization 2020 guidelines on physical activity and sedentary behaviour. *Br. J. Sports Med.* **2020**, *54*, 1451–1462. [CrossRef] [PubMed]
34. Ferrari, G.L.D.M.; Kovalskys, I.; Fisberg, M.; Gómez, G.; Rigotti, A.; Sanabria, L.Y.C.; García, M.C.Y.; Torres, R.G.P.; Herrera-Cuenca, M.; Zimberg, I.Z.; et al. Socio-demographic patterning of objectively measured physical activity and sedentary behaviours in eight Latin American countries: Findings from the ELANS study. *Eur. J. Sport Sci.* **2020**, *20*, 670–681. [CrossRef] [PubMed]
35. De Moraes Ferrari, G.L.; Kovalskys, I.; Fisberg, M.; Gómez, G.; Rigotti, A.; Sanabria, L.Y.C.; García, M.C.Y.; Torres, R.G.P.; Herrera-Cuenca, M.; Zimberg, I.Z.; et al. Methodological design for the assessment of physical activity and sedentary time in eight Latin American countries—The ELANS study. *MethodsX* **2020**, *7*, 100843. [CrossRef] [PubMed]
36. Slater, B.; Marchioni, D.L.; Fisberg, R.M. Estimando a prevalência da ingestão inadequada de nutrientes. *Rev. Saúde Pública* **2004**, *38*, 599–605. [CrossRef] [PubMed]
37. Mendes, A.; Gavioli, L.; Previdelli, A.N.; Fisberg, R.M.; Marchioni, D.M.L. The diet quality index evaluates the adequacy of energy provided by dietary macronutrients. *Rev. Nutr.* **2015**, *28*, 341–348. [CrossRef]
38. Araujo, M.C.; Bezerra, I.N.; Barbosa, F.D.S.; Junger, W.L.; Yokoo, E.M.; Pereira, R.A.; Sichieri, R. Consumo de macronutrientes e ingestão inadequada de micronutrientes em adultos. *Rev. Saúde Pública* **2013**, *47* (Suppl. S1), 177s–189s. [CrossRef]
39. Ley, S.H.; Hamdy, O.; Mohan, V.; Hu, F.B. Prevention and management of type 2 diabetes: Dietary components and nutritional strategies. *Lancet* **2014**, *383*, 1999–2007. [CrossRef] [PubMed]
40. Lutomski, J.E.; van den Broeck, J.; Harrington, J.; Shiely, F.; Perry, I.J. Sociodemographic, lifestyle, mental health and dietary factors associated with direction of misreporting of energy intake. *Public Health Nutr.* **2011**, *14*, 532–541. [CrossRef] [PubMed]
41. Rippin, H.L.; Hutchinson, J.; Greenwood, D.C.; Jewell, J.; Breda, J.J.; Martin, A.; Rippin, D.M.; Schindler, K.; Rust, P.; Fagt, S.; et al. Inequalities in education and national income are associated with poorer diet: Pooled analysis of individual participant data across 12 European countries. *PLoS ONE* **2020**, *15*, e0232447. [CrossRef]
42. Gómez, G.; Kovalskys, I.; Leme, A.C.B.; Quesada, D.; Rigotti, A.; Cortes Sanabria, L.Y.; Yepez Garcia, M.C.; Liria-Domínguez, M.R.; Herrera-Cuenca, M.; Fisberg, R.M.; et al. Socioeconomic Status Impact on Diet Quality and Body Mass Index in Eight Latin American Countries: ELANS Study Results. *Nutrients* **2021**, *13*, 2404. [CrossRef]
43. Shlisky, J.; Bloom, D.E.; Beaudreault, A.R.; Tucker, K.L.; Keller, H.H.; Freund-Levi, Y.; Fielding, R.A.; Cheng, F.W.; Jensen, G.L.; Wu, D.; et al. Nutritional Considerations for Healthy Aging and Reduction in Age-Related Chronic Disease. *Adv. Nutr.* **2017**, *8*, 17–26. [CrossRef]
44. Santos, P.V.; Sales, C.H.; Vieira, D.A.; de Mello Fontanelli, M.; Marchioni, D.M.; Fisberg, R.M. Family income per capita, age, and smoking status are predictors of low fiber intake in residents of São Paulo, Brazil. *Nutr. Res.* **2016**, *36*, 478–487. [CrossRef]
45. Lu, L.; Li, X.; Lv, L.; Xu, Y.; Wu, B.; Huang, C. Associations between omega-3 fatty acids and insulin resistance and body composition in women with polycystic ovary syndrome. *Front Nutr.* **2022**, *9*, 1016943. [CrossRef]
46. Carballo-Casla, A.; García-Esquinas, E.; Banegas, J.R.; Rodríguez-Artalejo, F.; Ortolá, R. Fish consumption, omega-3 fatty acid intake, and risk of pain: The Seniors-ENRICA-1 cohort. *Clin. Nutr.* **2022**, *41*, 2587–2595. [CrossRef] [PubMed]
47. Bhatt, D.L.; Steg, P.G.; Miller, M.; Brinton, E.A.; Jacobson, T.A.; Ketchum, S.B.; Doyle Jr, R.T.; Juliano, R.A.; Jiao, L.; Granowitz, C.; et al. Cardiovascular Risk Reduction with Icosapent Ethyl for Hypertriglyceridemia. *N. Engl. J. Med.* **2019**, *380*, 11–22. [CrossRef] [PubMed]
48. Castelló, A.; Rodríguez-Barranco, M.; Fernández de Larrea, N.; Jakszyn, P.; Dorronsoro, A.; Amiano, P.; Chirlaque, M.D.; Colorado-Yohar, S.; Guevara, M.; Moreno-Iribas, C.; et al. Adherence to the Western, Prudent and Mediterranean Dietary Patterns and Colorectal Cancer Risk: Findings from the Spanish Cohort of the European Prospective Investigation into Cancer and Nutrition (EPIC-Spain). *Nutrients* **2022**, *14*, 3085. [CrossRef]
49. Sisa, I.; Abeyá-Gilardon, E.; Fisberg, R.M.; Jackson, M.D.; Mangialavori, G.L.; Sichieri, R.; Cudhea, F.; Bannuru, R.R.; Ruthazer, R.; Mozaffarian, D.; et al. Impact of diet on CVD and diabetes mortality in Latin America and the Caribbean: A comparative risk assessment analysis. *Public Health Nutr.* **2021**, *24*, 2577–2591. [CrossRef]

50. IBGE. Instituto Brasileiro de Geografia e Estatística. *Pesquisa de Orçamentos Familiares 2017–2018: Avaliação Nutricional da Disponibilidade Domiciliar de Alimentos no Brasil*; IBGE: Rio de Janeiro, Brazil, 2020.
51. Institute of Medicine (US) Committee to Review Dietary Reference Intakes for Vitamin D and Calcium; Ross, A.C.; Del Valle, H.B.; Yaktine, A.L.; Taylor, C.L. *Dietary Reference Intakes for Calcium and Vitamin D*; Institute of Medicine: Washington, DC, USA, 2011.
52. Martini, L.A.; Verly Jr, E.; Marchioni, D.M.; Fisberg, R.M. Prevalence and correlates of calcium and vitamin D status adequacy in adolescents, adults, and elderly from the Health Survey—São Paulo. *Nutrition* **2013**, *29*, 845–850. [CrossRef] [PubMed]
53. De M Fontanelli, M.; Sales, C.H.; de Castro, M.A.; Fisberg, R.M. Healthful grain foods consumption by São Paulo residents: A 12-year analysis and future trends. *Public Health Nutr.* **2021**, *24*, 2987–2997. [CrossRef] [PubMed]
54. De Mello Fontanelli, M.; Arroyo, A.M.; Sales, C.H.; Seal, C.J.; Fisberg, R.M. Opportunities for diet quality improvement: The potential role of staple grain foods. *Public Health Nutr.* **2021**, *24*, 6145–6156. [CrossRef] [PubMed]
55. Steluti, J.; Selhub, J.; Paul, L.; Reginaldo, C.; Fisberg, R.M.; Marchioni, D.M.L. An overview of folate status in a population-based study from São Paulo, Brazil, and the potential impact of 10 years of national folic acid fortification policy. *Eur. J. Clin. Nutr.* **2017**, *71*, 1173–1178. [CrossRef]
56. Ministry of Health of Brazil. Secretariat of Health Care. Primary Health Care Department. *Dietary Guidelines for the Brazilian Population*; Ministry of Health of Brazil, Secretariat of Health Care: Brasília, Brazil, 2015.
57. The World Bank. Rural Population (% of Total Population)—Brazil. 2018. Available online: https://data.worldbank.org/indicator/SP.RUR.TOTL.ZS?locations=BR (accessed on 12 December 2023).

nutrients

MDPI

Article

Trends in Calcium Intake among the US Population: Results from the NHANES (1999–2018)

Zhongyi Yu [1,†], Yaqi Li [1,†], Djibril M. Ba [2], Susan J. Veldheer [3], Liang Sun [1], Tingting Geng [4,*] and Xiang Gao [1,*]

1 Department of Nutrition and Food Hygiene, Institute of Nutrition, School of Public Health, Fudan University, Shanghai 200032, China; zhongyi_yu@fudan.edu.cn (Z.Y.); yaqi_li@fudan.edu.cn (Y.L.); sun_liang@fudan.edu.cn (L.S.)

2 Department of Public Health Sciences, Penn State College of Medicine, Hershey, PA 17033, USA; djibrilba@pennstatehealth.psu.edu

3 Department of Family and Community Medicine, Penn State College of Medicine, Hershey, PA 17033, USA; sjv152@psu.edu

4 Department of Epidemiology and Biostatistics, School of Public Health, Tongji Medical College, Huazhong University of Science and Technology, Wuhan 430030, China

* Correspondence: tingting.geng@u.nus.edu (T.G.); xiang_gao@fudan.edu.cn (X.G.)

† These authors contributed equally to this work.

Abstract: Inadequate calcium intake is common in the US. Trends in calcium intake among the US population have been less studied, especially in more recent years. We used data from the National Health and Nutrition Examination Survey (NHANES) 1999–2000 to 2017–2018 to study trends in calcium derived from diet and dietary supplements among the US population aged 2 years, stratified by sex, age group, race, and ethnicity. Among the 80,880 participants included in our study, a substantial portion consistently lacked sufficient calcium intake, even when considering calcium from supplements. Concerning trends were observed over the more recent ten years (2009–2018), with decreased dietary calcium intake and no significant improvement in the prevalence of dietary calcium intake < Estimated Average Requirement (EAR) or the prevalence of taking calcium-containing dietary supplements among them. Decreasing trends in dietary calcium intake were more concerning among men, children, and non-Hispanic Whites. Attention should be given to subgroups with higher calcium intake requirements (e.g., 9–18 years and 60+ years), and subgroups with low levels of dietary calcium and a low prevalence of obtaining calcium from dietary supplements (e.g., the non-Hispanic Black subgroup). Concerning trends of calcium intake were observed among the US population from 2009 to 2018. Tailored guidance on dietary choices and dietary supplement use is required to change consumers' behaviors.

Keywords: calcium; trend; diet; dietary supplement

1. Introduction

Calcium plays a crucial role in many aspects of human health, including the formation and metabolism of bones, the activation of clotting factors, and the regulation of blood pressure and nerve functions [1–6]. Dietary calcium deficiency is a worldwide public health concern [7–11]. In the United States (US), it was reported that 42% of Americans failed to reach their estimated average requirements (EARs) for calcium, based on data from the National Health and Nutrition Examination Survey (NHANES) 2009–2010 [12]. Calcium was classified as one of the four dietary components of public health concern for the general US population [13].

While the insufficient intake of calcium has been emphasized in many previous studies [12–17], the trends of calcium intake and hence whether such a concerning situation has been improved are less studied. It was briefly mentioned in Dietary Data Brief No. 13 (2014) (https://www.ncbi.nlm.nih.gov/books/NBK589560/, accessed on 2 May 2023) that the dietary calcium intake among the US population increased to around 85 to 190 mg from 1994 to 2010, but no more detail was reported [12]. Previous reports on the trends observed in the consumption of ultra-processed food [18,19], water and beverages [20–25], and the intake of added sugar [26,27] have suggested changes in dietary choices among the US population over the past two decades. An assessment based on the NHANES 2003–2006 showed that dietary supplement use among the US population was not sufficient in helping them meet their recommended calcium intake levels [17]. Previous studies suggested that the prevalence of dietary supplement use among the US population increased from 1986 to 2018 [28–30]. Supplemental calcium intake was reported to increase from 1999 to 2007–2010 with a subsequent decrease until 2014, but the evaluation did not include supplemental and dietary intake together [31]. Consequently, it was unclear how many individuals with insufficient dietary calcium intake used supplements.

To address these research gaps, we aimed to assess the trends in calcium intake, with and without dietary supplements, over 20 years from 1999–2000 to 2017–2018 in the US population, using data from the NHANES. Data on such past trends among the population and subgroups of particular interest would be a critical prerequisite for policymakers to make scientific and successful communication strategies that could lead to behavioral changes to move toward healthier dietary patterns.

2. Materials and Methods

2.1. Data Source and Study Population

The NHANES is a repetitive cross-sectional survey with a complex, multistage probability sample design. It is conducted by the National Center for Health Statistics (NCHS) to obtain health-related information about the civilian, noninstitutionalized population in the US. Details of the study design, protocol, and data collection were described elsewhere [32]. The protocols were approved by the NCHS Ethics Review Board. For individuals aged 2–17 years old, parental/guardian written informed consent was obtained [33–35].

In the current study, we included individuals aged two years or older who had complete and valid data on the first-day 24-hour dietary recall during the ten cycles of the NHANES between 1999–2000 and 2017–2018. Previous studies showed disparity in dietary patterns by sex, age, race, and ethnicity [14,36–39]. Therefore, the potential differences in dietary patterns among subpopulations with different sociodemographic factors were investigated. To allow for tailored communication strategies, we examined the data overall and by age group, sex, race, and ethnicity. Considering that different dietary recommendations are given to people at different life stages, we defined the age groups according to *Dietary Guidelines for Americans 2020–2025* [13], with modification: Children aged 2–18 years old were divided into the age groups of 2–8 years old and 9–18 years old according to previous studies [26,40]. This resulted in four age groups: children aged 2–8 years old, children aged 9–18 years old, adults aged 19–59 years old, and older adults aged 60 years old or above. To reduce the impact of extreme records, the 82,534 sample persons were divided into eight subgroups by sex and age group. The top and bottom 1% for energy intake among each of the subgroups were further excluded from this study, resulting in 80,880 sample persons in total. The overall response rate was 86.2% (see Figure A1).

2.2. Dietary Calcium Intake Assessment

Dietary intake data and data on the calcium derived from individual foods were obtained from the 24 h dietary recall survey data "Dietary Interview—Individual Foods". For survey cycles from 2003–2004 to 2017–2018, when two 24-h dietary recalls were performed, only the first day's 24-h dietary recall data was included in this study to keep data consistent across all survey cycles [19,41,42]. Each sample person was assigned his/her EAR, recommended dietary allowance (RDA), and tolerable upper intake level (UL), based on his/her sex, age, and pregnancy and lactation status, according to dietary reference intakes (DRIs) determined by Institute of Medicine of the National Academies [43] (see

Table A1). Only sample persons clearly self-reported to be pregnant or breastfeeding a child were assigned pregnant/lactating DRIs. Those whose responses were reported as "refused", "don't know" or "missing" were assumed to be not pregnant/breastfeeding. The dietary and total calcium intake of each sample person was compared with his/her DRIs to classify the sample person's diet as "<EAR", "≥EAR, <RDA", "≥RDA, ≤UL", or ">UL". Seven subpopulations with different DRIs were defined based on age and sex: children aged 2–3 years old, 4–8 years old, and 9–18 years old; adults aged 19–50 years old; men aged 51–70 years old; men aged above 70 years old; and women aged above 50 years old.

2.3. Dietary Supplementation of Calcium

Each sample person was asked to report any dietary supplement taken within the last 30 days. For each dietary supplement reported, its ingredient list was screened for the keyword "calcium". Any supplement with any ingredient name with "calcium" (e.g., calcium, calcium phosphate, etc.) was considered a calcium-containing dietary supplement. This was then used to identify sample persons whose dietary calcium intake did not reach their EARs and who did not take calcium-containing supplements ("<EAR, no supplement" group).

From the 2007–2008 survey cycle and onward, data were available on the total calcium derived from dietary supplements on the day of the 24 h dietary recall. The total calcium intake (dietary and dietary supplement) was calculated and compared to DRIs to identify populations whose calcium intake was still insufficient, as well as those exceeding their ULs.

2.4. Statistical Analysis

All analyses were conducted according to the NHANES analytical guidelines, which include sampling weights, stratification, and clustering, to account for the complex NHANES sampling design and ensure nationally representative estimates [18–20,44]. For each survey cycle, the weighted percentage of the population falling into different categories (such as the categories established by comparing their intake with their DRIs) with 95% confidence intervals were calculated using Proc Surveyfreq (SAS Institute). The weighted mean daily calcium intake, quartiles, and their respective 95% confidence intervals were calculated using Proc Surveymeans (SAS Institute). The absolute difference was calculated by comparing the weighted mean daily calcium intake from 1999–2000 to 2017–2018. The p values for trends were estimated by making the survey cycle a continuous variable and testing it with a linear regression model using Proc Surveyreg (SAS Institute). The speed of the increasing/decreasing trend of calcium intake was presented using the point estimate with 95% confidence intervals of the coefficient of the linear regression and converted to mg/10 years. Day-one dietary sample weight was used for calculating the weighted mean calcium intake and the proportions of the population of each survey cycle. Appropriate weights for the combined NHANES survey cycles were used based on the NHANES analytic guidelines to calculate p values for trends over multiple survey cycles [45].

All analyses were conducted with SAS version 9.4 (SAS Institute Inc., Cary, NC, USA), and two-tailed $p < 0.05$ was considered statistically significant. Given the potential for type I error due to multiple comparisons, outcomes for stratified analyses should be interpreted as exploratory.

3. Results

After excluding 11,325 participants without valid first-day 24 h dietary recall and 1654 participants with extreme energy intake (those falling under the top and bottom 1% energy intake within each sex and age group), data from a total of 80,880 individuals were analyzed. There were 12,768 participants aged 2–8 years old, 19,196 aged 9–18 years old, 34,043 aged 19–59 years old, and 16,527 aged 60 years or above. Details of the unweighted sample sizes in each survey cycle and among each subgroup are listed in Table 1 and Figure A1.

3.1. Dietary Calcium Intake

The mean daily dietary calcium intake increased from 848 ± 28.6 mg/d in 1999–2000 to 1022 ± 13.7 mg/d in 2009–2010 but then slightly dropped to 966 ± 24.2 mg/d in 2017–2018 (Table 2, Figure 1). Both the increase in 1999–2008 (118 ± 56.4 mg/d·10 years^{-1}) and the decrease in 2009–2018 (−83.2 ± 36.3 mg/d·10 years^{-1}) were statistically significant, with an overall significantly increasing trend observed in the 1999–2018 period (59.0 ± 15.9 mg/d·10 years^{-1}) (Table 3).

When stratified by sex, age group, race, and ethnicity, men, children aged 9–18 years old, non-Hispanic Whites, and Mexican Americans had relatively higher dietary calcium intake. Across the ten survey cycles, women, adults aged 60+ years, and non-Hispanic Blacks consistently exhibited the lowest dietary calcium intake within their demographic subgroups. Among all age groups, adults aged 60+ years experienced the fastest increase in dietary calcium intake during 1999–2008 (136 ± 66.4 mg/d·10 years^{-1}), followed by the slowest decrease in 2009–2018 (−44.9 ± 67.6 mg/d·10 years^{-1}). The most significant decrease in 2009–2018 was observed among children aged 9–18 years (−135 ± 91.0 mg/d·10 years^{-1}), followed by children aged 2–8 years (−130 ± 61.0 mg/d·10 years^{-1}). From 1999 to 2008, the increase in dietary calcium intake was most significant among other Hispanic (183 ± 85.8 mg/d·10 years^{-1}) and non-Hispanic Black (182 ± 57.9 mg/d·10 years^{-1}) groups, followed by Mexican American (105 ± 73.9 mg/d·10 years^{-1}) and non-Hispanic White (104 ± 77.3 mg/d·10 years^{-1}) populations. A similar but not statistically significant increase was observed in other races and ethnicities (123 ± 175 mg/d·10 years^{-1}). From 2009 to 2018, a significant decrease in dietary calcium intake was only observed among non-Hispanic Whites (−111 ± 46.2 mg/d·10 years^{-1}) across all the races and ethnicities tested.

3.2. Proportion with Insufficient or Excessive Dietary Calcium Intake

From 1999 to 2018, the proportion of the US population (≥2 years old) not reaching their calcium EAR with their diet dropped from 60.1 ± 3.45% in 1999–2000 to 48.1 ± 2.60% in 2009–2010 but then remained stable until 49.8 ± 2.60% in 2017–2018 (Figure 1, for detailed data, see Table S1A). Similar trends were observed among most subpopulations when stratified by sex, age group, race, and ethnicity. Women, children aged 9–18 years old, adults aged 60+ years old, other Hispanics, non-Hispanic Blacks, and other races and ethnicities consistently had over 50% of the subpopulation with insufficient dietary calcium intake over the ten survey cycles tested. We did not observe notable improvement in the prevalence of dietary calcium less than EARs in any strata tested (by sex, age group, race, and ethnicity) since 2009–2010 (Table S1A). A small proportion of the population had dietary calcium above UL, fluctuating from 1.34 ± 0.35% in 1999–2000 to 3.48 ± 0.83% in 2009–2010, then to 2.54 ± 0.67% in 2017–2018. The quartiles of dietary calcium intake among subpopulations with different DRIs are presented in Figure A2, according to which children aged 9–18 years old, men aged above 70 years old, and women aged above 50 years old consistently had median dietary calcium intake below their EARs.

Among those whose dietary calcium intake failed to reach their EARs, the proportion of those with any calcium-containing dietary supplement taken within the past 30 days slightly increased from 37.0 ± 3.91% in 1999–2000 to 43.7 ± 2.79% in 2005–2006 but then declined to 33.3 ± 2.39% in 2017–2018 (Table S1B). This prevalence was lower among men, children aged 2–8 years old and 9–18 years old, Mexican Americans, other Hispanics, and non-Hispanic Blacks. Men, adults aged 60+ years, and non-Hispanic Whites consistently had the highest rate of dietary supplement use within their demographic subgroups.

Table 1. Demographic overview of the sample persons included.

Characteristics	No. of Participants (Weighted %) by NHANES Cycle [a]									
	1999–2000 (*n* = 7878)	2001–2002 (*n* = 8855)	2003–2004 (*n* = 8099)	2005–2006 (*n* = 8380)	2007–2008 (*n* = 8381)	2009–2010 (*n* = 8922)	2011–2012 (*n* = 7808)	2013–2014 (*n* = 7879)	2015–2016 (*n* = 7738)	2017–2018 (*n* = 6940)
Sex										
Men	3828 (48.6%)	4288 (48.7%)	3955 (49.1%)	4065 (48.8%)	4207 (47.9%)	4436 (48.7%)	3920 (49.4%)	3843 (49.3%)	3790 (48.7%)	3383 (48.7%)
Women	4050 (51.4%)	4567 (51.3%)	4144 (50.9%)	4315 (51.2%)	4174 (52.1%)	4486 (51.3%)	3888 (50.6%)	4036 (50.7%)	3948 (51.3%)	3557 (51.3%)
Age Group										
2–8 years	1113 (11.1%)	1399 (10.1%)	1175 (9.66%)	1372 (9.82%)	1379 (9.91%)	1419 (9.76%)	1415 (10.0%)	1189 (9.10%)	1157 (9.13%)	894 (8.90%)
9–18 years	2387 (14.7%)	2562 (15.3%)	2303 (15.0%)	2326 (14.6%)	1533 (14.1%)	1670 (14.2%)	1524 (13.3%)	1644 (13.8%)	1544 (13.6%)	1319 (13.6%)
19–59 years	2873 (57.6%)	3400 (58.8%)	2987 (57.5%)	3306 (57.4%)	3553 (58.4%)	3958 (57.6%)	3390 (57.4%)	3530 (57.0%)	3395 (56.0%)	2969 (55.4%)
≥60 years	1505 (16.6%)	1494 (15.8%)	1634 (17.9%)	1376 (18.2%)	1916 (17.6%)	1875 (18.5%)	1479 (19.4%)	1516 (20.1%)	1642 (21.2%)	1758 (22.1%)
Race and Ethnicity										
Mexican American	2665 (7.60%)	2218 (8.47%)	1985 (8.95%)	2204 (9.35%)	1686 (9.59%)	1941 (9.90%)	1052 (9.70%)	1334 (10.8%)	1468 (10.7%)	1011 (11.0%)
Other Hispanic	467 (7.58%)	398 (5.72%)	257 (3.30%)	269 (2.91%)	970 (5.37%)	945 (5.59%)	809 (6.66%)	745 (5.95%)	1007 (6.71%)	587 (6.88%)
Non-Hispanic White	2686 (67.9%)	3770 (69.5%)	3402 (70.5%)	3294 (69.6%)	3490 (67.7%)	3847 (65.9%)	2495 (63.3%)	2985 (62.8%)	2495 (61.3%)	2423 (59.3%)
Non-Hispanic Black	1784 (11.6%)	2133 (11.6%)	2119 (12.0%)	2207 (12.2%)	1878 (12.0%)	1657 (12.0%)	2167 (12.4%)	1697 (11.8%)	1653 (11.6%)	1600 (11.6%)
Other race or ethnicity [b]	276 (5.39%)	336 (4.68%)	336 (5.17%)	406 (5.89%)	357 (5.34%)	532 (6.63%)	1285 (7.94%)	1118 (8.69%)	1115 (9.74%)	1319 (11.2%)
Pregnancy [c]										
Pregnant	244 (5.58%)	261 (4.65%)	223 (4.76%)	315 (5.47%)	46 (2.25%)	48 (2.94%)	36 (2.15%)	43 (2.59%)	48 (3.06%)	38 (2.64%)
Not pregnant	492 (36.2%)	625 (39.7%)	675 (47.1%)	781 (50.3%)	702 (37.6%)	741 (35.2%)	542 (32.8%)	631 (35.6%)	621 (36.9%)	577 (39.2%)
Refused, do not know, or missing	1241 (58.2%)	1343 (55.7%)	1057 (48.1%)	1072 (44.2%)	1035 (60.1%)	1252 (61.9%)	1092 (65.1%)	1216 (61.8%)	1106 (60.1%)	898 (58.2%)
Lactation [c]										
Currently breastfeeding	42 (1.60%)	61 (2.74%)	50 (2.45%)	49 (2.23%)	30 (1.65%)	32 (1.11%)	21 (1.58%)	40 (2.73%)	41 (2.36%)	38 (2.65%)
Not breastfeeding	155 (7.28%)	175 (6.54%)	115 (4.79%)	162 (6.12%)	99 (4.95%)	113 (5.01%)	69 (3.27%)	101 (6.87%)	118 (7.36%)	102 (8.80%)
Refused, do not know, or missing	1780 (91.1%)	1993 (90.7%)	1790 (92.8%)	1957 (91.6%)	1654 (93.4%)	1896 (93.9%)	1580 (95.2%)	1749 (90.4%)	1616 (90.3%)	1373 (88.6%)

Abbreviations: NHANES, National Health and Nutrition Examination Survey. [a] Percentages were adjusted for NHANES weights to generate nationally representative percentages; [b] included multiracial/ethnic groups; [c] among women aged 14 to 50 years.

Table 2. Mean daily calcium intake among the US population, from 1999–2000 to 2017–2018.

	Mean Daily Dietary Calcium Intake (mg/d), (95% CI)									
	1999–2000	2001–2002	2003–2004	2005–2006	2007–2008	2009–2010	2011–2012	2013–2014	2015–2016	2017–2018
Total Diet										
Men	948 (919, 977)	1019 (977, 1061)	1024 (986, 1062)	1056 (1022, 1089)	1041 (996, 1085)	1141 (1116, 1165)	1135 (1093, 1177)	1091 (1066, 1116)	1060 (1024, 1096)	1079 (1044, 1114)
Women	753 (723, 782)	782 (755, 810)	804 (771, 837)	862 (824, 900)	843 (796, 890)	910 (896, 925)	888 (863, 913)	858 (837, 879)	856 (820, 891)	860 (834, 886)
2–8 years old	845 (791, 898)	950 (909, 991)	999 (938, 1061)	951 (913, 988)	951 (906, 995)	1022 (981, 1064)	1033 (989, 1076)	998 (943, 1052)	936 (896, 976)	941 (909, 973)
9–18 years old	902 (857, 947)	988 (920, 1057)	1028 (951, 1106)	999 (932, 1066)	989 (934, 1044)	1081 (1020, 1141)	1084 (1031, 1137)	1037 (987, 1088)	1012 (946, 1077)	981 (929, 1033)
19–59 years old	869 (834, 903)	910 (868, 952)	914 (874, 954)	987 (943, 1030)	961 (909, 1012)	1049 (1027, 1072)	1032 (996, 1068)	988 (959, 1016)	990 (951, 1029)	1005 (975, 1034)
≥60 years old	728 (689, 767)	730 (695, 765)	762 (728, 795)	831 (787, 876)	813 (768, 858)	894 (864, 925)	883 (835, 931)	876 (847, 905)	835 (784, 887)	872 (826, 918)
Mexican American	825 (793, 857)	920 (872, 967)	957 (885, 1029)	954 (913, 995)	925 (879, 971)	998 (951, 1046)	1098 (1050, 1145)	1038 (976, 1099)	986 (961, 1012)	1022 (985, 1059)
Other Hispanic	805 (740, 870)	842 (785, 899)	785 (714, 855)	875 (776, 975)	969 (933, 1006)	960 (922, 999)	955 (912, 998)	955 (900, 1011)	936 (873, 998)	951 (866, 1036)
Non-Hispanic White	894 (848, 941)	947 (906, 988)	955 (923, 986)	1001 (959, 1042)	972 (920, 1025)	1073 (1046, 1100)	1048 (1018, 1079)	1007 (980, 1034)	995 (957, 1032)	989 (961, 1017)
Non-Hispanic Black	666 (637, 695)	687 (658, 716)	716 (674, 759)	789 (752, 826)	796 (757, 836)	858 (825, 892)	860 (811, 908)	829 (793, 865)	794 (751, 837)	849 (816, 882)
Other race or ethnicity	740 (592, 888)	714 (649, 779)	791 (672, 910)	826 (763, 889)	809 (743, 875)	905 (846, 965)	877 (833, 921)	854 (812, 895)	879 (816, 942)	922 (867, 976)
Overall	848 (819, 876)	898 (868, 928)	912 (879, 945)	957 (923, 990)	938 (896, 980)	1022 (1009, 1036)	1010 (982, 1038)	973 (953, 993)	955 (920, 991)	966 (942, 991)
Diet and Dietary Supplements										
Men	NA *	NA *	NA *	NA *	1123 (1071, 1175)	1223 (1196, 1250)	1206 (1160, 1252)	1166 (1133, 1199)	1130 (1090, 1169)	1135 (1097, 1173)
Women	NA *	NA *	NA *	NA *	1042 (976, 1109)	1101 (1085, 1118)	1048 (1005, 1091)	1025 (996, 1055)	994 (945, 1042)	991 (960, 1021)
2–8 years old	NA *	NA *	NA *	NA *	965 (919, 1010)	1041 (995, 1087)	1044 (1000, 1087)	1008 (952, 1064)	943 (902, 984)	945 (914, 977)
9–18 years old	NA *	NA *	NA *	NA *	1019 (961, 1077)	1105 (1044, 1166)	1103 (1052, 1153)	1056 (1005, 1106)	1026 (956, 1096)	994 (940, 1047)
19–59 years old	NA *	NA *	NA *	NA *	1098 (1035, 1161)	1177 (1152, 1203)	1134 (1085, 1183)	1099 (1065, 1133)	1077 (1036, 1118)	1086 (1052, 1120)
≥60 years old	NA *	NA *	NA *	NA *	1139 (1055, 1223)	1214 (1179, 1249)	1161 (1107, 1215)	1148 (1107, 1189)	1088 (1019, 1156)	1086 (1030, 1141)
Mexican American	NA *	NA *	NA *	NA *	975 (930, 1021)	1051 (1001, 1101)	1141 (1090, 1192)	1078 (1013, 1144)	1032 (1010, 1053)	1064 (1020, 1108)
Other Hispanic	NA *	NA *	NA *	NA *	1038 (996, 1080)	1040 (993, 1087)	1028 (983, 1073)	1007 (950, 1063)	985 (915, 1056)	1011 (930, 1092)
Non-Hispanic White	NA *	NA *	NA *	NA *	1151 (1080, 1223)	1244 (1214, 1273)	1191 (1151, 1232)	1162 (1129, 1195)	1126 (1082, 1169)	1106 (1079, 1134)
Non-Hispanic Black	NA *	NA *	NA *	NA *	865 (828, 902)	930 (886, 974)	928 (873, 983)	893 (857, 930)	843 (802, 884)	899 (864, 935)
Other race or ethnicity	NA *	NA *	NA *	NA *	911 (831, 991)	1014 (944, 1084)	977 (934, 1021)	963 (920, 1007)	987 (919, 1055)	1014 (955, 1073)
Overall	NA *	NA *	NA*	NA *	1081 (1026, 1136)	1160 (1144, 1177)	1126 (1087, 1165)	1095 (1068, 1121)	1060 (1016, 1103)	1061 (1035, 1086)

Abbreviations: CI, confidence interval; NA, not applicable. The population might contain individuals with different dietary reference intake levels. * Data on calcium derived from dietary supplements was not collected.

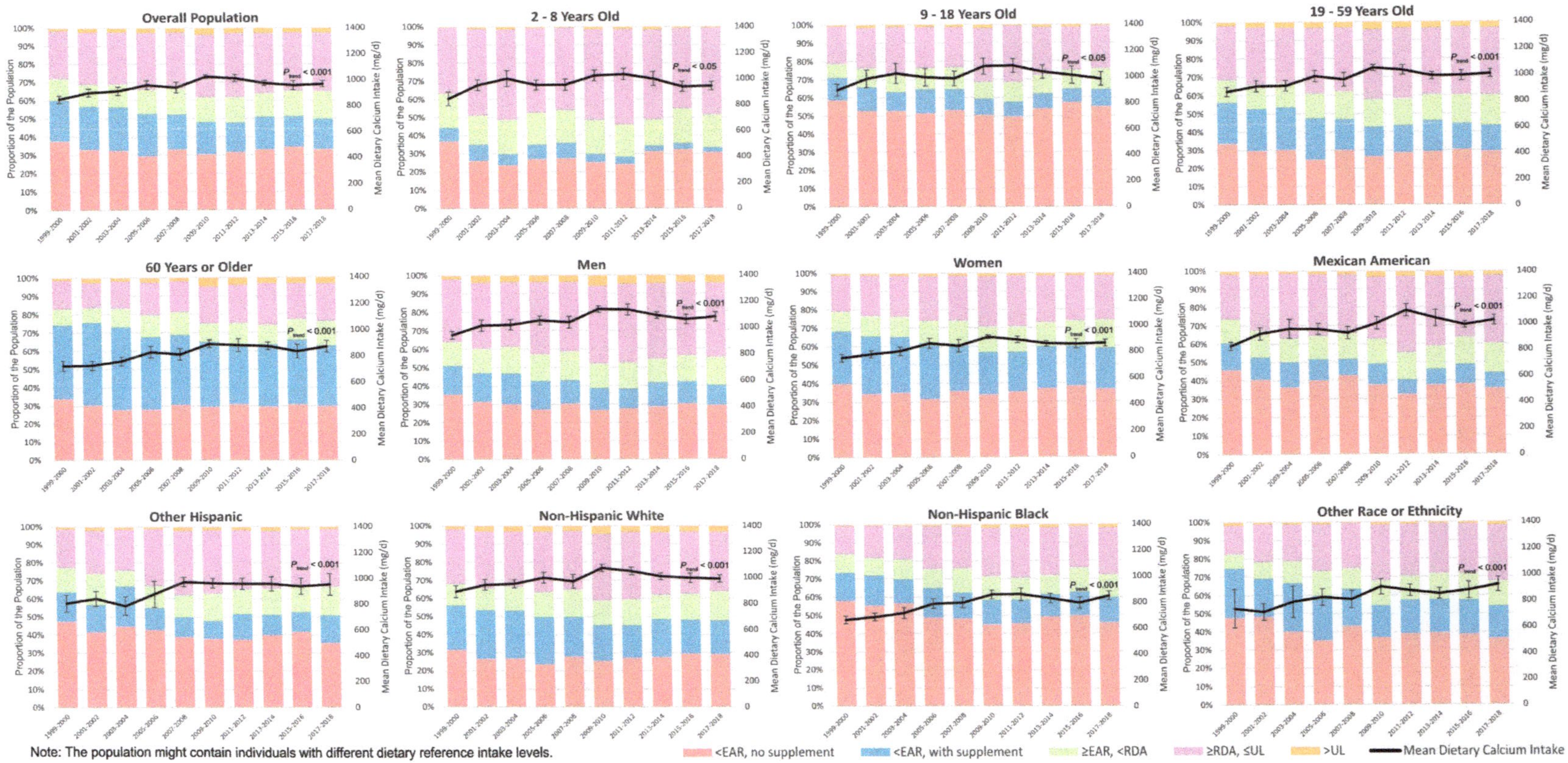

Figure 1. Dietary calcium intake and its distribution across DRIs among the US population, from 1999–2000 to 2017–2018.

Table 3. Trends of calcium intake among the US population.

	From 1999–2000 to 2017–2018		From 1999–2000 to 2007–2008		From 2009–2010 to 2017–2018	
	Coefficient Estimate (mg/d·10 years^{-1})	*p* for Trend	Coefficient Estimate (mg/d·10 years^{-1})	*p* for Trend	Coefficient Estimate (mg/d·10 years^{-1})	*p* for Trend
Total Diet						
Men	62.5 (43.5, 81.5)	<0.001	110 (49.7, 170)	<0.001	−99.0 (−152, −46.5)	<0.001
Women	55.2 (38.8, 71.7)	<0.001	129 (67.5, 190)	<0.001	−66.6 (−104, −29.6)	<0.001
2–8 years old	34.7 (8.23, 61.2)	<0.05	108 (28.6, 188)	<0.01	−130 (−191, −69.3)	<0.001
9–18 years old	36.7 (4.46, 68.8)	<0.05	90.5 (3.97, 177)	<0.05	−135 (−226, −44.1)	<0.01
19–59 years old	70.5 (50.8, 90.3)	<0.001	129 (59.3, 199)	<0.001	−65.5 (−112, −19.5)	<0.01
≥60 years old	80.1 (56.5, 104)	<0.001	136 (69.3, 202)	<0.001	−44.9 (−113, 22.7)	0.19
Mexican American	88.1 (61.3, 115)	<0.001	105 (30.9, 179)	<0.01	−33.5 (−113, 45.6)	0.40
Other Hispanic	84.9 (42.9, 127)	<0.001	183 (97.6, 269)	<0.001	−18.9 (−123.0, 85)	0.72
Non-Hispanic White	51.0 (30.3, 71.7)	<0.001	104 (26.4, 181)	<0.01	−111 (−157, −64.8)	<0.001
Non-Hispanic Black	95.8 (75.4, 116)	<0.001	182 (124, 240)	<0.001	−42.6 (−100, 15.3)	0.15
Other race or ethnicity	95.3 (47.5, 143)	<0.001	123 (−51.9, 299)	0.16	31.3 (−57.4, 120)	0.48
Overall	59.0 (43.1, 75.0)	<0.001	118 (61.9, 175)	<0.001	−83.2 (−119, −46.9)	<0.001
Diet and Dietary Supplements						
Men	NA *	NA *	NA *	NA *	−126 (−182, −69.9)	<0.001
Women	NA *	NA *	NA *	NA *	−137 (−184, −89.8)	<0.001
2–8 years old	NA *	NA *	NA *	NA *	−147 (−210, −83.2)	<0.001
9–18 years old	NA *	NA *	NA *	NA *	−150 (−242, −57.4)	<0.01
19–59 years old	NA *	NA *	NA *	NA *	−120 (−173, −66.2)	<0.001
≥60 years old	NA *	NA *	NA *	NA *	−163 (−244, −82.4)	<0.001
Mexican American	NA *	NA *	NA *	NA *	−42.1 (−126, 42.0)	0.32
Other Hispanic	NA *	NA *	NA *	NA *	−48.6 (−152, 54.9)	0.35
Non-Hispanic White	NA *	NA *	NA *	NA *	−170 (−220, −121)	<0.001
Non-Hispanic Black	NA *	NA *	NA *	NA *	−73.8 (−142, −5.81)	<0.05
Other race or ethnicity	NA *	NA *	NA *	NA *	17.7 (−80.7, 116)	0.72
Overall	NA *	NA *	NA *	NA *	−132 (−175, −90.0)	<0.001

Abbreviation: NA, not applicable. The population might contain individuals with different dietary reference intake levels. * Results not available due to absence of data on calcium derived from dietary supplement from 1999–2000 to 2005–2006.

3.3. Total Daily Calcium Intake

When the calcium intakes derived from diet and dietary supplements on the same day were combined (from 2007–2008 to 2017–2018 due to data availability), the overall daily calcium intake increased from 1081 ± 55.3 mg/d in 2007–2008 to 1160 ± 16.5 mg/d in 2009–2010 and then decreased to 1061 ± 25.5 mg/d in 2017–2018 (Table 2). Similar decreasing trends were observed among most strata, with the most significant decrease in 2009–2018 observed among non-Hispanic Whites (−170 ± 49.7 mg/d·10 years^{-1}). Men, adults aged 60+ years, and non-Hispanic Whites consistently had the highest calcium intake, while women, children aged 2–8 years, and non-Hispanic Blacks consistently had the lowest calcium intake among their demographic subgroups. The proportion of the US population whose daily calcium intake did not reach their EARs dropped from 43.7 ± 3.93% in 2007–2008 to 39.7 ± 1.29% in 2009–2010 but then increased again to 44.1 ± 2.45% in 2017–2018 (Figure 2, Table S2). Among the four age groups included in this study, children aged 9–18 years old consistently had the highest proportion with total calcium intake (from diet and dietary supplements) lower than their EARs, followed by adults aged 60+ years. Non-Hispanic Blacks, followed by other races and ethnicities, had the highest proportion of participants with insufficient calcium intake among the four racial groups studied. This proportion was consistently the lowest among men, children aged 2–8 years, and non-Hispanic Whites among all demographic subgroups across the ten survey cycles. The proportion of those who reached their UL fluctuated between 4.69 ± 1.18% in 2015–2016 and 6.99 ± 0.89% in 2009–2010. The quartiles of total calcium intake among subpopulations with different DRIs are presented in Figure A3.

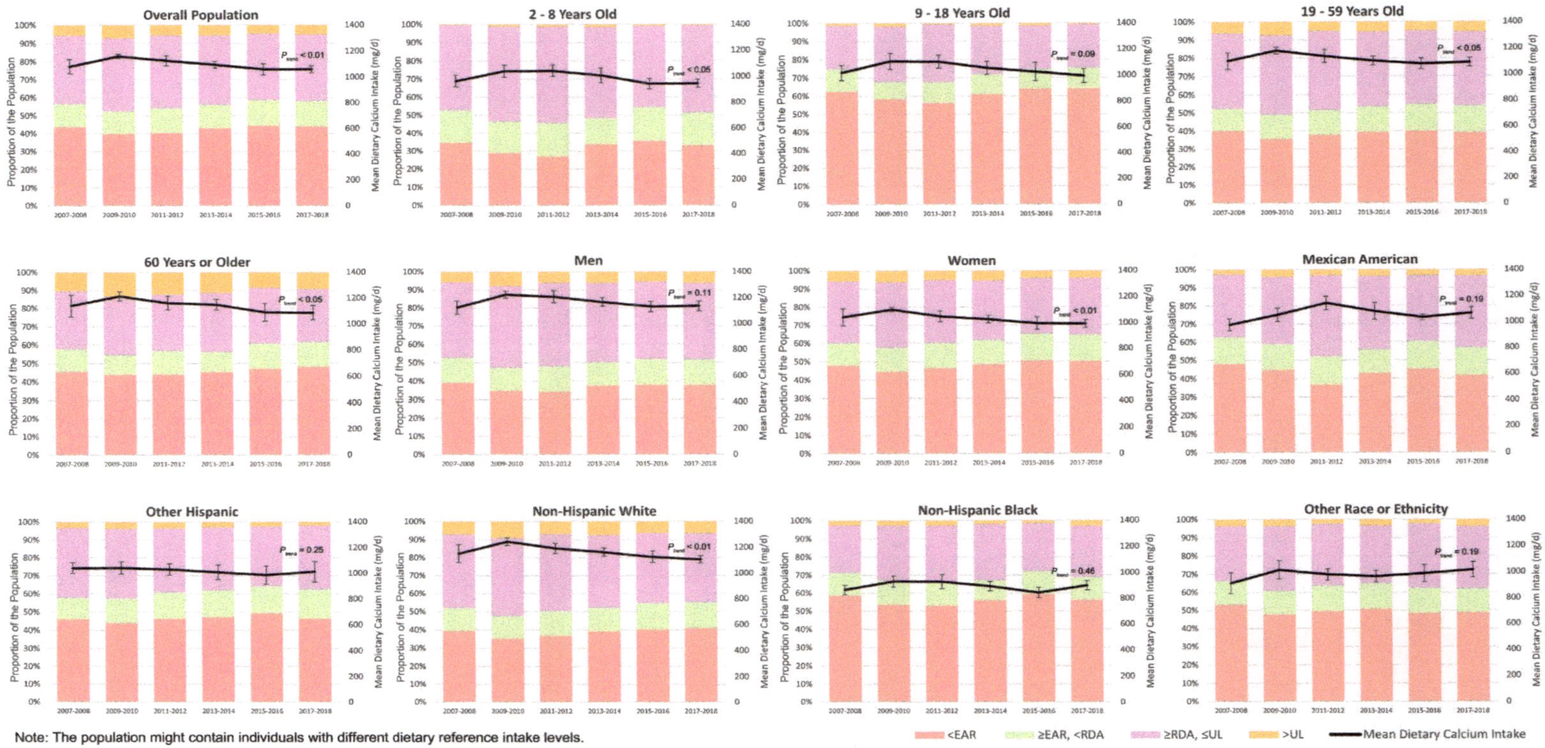

Figure 2. Calcium intake (dietary and supplement) and its distribution across DRIs among the US population, from 2007–2008 to 2017–2018.

4. Discussion

In this nationally representative sample of the US population with data from 1999 to 2018, a consistently large proportion of the population had insufficient dietary calcium intake, even after including the calcium derived from dietary supplements. From 1999 to 2018, the dietary calcium intake level increased but then decreased since it peaked in 2009–2010. The trends observed over the more recent ten-year period (2009–2018) are concerning: (1) no significant improvement was observed in the prevalence of dietary calcium intake < EAR; (2) the mean dietary calcium intake decreased significantly; and (3) no improvement was observed in the prevalence of calcium-containing dietary supplement use among those whose dietary calcium intake failed to reach their EARs.

Similar trends were observed among most of the strata tested (by age groups, sex, race, and ethnicity). The increasing trend from 1999–2000 to 2007–2008 was significant among all the strata tested, except for other races and ethnicities. Compared to men, women had relatively lower dietary calcium intake but were more likely to take calcium-containing dietary supplements when their dietary calcium intake alone was not sufficient for them to meet their EARs. Among the four age groups, the decreasing trends in calcium consumption from 2009 to 2018 were most notable among children (both aged 9–18 years old and 2–8 years old), which should be brought to attention. Although children aged 9–18 years old had relatively higher dietary calcium intake, they had the highest proportion of participants with insufficient calcium intake due to their high calcium requirements and lower rates of calcium-containing dietary supplement use. Adults aged 19–59 years old had the fastest increase from 1999 to 2008 and the slowest decrease from 2009 to 2018. However, this age group still consistently had the lowest dietary calcium intake. This age group also consistently had the highest rate of calcium-containing dietary supplement use, making them the subgroup with the highest values in terms of total calcium intake. However, this subgroup still had the second highest rate of insufficient calcium intake due to their higher EARs.

Non-Hispanic Blacks, followed by other races and ethnicities, consistently had the highest proportion of participants with insufficient calcium intake (from diet and dietary supplements) from 2007 to 2018. Non-Hispanic Blacks not only had low dietary calcium intake but also had a lower proportion of calcium-containing dietary supplement use among those with insufficient dietary calcium intake. Both Mexican Americans and non-Hispanic Whites had relatively higher dietary calcium intake across all racial groups, together with similar increasing rates in 1999–2008. However, dietary calcium intake significantly decreased in 2009–2018 among non-Hispanic Whites but not in other racial groups. Compared to non-Hispanic Whites, Mexican Americans were less likely to obtain additional calcium from dietary supplements when their dietary calcium intake was insufficient, which explained their higher rate of insufficient total calcium intake. Among the racial groups tested, the sharp decrease observed in dietary calcium intake from 2009–2010 to 2017–2018 among non-Hispanic Whites should also be brought to attention.

While concerns regarding calcium deficiency among the US population have been clearly established previously [12–17], the results reported in this study reveal a concerning decline in calcium intake among the US population since the 2009–2010 survey cycle, immediately after an increasing trend was reported according to a previous study [12]. This highlights the urgent need for effective measures to improve the dietary patterns of those who fail to reach their calcium EARs and to encourage the use of calcium-containing dietary supplements among those needed. The stratified analysis revealed different patterns across each demographic subgroup, which helps to identify those subgroups in need of better guidance on their food choices and/or dietary supplement use. This includes subpopulations not making enough effort to fulfill their increased need for calcium at critical life stages (such as children aged 9–18 years old), subpopulations with relatively lower proportions not reaching their EARs but showing concerning trends that need behavior adjustment (such as children aged 2–8 years old), and subpopulations with consistently lower proportion meeting their EARs who need urgent interventions (such as the non-Hispanic Black subgroup). This helps policymakers in making tailored messages and measures for targeted subgroups that might be more successful in changing people's perceptions and behaviors [46–48]. For example, messages given at certain events or places are more likely to reach certain subpopulations of interest. Social media has made it easier to push relevant messages to specific audiences. Calcium intake from diet and dietary supplements might be influenced by multiple factors such as culture, food preferences, health status, family income, education, environment, knowledge of nutrition science, and perception of certain foods and dietary supplements. Further analyses of trends in calcium-rich foods and the influence of potential factors are required to reveal the underlying changes in dietary choices that led to the trends observed in this study. Those who have difficulty in reaching their EARs with dietary calcium intake alone should be identified to support better guidance on dietary supplement use. This would further assist policymakers in understanding consumer food choices and deliver targeted and effective messages to guide different subpopulations. Even though dietary supplements were used by more US residents from 2007 to 2018, we did not observe any improvement in reducing calcium deficiency. Considering the coexistence of excessive calcium intake and supplement use among a small proportion of the population, individuals in this category should be carefully guided on their dietary supplement use to achieve better public health outcomes.

Limitations should be noted when interpreting the results of this study. As a cross-sectional study, the trends reported here could be partially explained by the cohort effect. For example, the generation falling under the 2–8-year-old age group in the 1999–2000 survey cycle would become part of the 19–59-year-old age group in the 2017–2018 survey cycle. Insufficient calcium intake was determined in this study as a calcium intake level that failed to reach the EAR level. It should be emphasized that the EAR level, by definition, reflects the estimated median requirement for a defined group of persons [43]. The mean calcium intake level reported in the subgroup analysis should not be compared with RNIs, as most of the subgroups presented in this study would have mixed RNIs. The subgroup including other races and ethnicities was less represented and was composed of many different races and ethnicities, which made their trends less clearly presented in this study. Considering that this subgroup had the second highest rate of insufficient calcium intake across all race and ethnicity strata, further study is required to identify minor races and ethnicities of concern. This study focused on calcium consumption alone but did not look at the bioavailability of the calcium consumed. Different forms of calcium and other nutrients consumed such as magnesium, phosphate, vitamin D, and casein phosphopeptides could all influence the health outcomes of calcium consumption and should be analyzed and discussed in future studies [49–57].

5. Conclusions

This study provides a nationally representative estimate of the calcium intake level and its sources among the US population aged 2 years or older over a 20-year period (1999 to 2018). A large proportion of the US population had insufficient calcium intake, but trends in more recent years were more concerning. Different trends were observed among certain subgroups, highlighting the need for tailored guidance.

Supplementary Materials: The following supporting information can be downloaded at: https://www.mdpi.com/article/10.3390/nu16050726/s1, Table S1A: Dietary calcium intake distribution (weighted) across DRIs among the US population, from 1999–2000 to 2017–2018; Table S1B: Prevalence of calcium-containing dietary supplement use among the US population with dietary calcium intake lower than their EARs, from 1999–2000 to 2017–2018; Table S2: Dietary and dietary supplement calcium intake distribution (weighted) across DRIs among the US population, from 2007–2008 to 2017–2018.

Author Contributions: Conceptualization, Z.Y. and X.G.; methodology, L.S. and D.M.B.; software, Z.Y. and D.M.B.; validation, Z.Y., Y.L. and S.J.V.; formal analysis, Z.Y.; data curation, Z.Y. and S.J.V.; writing—original draft preparation, Z.Y. and Y.L.; writing—review and editing, Y.L., D.M.B., S.J.V., L.S. and T.G.; visualization, Z.Y.; supervision, T.G. and X.G.; project administration, X.G.; funding acquisition, Y.L, T.G. and X.G. All authors have read and agreed to the published version of the manuscript.

Funding: This research was funded by the Startup Grant at Fudan University, grant numbers JIF201015Y and JIF201018Y. S. Veldheer is funded by the National Center for Advancing Translational Sciences, Grant KL2 TR002015 and Grant UL1 TR002014. The APC was funded by the Startup Grant at Fudan University.

Institutional Review Board Statement: Ethical review and approval were waived for this study because this study was a secondary analysis of public-use data available without personal identifiers. The survey data collected by the NHANES were approved under the NCHS Research Ethics Review Board (ERB), Protocol No 2011-17.

Informed Consent Statement: Informed consent was obtained from all subjects involved in the study.

Data Availability Statement: Publicly available datasets were analyzed in this study. These data can be found here: https://www.cdc.gov/nchs/nhanes/index.htm (accessed on 2 May 2023).

Acknowledgments: We are grateful to all those who contributed to the establishment and development of the NHANES database and all participants who responded to the survey.

Conflicts of Interest: The authors declare no conflicts of interest.

Appendix A

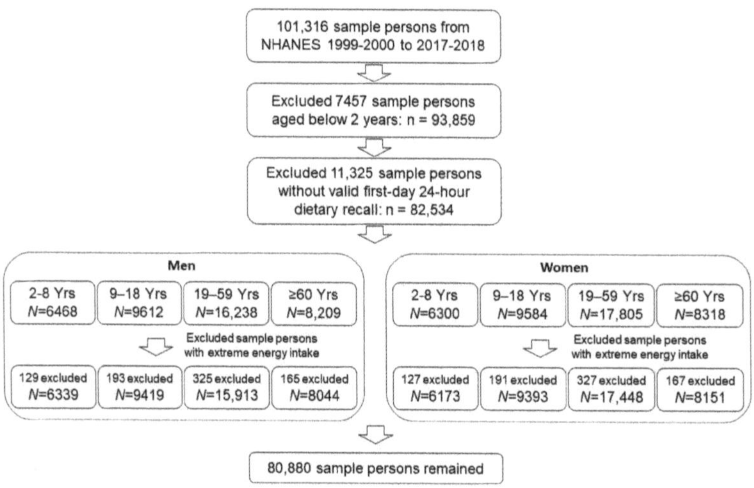

Figure A1. Participant flowchart of the study.

Appendix B

Table A1. Calcium dietary reference intakes (DRIs) by life stage (amount/day).

Life Stage Group	EAR	RDA	UL
2–3 years old	500 mg	700 mg	2500 mg
4–8 years old	800 mg	1000 mg	2500 mg
9–18 years old *	1100 mg	1300 mg	3000 mg
19–50 years old *	800 mg	1000 mg	2500 mg
Men			
51–70 years old	800 mg	1000 mg	2000 mg
>70 years old	1000 mg	1200 mg	2000 mg
Women			
>50 years old	1000 mg	1200 mg	2000 mg

Table A1. *Cont.*

Life Stage Group	EAR	RDA	UL
Pregnancy or Lactation *			
14–18 years old	1100 mg	1300 mg	3000 mg
19–50 years old	800 mg	1000 mg	2500 mg

Abbreviations: EAR, estimated average requirement; RDA, recommended dietary allowance; UL, tolerable upper intake level. * For women who are pregnant or breastfeeding a child, DRIs for pregnancy or lactation are applied.

Appendix C

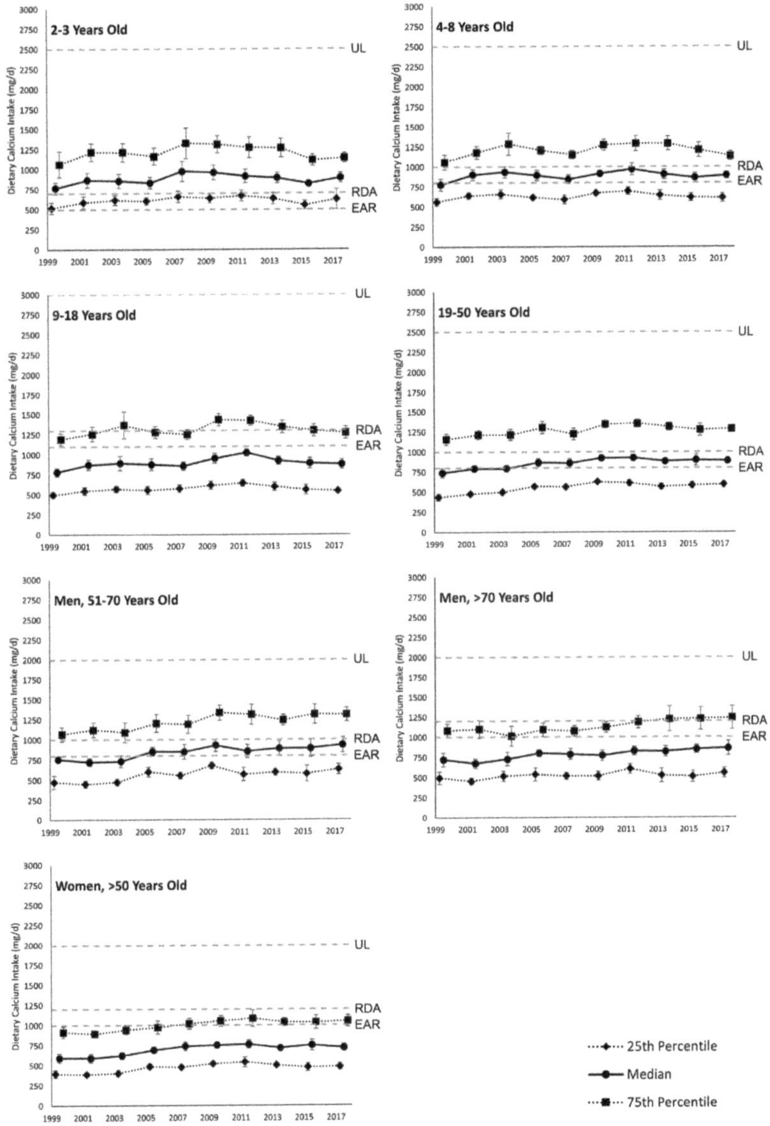

Figure A2. Weighted quartiles of dietary calcium intake among subpopulations with different dietary reference intake levels. Abbreviations: EAR, estimated average requirement; RDA, recommended dietary allowance; UL, tolerable upper intake level.

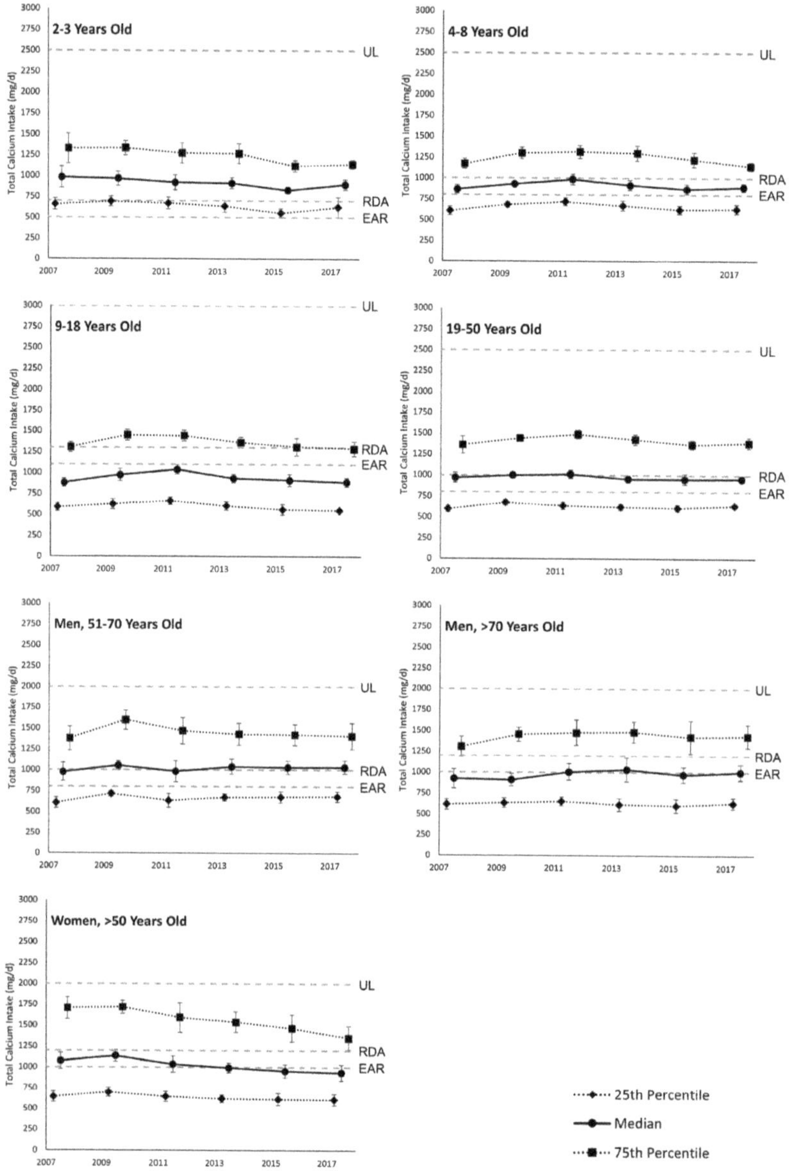

Figure A3. Weighted quartiles of total calcium intake (diet and dietary supplements) among subpopulations with different dietary reference intake levels. Abbreviations: EAR, estimated average requirement; RDA, recommended dietary allowance; UL, tolerable upper intake level.

References

1. Cormick, G.; Belizán, J.M. Calcium intake and health. *Nutrients* **2019**, *11*, 1606. [CrossRef]
2. Yao, P.; Bennett, D.; Mafham, M.; Lin, X.; Chen, Z.; Armitage, J.; Clarke, R. Vitamin D and calcium for the prevention of fracture: A systematic review and meta-analysis. *JAMA Netw. Open* **2019**, *2*, e1917789. [CrossRef] [PubMed]
3. Rizzoli, R.; Biver, E.; Brennan-Speranza, T.C. Nutritional intake and bone health. *Lancet Diabetes Endocrinol.* **2021**, *9*, 606–621. [CrossRef] [PubMed]
4. Shen, X.; Gu, X.; Liu, Y.-Y.; Yang, L.; Zheng, M.; Jiang, L. Association between dietary calcium and depression among American adults: National health and nutrition examination survey. *Front. Nutr.* **2023**, *10*, 1042522. [CrossRef] [PubMed]

5. Sllamniku Dalipi, Z.; Dragidella, F. Calcium and Vitamin D Supplementation as Non-Surgical Treatment for Periodontal Disease with a Focus on Female Patients: Literature Review. *Dent. J.* **2022**, *10*, 120. [CrossRef] [PubMed]
6. Subramaniam, T.; Fauzi, M.B.; Lokanathan, Y.; Law, J.X. The role of calcium in wound healing. *Int. J. Mol. Sci.* **2021**, *22*, 6486. [CrossRef] [PubMed]
7. Shlisky, J.; Mandlik, R.; Askari, S.; Abrams, S.; Belizan, J.M.; Bourassa, M.W.; Cormick, G.; Driller-Colangelo, A.; Gomes, F.; Khadilkar, A.; et al. Calcium deficiency worldwide: Prevalence of inadequate intakes and associated health outcomes. *Ann. N. Y. Acad. Sci.* **2022**, *1512*, 10–28. [CrossRef] [PubMed]
8. Fleming, K.H.; Heimbach, J.T. Consumption of calcium in the US: Food sources and intake levels. *J. Nutr.* **1994**, *124*, 1426S–1430S. [CrossRef] [PubMed]
9. Ajong, A.B.; Kenfack, B.; Ali, I.M.; Yakum, M.N.; Ukaogo, P.O.; Mangala, F.N.; Aljerf, L.; Telefo, P.B. Calcium supplementation in pregnancy: An analysis of potential determinants in an under-resourced setting. *PLoS ONE* **2023**, *18*, e0292303. [CrossRef]
10. Sutter, D.O.; Bender, N. Nutrient status and growth in vegan children. *Nutr. Res.* **2021**, *91*, 13–25. [CrossRef]
11. Beal, T.; White, J.M.; Arsenault, J.E.; Okronipa, H.; Hinnouho, G.-M.; Murira, Z.; Torlesse, H.; Garg, A. Micronutrient gaps during the complementary feeding period in South Asia: A Comprehensive Nutrient Gap Assessment. *Nutr. Rev.* **2021**, *79*, 26–34. [CrossRef]
12. Hoy, M.K.; Goldman, J.D. Calcium intake of the US population: What we eat in America, NHANES 2009–2010. In *FSRG Dietary Data Briefs*; United States Department of Agriculture (USDA): Beltsville, MD, USA, 2014.
13. U.S. Department of Agriculture; U.S. Department of Health and Human Services. *Dietary Guidelines for Americans, 2020–2025*; U.S. Department of Agriculture: Washington, DC, USA, 2020.
14. Cifelli, C.J.; Fulgoni, K.; Fulgoni, V.L., III; Hess, J.M. Disparity in Dairy Servings Intake by Ethnicity and Age in NHANES 2015–2018. *Curr. Dev. Nutr.* **2023**, *7*, 100010. [CrossRef] [PubMed]
15. Ma, J.; Johns, R.A.; Stafford, R.S. Americans are not meeting current calcium recommendations. *Am. J. Clin. Nutr.* **2007**, *85*, 1361–1366. [CrossRef]
16. Morgan, K.J.; Stampley, G.; Zabik, M.; Fischer, D.R. Magnesium and calcium dietary intakes of the US population. *J. Am. Coll. Nutr.* **1985**, *4*, 195–206. [CrossRef]
17. Mangano, K.M.; Walsh, S.J.; Insogna, K.L.; Kenny, A.M.; Kerstetter, J.E. Calcium intake in the United States from dietary and supplemental sources across adult age groups: New estimates from the National Health and Nutrition Examination Survey 2003–2006. *J. Am. Diet. Assoc.* **2011**, *111*, 687–695. [CrossRef]
18. Juul, F.; Parekh, N.; Martinez-Steele, E.; Monteiro, C.A.; Chang, V.W. Ultra-processed food consumption among US adults from 2001 to 2018. *Am. J. Clin. Nutr.* **2022**, *115*, 211–221. [CrossRef] [PubMed]
19. Wang, L.; Steele, E.M.; Du, M.; Pomeranz, J.L.; O'Connor, L.E.; Herrick, K.A.; Luo, H.; Zhang, X.; Mozaffarian, D.; Zhang, F.F. Trends in consumption of ultraprocessed foods among US youths aged 2–19 years, 1999–2018. *JAMA* **2021**, *326*, 519–530. [CrossRef]
20. Vieux, F.; Maillot, M.; Rehm, C.D.; Barrios, P.; Drewnowski, A. Trends in tap and bottled water consumption among children and adults in the United States: Analyses of NHANES 2011–16 data. *Nutr. J.* **2020**, *19*, 10. [CrossRef] [PubMed]
21. Marriott, B.P.; Hunt, K.J.; Malek, A.M.; Newman, J.C. Trends in intake of energy and total sugar from sugar-sweetened beverages in the United States among children and adults, NHANES 2003–2016. *Nutrients* **2019**, *11*, 2004. [CrossRef]
22. Drewnowski, A.; Rehm, C.D.; Constant, F. Water and beverage consumption among adults in the United States: Cross-sectional study using data from NHANES 2005–2010. *BMC Public Health* **2013**, *13*, 1068. [CrossRef]
23. Drewnowski, A.; Rehm, C.D.; Constant, F. Water and beverage consumption among children age 4–13y in the United States: Analyses of 2005–2010 NHANES data. *Nutr. J.* **2013**, *12*, 85. [CrossRef] [PubMed]
24. Della Corte, K.; Fife, J.; Gardner, A.; Murphy, B.L.; Kleis, L.; Della Corte, D.; Schwingshackl, L.; LeCheminant, J.D.; Buyken, A.E. World trends in sugar-sweetened beverage and dietary sugar intakes in children and adolescents: A systematic review. *Nutr. Rev.* **2021**, *79*, 274–288. [CrossRef] [PubMed]
25. Dai, J.; Soto, M.J.; Dunn, C.G.; Bleich, S.N. Trends and patterns in sugar-sweetened beverage consumption among children and adults by race and/or ethnicity, 2003–2018. *Public Health Nutr.* **2021**, *24*, 2405–2410. [CrossRef] [PubMed]
26. Ricciuto, L.; Fulgoni, V.L., III; Gaine, P.C.; Scott, M.O.; DiFrancesco, L. Trends in added sugars intake and sources among US children, adolescents, and teens using NHANES 2001–2018. *J. Nutr.* **2022**, *152*, 568–578. [CrossRef] [PubMed]
27. DiFrancesco, L.; Fulgoni, V.L., III; Gaine, P.C.; Scott, M.O.; Ricciuto, L. Trends in added sugars intake and sources among US adults using the National Health and Nutrition Examination Survey (NHANES) 2001–2018. *Front. Nutr.* **2022**, *9*, 897952. [CrossRef] [PubMed]
28. Kim, H.J.; Giovannucci, E.; Rosner, B.; Willett, W.C.; Cho, E. Longitudinal and secular trends in dietary supplement use: Nurses' health study and health professionals follow-up study, 1986–2006. *J. Acad. Nutr. Diet.* **2014**, *114*, 436–443. [CrossRef] [PubMed]
29. Kantor, E.D.; Rehm, C.D.; Du, M.; White, E.; Giovannucci, E.L. Trends in dietary supplement use among US adults from 1999–2012. *JAMA* **2016**, *316*, 1464–1474. [CrossRef]
30. Cowan, A.E.; Tooze, J.A.; Gahche, J.J.; Eicher-Miller, H.A.; Guenther, P.M.; Dwyer, J.T.; Potischman, N.; Bhadra, A.; Carroll, R.J.; Bailey, R.L. Trends in overall and micronutrient-containing dietary supplement use in US adults and children, NHANES 2007–2018. *J. Nutr.* **2022**, *152*, 2789–2801. [CrossRef]

31. Rooney, M.R.; Michos, E.D.; Hootman, K.C.; Harnack, L.; Lutsey, P.L. Trends in calcium supplementation, National Health and Nutrition Examination Survey (NHANES) 1999–2014. *Bone* **2018**, *111*, 23–27. [CrossRef]
32. National Center for Health Statistics. About the National Health and Nutrition Examination Survey. Available online: https://www.cdc.gov/nchs/nhanes/about_nhanes.htm (accessed on 2 May 2023).
33. Centers for Disease Control and Prevention. National Health and Nutrition Examination Survey—Survey Participants. Available online: https://www.cdc.gov/nchs/nhanes/participant/participant-confidentiality.htm (accessed on 2 May 2023).
34. Centers for Disease Control and Prevention. National Health and Nutrition Examination Survey—NCHS Ethics Review Board (ERB) Approval. Available online: https://www.cdc.gov/nchs/nhanes/irba98.htm (accessed on 2 May 2023).
35. Centers for Disease Control and Prevention. National Health and Nutrition Examination Survey—Examination Consent. Available online: https://www.cdc.gov/nchs/data/nhanes/nhanes_01_02/nh.cnstbrch.pdf (accessed on 2 May 2023).
36. Millen, B.E.; Quatromoni, P.A.; Gagnon, D.R.; Cupples, L.A.; Franz, M.M.; D'Agostino, R.B. Dietary patterns of men and women suggest targets for health promotion: The Framingham Nutrition Studies. *Am. J. Health Promot.* **1996**, *11*, 42–52. [CrossRef] [PubMed]
37. Rosinger, A.Y.; Patel, A.I.; Weaks, F. Examining recent trends in the racial disparity gap in tap water consumption: NHANES 2011–2018. *Public Health Nutr.* **2022**, *25*, 207–213. [CrossRef]
38. Agarwal, S.; Fulgoni, V.L., III. Association of Pork (All Pork, Fresh Pork and Processed Pork) Consumption with Nutrient Intakes and Adequacy in US Children (Age 2–18 Years) and Adults (Age 19+ Years): NHANES 2011–2018 Analysis. *Nutrients* **2023**, *15*, 2293. [CrossRef]
39. Overcash, F.; Reicks, M. Diet quality and eating practices among Hispanic/Latino men and women: NHANES 2011–2016. *Int. J. Environ. Res. Public Health* **2021**, *18*, 1302. [CrossRef] [PubMed]
40. Qin, Y.; Cifelli, C.J.; Agarwal, S.; Fugoni, V.L. Dairy food consumption is beneficially linked with iodine status in US children and adults: NHANES 2001–2018. *Public Health Nutr.* **2023**, *26*, 1828–1839. [CrossRef]
41. Murakami, K.; Livingstone, M.B.E. Prevalence and characteristics of misreporting of energy intake in US children and adolescents: National Health and Nutrition Examination Survey (NHANES) 2003–2012. *Br. J. Nutr.* **2016**, *115*, 294–304. [CrossRef] [PubMed]
42. Yang, P.; Rooney, M.R.; Wallace, A.S.; Kim, H.; Echouffo-Tcheugui, J.B.; McEvoy, J.W.; Ndumele, C.; Christenson, R.H.; Selvin, E.; Rebholz, C.M. Associations between diet quality and NT-proBNP in US adults, NHANES 1999–2004. *Am. J. Prev. Cardiol.* **2023**, *16*, 100528. [CrossRef] [PubMed]
43. Del Valle, H.B.; Yaktine, A.L.; Taylor, C.L.; Ross, A.C. *Dietary Reference Intakes for Calcium and Vitamin D*; National Academies Press (US): Washington, DC, USA, 2011.
44. Centers for Disease Control and Prevention. SAS Survey Procedure Tips. Available online: https://wwwn.cdc.gov/nchs/nhanes/tutorials/softwaretips.aspx (accessed on 2 May 2023).
45. Centers for Disease Control and Prevention. Weighting. Available online: https://wwwn.cdc.gov/nchs/nhanes/tutorials/Weighting.aspx (accessed on 2 May 2023).
46. Kaptein, M.; De Ruyter, B.; Markopoulos, P.; Aarts, E. Adaptive persuasive systems: A study of tailored persuasive text messages to reduce snacking. *ACM Trans. Interact. Intell. Syst. (TiiS)* **2012**, *2*, 10. [CrossRef]
47. Korda, H.; Itani, Z. Harnessing social media for health promotion and behavior change. *Health Promot. Pract.* **2013**, *14*, 15–23. [CrossRef]
48. Gough, A.; Hunter, R.F.; Ajao, O.; Jurek, A.; McKeown, G.; Hong, J.; Barrett, E.; Ferguson, M.; McElwee, G.; McCarthy, M. Tweet for behavior change: Using social media for the dissemination of public health messages. *JMIR Public Health Surveill.* **2017**, *3*, e6313. [CrossRef]
49. Liu, G.; Sun, S.; Guo, B.; Miao, B.; Luo, Z.; Xia, Z.; Ying, D.; Liu, F.; Guo, B.; Tang, J. Bioactive peptide isolated from casein phosphopeptides promotes calcium uptake in vitro and in vivo. *Food Funct.* **2018**, *9*, 2251–2260. [CrossRef]
50. Rosanoff, A.; Weaver, C.M.; Rude, R.K. Suboptimal magnesium status in the United States: Are the health consequences underestimated? *Nutr. Rev.* **2012**, *70*, 153–164. [CrossRef]
51. Bonjour, J.-P. Calcium and phosphate: A duet of ions playing for bone health. *J. Am. Coll. Nutr.* **2011**, *30*, 438S–448S. [CrossRef] [PubMed]
52. Veldurthy, V.; Wei, R.; Oz, L.; Dhawan, P.; Jeon, Y.H.; Christakos, S. Vitamin D, calcium homeostasis and aging. *Bone Res.* **2016**, *4*, 16041. [CrossRef] [PubMed]
53. Sun, S.; Liu, F.; Liu, G.; Miao, J.; Xiao, H.; Xiao, J.; Qiu, Z.; Luo, Z.; Tang, J.; Cao, Y. Effects of casein phosphopeptides on calcium absorption and metabolism bioactivity in vitro and in vivo. *Food Funct.* **2018**, *9*, 5220–5229. [CrossRef] [PubMed]
54. Liu, G.; Guo, B.; Sun, S.; Luo, M.; Liu, F.; Miao, J.; Tang, J.; Huang, Y.; Cao, Y.; Song, M. Promoting the Calcium-Uptake Bioactivity of Casein Phosphopeptides in vitro and in vivo. *Front. Nutr.* **2021**, *8*, 743791. [CrossRef] [PubMed]
55. Trailokya, A.; Srivastava, A.; Bhole, M.; Zalte, N. Calcium and calcium salts. *J. Assoc. Physicians India* **2017**, *65*, 100–103. [PubMed]
56. Zhang, Y.Y.; Stockmann, R.; Ng, K.; Ajlouni, S. Opportunities for plant-derived enhancers for iron, zinc, and calcium bioavailability: A review. *Compr. Rev. Food Sci. Food Saf.* **2021**, *20*, 652–685. [CrossRef]
57. Shkembi, B.; Huppertz, T. Calcium absorption from food products: Food matrix effects. *Nutrients* **2021**, *14*, 180. [CrossRef]

nutrients

MDPI

Article

Gender Differences in Body Satisfaction Perception: The Role of Nutritional Habits, Psychological Traits, and Physical Activity in a Strength-Training Population

Jorge Jimenez-Morcillo [1] and Vicente Javier Clemente-Suárez [1,2,*]

1 Faculty of Sports Sciences, Universidad Europea de Madrid, Tajo Street, s/n, 28670 Madrid, Spain; jorge.jimenez2@universidadeuropea.es

2 Grupo de Investigación en Cultura, Educación y Sociedad, Universidad de la Costa, Barranquilla 080002, Colombia

* Correspondence: vctxente@yahoo.es

Abstract: The objective of this study is to examine gender disparities in body satisfaction perception, emphasizing the influence of nutritional habits, psychometric assessments, levels of physical activity, and health-related metrics. Employing a sample of 605 strength-trained participants (385 males and 224 females), aged between 20 and 35 years, and regularly engaged in strength training, we conducted a thorough analysis using Google Forms. We evaluated variables including age, anthropometric data, resistance training frequency, food consumption patterns, and psychological profiles. Our findings indicate significant gender-based differences in body satisfaction perception. Females tend to overestimate their muscular size and express heightened concern regarding gluteal shape, while males exhibit a more realistic self-perception, primarily focused on hip width. Dietary patterns also display gender-specific tendencies; females prefer healthier options like vegetables, whereas males consume more milk, fermented products, and carbohydrates. Hydration practices diverge as well, with females showing higher water intake in contrast to males' preference for alcoholic and carbonated beverages. Psychologically, males demonstrate greater extroversion, while females exhibit higher conscientiousness, openness, and a tendency toward negative thoughts and anxiety. Regarding physical activity, females engage in training sessions with greater volume compared to males. This study highlights the intricate interplay of social, cultural, and personal factors shaping gender-specific perceptions of body satisfaction and their subsequent impact on health and lifestyle choices. These insights pave the way for future specialized interventions and research, underscoring the importance of understanding gender-specific nuances to promote healthy body satisfaction and self-perception.

Keywords: body satisfaction; gender differences; nutritional habits; psychological profiles; physical activity; societal norms

1. Introduction

In recent years, there has been a significant increase in the number of people using fitness centers and engaging in physical exercise for both aesthetic and health reasons [1]. Regular exercise is associated with a reduced risk of chronic diseases, such as type 2 diabetes, cardiovascular disease, and some types of cancer [2]. Moreover, the desire to achieve a fit body has become a cultural trend, as indicated by the growing popularity of social media influencers and fitness models [3]. This trend underscores the need for a deeper understanding of body satisfaction perception and its broader implications for strength-trained subjects. The concern for physical appearance and aesthetics is a phenomenon that is increasingly common today. In fact, dissatisfaction with physical appearance and the pursuit of aesthetic perfection can have serious consequences for individuals' health [4]. Body satisfaction plays a crucial role in mental health, contributing to self-esteem and overall well-being [5]. Dissatisfaction with physical appearance, on the other hand, is linked to negative mental health outcomes, including depression, anxiety, and eating disorders [6]. The pursuit of aesthetic perfection, fuelled by societal and media influences, can lead to unhealthy behaviors like excessive exercise or disordered eating [7]. Therefore, promoting a balanced and realistic body image is essential for both physical and mental health in strength-trained subjects [5].

The way people perceive their own bodies is strongly influenced by cultural and societal norms, as well as personal experiences. Negative body satisfaction, which involves a distorted and dissatisfied perception of one's own body, is associated with a variety of negative consequences. including low self-esteem, depression, and disordered eating behaviors [5]. Individuals with eating disorders, such as anorexia nervosa and bulimia nervosa, often have a distorted body satisfaction that leads them to engage in extreme weight loss behaviors, such as restrictive eating. Purging and over-exercising [6] highlight the importance of exploring these perceptions. Our study investigates the nuances of body satisfaction among different genders among strength-trained subjects. In addition, studies have found that poor body satisfaction is a risk factor for the development of disordered eating behaviors, particularly among strength-trained young women [7].

The relationship between body satisfaction and physical activity is complex and bidirectional. Strength-trained individuals who have positive body satisfaction are more likely to engage in physical activity and maintain an active lifestyle [8]. Conversely, regular physical activity can improve body satisfaction and self-esteem, particularly in individuals who engage in exercise for weight control [9]. However, body dissatisfaction and negative body satisfaction can also discourage strength-trained individuals from participating in physical activity, particularly in public or group settings [10]. This bidirectionality forms a crucial aspect of our study's focus. Therefore, interventions that address body satisfaction concerns may be beneficial in promoting physical activity and improving overall health and well-being [6].

Gender-specific nuances in body satisfaction perception form the cornerstone of our research. Research has consistently shown that strength-trained women tend to report more negative body satisfaction than strength-trained men, with higher levels of body dissatisfaction, appearance anxiety, and disordered eating behaviors. This gender difference may be partly explained by the greater emphasis placed on appearance and thinness in female socialization and media representations, as well as by the different sociocultural norms and expectations regarding body size and shape for men and women [11].

In contrast, strength-trained men are not immune to societal pressures concerning body satisfaction. While the idealized male physique has traditionally been associated with muscularity and strength, recent studies have revealed a growing emphasis on muscularity and leanness, indicating a shift in male body ideals [12]. Strength-trained men may encounter distinct challenges and experience body dissatisfaction when they perceive their bodies as falling short of these muscular ideals, potentially leading to behaviors such as excessive exercise or the utilization of anabolic steroids to enhance their physical appearance [13].

To thoroughly investigate gender disparities in body satisfaction, our study delves into the distinct perspectives and concerns of different genders. For strength-trained women, the primary focus of body satisfaction often aligns with societal standards of thinness and beauty, as evidenced by extensive research on the subject [5]. In contrast, strength-trained men's body satisfaction increasingly gravitates towards muscularity, reflecting a different set of societal expectations and norms [6]. Recognizing and dissecting these gender-specific concerns is essential. It allows for the development of targeted interventions and societal reforms aimed at fostering healthier body satisfaction and self-perception for individuals of all genders, thereby addressing the unique challenges each gender faces [14].

The primary objectives of this study were to examine disparities in body satisfaction perception between strength-trained males and females' perceptions based on a range of factors, including nutritional habits, psychometric measurements, physical activity levels, and health-related metrics. Specifically, we seek to elucidate the extent and nature of these disparities, focusing on the different ways strength-trained men and women perceive and react to body satisfaction pressures. We aimed to assess whether there are gender differences in the perception of body satisfaction, with a specific focus on strength-trained women's heightened vigilance toward their own body satisfaction as influenced predominantly by their nutritional consumption habits and specific psychological profile-related behaviors.

Our study is structured to systematically explore how these gender differences in body satisfaction perception, shaped by cultural, social, and personal factors, manifest distinctly in strength-trained men and women in terms of their nutritional habits and mental health-related behaviors. It is posited that strength-trained women may exhibit a greater tendency towards body dissatisfaction linked to socially promoted thinness ideals, impacting their dietary habits and psychological behaviors. Conversely, strength-trained men may experience dissatisfaction primarily related to musculature and strength, influencing their physical exercise practices and the adoption of extreme measures for muscle development. This investigation is pivotal in contributing to a more nuanced understanding of gender-specific body satisfaction perceptions and their impact on health and lifestyle choices.

2. Materials and Methods

In the current study, a total of 605 participants, of whom 385 are male and 224 are female, all engaged in strength training, were interviewed online. During the registration process, survey respondents were required to provide their full names and email addresses. These pieces of information were treated as strictly confidential and handled in accordance with data privacy regulations.

Study participants were invited to complete the survey by accessing a dedicated Google Forms link or scanning a provided QR code. Prior to their engagement in this study, all participants received comprehensive information concerning this research objectives and procedures. The inclusion criteria for this study required that both male and female participants be within the age range of 20 to 35 years and have engaged in strength training with a weekly frequency of 2 to 7 days, continuously for at least 6 months. To ensure the reliability of responses, each participant's submission was verified for consistency and completeness. Moreover, potential biases in responses were assessed through a preliminary analysis, identifying any patterns of skewed or unusual replies. It was explicitly communicated that their participation was entirely voluntary, and they retained the option to withdraw at any point during the study without incurring any penalties or consequences. "In order to participate, individuals were required to provide their digital consent by signing an informed consent form, thereby indicating their full understanding and willingness to participate in this research".

This research adhered to the principles outlined in the Helsinki Declaration (revised in Brazil in 2013) regarding human research ethics. Ethical approval for the study was obtained from the University Ethics Committee (CIPI/18/074), ensuring that this research was conducted in accordance with established ethical guidelines.

Through the Google Forms questionnaire. The following variables were analyzed:

Age and anthropometric variables: Gender, age (years), height (cm), weight (kg), and body mass index (BMI. kg/m^2) were obtained.

Resistance training frequency and intensity: These parameters were evaluated by quantifying weekly training sessions, categorized into aerobic and strength training: The volume of aerobic exercise was measured in minutes of weekly training to quantify strength training intensity. Subjects were asked what percentage of their weekly training was below 50% of their one-repetition maximum (1RM). Between 50% and 70%, between 70% and 85%, and above 85%. Lastly, percentages of 1RM for the back squat, deadlift, and bench press were also recorded.

Food consumption variables: We analyzed a food consumption frequency questionnaire that inquired about the frequency and quantities of various food items (juices 250 mL, water glasses 250 mL, alcoholic beverages 250 mL, fermented beverages 250 mL, soft drinks 250 mL, energy drinks 250 mL, milk glasses 250 mL, fruits 90 g, bakery/sweets 90 g, meat 150 g, fish 150 g, legumes 200 g, pasta or rice 150 g, vegetables 200 g, bread 50 g, fast food 180 g, whole foods 150 g, gel consumption 40 g, muesli bars 150 g, and protein drinks 300 mL). For this purpose, we utilized the European Prospective Investigation into Cancer and Nutrition Food Frequency Questionnaire (EPIC-FFQ), specifically adapted and validated for Spanish populations [15,16].

Nutritional habits: In terms of nutritional habits, measurements were taken for the number of takeout meals, the frequency of dining out, and the days when meals were prepared at home.

Psychological profile: The psychological profile was assessed using various scales and inventories. The Spanish version of the Big Five Inventory [17], with an alpha coefficient of 0.73, was employed to measure the five personality traits: openness to experience. conscientiousness. Extraversion, agreeableness, and neuroticism The reduced version of this inventory consisted of 44 items, with responses rated on a 5-point Likert scale ranging from 1 (completely disagree) to 5 (completely agree).

Anxiety levels were evaluated using the reduced version of the Spanish adaptation of the Spielberger State-Trait Anxiety Inventory, which had an alpha coefficient of 0.93 [18]. This version included 6 items assessing anxiety, with responses rated on a 4-point Likert scale ranging from 1 (not at all) to 4 (very much).

The Spanish version of the Acceptance and Action Questionnaire II [19] was utilized to measure experiential avoidance or psychological inflexibility. This questionnaire consisted of 7 items, with responses rated on a 7-point Likert scale ranging from 0 (never) to 7 (always). The alpha coefficient for this scale was 0.84 (ranging from 0.78 to 0.88).

Loneliness was measured using the Spanish version of the UCLA Loneliness Scale, which had an alpha coefficient of 0.94 [20]. The condensed version of this scale included 3 items, with responses rated on a 3-point Likert scale ranging from 1 (never) to 3 (frequently).

The Spanish version of the ZUNG Depression Scale [21], specifically adapted for assessing depression in the context of the COVID-19 crisis, was utilized. This self-report scale consisted of 20 items formulated in positive and negative terms. It demonstrated an alpha coefficient of 0.09 and had a high sensitivity and specificity of over 80%. The scale encompassed eight items each for somatic and cognitive symptoms, along with two items for mood and two for psychomotor symptoms.

To set differences in body satisfaction perception between strength-trained men and women, the following variables were measured using the eating disorder inventory [22], based on a numeric scale ranging from 1 (never) to 6 (always): satisfaction level with stomach size, muscle size, silhouette, buttock shape, thigh and hip size, body satisfaction, and body weight. Additionally, a scale ranging from 1 to 9 was employed, featuring figures representing different body silhouettes, with 1 being the thinnest and 9 the most voluminous. On this scale, subjects indicated which figure they identified with and which one they considered ideal.

Statistical Analysis

The authors used SPSS version 24.0 (SPSS Inc., Chicago, IL, USA) to conduct their statistical analyses. Descriptive statistics, such as means and standard deviations, were calculated for each variable. The normality and homogeneity of each variable were assessed using Kolmogorov-Smirnov tests. An independent *t*-test was used to analyze the differences in nutrition in the sociodemographic, academic, and psychological variables. The authors set the significance level at $p \leq 0.05$.

3. Results

In the analysis of the obtained results, substantial disparities in participant demographics came to light. Notably, it was evident that strength-trained female participants exhibited a statistically significant higher mean age in comparison to their strength-trained male counterparts. Furthermore, a marked contrast in body weight was observed, with strength-trained male participants displaying a statistically significant higher mean body weight (Table 1).

Table 1. Demographic, education, and employment data.

					95% Confidence Interval of the Difference	
Variable	**Male**	**Female**	**T**	***p***	**Lower**	**Upper**
Age (Years)	25.2 ± 8.6	27.4 ± 9.9	2.895	0.004	−3.79836	−0.72771
Heigh (cm)	145 ± 173.7	171.5 ± 19.0	1.573	0.116	−0.54486	4.92748
Weight (Kg)	76.3 ± 9.3	61.08 ± 10.4	18.241	0.000	13.61358	16.89863
Body Mass Index (Kg/m^2)	31.1 ± 3.5	21.8 ± 3.3	0.930	0.353	−8.73810	24.45937

Regarding nutritional data, it was observed that strength-trained men were more involved in food preparation compared to strength-trained women. Additionally, strength-trained women consumed a higher number of glasses of water daily than strength-trained men. Men, on the other hand, were found to consume more alcohol weekly, along with an increased consumption of soda. Similarly, men reported higher weekly consumption of glasses of milk, fermented foods, pastry sweets, cheese, and eggs compared to women. In terms of weekly food consumption, men reported higher consumption of processed meat, rice, pasta, bread, fast food, gels, and cereal bars compared to women. However, women reported consuming more cooked vegetables (Table 2).

Table 2. Nutritional data.

					95% Confidence Interval of the Difference	
Variable	**Male**	**Female**	**T**	***p***	**Lower**	**Upper**
Days eating out of home (weekly)	1.5 ± 1.3	1.3 ± 1.4	1.490	0.137	−0.05734	0.41794
Days of ordering takeout (weekly)	6.2 ± 5.3	5.3 ± 7.1	2.583	0.010	0.04555	0.33438
Cook most days (weekly)	1.7 ± 1.6	1.6 ± 0.9	1.896	0.058	−0.00568	0.32474
Satisfaction with the weigh	2.0 ± 0.8	2.1 ± 0.7	1.856	0.064	−0.25946	0.00736
Daily water glasses (250 mL)	3.4 ± 1.8	3.8 ± 1.8	2.267	0.024	−0.66028	−0.04726
Fruit juice consumption (mL) (weekly) (250 mL)	2.4 ± 0.9	2.3 ± 0.9	0.113	0.910	−0.15337	0.17201
Alcohol glass consumption (250 mL) (weekly)	2.6 ± 0.7	2.5 ± 0.6	0.742	0.458	−0.07478	0.16566
Beer consumption (25 mL) (weekly)	2.4 ± 0.8	2.4 ± 0.9	0.466	0.641	−0.11034	0.17897
Alcohol cup consumption (250 mL) (Weekly)	2.6 ± 0.7	2.5 ± 0.6	3.586	0.000	0.15199	0.52000
Cola/Soda consumption (250 mL) (weekly)	2.4 ± 0.8	2.4 ± 0.9	2.306	0.021	0.03481	0.43497
Energy drink consumption (250 mL) (weekly)	2.5 ± 1.0	2.1 ± 1.1	0.416	0.678	−0.24335	0.15833
Milk glasses consumption (250 mL) (weekly)	3.1 ± 2.3	2.7 ± 2.0	2.436	0.015	0.09129	0.85067
Fermented dairy consumption (125 g) (Weekly)	2.8 ± 2.0	2.5 ± 1.7	2.035	0.042	0.01185	0.66548

Table 2. *Cont.*

Variable	Male	Female	T	*p*	95% Confidence Interval of the Difference	
					Lower	Upper
Sweets/bakery consumption (90 g) (weekly)	2.3 ± 1.2	2.0 ± 1.1	3.146	0.002	0.12283	0.53084
Cheese consumption (5 g) (Weekly)	2.6 ± 1.7	2.1 ± 1.5	3.589	0.000	0.23172	0.79168
Egg consumption (Unity) (Weekly)	2.9 ± 2.4	2.5 ± 2.1	2.094	0.037	0.02595	0.81218
Meat consumption (150 g) (weekly)	3.0 ± 2.3	2.6 ± 2.1	2.194	0.029	0.04571	0.82665
Fish consumption (150 g) (weekly)	2.5 ± 1.7	2.3 ± 1.5	1.467	0.143	−0.07302	0.50439
Processed meat consumption (150 g) (weekly)	2.5 ± 1.6	2.2 ± 1.3	2.080	0.038	0.01594	0.55345
Legume consumption (200 g) (weekly)	2.3 ± 1.4	2.2 ± 1.2	0.560	0.576	−0.16993	0.30552
Rice consumption (80 g) (Weekly)	2.7 ± 2.1	2.3 ± 1.8	2.251	0.025	0.05079	0.74460
Weekly pasta (150 g) consumption	2.6 ± 2.0	2.2 ± 1.5	2.350	0.019	0.06221	0.69536
Weekly fruit consumption (90 g)	3.2 ± 2.5	3.5 ± 2.9	1.179	0.239	−0.73452	0.18337
Weekly raw vegetable (200 g) consumption	2.8 ± 2.2	3.0 ± 2.5	1.177	0.240	−0.63642	0.15955
Weekly cooked vegetable (200 g) consumption	2.8 ± 2.2	3.2 ± 2.6	1.956	0.051	−0.80284	0.00159
Weekly bread (50 g) consumption	3.0 ± 2.2	2.5 ± 1.8	2.628	0.009	0.12098	0.83602
Weekly whole food (150 g) consumption	2.8 ± 2.2	2.5 ± 2.0	1.553	0.121	−0.07497	0.64177
Weekly fast food (180 g) consumption	2.2 ± 1.0	2.1 ± 0.9	2.209	0.028	0.02115	0.36068
Weekly protein drink (300 mL) consumption	2.5 ± 1.4	2.5 ± 1.7	0.286	0.775	−0.22643	0.30364
Weekly gel consumption (40 g)	2.5 ± 1.0	2.3 ± 1.2	2.125	0.034	0.01589	0.40373
Weekly muesli bar (150 g) consumption	2.4 ± 1.1	2.2 ± 1.2	1.905	0.057	−0.00584	0.38625

Unity means one portion. A serving means one serving of a meal. The frequency with which each food/drink is consumed is indicated in each item.

In the context of variables influencing body satisfaction, several notable differences were observed. Men tended to perceive their muscle size as larger compared to women, whereas men exhibited a more objective self-assessment of their muscle size. Conversely, men perceived their hip width as wider than women. Furthermore, women expressed more concern about the size of their buttocks, considering it more significant than men did. Additionally, women exhibited a more favorable perception of others' silhouettes, engaging in fewer self-comparisons with others. In terms of psychological profiles, men demonstrated a higher degree of extroversion compared to women. Women, on the other hand, exhibited higher levels of conscientiousness and a greater openness to new experiences. Women reported a higher frequency of negative thoughts and displayed less effective coping mechanisms in response to stress. According to the ZUNG Score results, women showed a greater number of symptoms associated with depressive behaviors than men, and they also presented higher levels of anxiety compared to men (Table 3).

Table 3. Psychology and body satisfaction data.

					95% Confidence Interval of the Difference	
Variable	**Male**	**Female**	**T**	***p***	**Lower**	**Upper**
Extraversion (Big Five)	5.6 ± 1.7	4.9 ± 1.6	4.401	0.000	0.36435	0.95161
Pleasant (Big five)	5.7 ± 1.8	5.9 ± 1.9	1.321	0.187	−0.53582	0.10489
Scrupulous (Big five)	6.4 ± 1.8	6.8 ± 2.1	2.353	0.019	−0.74059	−0.06682
Neuroticism (Big five)	4.9 ± 1.9	5.9 ± 2.4	5.462	0.000	−1.36750	−0.64420
Openness to Experience (Big five)	6.5 ± 2.0	6.9 ± 2.2	2.173	0.030	−0.75389	−0.03813
ZUNG Score	47.4 ± 5.4	49.1 ± 5.5	3.504	0.000	−2.56506	−0.72262
AAQ II	20.7 ± 8.5	21.9 ± 9.5	1.624	0.105	−2.74040	0.26002
UCLA	4.3 ± 1.5	4.2 ± 1.7	1.092	0.275	−0.11971	0.41959
STAI	11.3 ± 3.4	11.4 ± 4.0	−3.473	0.001	−1.69633	−0.47094
Body Satisfaction (EDI)	18.2 ± 3.5	17.9 ± 3.5	1.113	0.266	−0.25846	0.93515

AAQ II (Acceptance and Action Questionnaire II); UCLA (UCLA Loneliness Scale); STAI (Spielberger State—Trait Anxiety Inventory); ZUNG (ZUNG Depression Scale).

Regarding health parameters, significant distinctions emerged. Men reported a higher frequency of experiencing a dry throat compared to women. Additionally, over the past year, men reported a longer duration of illness than women. Concerning weekly training intensity, it was noted that women engaged in training at a higher volume, below 50% intensity, compared to men (Table 4).

Table 4. Health and physical activity data.

					95% Confidence Interval of the Difference	
Variable	**Male**	**Female**	**T**	***p***	**Lower**	**Upper**
Days you have been injured in the last year	5.2 ± 6.0	3.8 ± 4.1	1.205	0.229	−1.08069	4.51267
Number of training sessions per week	4.9 ± 19.9	3.1 ± 5.6	0.248	0.804	−2.74999	3.54523
Average time in minutes of weekly training	25.4 ± 13.2	17.8 ± 25.9	0.563	0.574	−22.84060	12.66806
Minutes of weekly aerobic training	11.7 ± 100.2	9.8 ± 113.3	0.501	0.616	−40.87648	24.25635
Bench press PR (kg)	62.3 ± 201.7	40.6 ± 173.4	0.156	0.876	−14.22743	12.12950
Back squat PR (Kg)	45.0 ± 44.3	29.7 ± 36.1	0.828	0.408	−16.05149	6.54848
Percentage of the week below fifty percent of the maximum load	21.7 ± 40.4	30.5 ± 47.4	1.784	0.075	−18.39401	0.89632
Percentage of the week between fifty and seventy percent of the maximum load	12.7 ± 18.9	21.7 ± 0.9	1.506	0.133	−20.57099	2.72550

Table 4. *Cont.*

					95% Confidence Interval of the Difference	
Variable	**Male**	**Female**	**T**	***p***	**Lower**	**Upper**
Percentage of week between seventy and eighty-five percent of maximum load	9.6 ± 16.7	9.4 ± 18.2	0.151	0.880	−2.80138	3.26868
Percentage of training of week conducted above eighty-five percent	10.4 ± 19.0	13.1 ± 19.3	1.471	0.142	−7.66770	1.10683
Smoking	2.3 ± 0.8	2.2 ± 0.8	0.980	0.327	−0.07190	0.21525
Experience frequent gastritis or heartburn	1.9 ± 0.5	1.9 ± 0.7	0.812	0.417	−0.06238	0.15024
Frequent dry throat sensation	2.0 ± 0.6	1.9 ± 0.7	2.604	0.009	0.03777	0.26943
Frequent dental sensitivity	2.1 ± 0.6	1.9 ± 0.8	1.961	0.050	−0.00017	0.23821
Days sick throughout the year	3.6 ± 7.8	2.3 ± 3.4	2.388	0.017	0.24277	2.49120

The smoking frequency is daily.

4. Discussion

Our study investigated gender-related disparities in body satisfaction perception, shedding light on distinct patterns among strength-trained participants. Notable is the finding of substantial differences in demographic variables such as age and body weight, where female participants exhibited a higher mean age and lower body weight compared to males, as shown in Table 1. This may contribute to the observed differences in body satisfaction. Our results indicate that strength-trained men tend to perceive their hip width as wider than that of strength-trained women. In terms of size satisfaction, men showed more muscular size satisfaction compared to women, a phenomenon that can be attributed to the weight lifted in bench press and back squat exercises. This are consistent with the reported higher muscle mass and strength in men, as reflected in Table 4's data on bench press and back squat personal records. Our findings are consistent with those reported in the literature [23]. Furthermore, this study revealed that strength-trained women demonstrated increased concern regarding the size of their buttocks, deeming it to be of greater significance compared to the perception held by strength-trained men. This aligns with the nutritional data in Table 2, where women's dietary choices, like higher vegetable consumption, could be influenced by their body satisfaction concerns. Importantly, our findings also revealed that women exhibited a more favorable perception of others' silhouettes when compared to men, who engaged in fewer self-comparisons with their peers. This might be influenced by the psychological profiles presented in Table 3, where women showed higher levels of conscientiousness and openness to new experiences. These comprehensive insights contribute significantly to our understanding of how gender influences body satisfaction perception, offering valuable implications for research in psychology and the health sciences.

The initial hypothesis of our study contended that gender differences in body satisfaction are profoundly influenced by societal norms [24], which in turn significantly affect nutritional habits and psychological profiles. The significant differences in nutritional habits between genders, as shown in Table 2, support this hypothesis. Men's greater involvement in food preparation and higher consumption of processed foods and alcohol could reflect societal influences on dietary choices. We posited that women modify their diet to pursue a slim physique, while men tailor their eating habits towards achieving enhanced strength and muscle mass. Our findings corroborate that body satisfaction disparities are indeed conditioned by the pursuit of specific gender-based stereotypes driven by social and cultural influences. This is evidenced by the differences in dietary patterns, where men's higher consumption of carbohydrates and women's preference for vegetables (Table 2) reflect these societal norms [25]. However, this study also reveals that the psychological behaviors and nutritional practices undertaken to achieve these gender stereotypes challenge the prevailing dogma. Particularly, the higher levels of anxiety and depressive behaviors in women, as indicated by the ZUNG Score in Table 3, suggest a complex interplay between psychological factors and body satisfaction. This breakthrough provides novel avenues for research in the realm of body diversity, offering fresh perspectives on the distinctions and commonalities in body satisfaction among women and men.

In addition, the health parameters in Table 4, such as the longer duration of illness reported by men, may have implications for body satisfaction and perceived health. This could be influenced by their dietary and lifestyle choices, as indicated by their higher consumption of alcohol and processed foods. These distinctions align with prior findings in existing literature [26]. Such distinctions may offer perspective on the extended life expectancy observed among women. The contrast in hydration practices, with women showing a higher water intake, could be a contributing factor to this extended life expectancy. The contrast in hydration practices, with women showing a higher water intake, could be a contributing factor to this extended life expectancy. Our study delineates a contrast in hydration practices: women exhibit higher water intake, while men, conversely, tend toward excessive consumption of carbonated beverages and alcoholic drinks. Several scholars have proposed the presence of a gender disparity associated with these patterns of alcohol intake [27], suggesting a potential reason for the increased occurrence of renal diseases in men compared to women [28]. The detailed nutritional data in Table 2 corroborates these patterns, showing men's higher consumption of soda and alcohol. Regarding dietary patterns, consistent with prior research [29], our findings suggest that women tend to adhere to a significantly healthier dietary regimen compared to men, showing a preference for vegetable consumption over other food categories. This is further supported by the nutritional data in Table 2, where men reported higher consumption of processed meat, rice, pasta, bread, fast food, gels, and cereal bars compared to women. Further studies support this trend, indicating that women favor other healthful food categories, such as fruits, in comparison to men [30]. Additionally, our research findings illustrate that men tend to consume more carbohydrate-rich foods, including rice, pasta, confectioneries, and dairy products. This aligns with established literature that highlights the increased consumption of carbohydrates. [31] and dairy products [32] have been linked to ailments like type II diabetes and specific cancer types. In addition, other studies demonstrate that high consumption of dairy products and refined carbohydrates is associated with factors that can lead to metabolic syndrome, such as obesity and insulin resistance [33]. This disparity in dietary habits may elucidate the substantial contrast observed in the prevalence of metabolic syndrome between men and women, as proposed by certain researchers [34].

Certain studies suggest that [35], within the psychological domain, women tend to display greater extroversion during interpersonal interactions compared to men. This is reflected in our findings, where women demonstrated higher levels of conscientiousness and openness to new experiences (Table 3). Moreover, some researchers emphasize that, due to variations in the nervous system's composition, women are more adept at embracing novel experiences [36] and have access to a higher level of consciousness [37]. Our results support this assertion, showing that women in our study exhibited a greater degree of extroversion and openness to new experiences compared to men (Table 3). The cerebellum is larger in men than in women [38]. This difference, according to some authors, indicates that it is men who have better control over the levels of consciousness [39], although there is currently controversy in this aspect [40]. This information from previous research aligns with our study's outcomes, illustrating notable dissimilarities in how men and women engage in social interactions, with men exhibiting greater ease. Additionally, prior studies have suggested that interactions vary based on gender configurations, concluding that same-gender interactions may be comparatively more straightforward [41]. Our results indicate that regardless of which gender the subject interacts with, men have an easier time. Regarding stress, there is no clear consensus on which gender is more effective in managing it [42]; however, the results of our study show a significant difference, indicating that women handle stress worse than men and also have a greater predisposition to negative thoughts, in line with the scientific literature [43]. This aligns with the findings of [44], which show that women manage stress worse due to their higher exposure to negative thoughts. Likewise, other researchers have observed that women exhibit elevated levels of anxiety compared to men [45]. However, other studies show the opposite, demonstrating that men have a lower tolerance for anxiety [46]. Based on the outcomes derived from our ZUNG Score, it was evident that women exhibit higher levels of anxiety compared to men. Nevertheless, a correlation was observed between increased exposure to negative thoughts and reduced levels of stress and anxiety tolerance [47]. Men and women employ distinct neural resources in their management of stress and anxiety. These resources are linked to the activity of specific brain regions, including the dorsomedial prefrontal cortex, cerebellum, left parietal, temporal lobes, and occipital gyrus [48]. Nevertheless, other authors attribute these differences in stress and anxiety management to interindividual factors that go beyond merely belonging to one gender or another, such as external stressors, life expectations, family context, social support, or even learning based on behavioral imitation with other individuals [49].

In terms of body satisfaction, our findings suggest significant gender-based differences. Women perceive their muscle size as larger compared to men, which might be influenced by their nutritional and health concerns, as reflected in their higher consumption of cooked vegetables and lower intake of processed meats (Tables 1 and 2). Additionally, women are more aware of the size of their buttocks and demonstrate better emotional management regarding this aspect than men. This greater emotional control might also be related to the higher levels of consciousness and stress tolerance observed in women (Table 3). Furthermore, women exhibit greater tolerance for comparing themselves with other figures, whereas men show heightened sensitivity when making such comparisons. Extending these observations, other authors [50] link differences in body satisfaction perception to conditions like eating disorders or psychiatric patterns. In agreement with these observations, some studies [51] emphasize the importance of educating on the emotional management of body satisfaction perception to prevent dissatisfaction. Such dissatisfaction could lead to diseases associated with being overweight, including cancer or diabetes. According to our results, women exhibit better emotional management and, consequently, a lower predisposition to overweight-related disorders. Lastly, several studies [52] suggest that other cultural media factors drive behaviors leading to differences in body satisfaction between men and women. For instance, mass media and the idealization of a specific body type impact men more than women.

Regarding health parameters, some authors suggest that men experience more illnesses than women [53]. Our findings support this conclusion, showing that men tend to experience a longer duration of illness annually compared to women, which could be related to their dietary patterns and hydration practices (Table 4). However, alternative perspectives within existing literature emphasize a greater incidence of illness among women in contrast to men. This observation is attributed to three main factors: the extended longevity of women [54], which heightens the probability of higher illness rates; poorer mental health conditions [55]; and a more pronounced impact of cardiovascular diseases [56]. In contrast, other authors suggest that the prevalence of diseases among men and women is not straightforward and can be attributed to genetic, epigenetic, epidemiological, and geographical factors, as well as hormonal differences, all of which are interconnected with the social construct related to gender [57].

In relation to physical activity, the existing literature is not precise in elucidating gender differences in terms of training parameters. Some authors assert that women exhibit greater fatigue resistance than men [58], while others solely allude to the disparity in the utilization of energy substrates [59]. Our study goes further, establishing clear differences in how women train compared to men. The results of our study demonstrate that women train at a lower intensity than men. However, they tend to tolerate higher exercise volumes more effectively. It is noteworthy that other authors attribute gender-related differences in physical activity to differing objectives. On one hand, women aim for caloric reduction and a leaner silhouette, while on the other, men pursue greater muscle mass gain [60]. Apart from physiological variances, these differences align with the findings of our study. Lower-intensity, aerobic-oriented training aligns with the popular belief of 'weight loss', while high-intensity training is associated with strength gain. Nevertheless, these assertions have been extensively refuted by the scientific literature [61].

Our study's findings hold significant practical implications in public health, psychology, and nutrition. Understanding gender differences in body satisfaction perception can inform the design of tailored interventions to promote positive body satisfaction and healthy eating habits. For instance, educational programs focusing on emotional management and body satisfaction perception could be particularly beneficial for women, while campaigns to reduce the consumption of processed foods and carbonated beverages might have a more significant impact on men.

Our study presents limitations in analyzing the impact that these differences in body satisfaction perception have on specific psychological behaviors and particular nutritional habits. Furthermore, our research encounters constraints in effectively correlating our psychological, nutritional, and body image outcomes with the influences emanating from established societal and cultural norms. This limitation underscores the difficulty in drawing definitive links between individual perceptions and actions and the wider social and cultural frameworks. A future line of research could review the underlying causes determining these differences in body satisfaction perception, further exploring the complex interplay between individual and societal factors.

5. Conclusions

Our comprehensive investigation in a strength-trained population has unveiled significant gender disparities across various domains, encompassing body satisfaction, dietary patterns, hydration behaviors, health outcomes, psychological attributes, and levels of physical activity, aligning with established scientific literature [62]. Our observations indicate that females tend to overestimate their muscle size and exhibit heightened concern regarding the shape of their gluteal region, in contrast to males, who tend to possess a more realistic self-perception and a heightened focus on hip width, as substantiated by prior researchers [63]. Notably, women exhibit exceptional resilience in self-comparisons and excel in the emotional management of body satisfaction concerns, findings corroborated by previous studies [64].

Within the realm of dietary practices, our results suggest that women tend to favor healthier dietary choices, including increased consumption of vegetables, whereas men display a proclivity for higher intakes of milk, fermented products, pastries, cheese, and eggs. These dietary preferences concur with previous research findings [65]. With respect to hydration behaviors, our investigation reveals elevated water intake among women, while men display a preference for alcoholic and carbonated beverages. Additionally, men report longer durations of illness per year and a higher frequency of dry throat issues, consistent with earlier studies [66,67].

Psychologically, our study demonstrates that men exhibit greater extroversion, whereas women display higher levels of conscientiousness and openness to new experiences, consistent with the conclusions of prior research [68,69]. Nevertheless, women also experience more frequent negative thoughts, elevated anxiety levels, and a heightened predisposition toward depression. Our study contributes additional depth to this topic compared to earlier research, which primarily focused on the increased propensity for depression among women compared to men [70].

Lastly, in accordance with earlier research findings [71], women engage in training sessions of higher volume compared to men in the realm of physical activity. This comprehensive gender-specific analysis offers invaluable insights into the intricate interplay among physical, nutritional, and psychological factors in both genders, providing a solid foundation for future specialized interventions and studies in the field of nutritional science and health.

Author Contributions: Conceptualization, V.J.C.-S.; Methodology, V.J.C.-S.; Formal analysis, V.J.C.-S.; Investigation, V.J.C.-S.; Writing—original draft, J.J.-M. and V.J.C.-S. All authors have read and agreed to the published version of the manuscript.

Funding: This research received no external funding.

Institutional Review Board Statement: The study was conducted in accordance with the Declaration of Helsinki, and approved by the Institutional Ethics Committee of the Universidad Europea de Madrid (CIPI/21/082, 29/4/2021).

Informed Consent Statement: Informed consent was obtained from all subjects involved in the study.

Data Availability Statement: Data are contained within the article.

Conflicts of Interest: The authors declare no conflict of interest.

References

1. Fernández-Martínez, A.; Murillo-Lorente, V.; Sarmiento, A.; Álvarez-Medina, J.; Nuviala, A. Exercise Addiction and Satisfaction of Fitness Center Users as Precursors to the Intention of Continuing to Engage in Physical Activity. *Sustainability* **2020**, *13*, 129. [CrossRef]
2. Thyfault, J.P.; Bergouignan, A. Exercise and metabolic health: Beyond skeletal muscle. *Diabetologia* **2020**, *63*, 1464–1474. [CrossRef] [PubMed]
3. Durau, J.; Diehl, S.; Terlutter, R. Motivate me to exercise with you: The effects of social media fitness influencers on users' intentions to engage in physical activity and the role of user gender. *Digit. Health* **2022**, *8*, 205520762211027. [CrossRef] [PubMed]
4. Iff, S.; Fröhlich, S.; Halioua, R.; Imboden, C.; Spörri, J.; Scherr, J.; Butzke, I.; Seifritz, E.; Claussen, M.C. Training Patterns and Mental Health of Bodybuilders and Fitness Athletes During the First Lockdown of the COVID-19 Pandemic—A Cross-Sectional Study. *Front. Sports Act. Living* **2022**, *4*, 867140. [CrossRef] [PubMed]
5. Clemente-Suárez, V.J.; Ramírez-Goerke, M.I.; Redondo-Flórez, L.; Beltrán-Velasco, A.I.; Martín-Rodríguez, A.; Ramos-Campo, D.J.; Navarro-Jiménez, E.; Yáñez-Sepúlveda, R.; Tornero-Aguilera, J.F. The Impact of Anorexia Nervosa and the Basis for Non-Pharmacological Interventions. *Nutrients* **2023**, *15*, 2594. [CrossRef] [PubMed]
6. Griffiths, S.; Murray, S.B.; Krug, I.; McLean, S.A. Associations between body dissatisfaction and self-reported anxiety and depression in otherwise healthy men: A systematic review and meta-analysis. *PLoS ONE* **2020**, *15*, 0229268.
7. Rounsefell, K.; Gibson, S.; McLean, S.; Blair, M.; Molenaar, A.; Brennan, L.; Truby, H.; McCaffrey, T.A. Social media, body satisfaction and food choices in healthy young adults: A mixed methods systematic review. *Nutr. Diet.* **2020**, *77*, 19–40. [CrossRef] [PubMed]
8. Sabiston, C.M.; Pila, E.; Vani, M.; Thogersen-Ntoumani, C. Body satisfaction, physical activity, and sport: A scoping review. *Psychol. Sport Exerc.* **2019**, *42*, 48–57. [CrossRef]
9. Tylka, T.L. Refinement of the tripartite influence model for men: Dual body satisfaction pathways to body change behaviours. *Body Image* **2011**, *8*, 199–207. [CrossRef]
10. Mehnert, A.; Veers, S.; Howaldt, D.; Braumann, K.-M.; Koch, U.; Schulz, K.-H. Effects of a Physical Exercise Rehabilitation Group Program on Anxiety, Depression, Body Satisfaction, and Health-Related Quality of Life among Breast Cancer Patients. *Oncology* **2011**, *34*, 248–253. [CrossRef]
11. He, J.; Sun, S.; Zickgraf, H.F.; Lin, Z.; Fan, X. Meta-analysis of gender differences in body appreciation. *Body Image* **2020**, *33*, 90–100. [CrossRef] [PubMed]
12. Fatt, S.J.; Fardouly, J.; Rapee, R.M. #malefitspo: Links between viewing fitspiration posts, muscular-ideal internalisation, appearance comparisons, body satisfaction, and exercise motivation in men. *New Media Soc.* **2019**, *21*, 1311–1325. [CrossRef]
13. McCreary, D.R.; Hildebrandt, T.B.; Heinberg, L.J.; Boroughs, M.; Thompson, J.K. A Review of Body satisfaction Influences on Men's Fitness Goals and Supplement Use. *Am. J. Mens Health* **2007**, *1*, 307–316. [CrossRef] [PubMed]
14. Law, R.; Jevons, E.F. Exploring the perceived influence of social media use on disordered eating in nutrition and dietetics students. *J. Hum. Nutr. Diet.* **2023**, *36*, 2050–2059. [CrossRef] [PubMed]
15. EPIC Study Group. European Prospective Investigation into Cancer and Nutrition (EPIC): Study populations and data collection. *Public Health Nutr.* **2002**, *5*, 1113–1124. [CrossRef] [PubMed]
16. Gonzalez, C.A.; Riboli, E. Diet and cancer prevention: Contributions from the European Prospective Investigation into Cancer and Nutrition (EPIC) study. *Eur. J. Cancer* **2010**, *46*, 2555–2562. [CrossRef] [PubMed]
17. Gallardo-Pujol, D.; Rouco, V.; Cortijos-Bernabeu, A.; Oceja, L.; Soto, C.J.; John, O.P. Factor Structure, Gender Invariance, Measurement Properties, and Short Forms of the Spanish Adaptation of the Big Five Inventory-2. *Psychol. Test Adapt. Dev.* **2022**, *3*, 44–69. [CrossRef]

18. Van Knippenberg, F.; Duivenvoorden, H.; Bonke, B.; Passchier, J. Shortening the state-trait anxiety inventory. *J. Clin. Epidemiol.* **1990**, *43*, 995–1000. [CrossRef]
19. Paladines-Costa, B.; López-Guerra, V.; Ruisoto, P.; Vaca-Gallegos, S.; Cacho, R. Psychometric Properties and Factor Structure of the Spanish Version of the Acceptance and Action Questionnaire-II (AAQ-II) in Ecuador. *Int. J. Environ. Res. Public Health* **2021**, *18*, 2944. [CrossRef]
20. Russell, D. UCLA Loneliness Scale (Version 3): Reliability, Validity, and Factor Structure. *J. Pers. Assess.* **1996**, *66*, 20–40. [CrossRef]
21. Zung, W.W.K. A Self-Rating Depression Scale. *Arch. Gen. Psychiatry* **1965**, *12*, 63–70. [CrossRef] [PubMed]
22. Elosua, P.; López-Jáuregui, A. Internal structure of the Spanish adaptation of the eating disorder inventory-3. *Eur. J. Psychol. Assess.* **2012**, *28*, 25–31. [CrossRef]
23. Geer, E.B.; Shen, W. Sex differences in body composition and association with cardiometabolic risk. *Biol. Sex Differ.* **2021**, *12*, 38.
24. Pingitore, R.; Spring, B.; Garfieldt, D. Gender Differences in Body Satisfaction. *Obes. Res.* **1997**, *5*, 402–409. [CrossRef] [PubMed]
25. Austin, S.B.; Haines, J.; Veugelers, P.J. Body satisfaction and body weight: Gender differences and sociodemographic determinants. *BMC Public Health* **2009**, *9*, 313. [CrossRef] [PubMed]
26. Sudo, N.; Sekiyama, M.; Maharjan, M.; Ohtsuka, R. Gender differences in dietary intake among adults of Hindu communities in lowland Nepal: Assessment of portion sizes and food consumption frequencies. *Eur. J. Clin. Nutr.* **2005**, *60*, 469–477. [CrossRef] [PubMed]
27. Keyes, K.M.; Grant, B.F.; Hasin, D.S. Evidence for a closing gender gap in alcohol use, abuse, and dependence in the United States population. *Drug Alcohol Depend.* **2008**, *93*, 21–29. [CrossRef] [PubMed]
28. Rehm, J.; Shield, K.D.; Joharchi, N.; Shuper, P.A. Alcohol consumption and the intention to engage in unprotected sex: Systematic review and meta-analysis of experimental studies. *Addiction* **2011**, *107*, 51–59. [CrossRef]
29. Wardle, J.; Haase, A.M.; Steptoe, A.; Nillapun, M.; Jonwutiwes, K.; Bellisie, F. Gender differences in food choice: The contribution of health beliefs and dieting. *Ann. Behav. Med.* **2004**, *27*, 107–116. [CrossRef]
30. Rosenfeld, D.L.; Tomiyama, A.J. Gender differences in meat consumption and openness to vegetarianism. *Appetite* **2021**, *166*, 105475. [CrossRef]
31. Reynolds, A.; Mann, J.; Cummings, J.; Winter, N.; Mete, E.; Te Morenga, L. Carbohydrate quality and human health: A series of systematic reviews and meta-analyses. *Lancet* **2019**, *393*, 434–445. [CrossRef] [PubMed]
32. Knekt, P.; Järvinen, R.; Seppänen, R.; Pukkala, E.; Aromaa, A. Intake of dairy products and the risk of breast cancer. *Br. J. Cancer* **1996**, *73*, 687–691. [CrossRef] [PubMed]
33. Mozaffarian, D.; Hao, T.; Rimm, E.B.; Willett, W.C.; Hu, F.B. Changes in Diet and Lifestyle and Long-Term Weight Gain in Women and Men. *N. Engl. J. Med.* **2011**, *364*, 2392–2404. [CrossRef] [PubMed]
34. Grundy, S.M. Metabolic syndrome update. *Trends Cardiovasc. Med.* **2016**, *26*, 364–373. [CrossRef]
35. Evans, C.; McConnell, T.R. A New Measure of Introversion-Extroversion. *J. Psychol.* **1941**, *12*, 111–124. [CrossRef]
36. Weisberg, Y.J.; DeYoung, C.G.; Hirsh, J.B. Gender Differences in Personality across the Ten Aspects of the Big Five. *Front. Psychol.* **2011**, *2*, 178. Available online: http://journal.frontiersin.org/article/10.3389/fpsyg.2011.00178/abstract (accessed on 17 October 2023). [CrossRef]
37. Rueckert, L.; Naybar, N. Gender differences in empathy: The role of the right hemisphere. *Brain Cogn.* **2008**, *67*, 162–167. [CrossRef]
38. Zaidi, Z.F. Gender Differences in Human Brain: A Review. *Open Anat. J.* **2010**, *2*, 37–55. [CrossRef]
39. Raz, N.; Gunning-Dixon, F.; Head, D.; Williamson, A.; Acker, J.D. Age and Sex Differences in the Cerebellum and the Ventral Pons: A Prospective MR Study of Healthy Adults. *Am. J. Neuroradiol.* **2001**, *22*, 1161–1167.
40. Gurin, P. Women's Gender Consciousness. *Public Opin. Q.* **1985**, *49*, 143–163. [CrossRef]
41. Carli, L.L. Gender Differences in Interaction Style and Influence. *J. Personal. Soc. Psychol.* **1989**, *56*, 565–576. [CrossRef]
42. Matud, M. Gender differences in stress and coping styles. *Pers. Individ. Differ.* **2004**, *37*, 1401–1415. [CrossRef]
43. Costa, C.; Briguglio, G.; Mondello, S.; Teodoro, M.; Pollicino, M.; Canalella, A.; Fenga, C. Perceived stress in a gender perspective: A survey in a population of unemployed subjects of Southern Italy. *Front. Public Health* **2021**, *9*, 640454. [CrossRef] [PubMed]
44. Leach, L.S.; Christensen, H.; Mackinnon, A.J.; Windsor, T.D.; Butterworth, P. Gender differences in depression and anxiety across the adult lifespan: The role of psychosocial mediators. *Soc. Psychiatr. Epidemiol.* **2008**, *43*, 983–998. [CrossRef]
45. McLean, C.P.; Anderson, E.R. Brave men and timid women? A review of the gender differences in fear and anxiety. *Clin. Psychol. Rev.* **2009**, *29*, 496–505. [CrossRef]
46. Simonds, V. Are gender differences in depression explained by gender differences in co-morbid anxiety? *J. Affect. Disord.* **2003**, *77*, 197–202. [CrossRef]
47. Pirbaglou, M.; Cribbie, R.; Irvine, J.; Radhu, N.; Vora, K.; Ritvo, P. Perfectionism, Anxiety, and Depressive Distress: Evidence for the Mediating Role of Negative Automatic Thoughts and Anxiety Sensitivity. *J. Am. Coll. Health* **2013**, *61*, 477–483. [CrossRef]
48. Seo, D.; Ahluwalia, A.; Potenza, M.N.; Sinha, R. Gender differences in neural correlates of stress-induced anxiety. *J. Neurosci. Res.* **2016**, *95*, 115–125. [CrossRef]
49. Jick, T.; Mitz, L. Sex Differences in Work Stress. *Acad. Manag. Rev.* **1985**, *10*, 408–420. [CrossRef]
50. Hogan, M.J.; Strasburger, V.C. Body image, Eating Disorders, and the Media. *Adolesc. Med.* **2008**, *19*, 521–546.
51. Pelegrini, A.; Sacomori, C.; Santos, M.C.; Sperandio, F.F.; Cardoso, F.L. Percepção da imagem corporal em mulheres: Prevalência e associação com indicadores antropométricos. *Rev. Bras. Cineantropom. Desempenho. Hum.* **2013**, *16*, 58–65. [CrossRef]

52. Brennan, M.A.; Lalonde, C.E.; Bain, J.L. Body satisfaction Perceptions: Do Gender Differences Exist? *Psi Chi J.* **2010**, *15*, 130–138. [CrossRef]
53. Muennig, P.; Lubetkin, E.; Jia, H.; Franks, P. Gender and the Burden of Disease Attributable to Obesity. *Am. J. Public Health* **2006**, *96*, 1662–1668. [CrossRef] [PubMed]
54. Denton, M.; Prus, S.; Walters, V. Gender differences in health: A Canadian study of the psychosocial, structural and behavioural determinants of health. *Soc. Sci. Med.* **2004**, *58*, 2585–2600. [CrossRef] [PubMed]
55. Riecher-Rössler, A. Sex and gender differences in mental disorders. *Lancet Psychiatry* **2016**, *4*, 8–9. [CrossRef] [PubMed]
56. Peters, S.A.E.; Woodward, M.; Jha, V.; Kennedy, S.; Norton, R. Women's health: A new global agenda. *BMJ Glob. Health* **2016**, *1*, e000080. [CrossRef]
57. Mauvais-Jarvis, F.; Merz, N.B.; Barnes, P.J.; Brinton, R.D.; Carrero, J.-J.; DeMeo, D.L.; De Vries, G.J.; Epperson, C.N.; Govindan, R.; Klein, S.L.; et al. Sex and gender: Modifiers of health, disease, and medicine. *Lancet* **2020**, *396*, 565–582. [CrossRef]
58. Tornero-Aguilera, J.F.; Jimenez-Morcillo, J.; Rubio-Zarapuz, A.; Clemente-Suárez, V.J. Central and Peripheral Fatigue in Physical Exercise Explained: A Narrative Review. *Int. J. Environ. Res. Public Health* **2022**, *19*, 3909. [CrossRef]
59. Ruby, B.C.; Robergs, R.A. Gender Differences in Substrate Utilisation during Exercise. *Sports Med.* **1994**, *17*, 393–410. [CrossRef]
60. Hausenblas, H.A.; Fallon, E.A. Exercise and body satisfaction: A meta-analysis. *Psychol. Health* **2006**, *21*, 33–47. [CrossRef]
61. Tremblay, A.; Després, J.P.; Leblanc, C.; Craig, C.L.; Ferris, B.; Stephens, T.; Bouchard, C. Effect of intensity of physical activity on body fatness and fat distribution. *Am. J. Clin. Nutr.* **1990**, *51*, 153–157. [CrossRef] [PubMed]
62. Calzo, J.P.; Sonneville, K.R.; Haines, J.; Blood, E.A.; Field, A.E.; Austin, S.B. The development of associations among body mass index, body dissatisfaction, and weight and shape concern in adolescent boys and girls. *J. Adolesc. Health* **2012**, *51*, 517–523. [CrossRef] [PubMed]
63. Gualdi-Russo, E.; Rinaldo, N.; Masotti, S.; Bramanti, B.; Zaccagni, L. Sex Differences in Body Image Perception and Ideals: Analysis of Possible Determinants. *Int. J. Environ. Res. Public Health* **2022**, *19*, 2745. [CrossRef] [PubMed]
64. Padmanabhanunni, A.; Pretorius, T.B.; Khamisa, N. The role of resilience in the relationship between role stress and psychological well-being during the COVID-19 pandemic: A cross-sectional study. *BMC Psychol.* **2023**, *11*, 45. [CrossRef] [PubMed]
65. Fagerli, R.A.; Wandel, M. Gender differences in opinions and practices with regard to a "healthy diet". *Appetite* **1999**, *32*, 171–190. [CrossRef]
66. Gibson, S.; Shirreffs, S.M. Beverage consumption habits "24/7" among British adults: Association with total water intake and energy intake. *Nutr. J.* **2013**, *12*, 9. [CrossRef]
67. Ku, C.C.; MacPherson, P.; Khundi, M.; Nzawa Soko, R.H.; Feasey, H.R.; Nliwasa, M.; Dodd, P.J. Durations of asymptomatic, symptomatic, and care-seeking phases of tuberculosis disease with a Bayesian analysis of prevalence survey and notification data. *BMC Med.* **2021**, *19*, 298. [CrossRef]
68. Zopiatis, A.; Constanti, P. Extraversion, openness and conscientiousness: The route to transformational leadership in the hotel industry. *Leadersh. Organ. Dev. J.* **2012**, *33*, 86–104. [CrossRef]
69. Rodriguez-Besteiro, S.; Tornero-Aguilera, J.F.; Fernández-Lucas, J.; Clemente-Suárez, V.J. Gender Differences in the COVID-19 Pandemic Risk Perception, Psychology, and Behaviors of Spanish University Students. *Int. J. Environ. Res. Public Health* **2021**, *18*, 3908. [CrossRef]
70. Andersson, S.; Bathula, D.R.; Iliadis, S.I.; Walter, M.; Skalkidou, A. Predicting women with depressive symptoms postpartum with machine learning methods. *Sci. Rep.* **2021**, *11*, 7877. [CrossRef]
71. Holloway, J.B.; Baechle, T.R. Strength Training for Female Athletes. A review of selected aspects. *Sports Med.* **1990**, *9*, 216–228. [CrossRef] [PubMed]

nutrients MDPI

Article

An Assessment of Women's Knowledge of the Menstrual Cycle and the Influence of Diet and Adherence to Dietary Patterns on the Alleviation or Exacerbation of Menstrual Distress

Anna Ciołek [1], Malgorzata Kostecka [1,*], Julianna Kostecka [2], Paulina Kawecka [1] and Monika Popik-Samborska [3]

1 Department of Chemistry, Faculty of Food Science and Biotechnology, University of Life Sciences, Akademicka 15, 20-950 Lublin, Poland; anna.ciolek@up.lublin.pl (A.C.); paulina.kawecka@up.lublin.pl (P.K.)
2 Faculty of Medicine, Medical University of Lublin, Chodźki 19, 20-093 Lublin, Poland; kostecka.julianna@gmail.com
3 Dietetic Centre Project Health, Ametystowa 16, 20-576 Lublin, Poland
* Correspondence: malgorzata.kostecka@up.lublin.pl; Tel.: +48-814-456-846

Abstract: A growing number of women of reproductive age experience menstrual disorders. The menstrual cycle is considerably influenced by dietary habits, physical activity, and the use of stimulants. The main aim of this study was to assess women's knowledge about the menstrual cycle and the influence of diet and lifestyle factors on menstrual symptoms, and to identify dietary models that may alleviate or exacerbate menstrual distress. A total of 505 young women participated in the study. Nearly 90% of the respondents reported at least one menstrual disorder, mostly dysmenorrhea (70.7%), whereas secondary amenorrhea was least frequently reported (13.8%) (p = 0.002). In the study population, dysmenorrhea/menstrual distress was linked with higher consumption frequency of certain food groups. Women with severe dysmenorrhea consumed refined cereal products, processed meat, sugar, and water significantly more frequently than women with moderate menstrual pain. In turn, sweetened dairy products, animal fats, and fruit were consumed more frequently by women with low intensity of menstrual pain (mild pain). Significant differences in knowledge about the menstrual cycle and physiological changes in the body were observed between the compared dietary models.

Keywords: menstrual cycle; menstrual disorders; dysmenorrhea; visual analog scale (VAS); menstrual health; nutrition knowledge; anti-inflammatory diet; proinflammatory diet

1. Introduction

A growing number of women of reproductive age experience menstrual disorders. Menstrual symptoms such as dysmenorrhea, heavy menstrual bleeding, and perimenstrual mood disorders are known to be widespread among the general population [1]. Clinical trials have shown that menstrual symptoms can have a large impact on women's mental and physical well-being, personal relationships, education and career attainment, and can lead to long-standing impairments in the quality of life [2]. Furthermore, it is estimated that many women initially do not consult a doctor while facing menstrual symptoms [3,4]. However, dysmenorrhea, which is characterized by menstrual pain in the absence of pelvic pathology, is one of the main reasons for gynecological consultations among young women [5]. The annual economic burden due to menstrual symptoms in Japanese women was estimated at approximately 683 billion Japanese yen, and in more than 70% of cases, dysmenorrhea was associated with a decrease in work productivity [6,7]. Data indicate that more than one-quarter of women reduced their working hours or were absent from work for at least 1 day per 6 months as a result of menstrual pain [6]. Depending on their severity, menstrual distress symptoms can also negatively affect women's daily lives by preventing them from participating in social activities and maintaining social relations [7–9].

Research has also demonstrated that work or school absenteeism due to menstruation poses a significant economic, social, and health burden [9–12]. Despite the widespread prevalence of menstrual distress and the resulting decrease in the quality of life, including school and work absenteeism, this illness has received remarkably little scientific attention.

Dietary and lifestyle factors significantly affect the functioning of body organs and sex hormone levels. The menstrual cycle is considerably influenced by dietary habits, physical activity, and the use of stimulants. These factors affect the BMI and body fat percentage which are directly linked with ovulation disorders, and painful and irregular menstruation. The importance of dietary patterns for pain relief in women with dysmenorrhea is increasingly discussed in the literature [13]. However, too little attention has been paid to the role of specific food components in reducing menstrual distress. It is believed that healthy eating patterns may have pain-relieving properties. The development of an optimal diet for patients with dysmenorrhea constitutes a major challenge. Diets with low nutrient density, low in vitamins and minerals, and abundant in processed foods, may exert a negative impact on women's overall health and well-being, and increase the risk of diet-related diseases which, under certain circumstances, can lead to menstrual disorders and exacerbate menstrual distress symptoms [14,15].

In recent years, numerous attempts have been made to identify modifiable factors, including lifestyle factors, that potentially alleviate menstrual distress. Research findings could substantially contribute to an improvement in women's well-being by analyzing the relationship between dietary components and lifestyle factors that affect menstrual distress symptoms. The main aim of this study was to assess selected parameters associated with menstrual health and to correlate these parameters with the studied women's diet and nutrition knowledge. Potential correlations between adherence to an emergent dietary model and the severity of menstrual distress were also examined.

2. Materials and Methods

2.1. Study Design

A cross-sectional study was conducted in the city of Lublin and in Lublin voivodeship in eastern Poland between April 2022 and January 2023. The study involved a paper questionnaire and an online questionnaire that was completed independently by the participants with the use of Google Forms.

Participants

The minimal sample size for the study was calculated with the use of Cochran's formula [16] for the Polish population of women aged 18 to 40 years (N = 5,144,208 as of 31 December 2022) based on Statistical Yearbook data (Statistics Poland) [17]. The minimal sample size was determined at 384 persons at a significance level of 0.05, maximum error of 5%, and a sampling fraction of 0.5. The calculated sample size was adjusted for a 20% attrition rate to produce a total of 461 participants. A higher number of female respondents was achieved during recruitment, which decreased the maximum error and increased the power of the applied tests.

Inclusion criteria:

- Age: 18–40 years;
- Absence of serious illnesses that constitute exclusion criteria;
- Informed consent to participate in the study.

Exclusion criteria:

- Amenorrhea (absence of menstruation);
- Miscarriage in the previous 6 months;
- Pregnancy;
- Presence of biological offspring;
- Use of hormonal drugs (other than contraceptives), steroids, antidepressants, sleeping pills, or sedatives in the previous 6 months or directly before the trial;
- Chronic diseases and metabolic disorders, including type 1 and 2 diabetes, insulin resistance, polycystic ovary syndrome, endometriosis, sterility, infertility, hormonal

disorders, thyroid disorders, kidney disorders, asthma, Crohn's disease, anemia, eating disorders, epilepsy, rheumatoid arthritis, cancer, HPV infection;
- Diagnosed gynecological diseases or disorders, including congenital abnormalities of the reproductive tract;
- Pelvic floor disorders;
- Lack of consent to participate in the study.

2.2. Study Tools and Data Collection

Information about the study was posted on Facebook groups, posters at Lublin universities, and in gynecological clinics. The survey was completely voluntary and anonymous, and the participants did not provide any personal or sensitive information that could enable their identification. The study involved a conventional paper questionnaire and an online questionnaire that was completed with the use of Google Forms on a dedicated Facebook page. All participants were residents of Lublin voivodeship. Before the trial, all women were informed about the purpose of the study and the research protocol. Survey completion was regarded as an indication of consent to participate in the study. The main questionnaire contained questions about the menstrual cycle (duration; presence, type and prevalence of menstrual symptoms; heavy bleeding; pain; intermenstrual bleeding; secondary amenorrhea), as well as 7 questions analyzing the participants' knowledge about the physiology of the menstrual cycle and menstrual disorders. The participants received 1 point for every correct answer and 0 points for every incorrect answer. There were a maximum of 7 points in total, where 0–4 points denoted a low level of knowledge and >4 points denoted a high level of knowledge. Menstrual pain was rated on the visual analog scale (VAS). The participants were asked to indicate the average severity of menstrual pain by placing an "x" on a straight horizontal line with a length of 10 cm. The ends of the line represented the extreme limits of pain, where 0 points denoted a complete absence of pain, and 10 denoted severe pain. Pain intensity was self-assessed on the following scale: low (0–4.0 points), moderate (4.1–7.0 points), and severe (7.1–10 points), where 0.1 points was represented by 0.1 cm on the horizontal line. This part of the questionnaire also contained questions about the use of vitamin D supplements, dietary supplements (including herbal supplements), smoking, and alcohol consumption. The second part of the study involved a short food frequency questionnaire (FFQ). The questionnaire contained 37 food products divided into the following groups: cereal products; dairy products; meat and meat products; eggs and fish; fats and bread spreads; vegetables; pulses; fruit; nuts; sugar and confectionery products; beverages (including alcoholic beverages); and fast-food products. The respondents were asked to indicate the average consumption frequency of the products listed in the FFQ in the past year by selecting one of the seven options in the questionnaire: less than once a month; 1–3 times a month; 1–2 times a week; 3–4 times a week; 5–6 times a week; once daily; twice or more daily. The declared consumption frequency was converted into daily frequency using the appropriate conversion factors (Table 1). The participants' biographic data were collected, including age, place of residence, education, and marital status. The surveyed subjects were also asked to indicate their body height (cm) and body weight (kg) based on independently performed anthropometric measurements and to describe any changes in body weight in the previous 6 months. Based on the obtained anthropometric data, the body mass index (BMI) was calculated by dividing body weight (kilograms) by the square of the height (meters). The interpretation of BMI was based on the guidelines of the World Health Organization:

- <18.5 kg/m^2—underweight;
- 18.5–24.99 kg/m^2—normal weight;
- 25.0–29.99 kg/m^2—overweight;
- 30.0–34.99 kg/m^2—stage I obesity;
- >35 kg/m^2—stage II obesity.

Table 1. Conversion factors applied to the consumption frequency classes defined in the FFQ.

Frequency of Consumption as Defined in FFQ	Conversion Factor to Daily Frequency
Less than once a month	0.00
1–3 times a month	0.07
1–2 times a week	0.21
3–4 times a week	0.50
5–6 times a week	0.79
Once daily	1.00
Twice or more daily	2.00

Paper questionnaires were filled out independently at home. The questionnaires were revised, and missing information was provided during a meeting with a researcher. Online questionnaires were completed with the use of Google Forms, and the completeness of the answers was checked by the researchers. The paper questionnaire and the online questionnaire involved the same main questionnaire and the FFQ. A total of 571 women completed the questionnaire, and 505 correctly completed questionnaires were returned.

2.3. Dietary Patterns

Dietary patterns were derived by cluster analysis. The input variables were 14 dietary (in times/day) components of DPs. All input variables were standardized using our own database to achieve a mean equal to 0 and a standard deviation equal to 1. To identify the optimal number of clusters, the analysis was conducted several times. The K-means clustering algorithm was used, and the subjects were grouped based on the Euclidean distance. Finally, two clusters were selected (an anti-inflammatory model and a proinflammatory model). The correctness of cluster identification and labelling was verified by comparing the components of DPs between clusters in a one-way analysis of variance.

2.4. Data Processing and Statistical Analysis

Missing data were addressed by excluding incomplete questionnaires or sections from the analysis. The results were presented in tables and figures and were described. Categorical variables were presented as sample percentages (%), and continuous variables were expressed as the mean ± standard deviation. The differences between groups were analyzed in the chi-squared test (categorical variables) or the Mann–Whitney test (continuous variables). The Kruskal–Wallis test was applied to analyze the relationships between the variables in more than two mutually independent groups. Before statistical analysis, the data were checked for normal distribution in the Kolmogorov–Smirnov test. The odds ratios (ORs) and 95% confidence intervals (95% CIs) were calculated. The reference category (OR = 1.00) was mild intensity of menstrual pain. The significance of ORs was assessed by Wald's statistics. The results of all tests were regarded as statistically significant at $p < 0.05$. Data were processed in the Statistica program (version 13.1 PL; StatSoft Inc., Tulsa, OK, USA; StatSoft, Krakow, Poland) and in SPSS v. 27.

3. Results

The study involved 505 women with the mean age of 24.7 ± 4.5 years (range: 19–40 years). Nearly 50% of the participants resided in cities with a population of ≥250,000, and rural inhabitants accounted for 27.9% of the studied group (Table 2). Most of the surveyed women lived in informal relationships (49.9%), and a relatively high percentage of the population (23.0%) declared to be single. The vast majority of the studied subjects were professionally active or were students in paid employment (84.2%), and nearly 5% of the participants were unemployed.

Table 2. Sociodemographic characteristics of the studied group (N = 505).

Sociodemographic Parameters	N	N [%]	*p*-Value
Place of residence			
• City with a population of >250,000	254	50.3%	<0.05
• City with a population of <250,000	110	21.8%	
• Rural area	141	27.9%	
Age			
• <25 years	198	39.2%	<0.05
• >25 years	307	60.8%	
Marital status			
• Single	116	23.0%	<0.05
• Informal relationship	252	49.9%	
• Married	137	27.1%	
Education			
• Primary school	20	4%	
• Secondary school	165	32.7%	<0.05
• University	315	62.3%	
• Vocational school	5	1%	
Professional status			
• Student	57	11.3%	
• Student in paid employment	159	31.5%	<0.05
• Employed	266	52.7%	
• Unemployed	23	4.5%	

Differences are significant at $p < 0.05$.

The average BMI was 22.4 ± 4.2 kg/m^2. Most of the studied subjects (69.2%) had a healthy body weight. Overweight and obesity were determined in 23.5% of the surveyed population, where 51.3% of the participants were characterized by gynoid obesity (pear-shaped body), and 48.7% by android obesity (apple-shaped body). Only 5.2% of the subjects were underweight. Changes in body weight in the previous 6 months were reported by 52.0% of the participants, where 70% of the subjects declared weight gain, and 30% reported weight loss ($p = 0.013$). In both cases, the average change in body weight was 3.8 ± 1.6 kg. Changes in body weight were more frequently reported by women with excessive BMI ($p = 0.001$) and women with android obesity ($p = 0.021$).

3.1. Selected Menstrual Health Parameters

In the vast majority of the surveyed subjects, the length of the menstrual cycle ranged from 26 to 31 days, and cycles shorter than 26 days were reported by 10.7% of the participants. Most women had regular menstrual cycles (84.3%), and menstruation lasted 5.1 ± 1.0 days on average. Bleeding intensity was assessed as moderate by the vast majority of the participants (63.2%), whereas heavy or very heavy bleeding was reported by nearly every fourth respondent (26.1%). The average pain intensity measured on the VAS was 6.3 ± 2.8 points, and the results were used to divide women into three groups with different levels of pain intensity. The first group consisted of women with a VAS score of 0–4 points (mild pain), the second group comprised participants with a VAS score of 4.1–7 points (moderate pain), and the third group consisted of subjects with a VAS score of 7.1–10 points (severe pain).

Menstrual distress and disorders significantly affect overall health status. Nearly 90% of the respondents reported at least one menstrual disorder, mostly dysmenorrhea (70.7%), whereas secondary amenorrhea was least frequently reported (13.8%) ($p = 0.002$). The most frequent menstrual distress symptoms were abdominal pain, back pain, and generalized pain, and the prevalence of these symptoms increased with a rise in the menstrual pain score (Table 3).

Table 3. Menstrual disorders and distress symptoms relative to the self-reported intensity of menstrual pain (VAS).

	Mild Pain, N = 147 (29.1%)		Moderate Pain, N = 234 (46.4%)		Severe Pain, N = 124 (24.5%)		Kruskal–Wallis Test
	N	N%	N	N%	N	N%	
Abdominal pain	89	60.5	177	75.6	124	100	0.003
Anxiety	19	12.9	159	67.9	75	60.5	0.005
Generalized pain	23	15.6	173	73.9	117	94.3	0.002
Uterine contractions	106	72.1	170	72.6	95	76.6	ns
Back pain	91	61.2	178	76.0	97	78.2	ns
Headache	56	38.1	56	23.9	68	54.8	0.012
Fatigue	39	26.5	79	33.7	84	67.7	0.003
Leg pain	27	18.4	141	60.3	96	77.4	0.002
Nausea	11	7.5	17	7.3	10	8.0	ns
Insomnia	29	19.7	59	25.2	87	70.2	0.003
Loss of appetite	46	31.3	72	33.2	41	33.1	ns
Diarrhea/constipation	51	34.7	71	30.3	43	34.6	ns
Heart palpitations	12	8.2	24	10.3	27	21.8	0.041

ns—not statistically significant.

3.2. *The Influence of Diet and Eating Habits on the Menstrual Cycle*

Most of the subjects consumed four meals per day (N = 207, 41%), whereas the smallest number of women (N = 29, 5.7%) consumed two or fewer meals per day. In the studied group, 16.0% of the respondents adhered to a special diet, mostly a vegetarian diet (54.5% of the respondents adhered to a special diet). Light (low-calorie) food products were consumed by 73.3% of the surveyed subjects, and every tenth respondent consumed these products regularly or always. Dietary supplements were used by 84% of the surveyed population in the preceding 6 months. The most popular supplements were vitamin D, magnesium, vitamin B6, vitamin and mineral preparations, omega-3 fatty acids, and herbal supplements that alleviate menstrual pain and boost immunity. The phase of the menstrual cycle considerably affected food intake in more than half of the respondents ($p = 0.012$). During menstruation, 21.7% of the women ($p = 0.023$) experienced increased hunger, whereas 17.6% ($p = 0.031$) experienced food cravings, mainly sugar cravings.

On average, most women consumed 1730 mL of beverages per day, around 3.4 vegetable portions per day, 2.5 portions of cereal products per day, and 1.6 portions of sweets per day. The most frequently consumed food products were beverages, vegetables, fruit, sugar, and sweets, whereas fish, dry legumes, and nuts were consumed least frequently (Table 4). It should be noted that the consumption frequency of these groups of food products varied considerably from several times per day to several times per month. The following groups of food products were consumed least frequently: fermented dairy products, alcohol, fish, potatoes, and dry legumes. In this context, only reduced alcohol consumption can be regarded as a positive factor.

Table 4. Consumption frequency of selected groups of food products relative to the intensity of menstrual pain (tertile division, N = 505) and the odds ratios (95% confidence interval) in an analysis of the relationships between severe menstrual pain vs. mild menstrual pain and the consumption of particular food groups.

	Intensity of Menstrual Pain								*p*-Value	Severe Menstrual Pain (Ref. Mild Menstrual Pain)
	Total N = 505		Mild		Moderate		Severe			
	Daily Frequency		Daily Frequency		Daily Frequency		Daily Frequency			
Refined cereal products	1.4	(0–2)	1.2	(0–2)	1.5	(0–2)	1.7	(0–2)	0.0031	1.76 ** (1.06–1.98)
Whole-grain cereal products	0.81	(0–2)	0.94	(0–2)	0.83	(0–2)	0.67	(0–2)	0.023	0.88 * (0.64–1.02)
Milk	1.5	(0–2)	1.5	(0–2)	1.4	(0–2)	1.4	(0–2)	ns	0.92 (0.89–1.14)
Fermented milks	0.3	(0–2)	0.3	(0–2)	0.4	(0–2)	0.3	(0–2)	ns	0.94 (0.91–1.09)

Table 4. *Cont.*

	Intensity of Menstrual Pain								p-Value	Severe Menstrual Pain (Ref. Mild Menstrual Pain)
	Total N = 505		Mild		Moderate		Severe			
	Daily Frequency		Daily Frequency		Daily Frequency		Daily Frequency			
Sweetened dairy products	1.5	(0–2)	1.5	(0–2)	1.7	(0–2)	1.0	(0–2)	0.0016	0.73 (0.62–1.07)
Fresh meat	0.6	(0–2)	0.6	(0–2)	0.7	(0–2)	0.6	(0–2)	ns	1.02 (0.97–1.04)
Processed meat	1.5	(0–2)	1.3	(0–2)	1.3	(0–2)	1.7	(0–2)	0.002	1.54 * (1.12–1.87)
Fish	0.2	(0–1)	0.2	(0–1)	0.2	(0–1)	0.2	(0–1)	ns	1.03 (0.92–1.09)
Vegetable fats	0.4	(0–2)	0.4	(0–2)	0.5	(0–2)	0.3	(0–2)	ns	0.91 (0.81–1.01)
Animal fats	1.6	(0–2)	1.4	(0–2)	1.3	(0–2)	1.8	(0–2)	0.041	1.45 * (1.12–1.87)
Potatoes	0.3	(0–0.79)	0.3	(0–0.79)	0.3	(0–0.79)	0.3	(0–0.79)	ns	1.02 (0.97–1.04)
Vegetables	1.7	(0–2)	1.8	(0–2)	1.5	(0–2)	1.1	(0–2)	0.0027	0.53 ** (0.46–0.89)
Dry legumes	0.3	(0–1)	0.3	(0–1)	0.3	(0–1)	0.3	(0–1)	ns	1.02 (0.97–1.05)
Nuts	0.2	(0–2)	0.2	(0–2)	0.2	(0–2)	0.2	(0–2)	ns	1.02 (0.98–1.07)
Fruit	1.7	(0–2)	1.9	(0–2)	1.6	(0–2)	1.4	(0–2)	0.0027	0.71 * (0.64–0.89)
Sugar and sweets	1.6	(0–2)	1.1	(0–2)	1.4	(0–2)	1.9	(0–2)	0.001	2,19 ** (1.34–2.51)
Sweetened beverages	0.5	(0–2)	0.3	(0–2)	0.7	(0–2)	0.4	(0–2)	0.0031	1.19 (1.01–1.36)
Fast foods	0.7	(0–1)	0.7	(0–1)	0.8	(0–1)	0.7	(0–1)	ns	1.02 (0.97–1.08)
Alcohol	0.4	(0–2)	0.6	(0–2)	0.4	(0–2)	0.5	(0–2)	0.042	0.91 (0.76–1.09)
Water	1.7	(0–2)	1.6	(0–2)	1.1	(0–2)	1.8	(0–2)	0.0026	1.23 (1.01–1.46)

Statistically significant: ns—not statistically significant; * $p < 0.05$; ** $p < 0.01$.

In the study population, dysmenorrhea/menstrual distress was linked with a higher consumption frequency of certain food groups. Women with severe dysmenorrhea consumed refined cereal products, processed meat, sugar, and animal fats significantly more frequently than women with mild menstrual pain. In turn, sweetened dairy products, whole-grain cereal products, fruit, and vegetables were consumed more frequently by women with mild intensity of menstrual pain (mild pain) (Table 4).

3.3. Evaluation of Menstrual Health Parameters and Eating Habits in Women Adhering to Two Dietary Models

Two dietary models were developed based on the groups of food products and the frequency with which these products were consumed by the surveyed women. The first model, referred to as the anti-inflammatory model, is largely consistent with the planetary health diet which is composed mainly of vegetables, fruit, whole-grain cereal products, and legumes, and is characterized by reduced consumption of red meat, processed meat, refined cereal products, starchy vegetables, and added sugar. The second model, referred to as the proinflammatory model, involved higher consumption of processed foods, in particular refined cereal products, processed meat, animal fats, potatoes, sugar, sweets, sweetened beverages, and fast foods, and reduced consumption of vegetables, fruit, dairy products, and high-fiber cereal products. Based on the declared consumption of various groups of food products, 324 women (64.6%) were included in the first model, and 181 women (35.4%) were included in the second model ($p = 0.0231$). Smoking and alcohol consumption were the main health-related parameters that differentiated the participants. The number of women who had never smoked and consumed alcohol sporadically (less than several times per month) was significantly higher in model 1 than in model 2 (65.6% vs. 41.9%, $p = 0.027$, and 52.1% vs. 34.8%, $p = 0.031$, respectively).

No significant differences in average BMI values were observed between women following model 1 and model 2 (22.7 ± 4.6 vs. 22.3 ± 3.8 kg/m^2, respectively, $p = 0.236$). However, the number of women with a healthy BMI was significantly higher in model 1 than in model 2 (79.1% vs. 63.0%, $p = 0.004$). The percentage of overweight and obese women was significantly higher in model 2 than in model 1 (37.0% vs. 15.9%), but no significant differences in the percentage of women with gynoid and android obesity were noted between models.

The percentage of women experiencing low intensity of menstrual pain (mild pain) was significantly higher in model 1 (41.9%) than in model 2 (6%) (Table 5). Women adhering to the anti-inflammatory diet were also less affected by other menstrual distress symptoms.

Table 5. Menstrual health parameters, diet, and levels of knowledge in the compared dietary models.

	Model 1 (Anti-Inflammatory) N = 324	N%	Model 2 (Proinflammatory) N = 181	N%	p-Value in the Chi-Squared Test
Intensity of menstrual pain					
• mild	136	41.9%	11	6%	0.015
• moderate	167	51.5%	67	37%	
• severe	21	6.6%	103	57%	
Regular menstrual cycle					
• yes	289	89.2%	137	75.7%	0.041
• no	35	10.8%	44	24.3%	
Menstrual distress symptoms					
• <3	111	34.3	35	19.3%	0.017
• 3–8	186	57.4%	67	37%	
• >8	27	8.3%	79	43.6%	
Number of meals per day					
• 1–3	89	27.5%	46	25.5%	0.038
• 4	151	46.6%	56	30.9%	
• >5	84	25.9%	79	43.6%	
Adherence to a special diet					
• yes	33	10.2%	48	26.5%	0.028
• no	291	89.8%	133	73.5%	
Consumption of light food products					
• never	81	25%	54	29.8%	0.225
• rarely	212	65.4%	120	66.3%	
• regularly/always	31	9.6%	7	3.9%	
Use of dietary supplements in the previous 6 months					
• yes	263	81.2%	161	89%	0.317
• no	61	18.8%	25	11%	
Increased food intake during menstruation					
• yes	112	34.6%	106	58.6%	0.037
• no	212	65.4%	75	41.4%	
Increased hunger during menstruation					
• yes	79	24.4%	94	51.9%	0.028
• no	245	75.6%	87	48.1%	
Knowledge about dietary components that influence mood during menstruation					
• yes	247	76.2%	102	56.4%	0.021
• no	77	23.8%	79	43.6%	
Knowledge about the menstrual cycle					
• low	105	32.4%	98	54.1%	0.036
• high	219	67.6%	83	45.9%	
The influence of diet on the men-strual cycle					
• no influence	0	-	13	7.2%	0.029
• low influence	54	16.7%	36	19.9%	
• considerable influence	124	38.3%	75	41.4%	
• very high influence	146	45%	57	31.5%	

The use of dietary supplements, consumption of food products with a decreased content of one or more nutrients, and consumption of low-calorie foods did not differ significantly between the compared models ($p > 0.05$). Women adhering to the proinflammatory diet experienced hunger significantly more often ($p = 0.28$) and more frequently consumed a higher number of meals per day ($p = 0.038$) during menstruation. Women from the compared models differed significantly in their knowledge about the menstrual cycle and physiological changes in the body ($p < 0.05$). Women adhering to the anti-inflammatory diet had higher levels of knowledge.

Education was a factor that significantly influenced the participants' knowledge about the effect of dietary components such as saturated fatty acids (Figure 1), vitamin D (Figure 2), and simple sugars (Figure 3) on the menstrual cycle.

Most participants were of the opinion that a diet rich in unsaturated fatty acids (54.1%, $p = 0.0941$), vitamin D (68.9%, $p = 0.0231$), zinc, selenium, and iodine (68.9%, $p = 0.162$), B vitamins (76.4%, $p = 0.0712$), and antioxidants (66.7%, $p = 0.172$) contributes to a healthy menstrual cycle. Only 36.4% of the surveyed women identified saturated fatty acids and 35.4% identified simple sugars as dietary components that do not contribute to a healthy menstrual cycle.

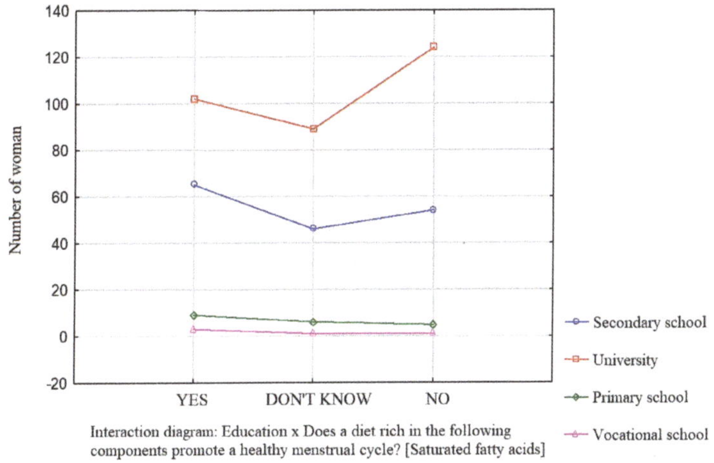

Figure 1. The relationship between education and the participants' knowledge about the influence of dietary components on the menstrual cycle (saturated fatty acids).

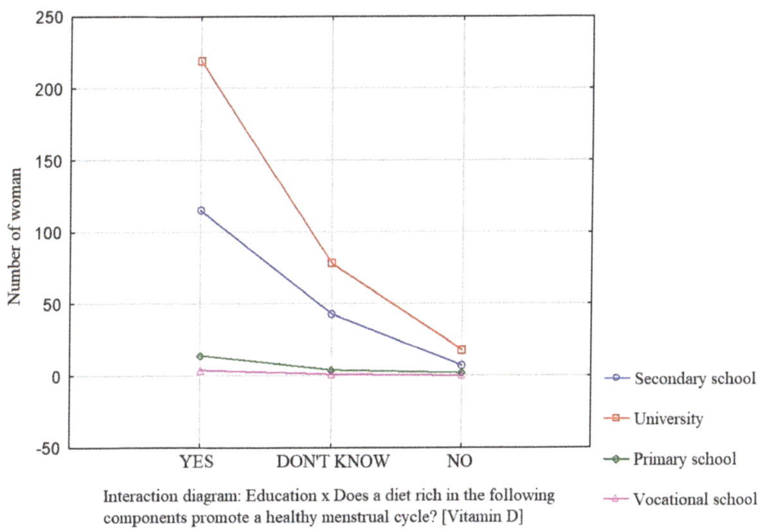

Figure 2. The relationship between education and the participants' knowledge about the influence of dietary components on the menstrual cycle (vitamin D).

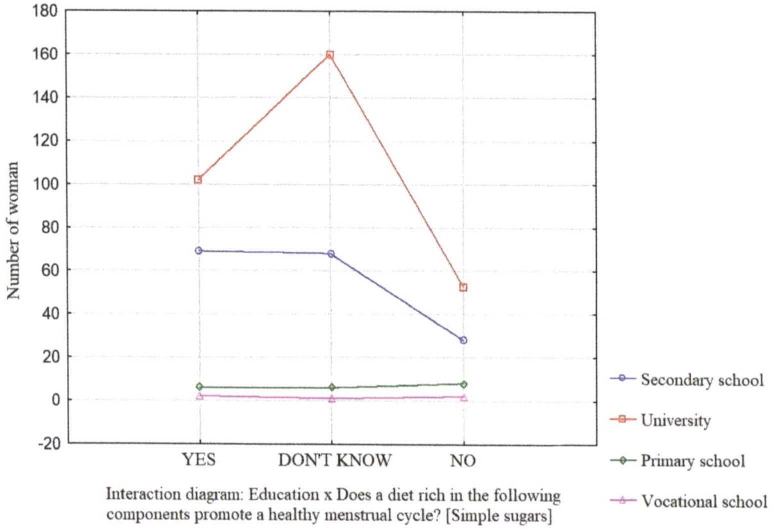

Figure 3. The relationship between education and the participants' knowledge about the influence of dietary components on the menstrual cycle (simple sugars).

4. Discussion

The literature on the relationship between diet and menstrual distress is selective and ambiguous. According to research, there is evidence to suggest that diet is linked with menstrual distress, including dysmenorrhea and/or other menstrual distress symptoms. However, most of the published studies are of low quality and rely on different methodologies (for diagnosing menstrual pain or collecting information about the participants' diets), which prevents a reliable comparison of data and the formulation of conclusions. Most studies on the subject were conducted in Asia and Africa, whereas only a handful of trials were carried out in Europe, including in Spain [18], Serbia [19], and Italy [20,21], which limits the scope of the available data. Two Polish epidemiological studies demonstrated that dysmenorrhea affects 65% of Polish women [22,23]. In the work of Barcikowska et al. [24], only 68 of the studied subjects (6.0%) did not report any symptoms of dysmenorrhea. In contrast, Szymańska et al. [13] assessed the influence of adherence to a dietary model on menstruation distress only in women with heavy and painful menstruation. The present study contributes new knowledge about the influence of diet and the proposed dietary models on the menstrual cycle and distress in a population of Polish women.

Recent studies have reported that in women who do not receive hormonal therapy (contraception, hormone replacement therapy), hormonal changes during the menstrual cycle have a significant impact on eating habits. An awareness of these changes can help women control their food intake and maintain normal weight [25,26]. The premenstrual syndrome (PMS) may predispose women to changes in appetite and food cravings [26,27]. In the population analyzed in this study, nearly a quarter of the surveyed women experienced increased appetite, including sugar cravings, during menstruation, and high pain intensity was significantly correlated with increased consumption of sweets ($p = 0.001$). Similar results were reported by Lefebvre et al. [28] who analyzed women's preferences for various groups of food products during the menstrual cycle. They found that most menstruating women craved fruit, sweets, and carbohydrates [28]. One of the hypotheses to be considered for the increase in carbohydrate intake during menstruation is the relationship between simple carbohydrates (high glycemic index) and a higher production of cerebral serotonin which reduces the negative mood effects [29]. It is believed that women unconsciously increase carbohydrate consumption in the days prior to menstruation to produce neurotransmitters that are related to mood improvement because carbohydrates, especially simple carbohydrates, increase the availability of tryptophan, a precursor of serotonin in the brain [29–31].

According to many researchers, dietary factors, lifestyle factors, and dietary models that potentially affect the intensity of menstrual pain should be identified. Research has shown that lifestyle habits, including the frequency of breakfast consumption, were associated with menstrual pain. In the present study, women with mild menstrual pain consumed regular meals (74.1% vs. 69.3%, $p = 0.0031$) and breakfasts (63.9% vs. 58.1%, $p = 0.046$) more frequently than women with severe menstrual pain. Similar results were noted in a study of Japanese women aged 18–20 years, where respondents who consumed breakfast 0–3 times per week experienced irregular menstrual cycles and severe menstrual pain significantly more often than women who consumed breakfast 4–7 days per week [32,33].

Menstrual health is integral to women's overall health and well-being. Despite the above, menstrual disorders remain insufficiently investigated, and some women have very little knowledge about the menstrual cycle. In the Western world, women tend to be more knowledgeable, and menstruation is no longer regarded as a taboo subject [34], but the physiological basis of menstruation, biological changes at puberty, the menstrual cycle, and infection risks posed by poor menstruation hygiene are hardly ever discussed openly [35,36]. A study conducted in Bangladesh revealed that most adolescent girls lacked scientific knowledge about menstruation and puberty, and adolescents were reluctant to address this topic or seek treatment for menstrual distress due to popular myths, misconceptions, and other cultural biases [37]. In a study of 125 American women, 52.8% of the participants had a high knowledge about the ovulatory cycle, whereas only 50.4% of the respondents were familiar with the average duration of menstrual flow [38]. Lungdsberg [39] investigated 1000 American women of various ethnicity, socioeconomic status, and educational background, and found that approximately 40% of the respondents were not fully familiar with the ovulatory cycle. A survey of 14- to 21-year-old girls and women conducted by Plan International UK in the United Kingdom and Ireland revealed that one in seven participants did not know what was happening during their first menstruation [40]. In 2020, a study carried out in Poland by the Kulczyk Foundation also demonstrated that nearly 40% of the surveyed girls and women aged 15–45 years had insufficient knowledge about the menstrual cycle, limited access to reliable information about menstruation, and a decreased quality of life and well-being [41]. In the present study, more than 60% of the participants had sufficient knowledge about the physiology of the menstrual cycle (education was a significantly differentiating factor, $p < 0.002$; 73% of university graduates vs. only 36% of women with secondary school education had adequate levels of knowledge), but more than a third of the respondents were not familiar with the length of the menstrual cycle, and 24% could not indicate the successive phases of the cycle.

Many women relied on alternative methods of self-care that were not always optimal. Similarly to this study, Fernández-Martínez [42] observed that non-steroidal anti-inflammatory drugs were the main self-care strategy of alleviating menstrual pain. In an epidemiological study of Danish women, the prevalence of menstrual pain (dysmenorrhea) was found to be inversely associated with the dietary intake of fish oil (n-3 fatty acid) and vitamin B12. These findings support the hypothesis that menstrual cramps, which are prostaglandin-mediated, can be influenced by dietary fatty acids, and that fish oil supplements could be potentially used to treat or prevent dysmenorrhea [43]. A high ratio of dietary omega-3 to omega-6 fatty acids could potentially alleviate dysmenorrhea. According to Hansen [44], diets rich in polyunsaturated fatty acids (PUFAs) can decrease the consumption of non-steroidal anti-inflammatory drugs during menstruation. In the current study, more than 80% of the surveyed women used dietary supplements, including remedies that alleviate menstrual pain and discomfort.

Adherence to a dietary pattern could be a factor that affects health, including menstrual health. However, this issue has been investigated by a small number of reliable studies [13,45,46]. Similarly to the present study, Szymanska et al. [13] found that adherence to an unprocessed diet based on the Mediterranean diet or the anti-inflammatory diet reduced pain intensity or decreased the incidence of menstrual distress. The cited authors analyzed the consumption frequency of selected food groups, such as vegetables, fruit, dairy, meat, legumes, fish, fast foods/salty products, and sweets. The presented findings can guide the development of new therapies for relieving menstrual pain.

Strengths and Limitations

Despite the fact that menstrual distress, in particular dysmenorrhea, affects a large portion of the female population, only a few studies have addressed the relationship between menstrual distress symptoms and diet. Most of the studies have been conducted in Asia on small population samples, and they investigated only a limited number of food products. The present study has several strengths. Above all, attempts were made to examine the complex relationship between menstrual distress symptoms, in particular dysmenorrhea, and Polish women's diets. In addition, the study sample was selected based on a narrow set of inclusion criteria, and validated tools were used assess menstrual pain and the participants' diets. The results can be used to draw reliable conclusions about the influence of diet on menstrual distress and to explore the underlying mechanisms of action. Two dietary models were identified and correlated with menstrual health factors, lifestyle factors, and women's knowledge about the menstrual cycle. The present findings can be used to formulate the objectives of health and nutrition education programs for women of reproductive age. Furthermore, moderate and severe menstrual pain was reported by a relatively high number of the surveyed women, which increased the power of statistical tests.

The main limitation of the study is that the study sample was not randomly selected, and that cross-sectional data were collected. As a result, the causes of menstrual distress could not be identified, and only the presence of correlations or relationships between the analyzed factors in the studied group of women could be determined.

5. Conclusions

Can menstrual health be linked to women's diet and nutritional knowledge? Can adherence to a dietary pattern confer potential benefits and influence the severity of menstrual discomfort? This study showed that in the analyzed population, menstrual pain/distress was associated with the consumption frequency of selected groups of food products. Two dietary models that potentially affect the menstrual cycle were identified. Consumption of a diet based on the principles of the planetary diet promoted a reduction in menstrual discomfort. Women consuming an anti-inflammatory diet containing low-processed products (vegetables, fruit, whole-grain cereals, dairy and legumes) experienced significantly less menstrual pain. In contrast, consumption of highly processed foods, including sweets, processed meat, foods high in saturated fat and low in fiber, was more frequently associated with increased menstrual pain and discomfort.

Significant differences in knowledge about the menstrual cycle and physiological changes in the body were observed between women adhering to the compared dietary models. The results indicate that an educational program targeting women of reproductive age and health professionals should be implemented to disseminate knowledge on the impact of diet and lifestyle factors on the alleviation of menstrual distress symptoms.

Author Contributions: A.C., M.K. and M.P.-S. were responsible for the concept and design of the main study. J.K., P.K. and A.C. were responsible for data cleaning and statistical analysis. M.K., P.K., M.P.-S. and J.K. were responsible for data interpretation for this particular paper, for writing the manuscript, and for data collection for the main study. M.K. and A.C. were responsible for revising the manuscript critically for important intellectual content. All authors have read and agreed to the published version of the manuscript.

Funding: The study was financially supported by the Polish Ministry of Science and Higher Education; the authors performed research with the help of volunteers (members of the Student Scientific Society of Dietetics).

Institutional Review Board Statement: The research plan was approved by the Ethics Committee of the Medical University of Lublin (KE-0254/273/2021, approval date: 16 December 2021).

Informed Consent Statement: Not applicable.

Data Availability Statement: Due to ethical restrictions and participant confidentiality, data cannot be made publicly available.

Acknowledgments: Thanks are expressed to the participants for their contributions to the study and the authors would like to thank Agnieszka Wójcik, Teresa Poniewozik, Aneta Milszmauedan and Milena Jaworska for their help with data collection.

Conflicts of Interest: The authors declare no conflict of interest.

References

1. Kocaoz, S.; Cirpan, R.; Degirmencioglu, A.Z. The prevalence and impacts heavy menstrual bleeding on anemia, fatigue and quality of life in women of reproductive age. *Pak. J. Med. Sci.* **2019**, *35*, 365–370. [CrossRef] [PubMed]
2. MacGregor, B.; Allaire, C.; Bedaiwy, M.A.; Yong, P.J.; Bougie, O. Disease Burden of Dysmenorrhea: Impact on Life Course Potential. *Int. J. Womens Health* **2023**, *15*, 499–509. [CrossRef] [PubMed]
3. Schoep, M.E.; Nieboer, T.E.; van der Zanden, M.; Braat, D.D.M.; Nap, A.W. The impact of menstrual symptoms on everyday life: A survey among 42,879 women. *Am. J. Obstet. Gynecol.* **2019**, *220*, 569. [CrossRef]
4. Yamada, K.; Kamagata, E. Reduction of quality-adjusted life years (QALYs) in patients with premenstrual dysphoric disorder (PMDD). *Qual. Life Res.* **2017**, *26*, 3069–3073. [CrossRef] [PubMed]
5. Fernández-Martínez, E.; Onieva-Zafra, M.D.; Parra-Fernández, M.L. The Impact of Dysmenorrhea on Quality of Life among Spanish Female University Students. *Int. J. Environ. Res. Public Health* **2019**, *16*, 713. [CrossRef] [PubMed]
6. Yoshino, O.; Takahashi, N.; Suzukamo, Y. Menstrual symptoms, health-related quality of life, and work productivity in Japanese women with dysmenorrhea receiving different treatments: Prospective observational study. *Adv. Ther.* **2022**, *39*, 2562–2577. [CrossRef] [PubMed]
7. Mizuta, R.; Maeda, N.; Tashiro, T.; Suzuki, Y.; Oda, S.; Komiya, M.; Urabe, Y. Quality of life by dysmenorrhea severity in young and adult Japanese females: A web-based cross-sectional study. *PLoS ONE* **2023**, *18*, e0283130. [CrossRef] [PubMed]
8. ACOG Committee Opinion No. 760: Dysmenorrhea and Endometriosis in the Adolescent. *Obstet. Gynecol.* **2018**, *132*, 249–258. [CrossRef]
9. Unnisa, H.; Annam, P.; Gubba, N.C.; Begum, A.; Thatikonda, K. Assessment of quality of life and effect of non-pharmacological management in dysmenorrhea. *Ann. Med. Surg.* **2022**, *81*, 104407. [CrossRef]
10. Kanchan, Y.; Rizwana, S.; Charu, S.; Kalpna, G.; Jitendra, J.; Goury, C. Menstrual pattern in medical students and their knowledge and attitude towards it. *Int. J. Med. Health Res.* **2018**, *4*, 19–22.
11. Bauman, D.; Sommer, A.; Hamer, T.; Noy, D.; Elami, M.; Yogev, S.S.; Magiel, E.; Revel-Vilk, S. Reduced Activity and Quality of Life in Women Soldiers with Heavy Menstrual Bleeding and Dysmenorrhea. *J. Pediatr. Adolesc. Gynecol.* **2022**, *35*, 53–58. [CrossRef] [PubMed]
12. Knopczyk, J.; Kaczorowska, A.; Mroczek, A. Influence of menstruation on pain of lumbar–sacra spine in women aged 20–35. In *Holistic Dimension of Modern Medicine*, 1st ed.; Krajewska-Kułak, E., Łukaszuk, C., Lewko, J., Kułak, W., Eds.; Uniwersytet Medyczny w Białymstoku: Białystok, Poland, 2021; Volume 8, pp. 973–982. ISBN 978-83-959846-8-6. (In Polish)
13. Szymańska, K.; Jaworski, M.; Gotlib, J.; Panczyk, M. Elements of eating pattern and intensity of dysmenorrhea—A cross-sectional study in sample of Polish women. *Med. Sci. Pulse* **2020**, *14*, 10–17. [CrossRef]
14. Graff, E.; Vedantam, S.; Parianos, M.; Khakoo, N.; Beiling, M.; Pearlman, M. Dietary Intake and Systemic Inflammation: Can We Use Food as Medicine? *Curr. Nutr. Rep.* **2023**, *12*, 247–254. [CrossRef] [PubMed]
15. Wohlgemuth, K.J.; Arieta, L.R.; Brewer, G.J.; Hoselton, A.L.; Gould, L.M.; Smith-Ryan, A.E. Sex differences and considerations for female specific nutritional strategies: A narrative review. *J. Int. Soc. Sports Nutr.* **2021**, *18*, 27–46. [CrossRef] [PubMed]
16. Cochran, W.G. *Sampling Techniques*, 3rd ed.; John Wiley & Sons: New York, NY, USA, 1977.
17. Główny Urząd Statystyczny. Available online: https://stat.gov.pl/ (accessed on 22 January 2023).
18. Onieva-Zafra, M.D.; Fernández-Martínez, E.; Abreu-Sánchez, A.; Iglesias-López, M.T.; García-Padilla, F.M.; Pedregal-González, M.; Parra-Fernández, M.L. Relationship between Diet, Menstrual Pain and other Menstrual Characteristics among Spanish Students. *Nutrients* **2020**, *12*, 1759. [CrossRef] [PubMed]
19. Pejčić, A.; Janković, S. Risk factors for dysmenorrhea among young adult female university students. *Ann. Dell'ist. Super. Di Sanita* **2016**, *52*, 98–103. [CrossRef]
20. Di Cintio, E.; Parazzini, F.; Tozzi, L.; Luchini, L.; Mezzopane, R.; Marchini, M.; Fedele, L. Dietary habits, reproductive and menstrual factors and risk of dysmenorrhoea. *Eur. J. Epidemiol.* **1997**, *13*, 925–930. [CrossRef]
21. Grandi, G.; Ferrari, X.; Cannoletta, P.; Volpe, C.A. Prevalence of menstrual pain in young women: What is dysmenorrhea? *J. Pain Res.* **2012**, *2012*, 169–174. [CrossRef]
22. Teul, I.; Kliś, K.; Jarzębak, K.; Wronka, I. The prevalence and correlates of menstrual pain in healthy university students. *Ann. Acad. Medicae Stetin.* **2014**, *60*, 89–94.

23. Zurawiecka, M.; Wronka, I. Association of primary dysmenorrhea with anthropometrical and socioeconomic factors in polish university students. *J. Obstet. Gynaecol. Res.* **2018**, *44*, 1259–1267. [CrossRef]
24. Barcikowska, Z.; Wójcik-Bilkiewicz, K.; Sobierajska-Rek, A.; Grzybowska, M.E.; Wąż, P.; Zorena, K. Dysmenorrhea and Associated Factors among Polish Women: A Cross-Sectional Study. *Pain Res. Manag.* **2020**, *2020*, 6161536. [CrossRef] [PubMed]
25. Hirschberg, A.L. Sex hormones, appetite and eating behaviour in women. *Maturitas* **2012**, *71*, 248–256. [CrossRef] [PubMed]
26. Kamemoto, K.; Yamada, M.; Matsuda, T.; Ogata, H.; Ishikawa, A.; Kanno, M.; Miyashita, M.; Sakamaki-Sunaga, M. Effects of menstrual cycle on appetite-regulating hormones and energy intake in response to cycling exercise in physically active women. *J. Appl. Physiol.* **2022**, *132*, 224–235. [CrossRef] [PubMed]
27. Saad, G.; Strenstron, E. Calories, beauty, and ovulation: The effects of the menstrual cycle on food and appearance-related consumption. *J. Cons. Psychol.* **2012**, *22*, 102–113. [CrossRef]
28. Lefebvre, M.; Hengartner, M.P.; Tronci, E.; Mancini, T.; Ille, F.; Röblitz, S.; Krüger, T.; Leeners, B. Food preferences throughout the menstrual cycle—A computer-assisted neuro-endocrino-psychological investigation. *Physiol. Behav.* **2022**, *255*, 113943. [CrossRef] [PubMed]
29. Murakami, K.; Sasaki, S.; Takahashi, Y.; Uenishi, K.; Watanabe, T.; Kohri, T.; Yamasaki, M.; Watanabe, R.; Baba, K.; Shibata, K.; et al. Dietary glycemic index is associated with decreased premenstrual symptoms in young Japanese women. *Nutrition* **2008**, *24*, 554–561. [CrossRef] [PubMed]
30. Tucci, S.A.; Murphy, L.E.; Boyland, E.J.; Dye, L.; Halford, J.C. Oral contra—Ceptive effects on food choice during the follicular and luteal phases of the menstrual cycle: A laboratory based study. *Appetite* **2010**, *55*, 388–392. [CrossRef]
31. Gorczyca, A.M.; Sjaarda, L.A.; Mitchell, E.M.; Mitchell, E.M.; Perkins, N.J.; Schliep, K.C.; Wactawski-Wende, J.; Mumford, S.L. Changes in macronutrient, micronutrient, and food group intakes throughout the menstrual cycle in healthy, premenopausal women. *Eur. J. Nutr.* **2016**, *55*, 1181–1188. [CrossRef]
32. Kazama, M.; Maruyama, K.; Nakamura, K. Prevalence of dysmenorrhea and its correlating lifestyle factors in Japanese female junior high school students. *Tohoku J. Exp. Med.* **2015**, *236*, 107–113. [CrossRef]
33. Naraoka, Y.; Hosokawa, M.; Minato-Inokawa, S.; Sato, Y. Severity of Menstrual Pain Is Associated with Nutritional Intake and Lifestyle Habits. *Healthcare* **2023**, *11*, 1289. [CrossRef]
34. Policy Brief: Women and Menstruation in the EU. Available online: https://eurohealth.ie/policy-brief-women-and-menstruation-in-the-eu-2/#_edn17 (accessed on 23 October 2023).
35. Tjon-A-Ten, V. (Ed.) *Menstrual Hygiene: A Neglected Condition for the Achievement of Several Millennium Development Goals*; Europe External Policy Advisors: Brussels, Belgium, 2007; pp. 1–24.
36. Mohammed, S.; Larsen-Reindorf, R.E. Menstrual knowledge, sociocultural restrictions, and barriers to menstrual hygiene management in Ghana: Evidence from a multi-method survey among adolescent schoolgirls and schoolboys. *PLoS ONE* **2020**, *15*, 0241106. [CrossRef] [PubMed]
37. Haque, S.; Rahman, M.; Itsukow, K.; Mutahara, M.; Sakisaka, K. The effect of a school-based educational intervention on menstrual health: An intervention study among adolescent girls in Bangladesh. *BMJ Open* **2014**, *4*, 004607. [CrossRef] [PubMed]
38. Ayoola, A.B.; Zandee, G.L.; Adams, Y.J. Women's knowledge of ovulation, the menstrual cycle, and its associated reproductive changes. *Birth* **2016**, *43*, 255–262. [CrossRef] [PubMed]
39. Lundsberg, L.S.; Pal, L.; Gariepy, A.M.; Xu, X.; Chu, M.C.; Illuzzi, J.L. Knowledge, attitudes, and practices regarding conception and fertility: A population-based survey among reproductive-age United States women. *Fertil. Steril.* **2014**, *101*, 767–774. [CrossRef] [PubMed]
40. Tingle, C.; Vora, S. Break the Barriers: Girls' Experiences of Menstruation in the UK Plan International UK. 2018. Available online: https://plan-uk.org/file/plan-uk-break-the-barriers-report-032018pdf/download?token=Fs-HYP3v (accessed on 20 October 2023).
41. Menstruation. Quantitative and Qualitative Research Report. Available online: https://kulczykfoundation.org.pl/uploads/media/default/0001/05/0fbe618f4aa748170c8b3f096367e2c607888eb8.pdf (accessed on 23 October 2023).
42. Fernández-Martínez, E.; Onieva-Zafra, M.D.; Abreu-Sánchez, A.; Fernández-Muñóz, J.J.; Parra-Fernández, M.L. Absenteeism during menstruation among nursing students in Spain. *Int. J. Environ. Res. Public Health* **2019**, *17*, 53. [CrossRef] [PubMed]
43. Deutch, B.; Bonefeld Jørgensen, E.; Hansen, J.C. Menstrual discomfort in Danish women reduced by dietary supplements of omega-3 PUFA and B12 (fish oil or seal oil capsules). *Nutr. Res.* **2000**, *20*, 621–631. [CrossRef]
44. Hansen, S.O.; Knudsen, U.B. Endometriosis, dysmenorrhoea and diet. *Eur. J. Obstet. Gynecol. Reprod. Biol.* **2013**, *169*, 162–171. [CrossRef]
45. Najafi, N.; Khalkhali, H.; Moghaddam Tabrizi, F.; Zarrin, R. Major dietary patterns in relation to menstrual pain: A nested case control study. *BMC Womens Health* **2018**, *18*, 69. [CrossRef]
46. Bajalan, Z.; Alimoradi, Z.; Moafi, F. Nutrition as a potential factor of primary dysmenorrhea: A systematic review of observational studies. *Gynecol. Obstet. Investig.* **2019**, *84*, 209–224. [CrossRef]

nutrients

MDPI

Article

Association between Cervical Cancer and Dietary Patterns in Colombia

Luz Adriana Meneses-Urrea [1,2], Manuel Vaquero-Abellán [3,4,*], Dolly Villegas Arenas [1,2], Narly Benachi Sandoval [1,5], Mauricio Hernández-Carrillo [6,7] and Guillermo Molina-Recio [4,8]

1 Research Group "Health Care (Recognized by Colciencias)", Universidad Santiago de Cali, Cali 760001, Colombia; luz.meneses00@usc.edu.co (L.A.M.-U.); dollyvillegas8@gmail.com (D.V.A.); nbenachi@clinic.cat (N.B.S.)
2 Department of Nursing, Universidad Santiago de Cali, Cali 760001, Colombia
3 IMIBIC GC12 Clinical and Epidemiological Research in Primary Care (GICEAP), 14014 Córdoba, Spain
4 Department of Nursing, Pharmacology and Physiotherapy, University of Córdoba, 14014 Córdoba, Spain; gmrsurf75@gmail.com
5 CAP Casanova, Consorci d'Atenció Primària de Salut Barcelona Esquerra, 08036 Barcelona, Spain
6 Health Faculty, Universidad del Valle, Cali 760001, Colombia; mauriciohc@gmail.com
7 Health Faculty, Escuela Nacional del Deporte, Cali 760001, Colombia
8 Lifestyles, Innovation and Health (GA-16), Maimonides Biomedical Research Institute of Córdoba (IMIBIC), 14014 Córdoba, Spain
* Correspondence: mvaquero@uco.es

Abstract: Cervical cancer is a global public health problem. It is the second leading cause of death among women of childbearing age worldwide. Several factors, including diet, have been shown to influence the risk of persistent HPV infection and tumor progression. This paper determines the relationship between dietary patterns and cervical cancer. It is an ecological study of multiple groups, based on two national sources: the High-Cost Account and the National Survey of Nutritional Situation of Colombia of 2015. The population consisted of 3472 women aged 35 to 64. The incidence of cervical cancer was used as the dependent variable while the independent variables included food consumption according to established patterns, area of residence, age, physical activity, and BMI, among other variables. The statistical analysis performed through associations between variables was evaluated by multiple linear regression using R2. 38.9% of the evaluated population belonged to the first quartile of wealth, and 76.5% resided in the municipal capital. The incidence of cervical cancer in Colombia was associated with being affiliated to a state-subsidized health regime and having diabetes mellitus. A conservative eating pattern, as well as belonging to a rural area, are evidenced as protective factors. These results invite the need to encourage public policies and promote healthy lifestyles.

Keywords: food consumption; cervix uterine; neoplasm; diet; risk factors

1. Introduction

Cervical cancer is a global public health problem, particularly in low- and middle-income countries (LMICs) [1]. It is the second most frequent and the second leading cause of death in women of reproductive age in the world [2]. In 2020, an incidence of 604,000 and 342,000 deaths was estimated [3]. According to GLOBOCAN data for 2020, Latin America and the Caribbean ranked second worldwide in incidence and mortality, with 59,439 new cases and 31,582 deaths [4]. It has been suggested that the incidence in these LMICs may be due to several factors, including lifestyle [5].

Human papillomavirus (HPV) is one of the causative agents of cervical cancer and precursor lesions [6]. Several causes have been shown to affect the risk of persistent HPV infection and the progression of neoplasms, including diet [7,8]. HPV survives in a cellular oxidative environment and has been shown to be more likely to evolve into neoplasms by increasing oxidative stress and DNA damage [9]. For these reasons, dietary intake of antioxidants appears to exert a protective effect on HPV infection and persistence [7,8]. According to the results of the EPIC (European Prospective Investigation into Cancer and Nutrition) study, there is a significant inverse association between invasive squamous cervical cancer and daily increases in fruit intake [10].

Regarding dietary patterns, a recent study has established that adhering to the Mediterranean diet reduces the risk of cervical cancer by 60%, while following a Western diet represents a risk factor for its appearance [11]. It is estimated that changes in dietary habits can contribute to preventing the onset of cancer by 30% to 40% [12].

For these reasons, this research was proposed to determine the relationship between dietary patterns and cervical cancer, considering other sociodemographic aspects of different regions in Colombia.

2. Methodology

A multi-group ecological study was conducted based on two national sources, HIGIA (High-Cost Account), and ENSIN 2015 (National Survey of Nutritional Situation of Colombia of 2015). The population consisted of 3472 women aged 35 to 64, distributed across six regions of Colombia: Atlántica, Central, Oriental, Pacífica, Orinoquía, and the Capital District of Bogotá.

The incidence of cervical cancer was used as the outcome variable, taken from the High-Cost Account. Independent variables were obtained from the National Survey of the Nutritional Situation (ENSIN) 2015, including: area of residence, affiliation regime, quartile of wealth, educational level, age ranges, compliance with the recommendations of physical activity, compliance with 30 min of physical exercise per day for at least 5 days, following the recommendations of vigorous physical activity, and BMI according to World Health Organization (WHO) categories [13]. In addition, information was collected on the suffering of hypertension, diabetes mellitus, following a special diet, and following a vegetarian diet. These variables were dichotomized.

The area of residence was structured as a categorical variable, including municipal seat (defined as the urban perimeter limited by agreements of the Municipal Council, where the administrative headquarters of the municipality is located), populated center (refers to the concentration of at least twenty contiguous houses, neighboring or attached to each other, located in the rural area of a municipality or a departmental corregimiento), and rural center, defined by dispersed dwellings with disaggregated farms [14].

The independent variable, consumption of dietary patterns, was taken from the work of Meneses et al., who established four dietary patterns: traditional, industrialized, conservative, and beverages/grilled foods. The traditional pattern was made up of the dairy group, potato/legume groups, cereal group, fried group, coffee/panela, and meat-sausages. The industrialized pattern was characterized by the consumption of soft drinks, fast foods, sweets, and package foods. The conservative pattern referred to individuals who based their diet on the group of vegetables, fruits, light foods, supplements, and whole foods. Finally, the beverages/grilled foods pattern was made up of the group of energy drinks, alcohol, and grilled foods [15]. To introduce the patterns into the statistical models, it was necessary to generate a new dichotomous dependent variable for each one, through the binomial distribution, as follows: those presenting some degree of consumption of the corresponding pattern were categorized as 1, while those who did not report any level of consumption of the pattern were categorized as 0.

The statistical analysis was performed through the association of contextual variables and was evaluated by multiple linear regression using R2 and the principle of statistical parsimony for multiple linear regression as a goodness of fit measure, which considers the minimum sum of squares [16]. 15 models were performed until the best one was obtained, representing the dietary patterns and accounting for possible confounding effects of the contextual variables on the incidence of cervical cancer. The statistical modeling used a stepwise method, with a criterion of eliminating probability values above 0.10.

Ethical Considerations

The study was endorsed by the Institutional Ethics Committee of the Universidad Santiago de Cali, Approval Act No. 11 of 29 May 2020. The database used was authorized by the Colombian Institute of Family Welfare (ICBF) to conduct the research, and it involved working with available anonymized data, with the consent (verbal or signed) of the participants in these national surveys to the interviewers of the national health system.

3. Results

Information was collected from a sample of 3472 women within the age range of 35 to 64. Through the evaluation of sociodemographic variables, relevant findings are highlighted, including the distribution of wealth, educational level, age, geographical location, and health insurance regime. The results indicate that 38.9% of the evaluated population belonged to the first quartile of wealth (Q1), and the region with the highest percentage in the first quartile of wealth (Q1) was Amazonia-Orinoquia, with 53.5%. 71.4% of respondents had an educational level up to high school, and 53% were in the age range of 35 to 49, occurring most frequently in the Atlantic region (64.7%). In addition, 76.5% resided in municipal capitals, with the Pacific region having the most reported living in rural areas at 32%. 58.1% of the participants belonged to the subsidized health care regime or were unaffiliated. It is important to note that this regime is used by the Colombian State to provide access to health services through granted subsidies for those without the ability to pay. The region with the highest percentage under this regime was the Amazonía-Orinoquia region, at 69.5% (Table 1).

Likewise, when considering the additional variables evaluated in the study, it was found that 12.6% of the population complied with the recommendations of physical activity, with 1.6% engaging with physical activity for at least 30 min, five times a week, and only 0.7% participating in vigorous physical activity. On the other hand, 100% of the sample did not follow a vegetarian diet or any kind of special diet. In relation to the prevalence of chronic diseases, 48.8% reported having hypertension, 2.7% had diabetes, 38.1% were overweight, and 76.3% were obese. Additional data structured by region are available in Table 2.

In relation to dietary patterns, 94.6% of the population had some consumption of pattern 1 (traditional), 92.9% of pattern 3 (conservative), 73.9% of pattern 2 (industrialized), and 57.7% had an intake linked to pattern 4 (food, beverages/grill). The traditional and conservative patterns stood out in the Pacific region, while the industrialized pattern was of higher consumption in the Atlantic region and the beverage/grill food pattern was reported more frequently in the Eastern region. The Department of Tolima, despite belonging to this region, reported no consumption. The Bogotá region was characterized by pattern 2 (industrialized) and the Amazonia-Orinoquia region, compared to the other regions, had the highest consumption of beverage/grilled foods (see Figure 1 and Table 3).

Table 1. Sociodemographic characteristics.

Variable	Category	Atlántico n = 762	Atlántico %	Oriental n = 609	Oriental %	Amazonia-Orinoquía n = 462	Amazonia-Orinoquía %	Region Bogotá n = 243	Region Bogotá %	Central n = 887	Central %	Pacífica n = 509	Pacífica %	Total n	Total %
Quartile of wealth	First quartile	363	47.6	208	34.2	247	53.5	6	2.5	286	32.2	241	47.3	1351	38.9
	Second quartile or more	399	52.4	401	65.8	215	46.5	237	98	601	19.8	268	52.7	2121	64.8
Educational level	Less than primary (0–4 years)	225	29.5	163	26.8	134	29	29	11.9	238	26.8	184	36.1	973	28
	Primary/Secondary complete	534	70.1	443	72.7	324	70.1	214	88.1	641	72.3	322	63.3	2478	71.4
Age ranges	35–39	198	26	118	19.4	90	19.5	49	20.2	163	18.4	86	16.9	704	20.3
	40–44	142	18.6	93	15.3	74	16	38	15.6	140	15.8	64	12.6	551	15.9
	45–49	153	20.1	91	14.9	73	15.8	42	17.3	169	19.1	68	13.4	596	17.2
	50–54	93	12.2	132	21.7	82	17.7	44	18.1	162	18.3	116	22.8	629	18.1
	55–59	97	12.7	92	15.1	86	18.6	41	16.9	132	14.9	87	17.1	535	15.4
	60–64	79	10.4	83	13.6	57	12.3	29	11.9	121	13.6	88	17.3	457	13.2
Area	City	585	76.8	409	67.2	441	95.5	243	100	663	74.7	315	61.9	2656	76.5
	Village/Rural	177	23.2	200	32.8	21	4.5	0	0	224	25.3	194	38.1	816	23.5
Health affiliation	Subsidized/nonaffiliated	500	65.6	320	52.5	321	69.5	71	29.2	478	53.9	326	64.0	2016	58.1
	Contributory	262	34.4	289	47.5	141	30.5	172	70.8	409	46.1	183	36	1456	41.9

Table 2. Lifestyle and health status.

Variable	Category	Atlántico n = 762 n(%)	Oriental n = 609 n(%)	Region Amazonia-Orinoquía n = 462 n(%)	Bogotá n = 243 n(%)	Central n = 887 n(%)	Pacífica n = 509 n(%)	Total n(%)
Meets physical activity recommendations	Complies	65(8.5)	86(14.1)	62(13.4)	49(20.2)	117(13.2)	59(11.6)	438(12.6)
	Does not comply	697(91.5)	523(85.9)	400(86.6)	194(79.8)	770(86.8)	450(88.4)	3034(87.4)
Physical activity 30 min per day (at least 5 days)	Complies	6(0.8)	15(2.5)	6(1.3)	6(2.5)	9(1.0)	12(2.4)	54(1.6)
	Does not comply	756(99.2)	594(97.5)	456(98.7)	237(97.5)	878(99.0)	497(97.6)	3418(98.4)
Meets recommendations for vigor	Complies	4(0.5)	4(0.7)	7(1.5)	2(0.8)	6(0.7)	3(0.6)	26(0.7)
	Does not comply	758(99.5)	605(99.3)	455(98.5)	241(99.2)	881(99.3)	506(99.4)	3446(99.3)
Overweight classification	Yes	284(37.3)	237(0.4)	167(36.1)	99(0.4)	331(37.3)	206(0.4)	1324(38.1)
	No	478(62.7)	372(0.6)	295(63.9)	144(0.6)	556(62.7)	303(59.5)	2148(61.9)
Obesity classification	Yes	222(29.1)	146(0.2)	153(33.1)	47(19.3)	253(28.5)	150(29.5)	971(28)
	No	540(70.9)	463(0.8)	456(98.7)	196(80.7)	634(71.5)	359(0.7)	2648(76.3)
Overweight/Obesity	No risk	174(25)	163(29.4)	104(24.2)	73(32.9)	224(25.3)	107(22.8)	845(24.3)
	At risk	523(75)	391(70.6)	326(75.8)	149(67.1)	592(72.5)	362(77.2)	2343(67.5)
Thinness	No risk	748(98.2)	608(99.8)	459(99.4)	243(100)	884(99.7)	506(99.4)	3448(99.3)
	At risk	12(1.6)	1(0.2)	3(0.6)	0(0)	3(0.3)	3(0.6)	22(0.7)

Table 2. *Cont.*

Variable	Category	Region Atlántico n = 762 n(%)	Oriental n = 609 n(%)	Amazonia-Orinoquía n = 462 n(%)	Bogotá n = 243 n(%)	Central n = 887 n(%)	Pacífica n = 509 n(%)	Total n(%)
Hypertension	No Yes	449(58.9) 313(41.1)	255(41.9) 354(58.1)	267(57.8) 195(42.2)	94(38.7) 149(61.3)	451 (50.8) 436(49.2)	262(51.5) 247(48.5)	1778 (51.2) 1694(48.8)
Diabetes	No Yes	746(97.9) 16(2.1)	594(97.5) 15(2.5)	437(94.6) 25(5.4)	236(97.1) 7(2.9)	870(98.1) 17(1.9)	494(97.1) 15(2.9)	3377(97.3) 95(2.7)
You follow a special diet	Yes No	0(0) 762(100)	0(0) 609(100)	0(0) 462(100)	0(0) 243(100)	0(0) 887(100)	0(0) 509(100)	0(0) 3472(100)
You are a vegetarian	Yes No	0(0) 762(100)	0(0) 609(100)	0(0) 462(100)	0(0) 243(100)	0(0) 887(100)	0(0) 509(100)	0(0) 3472(100)

Table 3. Eating patterns.

Variable	Category	Region Atlántico n = 762	%	Oriental n = 609	%	Amazonia-Orinoquía n = 462	%	Bogotá n = 243	%	Central n = 887	%	Pacífica n = 509	%	Total n	%
Pattern Consumption 1	Yes No	724 38	95 5.0	572 37	93.9 6.1	433 29	93.7 6.3	230 13	94.7 5.3	840 47	94.7 5.3	486 23	95.5 4.5	3285 187	94.6 5.4
Pattern Consumption 2	Yes No	618 144	81.1 18.9	465 144	76.4 23.6	315 147	68.2 31.8	191 52	78.6 21.4	634 253	71.5 28.5	342 167	67.2 32.8	2565 907	73.9 26.1
Pattern Consumption 3	Yes No	711 51	93.3 6.7	564 45	92.6 7.4	422 40	91.3 8.7	226 17	93 7	826 61	93.1 6.9	476 33	93.5 6.5	3225 247	92.9 7.1
Pattern Consumption 4	Yes No	317 445	41.6 58.4	289 320	47.5 52.5	218 244	47.2 52.8	79 164	32.5 67.5	357 530	40.2 59.8	209 300	41.1 58.9	1469 2003	42.3 57.7

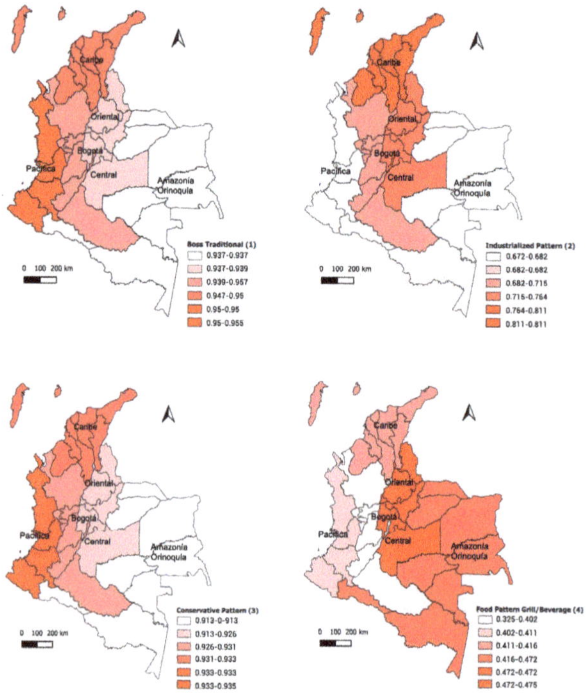

Figure 1. Dietary pattern by region.

Regarding the incidence of cervical cancer in people over 35 years of age in 2020, the highest rate was found in the Amazonia-Orinoquia region, with 23.8 cases per 100,000 habitants. This region is the one that reported the highest percentage of the population in Q1 of wealth, affiliation to the subsidized health regime, declarations of diabetes, and consumption of beverage foods/grill. The lowest incidence rate was reported in the Eastern region, with 12.8 per 100,000 hb. This region had the lowest prevalence of obesity (see Figure 2).

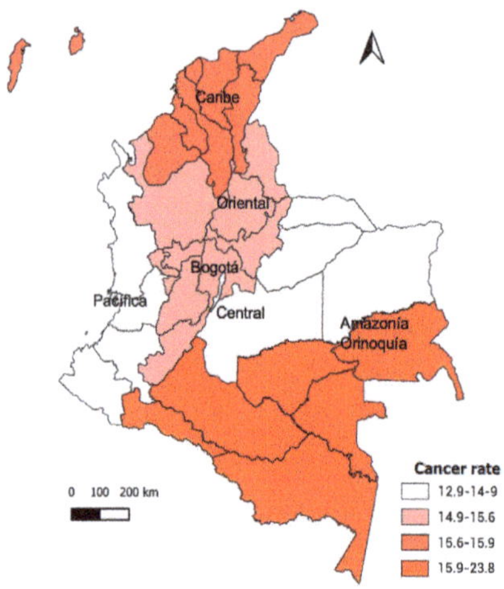

Figure 2. Incidence of cervical cancer by region.

Modelling was performed using an initial saturated model that contained all available explanatory variables [16]. After the variables in the multivariate model were adjusted, 15 models were generated. 68% of the incidence of cervical cancer can be explained by the explanatory variables of the multiple linear model (Table 4), showing a positive association with certain factors, including belonging to the subsidized regime or not being affiliated ($p = 0.002$), and having diabetes ($p = 0.07$). In addition, a negative association was found with the conservative dietary pattern ($p = 0.013$) and residing in a populated or dispersed rural center ($p = 0.003$), (Table 5).

Table 4. Comparison of ecological multiple linear regression models for cervical cancer incidence, adjusting for dietary patterns and other variables. Regions of Colombia. Year 2020.

Model	# Var	# Sig Var	R	R Square *	Adjusted R-Square	Standard Error of Estimation
1	19	0	0.889	0.78972641	0.54002652	3.35422758
2	18	0	0.889	0.78972435	0.56707953	3.25409468
3	17	1	0.889	0.78967934	0.59104315	3.16275003
4	16	1	0.889	0.78945918	0.61216165	3.08000556
5	15	1	0.888	0.78802338	0.62904091	3.01223699
6	14	1	0.886	0.78558842	0.64264736	2.95647781
7	13	2	0.884	0.7807387	0.65117521	2.92098817
8	12	3	0.880	0.7752289	0.65795703	2.89245402
9	11	4	0.878	0.77174234	0.66712424	2.85342993
10	10	4	0.874	0.76393546	0.66950964	2.84318767
11	9	5	0.868	0.75329098	0.6678917	2.85013866
12	8	4	0.864	0.74662941	0.67155664	2.83436886
13	7	3	0.856	0.73265115	0.66581394	2.85904041
14	6	2	0.840	0.70632243	0.64556155	2.94439819
15	5	4	0.825	0.6809907	0.62782248	3.01717983

Var: number of variables in the initial saturated model, # sig var: number of significant variables, Sig: significant. Adjusted for: does not meet physical activity recommendations, does not meet 30 min per day of exercise (at least 5 days), does not meet recommendations for vigorous physical activity, primary incomplete (0–4 years), first quartile of wealth, origin: urban or rural, BMI risk classification, consumption food pattern 1 (traditional), consumption dietary pattern 2 (industrialized), consumption dietary pattern 3 (preservative), consumption dietary pattern 4 (food drinks-grill, special diet, no vegetarian diet, subsidized affiliation regime/not affiliated, have high blood pressure, have diabetes). * R^2 avoids overestimation of goodness of fit.

Table 5. Model Factors of greatest influence on the incidence of cervical cancer.

Variable	Bivariate		Multivariate	
	R^2 (%)	p-Value	Standardized β	p-Value
Village/Rural	13.1	0.0300	−0.40	0.003
Conservative pattern consumption	18.5	0.0089	−0.28	0.013
Subsidized/Unaffiliated	18.1	0.0096	0.43	0.002
Have Diabetes	30.8	0.0004	0.37	0.007

Adjusted for: subsidized/unaffiliated affiliation, housing area town or rural center, consumption dietary pattern 3 (conservative), vegetarian diet, have diabetes.

4. Discussion

An ecological study was conducted using secondary data from the database of the National Survey of the Nutritional Situation (ENSIN) 2015 and the 2020 incidence rate of cervical cancer for people over 35 years of age, using the High-Cost Account as a source of information.

The incidence rate of cervical cancer has risen worldwide, especially in countries with a high Human Development Index (HDI). Colombia is considered a country with a high HDI [17]. This rate is influenced by aging, population growth, and changes in cancer risk factors, some of which are related to socioeconomic development [18].

The findings of this research showed associations between the incidence rate and variables including the area of residence, populated or rural center, subsidized health regime, having diabetes, and the consumption of the conservative pattern. The results of our study found no association with the quartile of wealth, despite the fact that 62.4% of the population was in quartiles 1 and 2 of wealth, which may be due to early detection and efficient treatment [19]. Several studies have reported that the probability of developing cancer is higher in socially vulnerable populations and that the risk of getting sick and dying is associated with lower levels of income, education, and higher degrees of social discrimination [20,21].

The lack of adequate health insurance coverage is a challenge in communities of poverty and is associated with reduced access to care, prevention, and diagnosis. Patel et al. conducted a study in California and reported that patients with *Medicaid*, insurance granted by the state, or those without any medical insurance had a higher incidence of cervical cancer [22], which coincides with the results of our research. Another study in the United States showed that *Medicaid* patients had a 38% increase in mortality (HR = 1.38; CI 95% 1.34–1.43), while uninsured patients had a 32% increase (HR = 1.32; CI 95%, 1.26–1.38), which may be associated with lower quality of care and reduced adherence to medical protocols in public hospitals [23]. On the other hand, the report on the situation of cancer in Colombia in 2021 reported that the incidence of cervical cancer was similar for both the contributory and subsidized regimes [24].

Regarding the area of residence, our research found that living in a populated/rural center decreases the incidence of cervical cancer, which coincides with the findings of Hall et al., who conducted a study in Florida, United States, using Cancer Data System data during the years 2014–2018. They sought to determine age-adjusted incidence and mortality for 22 types of cancer, including cervical cancer. These authors found that the incidence was significantly lower in rural areas than in urban areas [25]. In the same way, the study of Fantin et al., with cancer registries from 2011 to 2015 in Costa Rica, showed that cervical cancer was higher in urban areas [26]. In any case, it should be noted that the results of lower incidence in rural areas may be due to underreporting or poor accessibility to health services in these areas.

According to WHO recommendations, physical activity confers several benefits, including reducing mortality from any cause, cardiovascular diseases, hypertension, specific cancers, and type 2 diabetes, in addition to contributing to mental health. For these reasons, the WHO emphasizes that adults should perform moderate activity for two or more days a week, with a duration of 150–300 min of moderate to intense activity, or 75–150 min of vigorous activity to obtain these benefits [27]. In our research research, we found that only 8.5% meet these recommendations for physical activity, 0.8% meet the recommendations for 30 min of physical activity five times a week and 0.5% meet the recommendations for vigorous activity. These figures reflect a significant decrease, taking into account that in Colombia in 2010, the prevalence of moderate physical activity per week was 53.5% [28]. In high-income countries, the prevalence of physical inactivity was double (36.8%, 35–38) that of LMICs (16.2%, 14.2–17.9) [29]. Despite this, our study did not find an association between cervical cancer and physical activity, possibly due to the low percentage of the population that performs it regularly, which may have been decisive in finding a statistical relationship. Contrary to these findings, Lee et al. in their study in Korea, using cancer registries from 2006 to 2012 in women with intracervical neoplasia and cancer, showed that the risk of grade 2 and 3 intracervical neoplasia was inversely associated with physical activity [30].

With regard to BMI, our results showed no association with cervical cancer. Wise et al. and Emma et al. found an association between a BMI greater than 30 kg/m^2 and endometrial cancer [31,32]. Similarly, high BMI is considered one of the risk factors for all types of cancer, according to the Global Burden of Cancer [33]. The difference in results may be due to the ecological, pooled, and cross-sectional data used in this study, which has been able to reduce the measurement of the effect of obesity on the incidence of cervical cancer. However, the research discussed above [33,34] corresponds to longitudinal and individual studies, where such types of biases are usually controlled.

In relation to the disease declared in our study, diabetes was associated with an increased incidence of cervical cancer, which may be related to hyperglycemia and chronic inflammation caused by this pathology [34], in addition to the imbalance in the proteasome system among these patients, taking into account that the development of cancer requires high protein turnover and involves this system [35]. In a study by Garduño et al. in Mexico involving women with cervical cancer, an association with diabetes was found [36]. These results also coincide with those of Yang et al., who conducted a study in Taiwan with adults over 35 years diagnosed with several types of cancers, including cervical cancer, and found a similar association (adjusted RR 13.4; CI 95% 2.70–66.3) [37].

Regarding the incidence of cervical cancer, the highest rate in 2020 was found in the Amazon-Orinoquia region, in which the highest proportion of individuals was found in Q1, with affiliations to the subsidized health regime, a higher percentage of diabetes in relation to other regions, and more frequently reported consumption of beverage/grill foods. Studies have reported the presence of polycyclic aromatic hydrocarbons (PAHs) and heteroaromatic amines (HAAs) in meat that has been exposed to high temperatures during grilling [38,39]. One of the PAHs, benzo (a) pyrene (BaP), is known as a carcinogen, capable of modulating cellular processes including differentiation, proliferation, immune response, cancer promotion, and apoptosis [40,41].

On the other hand, according to the National Quality of Life Survey in 2018, in the Orinoquia-Amazon region, 69.9% of people aged 2 years and over reported consuming sugary drinks, a figure that exceeds the national record of 68.4% [42].

A diet high in sugar usually leads to weight gain and metabolic parameters associated with obesity, insulin resistance, the bioactivity of steroid hormones, oxidative stress, inflammation, and ultimately, the development and progression of cancer [43]. According to Choi et al., the consumption of sugary drinks is associated with type II endometrial cancer [44]. Therefore, the incidence of cervical cancer in this region may be associated with the consumption of sugary drinks.

In terms of dietary patterns, it was found that the conservative pattern is related to a lower incidence of cervical cancer. These results are consistent with Marziyeh et al., who showed that a high consumption of fruits and vegetables can reduce the risk of cervical cancer [45]. In addition, Barchitta et al., concluded that the risk of cervical cancer was lower in patients with high scores in the healthy diet pattern [8], while Mogge et al. found that patients with cervical cancer had a lower intake of fruits and vegetables [46]. In addition, Hwang et al. found that fruit and vegetable consumption reduces the risk of cervical cancer (OR = 2.84, 95% CI 1.26 to 6.42, p = 0.06 for vegetables; OR = 2.93, 95% CI 1.25 to 6.87, p = 0.01 for fruits) [47]. All of the above is possible because of the antioxidants that fruits and vegetables have, such as vitamin C and a- and b-carotene, which limit the damage caused by free radicals [48].

Limitations

Studies based on nutritional patterns rather than the measurement of dietary intakes do not allow us to know what type of foods or nutritional values could be more closely related with the development of this type of cancer. In any case, they are frequently used tools in ecological designs based on health surveys, as they represent food and nutrient consumption from a more comprehensive and community-based view on diet as a factor of exposure to a health event [49,50]. For these reasons, there is a need for longitudinal studies to establish a more precise association between dietary intakes and the development of cervical cancer. Another notable limitation is the lack of data on medical and gyneco-obstetrical factors, which were not collected in the health survey used for this secondary analysis. These factors could also be related to the development of this type of cancer. On the other hand, because it is a secondary source, the participants' responses may have recall bias. It should be noted that the sample size of the study decreases the probability of incurring type II errors.

5. Conclusions

It is concluded that, at the ecological level, the increase in the incidence of cervical cancer in Colombia was associated with affiliation to a health regime subsidized by the state and comorbidity with diabetes mellitus. In addition, the conservative dietary pattern, consisting of fruits and vegetables, as well as belonging to a rural area, were evidenced as protective variables. These results invite us to encourage public health policies that reduce population inequity and to make educational efforts for the promotion of healthy lifestyles to prevent cervical cancer.

Author Contributions: L.A.M.-U. and M.H.-C. conceptualized the study. L.A.M.-U. and M.H.-C. conducted the analysis and drafted the manuscript. L.A.M.-U., M.H.-C., D.V.A., N.B.S., G.M.-R. and M.V.-A. reviewed and revised the draft. All authors have read and agreed to the published version of the manuscript.

Funding: This study was funded by Dirección General de Investigaciones of Universidad Santiago de Cali under call No. 03-2020, call No. 10 of 2022 and call No. 02 of 2023.

Institutional Review Board Statement: This study was reviewed and approved by The Human Research Ethics Committee of Santiago of Cali University (Act N_11 from the May 29th session). Written informed consent for participation was not required for this study in accordance with national legislation (Resolution 8430 of 1993) and international requirements (Declaration of Helsinki and standards of Good Clinical Practice/Harmonized Tripartite Guide of the International Council for Harmonisation).

Informed Consent Statement: Informed consents are unavailable since the article was conducted through secondary analysis of databases corresponding to national health surveys in Colombia. However, all participants in these national surveys gave their consent (verbal or signed) to the interviewers of the national health system.

Data Availability Statement: The data will be made available to anyone who requests it from the corresponding author through a reasoned request.

Acknowledgments: This research has been funded by Dirección General de Investigaciones of Universidad Santiago de Cali under call No. DGI-02-2023. The authors thank the Colombian Institute of Family Welfare (ICBF) for providing the original database of the National Survey of Nutritional Situation of Colombia (ENSIN) and the University of Córdoba for providing the methodological tools for data analysis.

Conflicts of Interest: The authors declare no conflict of interest.

References

1. Bouvard, V.; Wentzensen, N.; Mackie, A.; Berkhof, J.; Brotherton, J.; Giorgi-Rossi, P.; Kupets, R.; Smith, R.; Arrossi, S.; Bendahhou, K.; et al. The IARC Perspective on Cervical Cancer Screening. *N. Engl. J. Med.* **2021**, *385*, 1908–1918. [CrossRef] [PubMed]
2. Arbyn, M.; Weiderpass, E.; Bruni, L.; de Sanjosé, S.; Saraiya, M.; Ferlay, J.; Bray, F. Estimates of incidence and mortality of cervical cancer in 2018: A worldwide analysis. *Lancet Glob. Health* **2019**, *8*, e191–e203. [CrossRef] [PubMed]
3. Organizacion Mundial de la Salud. Cancer Cervicouterino [Internet]. 2022. Available online: https://www.who.int/es/news-room/fact-sheets/detail/cervical-cancer (accessed on 1 March 2023).
4. International Agency for Research on Cancer; World Health Organization. Cervix Uteri. Source Globocan 2020 [Internet]. The Global Cancer Observatory. 2020, Volume 86. Available online: https://gco.iarc.fr/today/data/factsheets/cancers/23-Cervix-uteri-fact-sheet.pdf (accessed on 6 January 2023).
5. Cecilia, N.C.; Rosliza, A.M.; Suriani, I. Global Burden of Cervical Cancer: A literature Review. *Int. J Public Health Clin. Sci.* **2017**, *4*, 10–18.
6. Schiffman, M.H.; Brinton, L.A. The epidemiology of cervical carcinogenesis. *Cancer* **1995**, *76*, 1888–1901. [CrossRef]
7. García-Closas, R.; Castellsagué, X.; Bosch, X.; González, C.A. The role of diet and nutrition in cervical carcinogenesis: A review of recent evidence. *Int. J. Cancer* **2005**, *117*, 629–637. [CrossRef] [PubMed]
8. Barchitta, M.; Maugeri, A.; La Mastra, C.; La Rosa, M.C.; Favara, G.; Magnano San Lio, R.; Agodi, A. Dietary antioxidant intake and human papillomavirus infection: Evidence from a cross-sectional study in Italy. *Nutrients* **2020**, *12*, 1384. [CrossRef]
9. De Marco, F. Oxidative stress and HPV carcinogenesis. *Viruses* **2013**, *5*, 708–731. [CrossRef]

10. González, C.A.; Travier, N.; Luján-Barroso, L.; Castellsagué, X.; Bosch, F.X.; Roura, E.; Bueno-de-Mesquita, H.B.; Palli, D.; Boeing, H.; Pala, V. Dietary factors and in situ and invasive cervical cancer risk in the European prospective investigation into cancer and nutrition study. *Int. J. Cancer* **2011**, *129*, 449–459. [CrossRef]
11. Barchitta, M.; Maugeri, A.; Quattrocchi, A.; Agrifoglio, O.; Scalisi, A.; Agodi, A. The association of dietary patterns with high-risk human papillomavirus infection and cervical cancer: A cross-sectional study in Italy. *Nutrients* **2018**, *10*, 4046. [CrossRef]
12. World Cancer Research Fund; American Institute for Cancer Research. Diet, Nutrition, Physical Activity and Cancer: A Global Perspective [Internet]. 2018. Available online: https://www.wcrf.org/wp-content/uploads/2021/02/Summary-of-Third-Expert-Report-2018.pdf (accessed on 3 May 2023).
13. OMS. Obesidad y Sobrepeso [Internet]. 2021. Available online: https://www.who.int/es/news-room/fact-sheets/detail/obesity-and-overweight (accessed on 27 January 2023).
14. DANE. Conceptos Básicos. Análisis de Circuitos Eléctricos Estado Estable. Chrome. 2018. Available online: https://www.dane.gov.co/files/inf_geo/4Ge_ConceptosBasicos.pdf (accessed on 3 September 2023).
15. Meneses Urrea, L.A.; Vaquero Abellán, M.; Benachi Sandoval, N.; Villegas Arenas, D.; Osorio Murillo, O.; Molina-Recio, G. Dietary Patterns in Colombia: An Exploratory and Con fi rmatory Factor Analysis. *Front. Food Sci. Technol.* **2022**, *2*, 897877. [CrossRef]
16. Ohtani, K.; Tanizaki, H. Exact Distributions of R 2 and Ajusted r2 in a Linear Regression Model with Multivariate t Error Term. *J. Jpn. Stat. Soc.* **2004**, *34*, 101–109. [CrossRef]
17. Programa de Naciones Unidas para el Desarrollo (PNUD). Informe sobre Desarrollo Humano 2015: Trabajo al Servicio del desarrollo Humano. [Internet]. Informe. 2015, pp. 1–290. Available online: https://hdr.undp.org/system/files/documents/hdr2015reportsppdf.pdf (accessed on 1 June 2023).
18. Yi, M.; Li, T.; Niu, M.; Luo, S.; Chu, Q.; Wu, K. Epidemiological trends of women's cancers from 1990 to 2019 at the global, regional, and national levels: A population-based study. *Biomark. Res.* **2021**, *9*, 55. [CrossRef] [PubMed]
19. Pardo, C.; de Vries, E. Breast and cervical cancer survival at instituto nacional de cancerología, Colombia. *Colomb. Med.* **2018**, *49*, 102–108. [CrossRef]
20. Krieger, N. Defining and investigating social disparities in cancer: Critical issues. *Cancer Causes Control* **2005**, *16*, 5–14. [CrossRef] [PubMed]
21. López, F.E.; Pérez, P.T.; Murillo, E.N.; Quintero, G.C. Desigualdades sociales en la mortalidad por VIH y tumores malignos en municipios del departamento de Valle del Caua (Colombia) segun indicadores económicos 2009–2013. *Arch. Med.* **2018**, *18*, 373–384.
22. Parikh-Patel, A.; Morris, C.R.; Kizer, K.W. Disparities in quality of cancer care: The role of health insurance and population demographics. *Medicine* **2017**, *96*, e9125. [CrossRef]
23. Cherston, C.; Yoh, K.; Huang, Y.; Melamed, A.; Gamble, C.R.; Prabhu, V.S.; Li, Y.; Hershman, D.L.; Wright, J.D. Relative importance of individual insurance status and hospital payer mix on survival for women with cervical cancer. *Gynecol. Oncol.* **2022**, *166*, 552–560. [CrossRef]
24. de Alto, C.C. Situación del Cáncer en la Población Adulta Atendida en el SGSSS de Colombia 2021 [Internet]. Bogota-Colombia. 2021. Available online: https://cuentadealtocosto.org/site/wp-content/uploads/2022/08/01_agosto_libro_cancer_2021_final.pdf (accessed on 8 March 2022).
25. Hall, J.M.; Szurek, S.M.; Cho, H.; Guo, Y.; Gutter, M.S.; Khalil, G.E.; Licht, J.D.; Shenkman, E.A. Cancer disparities related to poverty and rurality for 22 top cancers in Florida. *Prev. Med. Rep.* **2022**, *29*, 101922. [CrossRef]
26. Fantin, R.; Ulloa, C.S.; Solís, C.B. Social gradient in cancer incidence in Costa Rica: Findings from a national population-based cancer registry. *Cancer Epidemiol.* **2020**, *68*, 101789. [CrossRef]
27. WHO. WHO Guidelines on Physical Activity and Sedentary Behaviour. *Routledge Handbook of Youth Sport.* 2016, pp. 1–582. Available online: https://iris.who.int/bitstream/handle/10665/336656/9789240015128-eng.pdf?sequence=1 (accessed on 8 June 2023).
28. Instituto Colombiano de Bienestar Familiar. Resumen Ejecutivo Encuesta Nacional de la Situacion Nutricional en Colombia. ENSIN 2010. 2011. Available online: https://www.icbf.gov.co/sites/default/files/resumenfi.pdf (accessed on 2 July 2023).
29. Guthold, R.; Stevens, G.A.; Riley, L.M.; Bull, F.C. Worldwide trends in insufficient physical activity from 2001 to 2016: A pooled analysis of 358 population-based surveys with 1·9 million participants. *Lancet Glob. Health* **2018**, *6*, e1077–e1086. [CrossRef]
30. Lee, J.K.; So, K.A.; Piyathilake, C.J.; Kim, M.K. Mild Obesity, Physical Activity, Calorie Intake, and the Risks of Cervical Intraepithelial Neoplasia and Cervical Cancer. *PLoS ONE* **2013**, *8*, e66555. [CrossRef] [PubMed]
31. Wise, M.R.; Jordan, V.; Lagas, A.; Showell, M.; Wong, N.; Lensen, S.; Farquhar, C.M. Obesity and endometrial hyperplasia and cancer in premenopausal women: A systematic review. *Am. J. Obstet. Gynecol.* **2016**, *214*, e1–e689. [CrossRef] [PubMed]
32. Crosbie, E.J.; Kitson, S.J.; McAlpine, J.N.; Mukhopadhyay, A.; Powell, M.E.; Singh, N. Seminar Endometrial cancer. *Lancet* **2022**, *399*, 1412–1428. [CrossRef] [PubMed]
33. Bill, F.; Foundation, M.G. The global burden of cancer attributable to risk factors, 2010–19: A systematic analysis for the Global Burden of Disease Study. *Lancet* **2019**, *2019*, 9–20. [CrossRef]
34. Tsilidis, K.K.; Kasimis, J.C.; Lopez, D.S.; Ntzani, E.E.; Ioannidis, J.P.A. Type 2 diabetes and cancer: Umbrella review of meta-analyses of observationlal studies. *BMJ* **2015**, *350*, g7607. [CrossRef]
35. Jang, H.H. Regulation of Protein Degradation by Proteasomes in Cancer. *J. Cancer Prev.* **2018**, *23*, 153–161. [CrossRef]

36. Garduño Orbe, B.; Hernández Wences, B.; Rayon Castañeda, C.J.; García Morales, G. Prevalencia de enfermedades crónicas en pacientes diagnosticadas con lesión intraepitelial del cérvix. *Atención Familiar* **2022**, *29*, 97. [CrossRef]
37. Yang, W.S.; Chen, P.C.; Lin, H.J.; Su, T.C.; Hsu, H.C.; Chen, M.F.; Lee, Y.T.; Chien, K.L. Association between type 2 diabetes and cancer incidence in Taiwan: Data from a prospective community-based cohort study. Acta Diabetol. *Acta Diabetol.* **2017**, *54*, 455–461. [CrossRef]
38. Zachara, A.; Gałkowska, D.; Juszczak, L. Contamination of smoked meat and fish products from Polish market with polycyclic aromatic hydrocarbons. *Food Control* **2017**, *80*, 45–51. [CrossRef]
39. Nor Hasyimah, A.K.; Jinap, S.; Sanny, M.; Ainaatul, A.I.; Sukor, R.; Jambari, N.N.; Nordin, N.; Jahurul, M.H.A. Effects of Honey-Spices Marination on Polycyclic Aromatic Hydrocarbons and Heterocyclic Amines Formation in Gas-Grilled Beef Satay. *Polycyclic. Aromat. Compd.* **2022**, *42*, 1620–1648. [CrossRef]
40. Sun, K.; Song, Y.; He, F.; Jing, M.; Tang, J.; Liu, R. A review of human and animals exposure to polycyclic aromatic hydrocarbons: Health risk and adverse effects, photo-induced toxicity and regulating effect of microplastics. *Sci. Total. Environ.* **2021**, *773*, 145403. [CrossRef] [PubMed]
41. Nagao, M.; Tsugane, S. Cancer in Japan: Prevalence, prevention and the role of heterocyclic amines in human carcinogenesis. *Genes Environ.* **2016**, *38*, 1–8. [CrossRef] [PubMed]
42. Departamento Administrativo Nacional de Estadística (DANE). Boletín Técnico. Encuesta Nacional de Calidad de Vida (ECV) [Internet]. 2019. Available online: https://www.dane.gov.co/files/investigaciones/condiciones_vida/calidad_vida/2018/Region-bt-ECV-18-amazonia-orinoquia.pdf (accessed on 2 May 2022).
43. Secretan, B.L.; Scoccianti, C.; Loomis, D. Special Rep or t Body Fatness and Cancer—Viewpoint of the IARC Working Group. *N. Engl. J. Med.* **2016**, *375*, 794–798. [CrossRef]
44. Inoue-Choi, M.; Robien, K.; Mariani, A.; Cerhan, J.R.; Anderson, K.E. Sugar-sweetened beverage intake and the risk of type I and type II endometrial cancer among postmenopausal women. *Cancer Epidemiol. Biomark. Prev.* **2013**, *22*, 2384–2394. [CrossRef] [PubMed]
45. Najafi, M.; Nazari, Z.; Shamsi, R.; Nikpayam, O.; Bahrami, A.; Hekmatdoost, A.; Hejazi, E. Dietary patterns and risk of cervical cancer: A case-control study. *Eur. J. Gynaecol. Oncol.* **2020**, *41*, 943–948. [CrossRef]
46. Hajiesmaeil, M.; Dahka, S.M.; Khorrami, R.; Rastgoo, S.; Bourbour, F.; Davoodi, S.H.; Shafiee, F.; Gholamalizadeh, M.; Torki, S.A.; Akbari, M.E.; et al. Intake of food groups and cervical cancer in women at risk for cervical cancer: A nested case-control study. *Casp. J. Intern. Med.* **2022**, *13*, 599–606. [CrossRef]
47. Hwang, J.H.; Lee, J.K.; Kim, T.J.; Kim, M.K. The association between fruit and vegetable consumption and HPV viral load in high-risk HPV-positive women with cervical intraepithelial neoplasia. *Cancer Causes Control* **2010**, *21*, 51–59. [CrossRef]
48. Coronado, H.M.; Vega, Y.; León, S.; Gutiérrez, T.R.; Marcela, V.F.; Radilla, V.C. Antioxidantes: Perspectiva actual para la salud humana. *Rev. Chil. Nutr.* **2015**, *42*, 206–212. [CrossRef]
49. Moeller, S.M.; Jill, R.; Millen, A.E.; Newby, P.K.; Tucker, K.L.; Krebs, S.M.; Muñoz, S.E.; Becaria Coquet, J.; Díaz, M.D. Dietary Patterns: Challenges and Opportunities in Evolution of dietary Patterns. *J. Am. Diet. Assoc.* **2007**, *107*, 1233–1239. [CrossRef]
50. Pou, S.A.; Niclis, C.; Aballay, L.R.; Tumas, N.; Román, M.D.; Muñoz, S.E.; Becaria Coquet, J.; del Pilar Díaz, M. Cáncer y Su Asociación Con Patrones Alimentarios En Córdoba (Argentina). *Nutr. Hosp.* **2014**, *29*, 618–628. [CrossRef]

nutrients

MDPI

Article

Lipid Profile in Children Born Small for Gestational Age

Justyna Zamojska [1,*], Katarzyna Niewiadomska-Jarosik [1], Beata Kierzkowska [1], Marta Gruca [1], Agnieszka Wosiak [2] and Elżbieta Smolewska [1]

1 Department of Pediatric Cardiology and Rheumatology, Medical University of Lodz, 90-419 Lodz, Poland; kasiajarosik@wp.pl (K.N.-J.); beata.kierzkowska@umed.lodz.pl (B.K.); marta.gruca@onet.eu (M.G.); elzbieta.smolewska@umed.lodz.pl (E.S.)

2 Institute of Information Technology, Lodz University of Technology, 90-924 Lodz, Poland; agnieszka.wosiak@p.lodz.pl

* Correspondence: j.zamojska@wp.pl

Abstract: Background: Lipid disorders are one of the risk factors for cardiovascular diseases. The aim of the study was to estimate the lipid profile in early childhood in the population of Polish children born small for gestational age (SGA). Materials and Methods: The study included 140 patients (93 SGA children and 47 controls) aged 5 to 11 years. All the subjects underwent a physical examination and blood laboratory tests for the glucose and lipid profiles. The SGA group was divided into subgroups, i.e., symmetrical and asymmetrical intrauterine growth restriction (IUGR). Results: Blood sample analysis revealed higher levels of total cholesterol (SGA group 190.61 ± 24.66 mg/dL vs. controls 143.23 ± 23.90; $p < 0.001$). The analysis of particular cholesterol fractions showed significantly higher mean values of triglycerides and LDL cholesterol as well as lower mean values of HDL cholesterol in SGA children. Children in both groups did not differ significantly in terms of weight or body mass index. A statistically significantly higher glucose concentration was observed in SGA patients with the symmetrical type of IUGR. Analyzing the differences regarding metabolic factors, we obtained a statistically significant difference only in fasting glucose concentration (asymmetrical IUGR = 90.56 ± 10.21 vs. symmetrical IUGR = 98.95 ± 14.79; $p < 0.001$). Conclusions: Children born SGA, even those not suffering from overweight or obesity in their early childhood, have an abnormal lipid profile, which may contribute to the development of cardiovascular diseases in adulthood.

Keywords: children; lipid profile; cholesterol; small for gestational age

1. Introduction

In the 1990s, the concept of fetal programming emerged as having a risk of developing type 2 diabetes, hypertension, and dyslipidemia in patients born small for gestational age (SGA) [1]. In the same year, Barker put forward a hypothesis suggesting that poor intrauterine growth caused by fetal malnutrition was associated with an increased incidence of cardiovascular diseases (CVDs) in adulthood. The hypothesis posited that fetuses receiving insufficient nutrition are more prone to develop abnormally high body weight. It is widely known that overweight and obesity contribute to the onset of cardiovascular and endocrine diseases (e.g., diabetes) in these individuals [2]. Moreover, the fetal origin hypothesis has expanded the conventional focus on adult health behaviors, such as smoking, appropriate levels of physical activity, and type of nutrition, to previously mentioned habitual factors that can influence prenatal welfare. Barker's hypothesis has inspired scientists to study the phenomenon of fetal programming in a more profound way. Birth weight is strongly correlated with the gender of the newborn, maternal and paternal anthropometric parameters, gestational age, and maternal comorbidities, i.e., diabetes, hypertension, or smoking [3].

The issue of low birth weight (LBW) remains a significant public health concern worldwide. Birth weight is regarded as one of the predictors of child mortality and morbidity. LBW newborns, as defined by the World Health Organization (WHO), are those weighing less than 2500 g (up to and including 2499 g) [4]. The term LBW refers to an absolute weight of <2500 g, independently of gestational age.

SGA is defined as birth weight below the tenth centile for gestational age and affects about 5 to 10% of neonates in developed countries [5]. The study revealed that 52% of unconfirmed stillbirths are caused by SGA, which also accounts for 10% of perinatal mortality. Furthermore, it is noteworthy that a significant proportion of unaccounted-for fetal deaths, namely, 72%, are attributed to low birth weight [6]. The "thrifty phenotype" hypothesis proposes that metabolic adaptations in early life support the survival of an organism by determining a proper growth trajectory in response to unfavorable intrauterine environmental simulation [7]. It is estimated that the global incidence of low birth weight ranges from 15% to 20% of all births, corresponding to more than 20 million births annually [8].

Children born small for gestational age can present two types of intrauterine growth restriction—symmetrical and asymmetrical. The conditions develop during organogenesis in the first or second trimester of pregnancy. The first type accounts for approximately 20–25% of all cases. In this type, all fetal dimensions are decreased in terms of anthropometrical dimensions as well as internal organs, which is usually accompanied by a permanent reduction in growth potential. The second type (asymmetrical IUGR) accounts for most cases, i.e., about 75–80%. This type is formed at the end of the second and third trimesters of pregnancy due to abnormal cell growth, not their amount. In the asymmetrical type, neonates are born with low weight, while other anthropometric parameters, such as body length, head circumference, and chest circumference, remain normal.

For this reason, the ponderal index (calculated based on the formula birth weight (g) $\times$ 100/length (cm^3)) is lower than in the symmetrical type [9–11]. According to the nomenclature, the two terms, i.e., intrauterine growth restriction and fetal growth restriction, are used interchangeably. They both refer to the prenatal diagnosis of growth restriction. Moreover, both these terms (IUGR and fetal growth restriction) are often used conversely with small for gestational age (SGA) [12]. A number of infants with SGA have IUGR, and indeed many infants with IUGR also have SGA. However, SGA cannot be used as a marker for IUGR because some infants with IUGR will have a birth weight greater than the 10th percentile [11]. Therefore, when distinguishing between SGA and IUGR, it is important to use fetal growth curves customized to constitutional factors to separate normal SGA infants from those with IUGR. It is important to highlight the differences between LBW, SGA, and IUGR. The term LBW is a separate nomenclature and should not be equivalently used with IUGR/SGA. This is because the definition of LBW is based on birth weight (less than 2500 g) regardless of gestational age, sex, race, and clinical features [11]. The definition of SGA refers to newborns whose birth weight is below the 10th percentile for a given gestational age or two standard deviations below population norms on growth charts. It should be mentioned that the definition of SGA only considers birth weight without taking into account intrauterine growth and physical characteristics at birth. Moreover, it must be added that we distinguish SGA and preterm SGA depending on the duration of pregnancy. The definition of IUGR is a typically clinical concept and applies to infants born with features of malnutrition and intrauterine growth retardation, independent of birth weight percentile [11]. To assess fetal growth, Roth's ponderal index (PI), a ratio of body weight to length, was used. In newborns with IUGR, where the accumulation of adipose tissue and muscle mass are reduced, the ponderal index is lower [13].

LBW is associated with many long-term complications. Numerous epidemiological studies show that low birth weight, regardless of other risk factors that appear later in life, can lead to cardiovascular diseases (especially hypertension and hyperlipidemia) and stroke, as well as increased mortality in adulthood [14,15]. Infants born with LBW may suffer from persistent neurological impairments, language development disorders, diminished academic performance, and a higher likelihood of chronic illnesses, such as the aforementioned cardiovascular diseases and diabetes [16]. In general, the occurrence of LBW can be triggered by fetal, placental, and maternal factors. Despite their different etiologies, these causes often share a common final pathway of inadequate uteroplacental perfusion and fetal nutrition [17]. Most children with SGA compensate for limited intrauterine growth by catching up early [18].

Catch-up growth (especially in terms of body weight) has been shown to increase the occurrence of some cardiometabolic risk factors, including resistance to insulin, overweight, and obesity, already in childhood [19]. The metabolic syndrome is a cluster of cardiovascular risk factors, including obesity, alterations in glucose-insulin metabolism, hypertension, and dyslipidemia [18]. The effect of birth weight on lipid levels in childhood is somewhat controversial. Low birth weight appears to be associated with unfavorable lipid levels [20]. It is considered that poor catch-up growth in height may increase the risk of high total cholesterol [21].

Studies have also revealed a positive correlation between elevated levels of total cholesterol, LDL cholesterol, and apolipoprotein B in adults born SGA and a small abdominal circumference observed in newborns after birth [22]. There are relatively few reports referring to research on lipids and lipoproteins in the blood serum of SGA children [21,23–29]. Although their results vary depending on the studied population, it is worth emphasizing that assessing of the lipid profile in SGA children is recommended in certain regions [30].

The long-term effects of low birth weight have been analyzed in many publications [2, 16,18,19,31–34]. As we mentioned earlier, low birth weight in the long perspective is most related to cardiovascular and metabolic diseases in adulthood [2]. It has been shown that adults born SGA had higher systolic and diastolic blood pressure compared to adults born AGA [31]. According to an article published in the European Journal of Endocrinology, SGA adults had higher fat mass with central adiposity, insulin resistance, and an improper lipid profile [32]. In addition, it was found that carotid intima-media thickness (cIMT) was higher in SGA-born adults with spontaneous catch-up growth compared to adults born with AGA [31]. Regarding the catch-up growth phenomenon, it was also revealed that in SGA girls, during growth and development, adipose deposition and insulin resistance can develop, leading to metabolic syndrome in adulthood [33]. It is also shown that young adults born with SGA are more frequently obese and have lower serum leptin levels compared to AGA controls [34].

Cardiovascular disease prevention is a comprehensive set of measures undertaken at the population level or targeted at individuals to eliminate or minimize the adverse effects of cardiovascular disease and its associated impairments [35]. The preventive efficacy of such measures has been demonstrated in numerous population-based studies, including the CARDIA study [36].

Despite many studies on SGA patients currently [5,6,18,21,23–30], the increased exposure of children to risk factors for the development of CVD sheds new light on this patient group. A sedentary lifestyle, abnormal dietary habits, and their consequent lipid metabolism disorders contribute to the development of cardiovascular disease in the pediatric population [37]. Patients with SGA are at higher risk of developing CVD than their healthy peers [18]. Therefore, it is important to conduct research in this group of patients in order to detect any metabolic disorders that may develop early.

This study is a retrospective work to determine whether children from the Polish population born small for gestational age are affected by abnormalities in the lipid profile in their early years.

2. Materials and Methods

The study included 93 children (50 girls, 43 boys) aged 5–11 years, randomly selected from an outpatient clinic at the Pediatric Cardiology and Rheumatology Department of the Medical University of Lodz, born on time and small for gestational age, i.e., with birth weight below the tenth centile according to gestational age (SGA—small for gestational age), assessed prenatally based on fetal ultrasound parameters. The control group comprised 47 healthy children (24 girls, 23 boys), born with normal birth weight (appropriate for gestational age—AGA), age- and sex-matched to the analyzed group. Gestational age was calculated based on the date of the mother's last menstrual period.

The small for gestational age subjects were divided into two subgroups, i.e., symmetrical ($N = 43$) and asymmetrical IUGR ($N = 50$). The division into subgroups was made based on data from the prenatal history—according to ultrasound measurements of the head, abdominal, and chest circumference; biparietal diameter; and femur length. Then, it was based on the analysis of anthropometric measurements at birth and the ponderal index. The following formula was used to calculate the ponderal index: birth weight (g) $\times$ 100/length (cm^3). Symmetrical IUGR had all parameters reduced and a normal ponderal index, i.e., more than 2. Asymmetrical IUGR had reduced weight and length, normal head circumference, and a ponderal index less than 2.

Mothers who had multiple pregnancies; high blood pressure during pregnancy; diabetes before pregnancy; liver problems during pregnancy; infection with syphilis or HIV; or systemic diseases like hypertension, diabetes, rheumatism, thyroid disease, chronic kidney disease, and obesity were not qualified for our study. Furthermore, the exclusion criteria in the study were illicit drug use during pregnancy, maternal smoking, or alcohol consumption. Evidence for chromosomal or infectious etiology of SGA, hypothyroidism, and systemic or acute disease (e.g., kidney or liver dysfunction, hypertension, gastrointestinal, nephrological, neurological, or cardiac diseases) were also exclusion criteria for pediatric participants. Children who had a history of taking antibiotics or other symptomatic drugs used for infections were not excluded. Only pediatric patients receiving other pharmacotherapies were not included. Informed consent was obtained from all the children's parents. All the subjects underwent a physical examination, during which demographic and anthropometric data were collected. The data included information about birth weight and gestational age. Current weight, height, and body mass index (BMI) were measured. When measuring body mass using a calibrated scale, each participant was dressed in light clothing and barefoot. For the calculation of BMI, the formula weight (kg)/height (m^2) was applied. Blood samples were collected from all the patients for fasting glucose and the lipid profile, including individual lipoprotein fractions, i.e., overall cholesterol, high-density lipoprotein cholesterol (HDL-cholesterol), low-density lipoprotein cholesterol (LDL-cholesterol), and triglycerides.

The blood samples were collected in the morning from the children who had fasted for at least 12 h.

The distribution of parameters was tested for normality using the Shapiro–Wilk W test. Differences in characteristics between the control group and patients with SGA, as well as between symmetrical and asymmetrical SGA cases, were assessed using the Mann–Whitney U test. Relationships were evaluated using Spearman's correlation coefficient. Scatterplots were drawn to illustrate the correlations between fasting glucose levels and birth weight as well as actual body weight. Results were considered statistically significant if the p-value was less than 0.05.

The study was approved by the Medical Ethical Committee of the Faculty of Health Sciences, Lodz University (No. RNN/150/09/KB).

3. Results

All the children were examined at the Pediatric Cardiology and Rheumatology Department of the Medical University of Lodz. At the time of the study, they were in good condition, without any chronic illnesses or drug-taking history.

The medical history investigation showed a statistically significant distinction regarding birth weight (SGA group—2545.22 $\pm$ 209.07 g vs. control group—3370.29 $\pm$ 503.11 g; $p < 0.001$). However, there was no significant difference between the groups regarding gestational age. The physical examination revealed no statistically significant differences between the mean values of body weight and body mass index (BMI), while the SGA group subjects were significantly smaller than the control peers (Table 1).

Table 1. Characteristics of the patients.

	SGA Group (N = 93) Mean ± SD	Control Group (N = 47) Mean ± SD	p Value
Sex (Male/Female)	43/50	23/24	0.76 (NS)
Age on examination	7.53 ± 1.35	7.4 ± 1.77	0.67 (NS)
Birth weight (g)	2545.22 ± 209.07	3370.29 ± 503.11	$p < 0.001$
Birth height (cm)	51.43 ± 2.61	54.51 ± 3.20	$p < 0.001$
Gestational age (hbd)	38.98 ± 0.86	39.09 ± 0.74	0.52 (NS)
Actual height (cm)	123.78 ± 10.06	128.11 ± 10.18	$p < 0.05$
Actual weight (kg)	24.79 ± 8.54	26.53 ± 7.78	0.30 (NS)
BMI	15.80 ± 2.83	15.97 ± 2.43	0.76 (NS)

SGA—small for gestational age, N—number of children, SD—standard deviation, NS—not significant, hbd—weeks of gestation, BMI—body mass index.

We divided the children with SGA into the symmetrical (N = 43) and asymmetrical (N = 50) types of intrauterine growth restriction (Table 2). We found a significant difference in the ponderal index value between these groups (mean symmetrical 2.02 ± 0.23 g/cm^3 vs. mean asymmetrical 1.75 ± 0.16 g/cm^3; $p < 0.00001$). In the symmetrical SGA group, the current height (121.51 ± 9.34 vs. 125.73 ± 10.34; $p < 0.05$) and body weight (23.22 ± 7.59 vs. 26.14 ± 9.13; $p < 0.05$) were statistically significantly lower than in the group of children with the asymmetrical SGA.

Table 2. Characteristics of the SGA patients.

	SGA Symmetrical (N = 43) Mean ± SD	SGA Asymmetrical (N = 50) Mean ± SD	p Value
Sex (Male/Female)	22/21	21/29	0.38 (NS)
Age on examination	7.72 ± 1.15	7.79 ± 1.46	0.16 (NS)
Birth weight (g)	2506.74 ± 256.66	2578.30 ± 152.28	0.51 (NS)
Birth height (cm)	49.79 ± 2.65	52.84 ± 1.53	$p < 0.001$
Gestational age (hbd)	38.94 ± 0.82	39.02 ± 0.91	0.62 (NS)
Current height (cm)	121.51 ± 9.34	125.73 ± 10.34	$p < 0.05$
Current weight (kg)	23.22 ± 7.59	26.14 ± 9.13	$p < 0.05$
BMI	15.35 ± 2.63	16.19 ± 2.97	0.12 (NS)
Ponderal index (g/cm^3)	2.02 ± 0.23	1.75 ± 0.16	$p < 0.00001$

SGA—small for gestational age, N—number of children, SD—standard deviation, NS—not significant, hbd—weeks of gestation, BMI—body mass index.

The analysis of blood samples revealed statistically significantly higher fasting glucose levels ($p < 0.001$) in the SGA group. Similar findings were observed for the mean total cholesterol levels (SGA group 190.61 ± 24.66 mg/dL vs. control subjects 143.23 ± 23.90; $p < 0.001$). The analysis of particular cholesterol fractions showed significantly higher mean values of triglycerides, LDL cholesterol, and HDL cholesterol in the children born SGA (Table 3).

Table 3. Glucose and lipid profile in examined patients.

Parameter	SGA Group (N = 93) Mean ± SD	Control Group (N = 47) Mean ± SD	p Value
Glucose (mg/dL)	94.51 ± 12.47	84.64 ± 6.39	<0.001
Total cholesterol (mg/dL)	190.61 ± 24.66	143.23 ± 23.90	<0.001
HDL cholesterol (mg/dL)	71.46 ± 13.31	57.94 ± 18.50	<0.001
LDL cholesterol (mg/dL)	105.35 ± 20.96	82.67 ± 16.92	<0.001
Triglycerides	112.32 ± 38.10	55.89 ± 18.31	<0.001

SGA—small for gestational age, N—number of children, SD—standard deviation.

Analyzing the differences regarding metabolic factors between the subgroups of children with asymmetrical and symmetrical IUGR (Table 4), we obtained a statistically significant difference only in fasting glucose concentration (mean glucose level for asymmetrical IUGR = 90.56 ± 10.21 vs. symmetrical IUGR = 98.95 ± 14.79; $p < 0.001$). Total cholesterol, HDL cholesterol, LDL cholesterol, and triglycerides were not statistically significantly different in the IUGR subgroups. However, when analyzing the SGA group according to sex, our study showed statistically significant higher HDL cholesterol levels in males compared to females (SGA males = 75.55 ± 12.80 vs. SGA females = 67.91 ± 12.91; $p < 0.05$). Comparably, we also obtained significantly higher HDL cholesterol values in the group of boys, taking into consideration the division into symmetric and asymmetric hypotrophy. However, we achieved statistical significance only in the group of boys with asymmetric hypotrophy (77.38 ± 14.30 vs. 67.87 ± 12.07, $p < 0.05$). As for the remaining metabolic parameters, the values of total cholesterol and LDL cholesterol were higher in the SGA group in boys, and triglycerides were higher in girls, but without statistical significance.

Table 4. Glucose and lipid profile in SGA patients.

Parameter	SGA Symmetrical (*N* = 43) Mean ± SD	SGA Asymmetrical (*N* = 50) Mean ± SD	*p* Value
Glucose (mg/dL)	98.95 ± 14.79	90.56 ± 10.21	<0.001
Total cholesterol (mg/dL)	190.90 ± 27.26	188.64 ± 23.70	0.73 (NS)
HDL cholesterol (mg/dL)	70.95 ± 13.00	71.86 ± 13.76	0.85 (NS)
LDL cholesterol (mg/dL)	104.65 ± 23.71	103.03 ± 19.49	0.87 (NS)
Triglycerides	109.09 ± 38.42	111.4 ± 39.31	0.91 (NS)

SGA—small for gestational age, *N*—number of children, SD—standard deviation, NS—not significant.

We studied numerous correlations in both groups of patients. Surprisingly, few correlations reached statistical significance (see Tables 5 and 6).

Table 5. Correlation coefficient between selected parameters—control group.

Parameter	Glucose	Total Cholesterol	HDL Cholesterol	LDL Cholesterol	Triglycerides
Birth weight	0.33	0.03	0.16	−0.01	0.02
Birth height	0.26	0.31	0.19	−0.11	−0.02
Actual weight	0.18	0.05	−0.24	−0.17	−0.18
BMI	0.10	0.04	−0.38 *	0.05	−0.17

* $p < 0.05$ (statistically significant).

Table 6. Correlation coefficient between selected parameters—SGA group.

Parameter	Glucose	Total Cholesterol	HDL Cholesterol	LDL Cholesterol	Triglycerides
Birth weight	−0.17	−0.01	0.08	−0.13	−0.03
Birth height	−0.40 *	0.09	0.09	0.13	−0.04
Actual weight	−0.22 *	−0.01	−0.002	−0.03	0.08
BMI	−0.16	−0.09	−0.06	−0.08	0.10

* $p < 0.05$ (statistically significant).

In the SGA group children, there was a negative correlation between birth weight and fasting glucose levels (r = −0.17; p = 0.033), total cholesterol levels (r = −0.01; p = 0.921), LDL cholesterol levels (r = −0.02; p = 0.848), and triglyceride levels (r = −0.04; p = 0.734), and there was a positive correlation between birth weight and HDL cholesterol levels (r = 0.09; p = 0.415). None of these correlations were statistically significant. In the AGA group, the correlation results were slightly different. There were positive correlations between birth weight and fasting glucose levels (r = 0.33; p = 0.054), total cholesterol levels (r = 0.03; p = 0.861), HDL cholesterol levels (r = 0.16; p = 0.352), and triglyceride levels

($r = 0.02$; $p = 0.894$), and there were negative correlations between birth weight and LDL cholesterol levels ($r = -0.01$; $p = 0.946$). In this group, the correlations did not reach the level of statistical significance either.

The statistically significant negative correlations in the SGA group of children were found between the fasting glucose level and birth height ($r = -0.40$; $p < 0.001$) (Figure 1), as well as between the fasting glucose level and current body weight ($r = -0.22$; $p = 0.034$) (Figure 2).

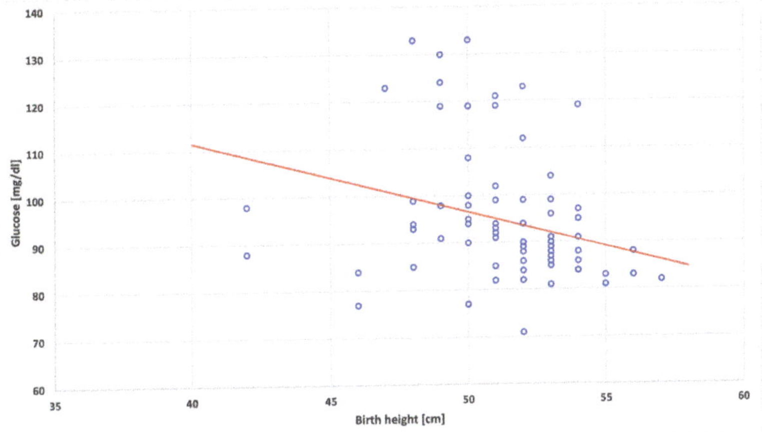

Figure 1. Correlation between fasting glucose level and actual birth height in the children born as small for gestational age.

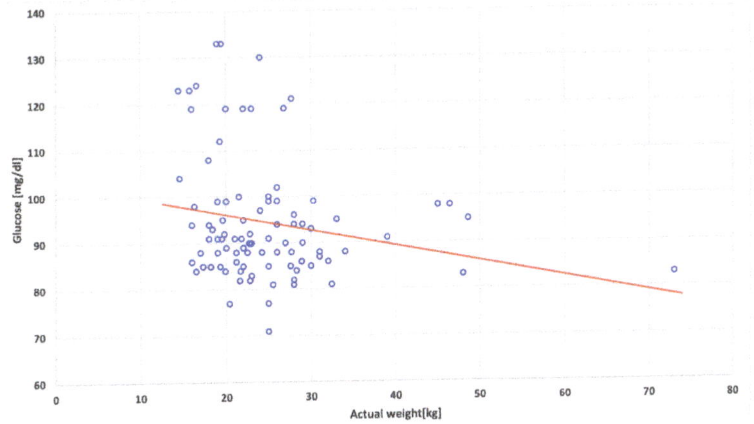

Figure 2. Correlation between fasting glucose level and actual body weight in the children born small for gestational age.

In the AGA group, we found this correlation to be positive, however, with no statistical significance ($r = 0.18$; $p = 0.305$). Contrary to our expectations, we found a negative correlation between total cholesterol and actual body weight as well as BMI in the SGA group, but it was not statistically significant ($r = -0.01$; $p = 0.922$ and $r = -0.09$; $p = 0.393$, respectively). In the AGA group, these correlations were different. We observed a positive, insignificant correlation between total cholesterol levels and the patient's actual weight ($r = 0.05$; $p = 0.785$) and BMI ($r = 0.04$; $p = 0.839$).

In the SGA group, current body weight also correlated negatively with LDL cholesterol (r = −0.03; p = 0.811) and HDL cholesterol levels (r = −0.002; p = 0.979), whereas with triglyceride levels, the correlation was positive (r = 0.08; p = 0.462). These correlations were not statistically significant.

In terms of BMI in the SGA group, and for fasting glucose level (r = −0.16; p = 0.118), LDL cholesterol (r = −0.08; p = 0.448), and HDL cholesterol levels (r = −0.06; p = 0.545), we found statistically insignificant negative correlations, whereas a positive correlation was observed for triglycerides (r = 0.10; p = 0.320). In the AGA group, we found a negative correlation with BMI for HDL cholesterol (r = −0.381; p = 0.023) and, unlike in the SGA group, a negative correlation for triglycerides (r = −0.17; p = 0.329). In the AGA group, a positive correlation was revealed between BMI and fasting glucose (r = 0.10; p = 0.577) as well as LDL cholesterol (0.06; p = 0.746). All the correlations mentioned above were not statistically significant.

Regarding metabolic parameters and the subgroup of SGA patients (Tables 7 and 8), we found a statistically significant negative correlation in the patients with the asymmetrical type of IUGR between birth length and fasting glucose concentration (r = −0.27; p = 0.05). For both types of IUGR, we observed a downward correlation between birth weight and current body weight (r = −0.06; p = 0.66 and r = −0.008; p = 0.59)—however, this was not statistically significant. Also, the BMI of the patients correlated positively with the glucose level in the subjects with asymmetrical IUGR and negatively in the subjects with the symmetrical type (r = 0.03; p = 0.84 and r = −0.15; p = 0.33). These correlations were not statistically significant. As regards total cholesterol levels and concentrations of HDL cholesterol, LDL cholesterol, and triglycerides, we found statistically significant positive correlations between birth length as well as total cholesterol levels and the HDL cholesterol level (r = 0.45; p = 0.003) in asymmetrical IUGR patients. There were no other statistically significant correlations between the lipid profile and BMI, birth, and actual weight in the two IUGR subgroups.

Table 7. Correlation coefficient between selected parameters—SGA symmetrical group.

Parameter	Glucose	Total Cholesterol	HDL Cholesterol	LDL Cholesterol	Triglycerides
Birth weight	−0.14	−0.14	0.09	−0.07	−0.11
Birth height	−0.18	0.27	0.45 *	0.23	−0.002
Actual weight	−0.26	−0.05	−0.05	−0.14	0.01
BMI	−0.15	−0.18	−0.19	−0.22	0.08

* $p < 0.05$ (statistically significant).

Table 8. Correlation coefficient between selected parameters—SGA asymmetrical group.

Parameter	Glucose	Total Cholesterol	HDL Cholesterol	LDL Cholesterol	Triglycerides
Birth weight	−0.06	0.03	0.01	0.07	0.001
Birth height	−0.27 *	0.10	−0.06	0.16	−0.04
Actual weight	−0.08	0.11	−0.01	0.09	0.11
BMI	0.03	−0.05	−0.04	−0.04	−0.006

* $p < 0.05$ (statistically significant).

4. Discussion

Our results show significant differences in the lipid profile between the SGA group and the AGA controls. As it is known from the literature, prenatal development can affect CVD outcomes. Factors influencing prenatal and postnatal growth may affect future lipid profiles and their clinical manifestations in adulthood [38].

Since the 1990s, several controversial studies have supported the hypothesis that low birth weight can lead to metabolic changes in these individuals in later life.

In their observational studies, Howe et al. found a correlation between postnatal growth and the lipid profile [39]. The Avon Longitudinal Study of Study of Parents and Children, ALSPAC, conducted since 1991, has revealed a positive correlation between the ponderal index in infancy and levels of triglycerides and LDL cholesterol in patients at 15 years of age. These authors also revealed a negative correlation between this index and HDL cholesterol levels in the same group. Other researchers, in their prospective study (Amsterdam Born Children and their Development), also showed a negative correlation for HDL cholesterol levels and a positive correlation for triglycerides and postnatal weight gain in children aged 5–6 years. The postnatal weight was observed to change over one to three months [40]. In our study, we obtained similar results regarding HDL cholesterol but opposite results regarding triglycerides. This may be due to the older age of the children we examined or a different type of diet also due to age. Similar to other researchers, our analysis showed significantly higher mean values of fasting glucose levels in the children born SGA [29].

Yu et al., whose study only concerned 8-year-old girls, showed, like us, a statistically significant lower height and body weight in SGA patients. Contrary to our results, BMI was significantly lower. This difference may result from examining only the female population [33]. Our results are also consistent with the ponderal index. We found a significantly lower value of the ponderal index in the patients with the asymmetrical type of IUGR [9–11].

Nevertheless, some previous works are not directly comparable with our paper because of differences in age, weight, and height of the examined children.

Our results correspond to reports of Donker et al., who found a relationship between higher triglyceride levels and low birth weight in children in a similar age group (7–11 years) [23]. Prevalence rates in the upper decile of serum lipid concentrations for children with a low birth weight ($\pm$2500 g) compared to children with a birth weight > 2500 g were calculated for each race–gender group. Based on a study by American researchers, it was shown that white boys with a low birth weight were, in a higher percentage than expected, in the highest range of triglyceride concentrations ($0.01 \pm p \pm 0.05$) [23]. This study was the first to demonstrate an association between low birth weight of children and their high triglyceride levels in the future. In our study, we did not observe statistically significant differences according to triglyceride levels between boys and girls, but interestingly, we obtained higher values of HDL cholesterol in male SGA patients. This difference was also statistically significant in male group with asymmetrical SGA. For patients with symmetrical SGA, this value was without statistical meaning.

Antal et al., on the other hand, when analyzing children aged 14–16 years, found no differences in lipid concentrations between individuals with insufficient birth weight and those with normal birth weight. It should be mentioned that the examined children differ according to fetal age, including those born prematurely [24]. Findings similar to ours were presented by Koklu et al. in a group of infants with SGA of different ages than our subjects. The authors observed notably elevated levels of triglycerides compared to the AGA group. In our analysis, this difference was also noticeable. They also assessed aortic intima-media thickness, showing higher values for SGA patients and a strong correlation with triglyceride levels [41]. We did not assess cIMT in our study, but the association between carotid artery IMT complex thickness and lipid disorders has been increasingly reported in scientific studies [42].

Spanish researchers studied 135 newborns with intrauterine growth delay and 116 newborns born on time, between 38 and 41 weeks of gestation. They concluded that triglyceride concentrations were higher in the study group than in neonates born on time (45 ± 27 and 36 ± 19 mg/dL, respectively, $p < 0.001$). The findings of asymmetric growth restriction in male and female newborns revealed disparities in serum triglyceride values compared to healthy individuals. However, no differences were reported among the SGA and AGA groups concerning total cholesterol, LDL cholesterol, or HDL cholesterol [43]. In another work, Chinese researchers evaluated metabolic changes in young rats born SGA. They obtained results that corresponded to our findings, i.e., that rats born with low birth weight demonstrated significantly higher levels of total cholesterol, triglycerides, and LDL cholesterol [44]. A team of Spanish researchers, Ibanez et al., evaluated female children with precocious puberty aged 5–18 years. They noted a relationship between the occurrence of dyslipidemia and low birth weight, suggesting that detected metabolic disorders originate from the prenatal period [25]. Tenhola et al., in a Finnish population study of SGA children aged 5–12-years, found no association between body mass index (BMI) and serum lipid levels, but almost as many as half of the subjects with SGA (47.3%) were in the highest quartile for serum total cholesterol, which was adequate for children of gestational age ($p = 0.038$) [21]. Our results correspond to this study—we also did not show such differences. We obtained only a negative correlation between glucose concentration and birth length and current body weight in the SGA group. This may be due to the age of the examined children, in which the lipid profile itself does not yet clearly reflect developing metabolic disorders.

Interestingly, it was not body mass but weak dynamics of catch-up height in SGA children that increased the risk of elevated triglyceride levels at the age of 12 years almost 14 times more as compared to SGA children who had a good catch-up growth in height [21]. Krochik et al. evaluated early risk factors of metabolic syndrome occurrence in SGA children in the period prior to puberty. Although the study group showed significantly higher levels of basal insulin, basal cortisol, and uric acid, there was no statistically significant difference between the examined groups in LDL and HDL cholesterol levels [27]. Also, Umer et al. noticed that low birth weight was related to higher levels of LDL, non-HDL, and triglycerides and lower HDL levels in 11-year-old children [28]. Huang et al. studied a population of prepubertal short SGA children (aged six years). The results showed that serum concentrations of total cholesterol, triglycerides, Apo B, and Apo B/Apo A-I in this group were significantly higher. It was observed that more than 33% of short SGA children had hypercholesterolemia and 23% had hypertriglyceridemia compared to a short AGA group [45].

However, contrary to the results of this study, Evangelidou et al. [46] did not observe any significant differences in the serum total cholesterol, LDL cholesterol, triglycerides, Apo-A-1, Apo-B, and Lp(a) between an SGA group and AGA controls. The levels of Lp(a), nevertheless, were significantly higher in the SGA <3rd percentile subgroup than in the SGA 3rd-10th percentile subgroup ($p < 0.05$). In our work, we compared glucose levels between the SGA and AGA groups, demonstrating a significantly higher level in the former and a negative correlation with birth length and the current body weight.

Similar observations were made by Italian researchers [47]. Long-term studies on SGA children in two age groups (8.4 ± 1.4 years and 13.3 ± 1.8 years) evaluated lipids and glucose levels. As for glucose levels, our results corresponded to those obtained by the authors mentioned above, i.e., glucose values were noticeably higher in the two SGA groups vs. the AGA group. There were no changes found, however, in the lipid profile. It is difficult to draw conclusions about the origin of these differences. Perhaps an analysis of diet and catch-up growth, as well as ethnic differences, could help in their interpretation.

Swedish researchers conducted a prospective, longitudinal cohort study that enrolled 285 Swedish children with low birth weight and 95 children with normal birth weight (2501–4500 g). In children aged three-and-a-half and seven years, blood samples were tested and compared between the groups for the lipid profile (HDL cholesterol and LDL cholesterol) with the evaluation of apolipoproteins (ApoA1 and ApoB) as well as glucose, insulin, and homeostatic model assessment of insulin resistance (HOMA-IR). The results showed that the SGA group demonstrated a significantly higher level of mean fasting glucose than the control group. However, there were no considerable differences in levels of insulin, HOMA-IR (homeostatic model assessment for insulin resistance), or blood lipids between the SGA and AGA groups [29].

On the other hand, a study by Hong Zu Deng et al. [48] showed no differences between SGA and AGA levels of glucose and insulin, although it should be emphasized that it was conducted on a younger pediatric group.

However, attention should be paid to the limitations regarding the interpretation of our paper results. Firstly, it was a single-center study. Hence, it was carried out on a relatively small group of patients, which was its major limitation. Secondly, the study design was based on collected retrospective data, which was another limitation.

The limitations mentioned above might suggest that the derived conclusions are not readily applicable to the entire population of prepubescent SGA children.

5. Limitations

The main limitations of the study include recall error (part of the analysis was based on parental responses) and selection bias (only patients who agreed to participate in the study during the recruitment period were included in the research). Moreover, another limitation of this work was the relatively small group of patients and a population of only Polish children (Caucasian race). However, this was a single-center study. Future re-analysis and objective follow-up would be possible once the study group has been enlarged.

6. Conclusions

This study contributes to the professional literature by demonstrating that children born SGA, with no differences in weight and BMI, have an abnormal lipid profile compared to AGA children. This could be a potential risk factor for cardiovascular diseases in adulthood. Therefore, it is justified to conduct a study on a larger group of patients born SGA. Moreover, it would be valuable to investigate in SGA patients the correlation between the results of metabolic tests and assessment of the intima-media complex, as an independent marker of cardiovascular risk.

To prevent cardiovascular complications, this group should be closely monitored by a team of specialists, including pediatricians, cardiologists, pediatric cardiologists, endocrinologists, and pediatric nutritionists.

Author Contributions: Conceptualization: J.Z. and K.N.-J.; methodology, J.Z. and K.N.-J.; software, A.W.; validation, J.Z., K.N.-J. and A.W.; formal analysis, J.Z., K.N.-J. and A.W.; investigation, J.Z. and K.N.-J.; resources, M.G. and B.K.; data curation, J.Z. and K.N.-J.; writing—original draft preparation, J.Z., K.N.-J., B.K. and M.G.; writing—review and editing, J.Z. and M.G.; visualization, M.G.; supervision, E.S.; project administration, E.S. The authors are solely responsible for the content of the article. All authors have read and agreed to the published version of the manuscript.

Funding: This work was supported by a grant from the Medical University of Lodz, Poland (No. 503/1-000-01/503-11-001).

Institutional Review Board Statement: The study was conducted in accordance with the Declaration of Helsinki and approved by the Medical Ethical Committee of the Faculty of Health Sciences, Lodz University (No. RNN/150/09/KB).

Informed Consent Statement: Informed consent was obtained from all the subjects involved in the study.

Data Availability Statement: Data are contained within the article.

Acknowledgments: We thank all the participants who contributed to this study. We gratefully acknowledge the contribution of the children whose data were used in this analysis, their caregivers, and the team from the Immunopathology and Genetics Laboratory at the University Pediatric Centre, Medical University of Lodz, Poland.

Conflicts of Interest: The authors declare no conflict of interest.

References

1. Hong, Y.H.; Chung, S. Small for gestational age and obesity related comorbidities. *Ann. Pediatr. Endocrinol. Metab.* **2018**, *23*, 4–8. [CrossRef]

2. Barker, D.J. The fetal and infant origins of adult disease. *Br. Med. J.* **1990**, *301*, 1111. [CrossRef]
3. Thomas, P.; Peabody, J.; Turnier, V.; Clark, R.H. A new look at intrauterine growth and the impact of race, altitude, and gender. *Pediatrics* **2000**, *106*, E21. [CrossRef]
4. World Health Organization. *International Statistical Classification of Diseases and Related Health Problems*, 10th revision, 2nd ed.; World Health Organization: Geneva, Switzerland, 2004.
5. Figueras, F.; Eixarch, E.; Gratacos, E.; Gardosi, J. Predictiveness of antenatal umbilical artery Doppler for adverse pregnancy outcome in small-for-gestational-age babies according to customised birthweight centiles: Population-based study. *BJOG* **2008**, *115*, 590–594. [CrossRef]
6. Alisi, A.; Panera, N.; Agostoni, C.; Nobili, V. Intrauterine growth retardation and nonalcoholic Fatty liver disease in children. *Int. J. Endocrinol.* **2011**, *2011*, 269853. [CrossRef] [PubMed]
7. Hofman, P.L.; Cutfield, W.S.; Robinson, E.M.; Bergman, R.N.; Menon, R.K.; Sperling, M.A.; Gluckman, P.D. Insulin resistance in short children with intrauterine growth retardation. *J. Clin. Endocrinol. Metab.* **1997**, *82*, 402–406. [CrossRef] [PubMed]
8. Desta, M.; Tadese, M.; Kassie, B.; Gedefaw, M. Determinants and adverse perinatal outcomes of low birth weight newborns delivered in Hawassa University Comprehensive Specialized Hospital, Ethiopia: A cohort study. *BMC Res. Notes* **2019**, *12*, 118. [CrossRef]
9. Lubchenco, L.O.; Hansman, C.; Boyd, E. Intrauterine growth in length and head circumference as estimated from live births at gestational ages from 26 to 42 weeks. *Pediatrics* **1966**, *37*, 403–408. [CrossRef]
10. Suhag, A.; Berghella, V. Intrauterine growth restriction (IUGR): Etiology and diagnosis. *Curr. Obstet. Gynecol. Rep.* **2013**, *2*, 102–111. [CrossRef]
11. Sharma, D.; Shastri, S.; Sharma, P. Intrauterine growth restriction: Antenatal and postnatal aspects. *Clin. Med. Insights Pediatr.* **2016**, *10*, 67–83. [CrossRef]
12. Bakketeig, L.S. Current growth standards, definitions, diagnosis and classification of fetal growth retardation. *Eur. J. Clin. Nutr.* **1998**, *52* (Suppl. S1), S1–S4. [PubMed]
13. Hwang, J.K.; Kang, H.N.; Ahn, J.H.; Lee, H.J.; Park, H.K.; Kim, C.R. Effects of Ponderal Index on Neonatal Mortality and Morbidities in Extremely Premature Infants. *J. Korean Med. Sci.* **2022**, *37*, e198. [CrossRef] [PubMed]
14. Mohseni, R.; Mohammed, S.H.; Safabakhsh, M.; Mohseni, F.; Monfared, Z.S.; Seyyedi, J.; Mejareh, Z.N.; Alizadeh, S. Birth Weight and Risk of Cardiovascular Disease Incidence in Adulthood: A Dose-Response Meta-analysis. *Curr. Atheroscler. Rep.* **2020**, *22*, 12. [CrossRef] [PubMed]
15. Wang, T.; Tang, Z.; Yu, X.; Gao, Y.; Guan, F.; Li, C.; Huang, S.; Zheng, J.; Zeng, P. Birth Weight and Stroke in Adult Life: Genetic Correlation and Causal Inference with Genome-Wide Association Data Sets. *Front. Neurosci.* **2020**, *14*, 479. [CrossRef] [PubMed]
16. Zerbeto, A.B.; Cortelo, F.M.; CFilho, É.B. Association between gestational age and birth weight on the language development of Brazilian children: A systematic review. *J. Pediatr.* **2015**, *91*, 326–332. [CrossRef] [PubMed]
17. Cutland, C.L.; Lackritz, E.M.; Mallett-Moore, T.; Bardají, A.; Chandrasekaran, R.; Lahariya, C.; Nisar, M.I.; Tapia, M.D.; Pathirana, J.; Kochhar, S.; et al. Low birth weight: Case definition & guidelines for data collection, analysis, and presentation of maternal immunization safety data. *Vaccine* **2017**, *35*, 6492–6500. [CrossRef]
18. Nordman, H.; Jääskeläinen, J.; Voutilainen, R. Birth Size as a Determinant of Cardiometabolic Risk Factors in Children. *Horm. Res. Paediatr.* **2020**, *93*, 144–153. [CrossRef]
19. Lurbe, E.; Aguilar, F.; Álvarez, J.; Redon, P.; Torró, M.I.; Redon, J. Determinants of Cardiometabolic Risk Factors in the First Decade of Life: A Longitudinal Study Starting at Birth. *Hypertension* **2018**, *71*, 437–443. [CrossRef]
20. Mullett, M.D.; Cottrell, L.; Lilly, C.; Gadikota, K.; Dong, L.; Hobbs, G.; Neal, W.A. Association between birth characteristics and coronary disease risk factors among fifth graders. *J. Pediatr.* **2014**, *164*, 78–82. [CrossRef]
21. Tenhola, S.; Martikainen, A.; Rahiala, E.; Herrgård, E.; Halonen, P.; Voutilainen, R. Serum lipid concentrations and growth characteristics in 12-year-old children born small for gestational age. *Pediatr. Res.* **2000**, *48*, 623–628. [CrossRef]
22. Barker, D.J.; Martyn, C.N.; Osmond, C.; Hales, C.N.; Fall, C.H. Growth in utero and serum cholesterol concentrations in adult life. *BMJ* **1993**, *307*, 1524–1527. [CrossRef] [PubMed]
23. Donker, G.A.; Labarthe, D.R.; Harrist, R.B.; Selwyn, B.J.; Srinivasan, S.R.; Wattigney, W.; Berenson, G.S. Low birth weight and serum lipid concentrations at age 7–11 years in a biracial sample. *Am. J. Epidemiol.* **1997**, *145*, 398–407. [CrossRef] [PubMed]
24. Antal, M.; Agfalvi, R.; Nagy, K.; Szepvölgyi, J.; Banto, E.; Regöly-Merei, A.; Biro, L.; Biro, G. Lipid status in adolescents born with low birth weight. *Z. Ernahrungswiss.* **1998**, *37* (Suppl. S1), 131–133. [PubMed]
25. Ibanez, L.; Potau, N.; de Zegher, F. Precocious pubarche, dyslipidemia, and low IGF binding protein-1 in girls: Relation to reduced prenatal growth. *Pediatr. Res.* **1999**, *46*, 320–322. [CrossRef]
26. Okosun, I.S.; Dever, G.E.; Choi, S.T. Low birth weight is associated with elevated serum lipoprotein(a) in white and black American children ages 5-11 y. *Public. Health* **2002**, *116*, 33–38. [CrossRef]
27. Krochik, A.G.; Chaler, E.A.; Maceiras, M.; Aspres, N.; Mazza, C.S. Presence of early risk markers of metabolic syndrome in prepubertal children with a history of intrauterine growth restriction. *Arch. Argent. Pediatr.* **2010**, *108*, 10–16.
28. Umer, A.; Hamilton, C.; Cottrell, L.; Giacobbi, P.; Innes, K.; Kelley, G.A.; Neal, W.; John, C.; Lilly, C. Association between birth weight and childhood cardiovascular disease risk factors in West Virginia. *J. Dev. Orig. Health Dis.* **2020**, *11*, 86–95. [CrossRef]
29. Starnberg, J.; Norman, M.; Westrup, B.; Domellöf, M.; Berglund, S.K. Cardiometabolic risk factors in children born with marginally low birth weight: A longitudinal cohort study up to 7 years-of-age. *PLoS ONE* **2019**, *14*, e0215866. [CrossRef]

30. Boguszewski, M.C.; Mericq, V.; Bergada, I.; Damiani, D.; Belgorosky, A.; Gunczler, P.; Ortiz, T.; Llano, M.; Domené, H.M.; Calzada-León, R.; et al. Latin American consensus: Children born small for gestational age. *BMC Pediatr.* **2011**, *11*, 66. [CrossRef]
31. Finken, M.J.; van der Steen, M.; Smeets, C.C.; Walenkamp, M.J.; de Bruin, C.; Hokken-Koelega, A.C.; Wit, J.M. Children Born Small for Gestational Age: Differential Diagnosis, Molecular Genetic Evaluation, and Implications. *Endocr. Rev.* **2018**, *39*, 851–894. [CrossRef]
32. Goedegebuure, W.J.; Van der Steen, M.; Smeets, C.C.J.; Kerkhof, G.F.; Hokken-Koelega, A.C.S. SGA-born adults with postnatal catch-up have a persistently unfavourable metabolic health profile and increased adiposity at age 32 years. *Eur. J. Endocrinol.* **2022**, *187*, 15–26. [CrossRef] [PubMed]
33. Yu, X.; Yang, X.; Zhao, Y.; Luo, X.P.; Liang, Y.; Wu, W.; Ying, Y.Q.; Ye, F.; Hou, L. A comparison of the growth status, level of blood glucose, and lipid metabolism in small for gestational age and appropriate for gestational age girls with central precocious puberty: A retrospective study. *Transl. Pediatr.* **2021**, *10*, 783–789. [CrossRef] [PubMed]
34. Dunger, D.; Darendeliler, F.; Kandemir, N.; Harris, M.; Rabbani, A.; Kappelgaard, A.M. What is the evidence for beneficial effects of growth hormone treatment beyond height in short children born small for gestational age? A review of published literature. *J. Pediatr. Endocrinol. Metab.* **2020**, *33*, 53–70. [CrossRef]
35. Porta, M. (Ed.) *A Dictionary of Epidemiology*, 6th ed.; Oxford University Press: New York, NY, USA, 2014; pp. 33–225.
36. Liu, K.; Daviglus, M.L.; Loria, C.M.; Colangelo, L.A.; Spring, B.; Moller, A.C.; Lloyd-Jones, D.M. Healthy lifestyle through young adulthood and the presence of low cardiovascular disease risk profile in middle age: The Coronary Artery Risk Development in (Young) Adults (CARDIA) study. *Circulation* **2012**, *125*, 996–1004. [CrossRef] [PubMed]
37. Rodrigues, A.N.; Abreu, G.R.; Resende, R.S.; Goncalves, W.L.; Gouvea, S.A. Cardiovascular risk factor investigation: A pediatric issue. *Int. J. Gen. Med.* **2013**, *6*, 57–66. [CrossRef] [PubMed]
38. Zouridis, A.; Manousopoulou, A.; Potiris, A.; Sarli, P.M.; Aravantinos, L.; Pervanidou, P.; Deligeoroglou, E.; Garbis, S.D.; Eleftheriades, M. Impact of Maternal Food Restriction on Heart Proteome in Appropriately Grown and Growth-Restricted Wistar-Rat Offspring. *Nutrients* **2021**, *13*, 466. [CrossRef]
39. Howe, L.D.; Tilling, K.; Benfield, L.; Logue, J.; Sattar, N.; Ness, A.R.; Smith, G.D.; Lawlor, D.A. Changes in ponderal index and body mass index across childhood and their associations with fat mass and cardiovascular risk factors at age 15. *PLoS ONE* **2010**, *5*, e15186. [CrossRef] [PubMed]
40. Oostvogels, A.J.; Stronks, K.; Roseboom, T.J.; van der Post, J.A.; van Eijsden, M.; Vrijkotte, T.G. Maternal prepregnancy BMI, offspring's early postnatal growth, and metabolic profile at age 5-6 years: The ABCD Study. *J. Clin. Endocrinol. Metab.* **2014**, *99*, 3845–3854. [CrossRef]
41. Koklu, E.; Kurtoglu, S.; Akcakus, M.; Koklu, S.; Buyukkayhan, D.; Gumus, H.; Yikilmaz, A. Increased aortic intima-media thickness is related to lipid profile in newborns with intrauterine growth restriction. *Horm. Res.* **2006**, *65*, 269–275. [CrossRef]
42. Guo, H.J.; Li, C.C.; Bian, X.Y.; Hao, Q. Correlation study on the relationship between dyslipidemia and carotid intima-media thickness in patients with diabetes mellitus. *Pak. J. Med. Sci.* **2023**, *39*, 875–879. [CrossRef]
43. Molina, M.; Casanueva, V.; Cid, X.; Ferrada, M.C.; Pérez, R.; Dios, G.; Reyes, M.; Venegas, H.; Cid, L. Lipid profile in newborns with intrauterine growth retardation. *Rev. Med. Chil.* **2000**, *128*, 741–748. [PubMed]
44. Zheng, R.D.; Wang, W.J.; Ying, Y.Q.; Luo, X.P. Effects of intrauterine growth retardation with catch-up growth on sugar-lipid metabolism and adipocyte function in young rats. *Chin. J. Contemp. Pediatr.* **2015**, *17*, 1124–1130.
45. Huang, Y.; Li, Y.; Chen, Q.; Chen, H.; Ma, H.; Su, Z.; Du, M. Low serum adiponectin levels are associated with reduced insulin sensitivity and lipid disturbances in short children born small for gestational age. *Clin. Endocrinol.* **2015**, *83*, 78–84. [CrossRef] [PubMed]
46. Evagelidou, E.N.; Giapros, V.I.; Challa, A.S.; Kiortsis, D.N.; Tsatsoulis, A.A.; Andronikou, S.K. Serum adiponectin levels, insulin resistance, and lipid profile in children born small for gestational age are affected by the severity of growth retardation at birth. *Eur. J. Endocrinol.* **2007**, *156*, 271–277. [CrossRef] [PubMed]
47. Chiavaroli, V.; Marcovecchio, M.L.; de Giorgis, T.; Diesse, L.; Chiarelli, F.; Mohn, A. Progression of cardio-metabolic risk factors in subjects born small to karge for gestational age. *PLoS ONE* **2014**, *9*, e104278. [CrossRef]
48. Deng, H.Z.; Deng, H.; Su, Z.; Li, Y.H.; Ma, H.M.; Chen, H.S.; Du, M.L. Insulin resistance and adiponectin levels are associated with height catch-up growth in pre-pubertal Chinese individuals born small for gestational age. *Nutr. Metab.* **2012**, *9*, 107. [CrossRef]

nutrients MDPI

Article

Room for Improvement in Sports Nutrition Knowledge amongst Parents and Caregivers of Male Academy Soccer Players in the UK: A Cross-Sectional Study

Luke Callis [1], Mark Russell [2], Howard Hurst [3], Jack Hardwicke [4] and Charlie Jon Roberts [1,*]

[1] Faculty of Arts, Science and Technology, University of Northampton, Northampton NN1 5PH, UK; luke.callis@northampton.ac.uk
[2] School of Sport and Wellbeing, Leeds Trinity University, Leeds LS18 5HD, UK; m.russell@leedstrinity.ac.uk
[3] Centre for Applied Sport Physical Activity and Performance, University of Central Lancashire, Preston PR1 2HE, UK; hthurst@uclan.ac.uk
[4] Department of Sport Science, Nottingham Trent University, Nottingham NG11 8NS, UK; jack.hardwicke@ntu.ac.uk
* Correspondence: charlie.roberts@northampton.ac.uk

Abstract: In professional soccer clubs in the UK, nutrition support is often polarised towards senior players or those in the senior academy age groups seeking first team selection/involvement. Accordingly, there is an increased reliance on parents and caregivers to provide support regarding nutritional intake. Therefore, the aim of this study was to evaluate the quality of nutrition knowledge of parents and caregivers of male youth soccer players within developmental academies in the UK. Across a single competitive season, 360 registered parents and caregivers of male soccer players from English Premier League under 9–11 (Foundation Phase) and under 12–16 (Youth Development Phase) age group academies completed an online version of the 88-item validated Nutrition for Sport Knowledge Questionnaire. Nutrition knowledge scores were classified as "poor" (43 ± 23%). Nutrition knowledge scores were significantly greater in respondents with dependents representing Category 1 (45 ± 13%) vs. Category 2 (39 ± 15%) academies and in Foundation Phase (44 ± 13%) vs. Youth Development Phase (41 ± 15%). These results demonstrate that there is room for improvement in the nutrition knowledge levels of parents and caregivers of male soccer academy players. We recommend that club academies provide appropriate resources towards nutritional education for parents and caregivers.

Keywords: nutrition knowledge; academy soccer; nutrition support; sports nutritionist; youth nutrition; youth athlete

1. Introduction

The Elite Player Performance Plan (EPPP) is a strategy introduced in 2012 by the English Premier League to develop high-quality homegrown male soccer players by increasing investment in youth development [1]. Age ranges of youth academy players in the EPPP Foundation Phase (FP), Youth Development Phase (YDP), and Player Development Phase (PDP) are under (U) 9–11 years, U12–16 years, and U17–23 years, respectively. In the 21/22 season, there were 14,226 players enrolled in the EPPP system, with FP and YDP players totalling 3741 and 7226, respectively [2]. Clubs are categorized from Categories 1 to 4, with Category 1 clubs providing more comprehensive services and receiving the most funding [1].

Soccer players require careful manipulation of their overall energy, macronutrient, and micronutrient intakes, along with consideration for daily and weekly variability in food intake in relation to training and matches [3]. English academy players exhibit large but variable energy expenditures due to the high-intensity, intermittent nature of play [4], high weekly distances covered during training and matches [5], and total activity duration [4,5]. The number of training sessions and match events players engage in weekly increases from four in Under-9s to nine in under-16s age groups, with some days containing $\geq$ two sessions [4]. Using the doubly labelled water method, total energy expenditure of Category 1 academy players was measured over a 14-day in-season period [5]. The authors observed energy expenditures of 2859 ± 265 kcal·d^{-1} and 3029 ± 262 kcal·d^{-1} in the U12/13 and U15 age groups, respectively. High daily energy expenditures may increase susceptibility to negative energy balance unless matched with appropriate nutritional intake, with mean daily deficits of -311 ± 397 kJ reported in U16 male Premier League academy players [6]. Furthermore, youth academy players will likely have attendance at school, social obligations, and rest periods as priorities alongside training and matches [7]. Therefore, youth academy soccer players not only have high-energy demand due to sporting commitments but also have congested schedules that can lead to difficulty in meeting energy requirements; thus, nutritional support from clubs and/or stakeholders is important in this context.

There is variability in the type and depth of nutrition services required by clubs. Notably, the EPPP stipulates that Category 1 clubs are required to employ a SENr accredited nutritionist or be under the management of an individual with this accreditation on at least a part-time basis, with Category 2–4 clubs not having any requirement for nutrition support personnel [8]. Full-time nutritionists are provided by 64%, 0%, and 14% of Category 1, Category 2, and Category 3 academies, respectively [9]. The types of nutrition support offered include individual consultations and group seminars, support for stakeholders including support staff and caregivers, and cooking sessions across Category 1–3 academies [9]. Some clubs provide main meals, snacks, and beverages to all players, some offer meals sporadically, some providing meals to older players enrolled in the PDP to a much greater extent than younger players, whilst some provide no meals at all [9]. Collectively, it is clear there is a skewed approach to nutrition support provision, with efforts focused on higher age groups overall but with more concentrated effort in Category 1 academies.

Sports nutritionists indicate that limited time is often a barrier to providing adequate support, particularly given that full-time roles are rare and that the number of hours practitioners are employed does not translate to contact time with players and key stakeholders [10]. As the dietary habits of children in the FP and YDP age groups are heavily influenced by the parents' and caregivers' ("caregivers" hereafter) purchasing, provision, and preparation of food and meals [11–13] on an almost full-time, exclusive basis, such stakeholders are key influencers of the quality of food provided.

Dietary habits are multifactorial and are influenced by socioeconomic status, education, cultural background, appetite, cost, convenience, and knowledge [14,15]. Nutrition knowledge is described as an important factor in the food choice process of athletes as this can influence not only an awareness of nutrition but also the ability to apply this practically when choosing appropriate food and meals [16]. Those possessing greater levels of knowledge tend to consume more fruit and vegetables [17,18], and athletes with higher nutrition knowledge scores demonstrate more favourable body composition values [19]. Whilst described previously in elite youth mixed athletes [20,21], the nutrition knowledge levels of the caregivers are likely of major importance. Lack of nutrition knowledge in caregivers was identified as a barrier for adolescents receiving healthy meals [22], and adolescents described family members as important sources of information on nutrition, with their support also one of the most helpful factors for promoting dietary change [23]. Furthermore, older academy players highlighted that caregivers can be enablers to good dietary habits if their nutrition knowledge is good; however, the requirement to eat what is provided for the family may be a barrier to players-specific nutrition requirements being met [24]. Despite the important role caregivers play in helping children and adolescents adopt appropriate nutritional practices, a recent audit into nutrition services provided by English soccer academies indicates that although 50–90% of clubs in Categories 1–3 reported providing "parent education", collective FP and YDP nutrition support totalled <20 h per month [9].

It was previously highlighted that clubs should allow adequate time for sports nutritionists, ideally on a full-time basis, to provide sufficient support for all age groups in academies beginning at a young age [24]. With a part-time nutritionist being required only when academies possess Category 1 status, ensuring adequate nutrition support is provided to all players enrolled from U9–U23 and key stakeholders may be unfeasible. Given the importance of nutrition for health and well-being and athletic success and development in youth players and the critical role caregivers play in supporting this, it is important to understand whether these individuals are best equipped to facilitate optimal dietary practices. As such, the purpose of the present study was to quantify the nutrition knowledge of the caregivers of elite FP and YDP male academy soccer players, compare overall scores from Categories 1 to 3 academies and age-stratified phases, and report overall question-specific responses relevant to the population. We hypothesised that caregivers would present "poor" nutrition knowledge levels due to the limited nutrition support offered to caregivers in academy environments.

2. Materials and Methods

2.1. Study Design

A total of 364 individuals who were registered as parents or primary caregivers to male players within the FP (U9–U11) or YDP (U12–U16) were invited to participate in this study. Clubs involved were of Category 1, Category 2, and Category 3 status (as per 22/23 season classifications). Data collection was conducted between November 2022 and April 2023. Ethical approval was obtained from the University of Northampton Faculty of Arts, Science and Technology Research Ethics Committee (FAST-REC approval number: 212211).

This study utilized a cross-sectional design. Member(s) of support staff at clubs were contacted to explain the purpose and requirements of this study. If interested, the member(s) of staff were asked to distribute the questionnaire, which was accessible via a link or QR code, to caregivers of players enrolled in the EPPP academy. Prior to the questionnaire, participants were presented with the participant information sheet and consent form, with contact details of the research team if they wished to ask any questions about this study. If participants selected that they did not provide informed consent, they were taken out of the questionnaire and were not asked to provide any further information.

2.2. Instruments

General and sport-specific nutrition knowledge levels were assessed using the Sport Nutrition Knowledge Questionnaire (SNKQ) [25]. Demographic and general subject-specific information was enquired about prior to the SNKQ. The SNKQ comprises 88 questions covering a range of topics related to weight management, macronutrients and micronutrients, sport- and athletic-specific information, supplements, and alcohol. A correct answer received one point whilst an incorrect or "not sure" response received zero points. Overall scoring was assessed as described previously [26], being "poor" knowledge (0–49%), "average" knowledge (50–65%), "good" knowledge (66–75%), and "excellent" knowledge (75–100%). The questionnaire demonstrated both construct and content validity, and all sections except for the "supplementation" section demonstrating acceptable test–retest reliability [25]. Small modifications were made to some questions to ensure relevance to a UK population. For example, questions related to alcohol consumption were amended to reflect the UK government recommendations regarding alcohol units [27]. The item response formats include agree/disagree/not sure, multiple choice, and effective/not effective/not sure. The questionnaire was inputted and completed on an online survey-hosting website (Microsoft Forms, Microsoft, Redmond, WA, USA).

2.3. Statistical Analysis

Descriptive statistics were presented as mean ± standard deviation. Data were analysed using SPSS Statistics (version 28.0.1.1, IBM, Armonk, NY, USA). Shapiro–Wilks testing was applied to test for normality, with data deemed parametric. Homogeneity of variance was assessed using a Levene test. Differences in nutrition knowledge scores between academy categories were analysed using a one-way analysis of variance, with post hoc testing conducted using a Tukey HSD and n^2 effect sizes interpreted as small ($n^2 = 0.010$), medium ($n^2 = 0.060$), and large ($n^2 = 0.140$) [28]. An independent samples t-test was applied to explore differences in nutrition knowledge scores between age-stratified phases, with Cohen's d effect sizes interpreted as small ($d = 0.2$), medium ($d = 0.5$), and large ($d = 0.8$) [28]. Confidence was set at $p < 0.05$ for all tests.

3. Results

The questionnaire was accessed by 364 individuals. Of these, three did not provide informed consent and one participant did not provide adequate information related to the academy that they were registered with and were subsequently removed from the analysis. As such, 360 participants from eleven academies (three Category 1, three Category 2, and five Category 3) completed the full questionnaire. The questionnaire was completed in an average of 27 min 36 s. Participant demographics are displayed in Table 1.

Table 1. Participant demographics.

	Categories	Responses (n)
Sex	Male	232
	Female	129
Academy category	Category 1	75
	Category 2	75
	Category 3	210
Age group	FP	142
	YDP	218
"On average, how many hours does your child/dependent train per week? (include all fitness related activities, both at and away from the sporting club)"	<3 h	0
	3–4 h	2
	4–5 h	20
	5–6 h	28
	6–7 h	51
	7–8 h	58
	>8 h	201
"Does the sporting organization your child/dependent is with provide access to nutrition support for you and/or your child/dependent? Select all that apply"	Access to nutrition information relevant to healthy eating	154
	Access to nutrition information relevant to sports/training nutrition	152
	Access to group presentations by nutritionists/dieticians	88
	Individual consultations with nutritionists/dieticians	12
	Cooking classes	4
	Hand-outs	25
	Recipes	14
	None	126
"If not provided, what would you find beneficial for the sporting organization your child/dependent is with provide access to nutrition support for you and/or your child/dependent? Select all that apply".	Access to nutrition information relevant to healthy eating	140
	Access to nutrition information relevant to sports/training nutrition	204
	Access to group presentations by nutritionists/dieticians	122

Table 1. *Cont.*

	Categories	Responses (*n*)
	Individual consultations with nutritionists/dieticians	155
	Cooking classes	46
	Hand-outs	85
	Recipes	136
	None	21

Collectively, nutrition knowledge scores were 42.8 ± 23.4%, classified as "poor" [26]. Thirty-six (10%) respondents indicated that they had previously received formal human nutrition education. Participants indicated that "family" (*n* = 162), "coach" (*n* = 125), and "friends" (*n* = 80) had previously given their child/dependent advice regarding their diet. The top sources of information participants relied on regarding nutrition were selected as "internet search" (*n* = 211), "family" (*n* = 183), and "coach" (*n* = 103). The organisation their child/dependent is with providing no access to nutrition support for either themselves or their child/dependent was reported by 126 participants. Collective responses for population-specific questions are displayed in Figure 1.

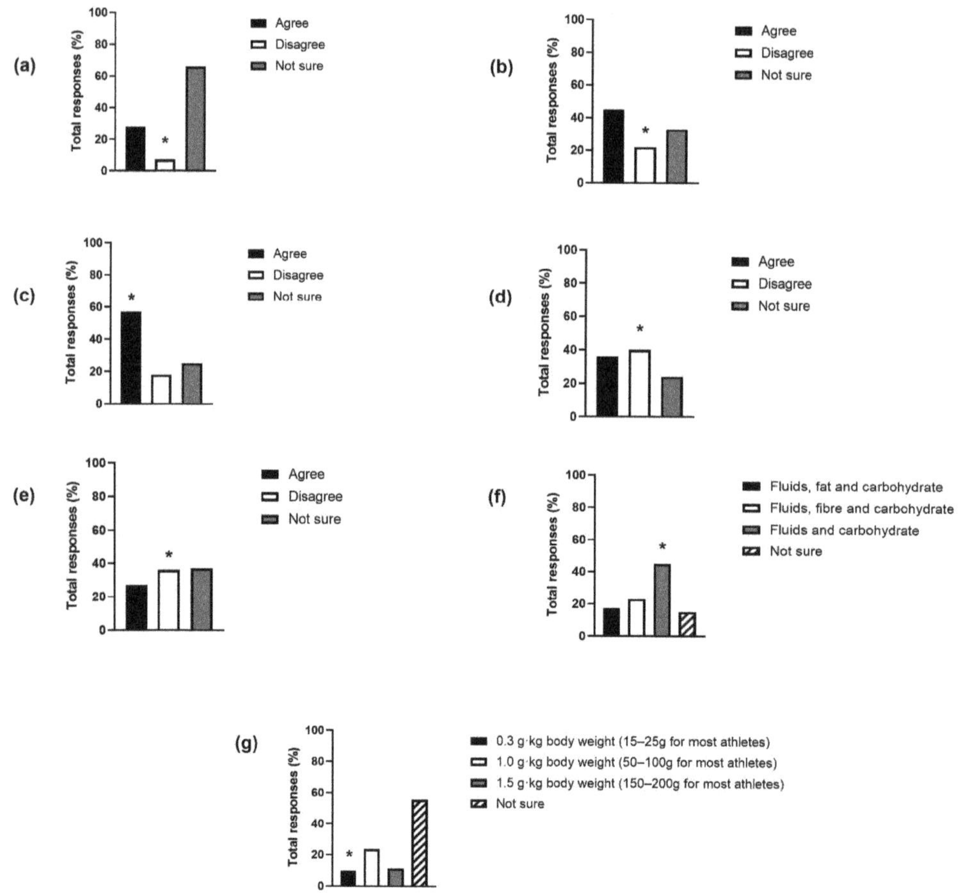

Figure 1. Responses (%) to questions and statements of population relevance from the SNKQ. * denotes correct response. (**a**) Athletes aged 15 to 24 years need 500 mg of calcium each day; (**b**) Iron

tablets should be taken by all athletes who feel tired and are pale; (**c**) Supplement labels may sometimes say things that are not true; (**d**) All supplements are tested to make sure they are safe and don't have any contamination; (**e**) Athletes should not eat more than 20 g of fat per day; (**f**) Before competition, athletes should eat foods that are high in; (**g**) How much protein do you think experts say athletes should eat after resistance exercise?

One-way ANOVA testing revealed a significant difference in nutrition knowledge scores between academy categories ($F = 3.018$; $p = 0.05$; $n^2 = 0.017$; Figure 2). Post hoc analysis indicated that the caregivers of players enrolled in Category 1 academies demonstrated significantly greater nutrition knowledge scores than those enrolled in Category 2 academies (mean difference = 5.76%; $p = 0.039$). No significant differences were observed between Category 1 and Category 3 (mean difference = 2.66%; $p = 0.355$) and Category 2 and Category 3 academies (mean difference = 3.10%; $p = 0.246$).

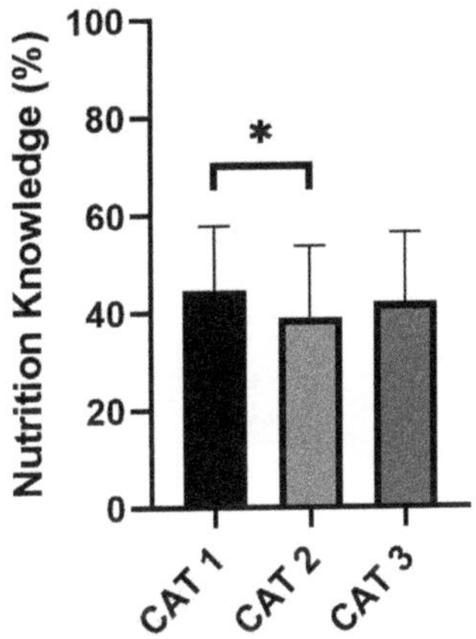

Figure 2. SNKQ scores between academy categories. * denotes significant difference between conditions ($p < 0.05$). CAT: category.

Independent samples *t*-testing revealed a significant difference in nutrition knowledge scores between caregivers of players representing YDP and FP academies ($t = 2.015$; $p = 0.045$; $d = 0.217$; Figure 3).

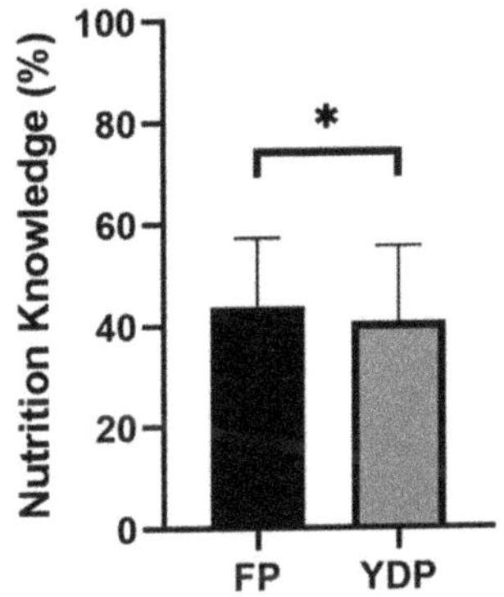

Figure 3. SNKQ scores between age-stratified phase. * denotes significant difference between conditions ($p < 0.05$). FP: Foundation Phase (Under 9–Under 11); YDP: Youth Development Phase (Under 12–Under 16).

4. Discussion

The aims of the present study were to quantify and compare nutrition knowledge of the caregivers of EPPP male academy players, compare overall scores from Categories 1 to 3 academies and age-stratified phases, and report overall question-specific responses relevant to the population. In line with our hypothesis, collective responses indicate a "poor" level of nutrition knowledge in this population. Nutrition knowledge scores were greater in caregivers of Category 1 compared to Category 2 players, while responses between Category 1 and Category 3 and Category 2 and Category 3 were not statistically different. Furthermore, caregivers of FP players demonstrated significantly greater nutrition knowledge scores than caregivers of YDP players.

Overall, category-specific and age phase-specific nutrition knowledge scores were classified as "poor" [26]. Similar results using the validated 88-item NSKQ were observed in female collegiate volleyball [29], female [30] and male Australian rules football [26], and elite and nonelite Gaelic football [31] players. Professional soccer players from a variety of countries previously demonstrated an average nutrition knowledge score of 52% [32]. Despite numerous studies exploring nutrition knowledge, the present study is the first to explore the nutrition knowledge levels of caregivers of academy players aged U16, who act as key stakeholders in the delivery of nutrition practices and development of nutrition behaviours for young players.

These results are not unexpected, given the limited collective support provided within YDP and FP academies when compared to within PDP programs [9]. In the present study, 35% of respondents reported that they or their child/dependent received no nutritional support from the club. It was indicated that overall, monthly support provided from an accredited nutritionist was reported as 62 ± 57 h for Category 1 academies, 12 ± 9 h for Category 2 academies, and 14 ± 26 h for Category 3 academies [9]. Within this, "parent education" was provided within FP (Category 1: 85%; Category 2: 67%; Category 3: 56%) and YDP (Category 1: 85%; Category 2: 72%; Category 3: 59%) clubs in a skewed fashion. At the FP and YDP levels, 20 h per month of nutrition support was reported from accredited nutritionists in Category 1 academies, < 10 h per month in Category 2 academies, and <15 h per month in Category 3 academies. The support available for PDP players was reportedly greater than that for players in U9–U16 age categories both overall and with consideration to specific services such as one-to-one support and cooking workshops [9]. Whilst expected due to players in the PDP being supported to transition into senior teams, the limited support available to younger players may compromise their biological and sport-specific development and therefore their progression through adolescence towards professional contracts [33].

Ensuring energy and nutrient intake is sufficient to support optimal health, growth, development, performance, and recovery is of the utmost importance; however, academy players are likely to face challenges in meeting elevated energy requirements. Congested schedules due to sporting, academic, and life commitments resulting in limited time; as well, financial barriers were identified as challenges for athletes' adequately fuelling by both players and coaches [34]. Furthermore, knowledge regarding appropriate dietary practices for high-level players was reported to be limited [34]. It was demonstrated that a moderate positive correlation between sport nutrition knowledge, energy ($rho = 0.31$, $p = 0.04$), and carbohydrate intake ($rho = 0.32$, $p = 0.04$) exists in professional and semiprofessional male soccer players in Australia [35]. Whilst the current study assessed the nutrition knowledge levels of caregivers, as key stakeholders in the provision of food and beverages to youth players, establishing a relationship between nutrition knowledge levels in this population and adequate dietary intake to support optimal health and well-being, performance, and recovery warrants further investigation.

Daily macronutrient requirements are elevated in youth players to provide energy and substrates for growth, development, and activity. Whilst protein and carbohydrate intake receives considerable attention in players, dietary fat is necessary for meeting essential fatty acid and fat-soluble vitamin requirements, providing energy during growth [36] and due to the greater fat oxidation rates exhibited in youth compared to adults [37]. In the present study, the statement "athletes should not eat more than 20 g of fat per day" was incorrectly answered by 64% of respondents. The UK government recommend that males aged 11–18 consume 35% of total energy intake as dietary fat, equating to an average of up to 97 g per day [38]. Additionally important is the periodization of food intake prior to matches to ensure adequate glycogen stores and hydration status [39–41] and following matches and training to facilitate optimal glycogen repletion, muscle damage repair, and adaptation [41,42]. Consuming foods that are high in fluids and carbohydrates before competition and protein recommendations of 0.3 $g \cdot kg^{-1}$ body weight after resistance exercise were correctly selected by 45% and 10% respondents, respectively. Whilst these results in isolation cannot be used to suggest that academy soccer players are observing suboptimal fuelling and recovery practices, they may highlight areas for nutrition practitioners to consider when working with players and key stakeholders such as caregivers.

Calcium requirements are elevated during adolescence to compensate for the greater bone remodelling that occurs during this life stage, with 26% of adult total bone mineral accretion expected in the two years around peak bone mineral velocity age of 14.1 ± 0.95 years in males [43]. As such, it is recommended that adolescent athletes consume 1000–1300 mg calcium daily [3,44,45]. In the present study, 7% of respondents were able to correctly identify that "athletes aged 15 to 24 years of age require 500 mg calcium per day" is incorrect. Soccer players are at an increased risk of injury due to the high-intensity, intermittent style of play and potential impacts encountered during match-play. Higher incidence of injury has been reported in youth soccer players between the ages of 13.5 and 14.5 years old, in line with athletes entering a period of rapid growth known as peak height velocity [46]. This window of increased injury risk further highlights the need to optimise nutritional strategies, particularly in the YDP age groups. Low calcium intake has been identified as a predictor for low bone mineral density in male adolescent athletes and demonstrates a cumulative effect of low bone mineral density risk when present with other risk factors such as stress fracture history and <85% expected body mass [47]. Low bone mineral density is a risk factor for fractures [48], and fractures represent 3–7% of injury occurrence within English academy environments [49,50]. Despite the low incidence compared to other injuries, fracture recovery required a median of 32 days recovery before return to play is observed in professional soccer players [51]. As such, ensuring nutritional practices are appropriate to support healthy growth and development and reduce the risk of injury is of importance for key stakeholders of academy soccer players.

The use of dietary supplements is commonplace in athletic populations [52]; however, sporting organisations including the International Olympics Committee [45] and Sports Dieticians Australia [44] discourage the use of ergogenic supplementation in adolescent athletes due to limited data, with UK Anti-Doping stating that "there are no guarantees that any supplement product is free from banned substances" [53] with 38% of 66 sports supplements sold online containing undeclared doping substances [54]. Contamination of sports supplements is unlikely to be intentional [55]; however, UK Anti-Doping rules stipulate that it is the athletes' responsibility if they receive a positive test for a prohibited substance and recommend only purchasing batch-tested supplements to mitigate the risk of ingesting a contaminated product [53]. In the present study, 60% of caregivers did not correctly identify that not all supplements are tested to make sure they are safe and do not have any contamination. It is crucial that caregivers are aware of their responsibilities and those of their child or dependent, given that youth players registered with the Football Association in the UK are subject to strict antidoping testing regulations [56].

4.1. Strengths and Limitations

To our knowledge, this is the first time the validated NSKQ was distributed to caregivers of youth academy athletes; however, it is noteworthy that the questionnaire is not validated within an English population [25]. Despite its novelty and contribution to knowledge, there are limitations to this work which we acknowledge. First, we were unable to collect data on the number of registered caregivers at clubs. As such, we are not able to determine the overall response rate from those whom the questionnaire was initially presented to. Second, due to the cross-sectional nature of this study, our results only represent a specific cohort of caregivers during one competitive season. Third, the self-report nature of the questionnaire inherently leaves a possible margin of error in participant responses due to misunderstandings of the questions and social desirability bias. Fourth, despite the large sample size and recruitment of participants from 11 academies, there is the potential for selection bias due to the sampling strategy adopted. Finally, the quantitative nature of the data also means that we provide a cursory but not a rich set of data on caregivers' nutrition knowledge. Human knowledge, and subsequent behaviour based on that knowledge, is a complex social process that cannot be effectively understood through quantitative measures alone. Future research is required to understand more fully the nutrition knowledge and behaviours of caregivers in soccer environments.

4.2. Practical Considerations

Whilst data collected via the SNKQ suggests poor nutritional knowledge in caregivers, we cannot unequivocally conclude a direct translation into a lack of best-practice sports nutrition information by caregivers of youth soccer players or an inability to apply this when providing food, beverages, and meals to their dependent. Additionally, the lack of uniform responses means the practical relevance of significant differences in service provision between age groups or categories is unlikely. Despite this, our results do provide a basic insight that practitioners can consider within their practice. For example, ensuring that caregivers of YDP and FP players are provided with information about the dietary requirements of calcium for an adolescent player, alongside ways this can be incorporated into daily dietary intake, may contribute to optimal growth and development, and reduce the risk of growth and bone-related injuries. Given the negative correlation between injury to young players and progression into a first team environment [57], any strategies with potential to reduce injury risk in elite youth soccer deserve great consideration.

During childhood and adolescence, humans experience significant physiological, metabolic, and hormonal changes, with dietary intake playing a major role in the biological maturation of physiological systems that can influence health in later life [58]. Nutrition support in elite environments is often about improving performance and providing food, not supporting behaviour change or promoting optimal long-term health and well-being [10]. Relationships and behaviours with food are developed during childhood and adolescence [36], and ensuring that players and key stakeholders are provided with holistic nutrition support can help promote life skills; this is noteworthy, as the Youth Development Rules indicate that Category 1 and Category 2 academies in the EPPP are required to provide, independent of a registered nutritionist, individuals on a full-time and part-time basis, respectively, to develop life skills such as those surrounding food and nutrition [2]. This is important to consider not only due to the immediate impact that suboptimal dietary intake can have on growth and development during childhood and adolescence but also given how few players will proceed to first teams [59], with 10% progression rates being reported from academy systems to senior teams [33,60]. Providing individualised support to caregivers and working within their sociocultural environment is crucial for facilitating appropriate nutritional practices in children and dependents [15]. Providing support to reenforce or improve the health and nutrition literacy of caregivers can thus extend to their dependents, promoting health behaviours over the lifespan [61].

Parents, caregivers, and wider family networks have been identified as both barriers and enablers to optimising eating patterns in academy soccer [24] and high-level rugby players [13,62]. As such, we recommend that club academies provide appropriate resources towards nutritional education for caregivers, within the means available.

5. Conclusions

In conclusion, these results suggest that there is room for improvement in the nutrition knowledge in the caregivers of EPPP FP and YDP academy players. Our findings highlight the importance of providing holistic nutritional support to both youth academy players and key stakeholders, as the gaps in knowledge are not only sport-specific but also pertain to nutrition for general health and growth. Despite the focus of this study on soccer, these findings have implications across any developmental athletic environments. Future research should aim to build upon these findings, using a range of methodological approaches, such as interventions designed to upskill caregiver nutrition knowledge and qualitative data collection to gain a deeper understanding of current service provision within elite soccer developmental environments from the perspective of players, caregivers, practitioners, and support staff.

Author Contributions: Conceptualization, L.C. and C.J.R.; methodology, L.C. and C.J.R.; data curation, C.J.R., M.R., H.H., J.H. and C.J.R.; writing—original draft preparation, L.C. and C.J.R.; writing—review and editing, L.C., M.R., H.H., J.H. and C.J.R.; project administration, C.J.R. All authors have read and agreed to the published version of the manuscript.

Funding: This research received no external funding.

Institutional Review Board Statement: This study was conducted in accordance with the Declaration of Helsinki and approved by the Institutional Review Board (or Ethics Committee) of University of Northampton (FAST-REC approval number: 212211; approved 30 September 2022).

Informed Consent Statement: Informed consent was obtained from all participants involved in this study.

Data Availability Statement: All data underpinning this publication are openly available from the University of Northampton Research Explorer at doi:10.24339/9b98137d-70c7-4f96-a332-527bb99a4d46.

Acknowledgments: The authors acknowledge all support staff at clubs who supported this study.

Conflicts of Interest: The authors declare no conflict of interest.

References

1. Premier League. Premier League Elite Player Performance Plan. 2011. Available online: https://www.premierleague.com/youth/EPPP (accessed on 26 May 2023).
2. Premier League. Youth Development Rules. 2020. Available online: https://resources.premierleague.com/premierleague/document/2020/09/23/9af878e5-d485-4683-87d9-4e4c3834d3bf/PL-2020-21-YD-Rules.pdf (accessed on 26 May 2023).
3. Collins, J.; Maughan, R.J.; Gleeson, M.; Bilsborough, J.; Jeukendrup, A.; Morton, J.P.; Phillips, S.M.; Armstrong, L.; Burke, L.M.; Close, G.L.; et al. UEFA expert group statement on nutrition in elite football. Current evidence to inform practical recommendations and guide future research. *Br. J. Sports Med.* **2021**, *55*, 416. [CrossRef] [PubMed]
4. Bangsbo, J.; Mohr, M.; Krustrup, P. Physical and metabolic demands of training and match-play in the elite football player. *J. Sports Sci.* **2006**, *24*, 665–674. [CrossRef] [PubMed]
5. Hannon, M.; Parker, L.; Carney, D.; McKeown, J.; Speakman, J.; Hambly, C.; Drust, B.; Unnithan, V.; Close, G.; Morton, J. Energy Requirements of Male Academy Soccer Players from the English Premier League. *Med. Sci. Sports Exerc.* **2021**, *53*, 200–210. [CrossRef] [PubMed]
6. Briggs, M.A.; Cockburn, E.; Rumbold, P.L.; Rae, G.; Stevenson, E.J.; Russell, M. Assessment of energy intake and energy expenditure of male adolescent academy-level soccer players during a competitive week. *Nutrients* **2015**, *7*, 8392–8401. [CrossRef] [PubMed]
7. Roberts, C.J.; Gill, N.D.; Beaven, C.M.; Posthumus, L.R.; Sims, S.T. Application of a nutrition support protocol to encourage optimisation of nutrient intake in provincial academy rugby union athletes in New Zealand: Practical considerations and challenges from a team-based case study. *Int. J. Sports Sci. Coach.* **2022**. [CrossRef]
8. EFL. 2023. Available online: https://www.efl.com/siteassets/efl-documents/youth-development-academy-parents-carers-handbook-2022-23-e-book-version.pdf (accessed on 26 May 2023).
9. Carney, D.J.; Hannon, M.P.; Coleman, N.M.; Murphy, R.C.; Close, G.L.; Morton, J.P. An audit of performance nutrition services in English soccer academies: Implications for optimising player development. *Sci. Med. Footb.* **2023**, *7*, 146–156. [CrossRef]
10. Bentley, M.R.; Mitchell, N.; Sutton, L.; Backhouse, S.H. Sports nutritionists' perspectives on enablers and barriers to nutritional adherence in high performance sport: A qualitative analysis informed by the COM-B model and theoretical domains framework. *J. Sports Sci.* **2019**, *37*, 2075–2085. [CrossRef]

11. Iglesias-Gutiérrez, E.; García-Rovés, P.M.; Rodríguez, C.; Braga, S.; García-Zapico, P.; Patterson, Á.M. Food habits and nutritional status assessment of adolescent soccer players. A necessary and accurate approach. *Can. J. Appl. Physiol.* **2005**, *30*, 18–32. [CrossRef]
12. Fitzgerald, A.; Heary, C.; Nixon, E.; Kelly, C. Factors influencing the food choices of Irish children and adolescents: A qualitative investigation. *Health Promot. Int.* **2010**, *25*, 289–298. [CrossRef]
13. Sharples, A.M.; Galloway, S.D.; Baker, D.; Smith, B.; Black, K. Barriers, attitudes, and influences towards dietary intake amongst elite Rugby union players. *Front. Sports Act. Living* **2021**, *3*, 369. [CrossRef]
14. Trakman, G.L.; Forsyth, A.; Devlin, B.L.; Belski, R. A systematic review of athletes' and coaches' nutrition knowledge and reflections on the quality of current nutrition knowledge measures. *Nutrients* **2016**, *8*, 570. [CrossRef] [PubMed]
15. Delbosq, S.; Velasco, V.; Vercesi, C. Gruppo Regionale HBSC Lombardia 2018, Vecchio LP. Adolescents' Nutrition: The Role of Health Literacy, Family and Socio-Demographic Variables. *Int. J. Environ. Res. Public Health* **2022**, *19*, 15719. [CrossRef] [PubMed]
16. Birkenhead, K.L.; Slater, G. A review of factors influencing athletes' food choices. *Sports Med.* **2015**, *45*, 1511–1522. [CrossRef] [PubMed]
17. Spronk, I.; Kullen, C.; Burdon, C.; O'Connor, H. Relationship between nutrition knowledge and dietary intake. *Br. J. Nutr.* **2014**, *111*, 1713–1726. [CrossRef]
18. Spronk, I.; Heaney, S.E.; Prvan, T.; O'Connor, H.T. Relationship between general nutrition knowledge and dietary quality in elite athletes. *Int. J. Sport Nutr. Exerc. Metab.* **2015**, *25*, 243–251. [CrossRef]
19. Jagim, A.R.; Fields, J.B.; Magee, M.; Kerksick, C.; Luedke, J.; Erickson, J.; Jones, M.T. The influence of sport nutrition knowledge on body composition and perceptions of dietary requirements in collegiate athletes. *Nutrients* **2021**, *13*, 2239. [CrossRef]
20. Bird, S.P.; Rushton, B.D. Nutritional knowledge of youth academy athletes. *BMC Nutr.* **2020**, *6*, 35. [CrossRef]
21. Heydenreich, J.; Carlsohn, A.; Mayer, F.; Heydenreich, J. Nutrition knowledge and food choice in young athletes. *Int. J. Pediatr. Res.* **2014**, *2014*, 974700.
22. Liu, K.S.; Chen, J.Y.; Ng, M.Y.; Yeung, M.H.; Bedford, L.E.; Lam, C.L. How does the family influence adolescent eating habits in terms of knowledge, attitudes and practices? A global systematic review of qualitative studies. *Nutrients* **2021**, *13*, 3717. [CrossRef]
23. Shepherd, J.; Harden, A.; Rees, R.; Brunton, G.; Garcia, J.; Oliver, S.; Oakley, A. Young people and healthy eating: A systematic review of research on barriers and facilitators. *Health Educ. Res.* **2006**, *21*, 239–257. [CrossRef]
24. Carter, J.L.; Lee, D.J.; Ranchordas, M.K.; Cole, M. Perspectives of the barriers and enablers to nutritional adherence in professional male academy football players. *Sci. Med. Footb.* **2022**, 1–2. [CrossRef] [PubMed]
25. Trakman, G.L.; Forsyth, A.; Hoye, R.; Belski, R. The nutrition for sport knowledge questionnaire (NSKQ): Development and validation using classical test theory and Rasch analysis. *J. Int. Soc. Sports Nutr.* **2017**, *14*, 26. [CrossRef] [PubMed]
26. Jenner, S.L.; Trakman, G.; Coutts, A.; Kempton, T.; Ryan, S.; Forsyth, A.; Belski, R. Dietary intake of professional Australian football athletes surrounding body composition assessment. *J. Int. Soc. Sports Nutr.* **2018**, *15*, 43. [CrossRef]
27. GOV.UK. Chapter 12: Alcohol. Available online: https://www.gov.uk/government/publications/delivering-better-oral-health-an-evidence-based-toolkit-for-prevention/chapter-12-alcohol (accessed on 3 March 2023).
28. Cohen, J. *Statistical Power Analysis for the Behavioral Sciences*; Lawrence Erlbaum: Hillsdale, NJ, USA, 1988.
29. Danh, J.P.; Nucci, A.; Andrew Doyle, J.; Feresin, R.G. Assessment of sports nutrition knowledge, dietary intake, and nutrition information source in female collegiate athletes: A descriptive feasibility study. *J. Am. Coll. Health* **2021**, 1–9. [CrossRef]
30. Jenner, S.L.; Devlin, B.L.; Forsyth, A.K.; Belski, R. Assessing the nutrition knowledge of professional female Australian football (AFLW) athletes. *Sci. Med. Footb.* **2020**, *4*, 240–245. [CrossRef]
31. Renard, M.; Anton-Solanas, A.; Kelly, D.T.; Ó Catháin, C. Evaluation of nutrition knowledge in elite and sub-elite Gaelic football players. *Sci. Med. Footb.* **2022**, *6*, 82–88. [CrossRef] [PubMed]
32. Staśkiewicz, W.; Grochowska-Niedworok, E.; Zydek, G.; Białek-Dratwa, A.; Grajek, M.; Jaruga-Sękowska, S.; Kowalski, O.; Kardas, M. Changes in body composition during the macrocycle of professional football players in relation to sports nutrition knowledge. *Front. Nutr.* **2022**, *9*, 981894. [CrossRef] [PubMed]
33. Dugdale, J.H.; Sanders, D.; Myers, T.; Williams, A.M.; Hunter, A.M. Progression from youth to professional soccer: A longitudinal study of successful and unsuccessful academy graduates. *Scand. J. Med. Sci. Sports* **2021**, *31*, 73–84. [CrossRef]
34. Logue, D.M.; Mahony, L.; Corish, C.A.; Tobin, D.; Doherty, R.; O'Higgins, G.; Madigan, S.M. Athletes' and coaches' perceptions of nutritional advice: Eating more food for health and performance. *Nutrients* **2021**, *13*, 1925. [CrossRef]
35. Andrews, M.C.; Itsiopoulos, C. Room for improvement in nutrition knowledge and dietary intake of male football (soccer) players in Australia. *Int. J. Sport Nutr. Exerc. Metab.* **2016**, *26*, 55–64. [CrossRef]
36. Desbrow, B. Youth athlete development and nutrition. *Sports Med.* **2021**, *51* (Suppl. S1), 3–12. [CrossRef] [PubMed]
37. Hannon, M.P.; Close, G.L.; Morton, J.P. Energy and macronutrient considerations for young athletes. *Strength Cond. J.* **2020**, *42*, 109–119. [CrossRef]
38. Public Health England. Government Recommendations for Energy and Nutrients for Males and Females Aged 1–18 Years and 19+ Years. 2016. Available online: https://assets.publishing.service.gov.uk/government/uploads/system/uploads/attachment_data/file/618167/government_dietary_recommendations.pdf (accessed on 26 May 2023).
39. Maughan, R.J.; Shirreffs, S.M. Development of hydration strategies to optimize performance for athletes in high-intensity sports and in sports with repeated intense efforts. *Scand. J. Med. Sci. Sports* **2010**, *20*, 59–69. [CrossRef] [PubMed]

40. Williams, C.; Serratosa, L. Nutrition on match day. *J. Sports Sci.* **2006**, *24*, 687–697. [CrossRef] [PubMed]
41. Williams, C.; Rollo, I. Carbohydrate nutrition and team sport performance. *Sports Med.* **2015**, *45*, 13–22. [CrossRef]
42. Heaton, L.E.; Davis, J.K.; Rawson, E.S.; Nuccio, R.P.; Witard, O.C.; Stein, K.W.; Baar, K.; Carter, J.M.; Baker, L.B. Selected in-season nutritional strategies to enhance recovery for team sport athletes: A practical overview. *Sports Med.* **2017**, *47*, 2201–2218. [CrossRef]
43. Bailey, D.A.; McKay, H.A.; Mirwald, R.L.; Crocker, P.R.; Faulkner, R.A. A six-year longitudinal study of the relationship of physical activity to bone mineral accrual in growing children: The university of Saskatchewan bone mineral accrual study. *J. Bone Miner. Res.* **1999**, *14*, 1672–1679. [CrossRef]
44. Desbrow, B.; McCormack, J.; Burke, L.M.; Cox, G.R.; Fallon, K.; Hislop, M.; Logan, R.; Marino, N.; Sawyer, S.M.; Shaw, G.; et al. Sports Dietitians Australia position statement: Sports nutrition for the adolescent athlete. *Int. J. Sport Nutr. Exerc. Metab.* **2014**, *24*, 570–584. [CrossRef]
45. Bergeron, M.F.; Mountjoy, M.; Armstrong, N.; Chia, M.; Côté, J.; Emery, C.A.; Faigenbaum, A.; Hall, G.; Kriemler, S.; Léglise, M.; et al. International Olympic Committee consensus statement on youth athletic development. *Br. J. Sport Med.* **2015**, *49*, 843–851. [CrossRef]
46. Van der Sluis, A.; Elferink-Gemser, M.T.; Brink, M.S.; Visscher, C. Importance of peak height velocity timing in terms of injuries in talented soccer players. *Int. J. Sport Med.* **2015**, *36*, 327–332.
47. Barrack, M.T.; Fredericson, M.; Tenforde, A.S.; Nattiv, A. Evidence of a cumulative effect for risk factors predicting low bone mass among male adolescent athletes. *Br. J. Sport Med.* **2017**, *51*, 200–205. [CrossRef] [PubMed]
48. Jonvik, K.L.; Torstveit, M.K.; Sundgot-Borgen, J.; Mathisen, T.F. Do we need to change the guideline values for determining low bone mineral density in athletes? *J. Appl. Phys.* **2022**, *132*, 1320–1322. [CrossRef] [PubMed]
49. Read, P.J.; Oliver, J.L.; De Ste Croix, M.B.; Myer, G.D.; Lloyd, R.S. An audit of injuries in six English professional soccer academies. *J. Sport Sci.* **2018**, *36*, 1542–1548. [CrossRef]
50. Light, N.; Johnson, A.; Williams, S.; Smith, N.; Hale, B.; Thorborg, K. Injuries in youth football and the relationship to player maturation: An analysis of time-loss injuries during four seasons in an English elite male football academy. *Scand. J. Med. Sci. Sport* **2021**, *31*, 1324–1334. [CrossRef]
51. Larsson, D.; Ekstrand, J.; Karlsson, M.K. Fracture epidemiology in male elite football players from 2001 to 2013: 'How long will this fracture keep me out?'. *Br. J. Sport Med.* **2016**, *50*, 759–763. [CrossRef] [PubMed]
52. Knapik, J.J.; Steelman, R.A.; Hoedebecke, S.S.; Austin, K.G.; Farina, E.K.; Lieberman, H.R. Prevalence of dietary supplement use by athletes: Systematic review and meta-analysis. *Sport Med.* **2016**, *46*, 103–123. [CrossRef]
53. UK Anti Doping. Managing Supplement Risks. 2023. Available online: https://www.ukad.org.uk/playerss/managing-supplement-risks (accessed on 26 May 2023).
54. Duiven, E.; van Loon, L.J.; Spruijt, L.; Koert, W.; de Hon, O.M. Undeclared doping substances are highly prevalent in commercial sports nutrition supplements. *J. Sport Sci. Med.* **2021**, *20*, 328. [CrossRef] [PubMed]
55. Maughan, R.J. Contamination of dietary supplements and positive drug tests in sport. *J. Sport Sci.* **2005**, *23*, 883–889. [CrossRef] [PubMed]
56. The Football Association. The Drug Testing Process. 2023. Available online: https://www.thefa.com/football-rules-governance/anti-doping/the-drug-testing-process#:~:text=You%20can%20be%20drug%20tested,multiple%20times%20during%20the%20season (accessed on 26 May 2023).
57. Larruskain, J.; Lekue, J.A.; Martin-Garetxana, I.; Barrio, I.; McCall, A.; Gil, S.M. Injuries are negatively associated with player progression in an elite football academy. *Sci. Med. Footb.* **2022**, *6*, 405–414. [CrossRef]
58. Norris, S.A.; Frongillo, E.A.; Black, M.M.; Dong, Y.; Fall, C.; Lampl, M.; Liese, A.D.; Naguib, M.; Prentice, A.; Rochat, T.; et al. Nutrition in adolescent growth and development. *Lancet* **2022**, *399*, 172–184. [CrossRef]
59. Russell, M. Food for Thought: Levelling the Playing Field for Academy Nutritionists in English Youth Soccer. 2018. Available online: https://blogs.bmj.com/bjsm/2018/01/26/food-thought-levelling-playing-field-academy-nutritionists-english-youth-soccer/ (accessed on 20 May 2023).
60. Grossmann, B.; Lames, M. From talent to professional football–youthism in German football. *Int. J. Sport Sci. Coach.* **2015**, *10*, 1103–1113. [CrossRef]
61. de Buhr, E.; Tannen, A. Parental health literacy and health knowledge, behaviours and outcomes in children: A cross-sectional survey. *BMC Public Health* **2020**, *20*, 1096. [CrossRef] [PubMed]
62. Stokes, E.G.; Hughes, R.; Shaw, D.M.; O'Connor, H.T.; Beck, K.L. Perceptions and determinants of eating for health and performance in high-level male adolescent rugby union players. *Sports* **2018**, *6*, 49. [CrossRef] [PubMed]

MDPI AG
Grosspeteranlage 5
4052 Basel
Switzerland
Tel.: +41 61 683 77 34

Nutrients Editorial Office
E-mail: nutrients@mdpi.com
www.mdpi.com/journal/nutrients

www.ingramcontent.com/pod-product-compliance
Lightning Source LLC
Chambersburg PA
CBHW061547220926
51850CB00005B/273
* 9 7 8 3 7 2 5 8 6 4 0 8 9 *